HIGH ALTITUDE MEDICINE

HIGH ALTITUDE MEDICINE

Herbert N. Hultgren, M.D.

Professor of Medicine, Emeritus
Stanford University School of Medicine

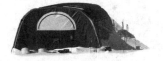

Stanford, California

HIGH ALTITUDE MEDICINE

For information, address
Hultgren Publications,
827 San Francisco Court,
Stanford, California 94305-1021
or
hultgren@highaltitudemedicine.com

**Library of Congress Catalog Card Number
97-93140**

ISBN 0-9655183-0-2

Cover Photo

Denali Medical Research Projects tents in the Sheldon Amphitheater
at 14,000 feet on Mt. McKinley. Here for nine seasons Peter Hackett
and his colleagues carried out important research on many
acute altitude medical problems.

Photo: Courtesy of Peter Hackett, M.D.

To Barbara, Peter, Bruce and John

Table of Contents

Foreword

One hundred and fifty years ago the Golden Age of mountaineering began, and soon all the summits in the Alps and a few in the Andes and Himalayas had been reached. Climbers described unpleasant symptoms on high peaks like those a few daring mountain travelers had in the distant past blamed on pestilential vapors.

Then, toward the end of the nineteenth century Paul Bert proved conclusively what a few scientists had already suggested — that lack of oxygen due to decreased barometric pressure was the primary cause of mountain sickness. Since then research in the clinical aspects of hypoxia has increased rapidly, not only on mountains but in many illnesses at sea level.

Among the leaders of this research and its application is the author of this book, Herb Hultgren, who has been my friend for more than thirty years. Few are as qualified to explain the effects of hypoxia on high mountains or due to sea level illness.

Herb is an experienced cardiologist, clinician and mountaineer. He has done pioneering research in the Peruvian Andes and in North America and probably knows and has observed as much about high altitude illnesses as any physician in the world. He has published extensively and has an encyclopedic knowledge of the work of others.

As the table of contents shows, his book is written primarily for practicing physicians, but there is much to interest researchers as well. Herb describes the clinical aspects of high altitude illnesses and explains what is known today of their causative mechanisms and pathophysiology. He writes sparsely and without long complicated discussions; he is skeptical of anecdotes, but nevertheless shows how they have helped us to learn, and how to evaluate them carefully.

The combination of his clinical experience, his years of high altitude research, his own climbs, and his prodigious knowledge of the literature makes this book essential reading for all physicians interested in hypoxic medical problems.

Charles S. Houston, M.D.
Burlington, Vermont
January 21, 1997

Acknowledgments

I am indebted to many people who assisted in the preparation of this volume, including those who participated in my research studies in Peru and the U.S., investigators who generously reviewed sections of the manuscript, and friends and colleagues who offered advice and suggestions. They include: James Alexander, M.D., Ann Bolger, M.D., Howard Burchell, M.D., Gail Butterfield, Ph.D., Hon. Judge Kenneth Eymann, Robert Grover, M.D., Peter Hackett, M.D., Ben Honigman, M.D., Tom Hornbein, M.D., Ben Levine, M.D., Julie Ann Lickteig, M.S., Emilio Marticorena, M.D., Dick Nicholas, M.D., John Reeves, M.D., Rob Roach, Ph.D., Gil Roberts, M.D., Robert Schoene, M.D., John Severinghaus, M.D., the late John Sutton, M.D., John West, M.D., and Eugene Wolfel, M.D.

Charles Houston, M.D., was of invaluable help in his critique of each chapter and in providing additional information gained through his many years of experience in the field of high altitude medicine.

Special appreciation is due Bonita Bell, who professionally word processed my manuscript; Shirley Taylor who provided a wealth of editorial assistance and Janet Perlman who performed the arduous task of indexing.

Many of the illustrations were expertly prepared by the Medical Illustration staff of the Palo Alto, California Veteran Affairs Medical Center. Preparation of the volume was supported in part by grants from the Ford Foundation to Stanford University, the American Physiological Society and the Palo Alto Institute for Research and Education.

I would be remiss if I did not acknowledge my wife, Barbara, who painstakingly has kept track of innumerable details contributing to the completion of this volume.

Finally, I thank my son Peter, the successful businessman in the family, for his management of the many business details including marketing of the volume. His business acumen and marketing savvy have no limits.

Introduction

The purpose of this volume is to present a summary of current knowledge regarding the effects of acute and chronic exposure to high altitude upon physiological functions in man as well as to review the important medical problems associated with high altitude. By presenting this summary and review in a convenient form, I hope to assist physicians and paramedical personnel in recognizing the various forms of high altitude illness so that prevention and treatment can be appropriately employed.

During the past thirty years numerous well-planned studies have been made of the various effects of high altitude upon human physiology. These investigations have been carried out on Mount Logan, Mount McKinley, and Mount Everest as well as in the Rocky Mountains and at the White Mountain Research Station in California. In a study called Operation Everest II, eight young men spent 40 days in a hypobaric chamber at Natick, Massachusetts, with a gradual decrease in pressure to an equivalent altitude of 29,000 feet (8,839 m). This study permitted the use of specialized methods of investigation that would not have been possible under field conditions.

The results of these various investigations have so far not been available in a single presentation but have appeared in numerous papers and abstracts in scientific journals and symposia. One of the chief purposes of this book is to summarize the observations and place the results in the context of earlier studies. I do not presume to have covered the field completely: some studies have been omitted for the sake of brevity, and some, also, have perhaps been misquoted or misinterpreted, for which I apologize.

The importance of medical problems of high altitude exposure can be illustrated by the following brief case reports.

A young executive in a computer firm was sent to Lima, Peru, as a consultant. His wife and two teenage sons accompanied him, and they planned a week's visit to Cuzco and Machu Picchu. They flew from Lima to Cuzco, 11,380 feet (3,470 m)— a fairly short flight—and spent the remainder of the day on a strenuous tour of the ruins at Sacsahuaman. That night they slept poorly, and the next morning all experienced severe headache, loss of appetite, weakness, and shortness of breath on slight effort, a condition known locally as *soroche*. The following night the symptoms were worse and they could only sleep for short periods because of difficulty in breathing, severe headache, and a sense of suffocation. During fretful periods of sleep they experienced strange nightmares. The following day they cancelled their trip and returned to Lima, where their symptoms subsided in a few hours.

A 37-year-old architect who is a capable skier went to a ski lodge at 8,900 feet (2,715 m) in the Rockies with his wife for the Christmas holiday. He had skied previously only in the Lake Tahoe area of California. The day after he arrived, he skied on all except the most advanced runs. The second day, after a strenuous morning on the slopes, he noticed progressive weakness, chest congestion, shortness of breath, and a persistent cough. He felt so weak that he could barely climb the ramp to get on the chair lift. At three o'clock in the afternoon he went to his room to rest. At six, his wife came to the room and found him semiconscious; he was breathing in a rapid, labored manner, and he had an unusual blue color to his lips that she had never seen before. She could barely arouse him and noticed unusual sounds with each breath that suggested fluid in his lungs. An ambulance was called, oxygen was administered, and he was rushed to a nearby hospital. He recovered after two days of bed rest and oxygen therapy.

A 21-year-old mountaineer from Los Angeles joined his father and six other climbers on a climb of Mount Aconcagua in Argentina. He had not previously climbed higher than 14,000 feet (4,280 m) nor slept higher than 10,000 feet (3,050 m). The trip was a regular tour organized by a well-known travel company and led by an experienced guide and climber. The party drove to the end of the road at 13,000 feet (3,965 m) and climbed to a hut at 15,000 feet (4,575 m) in one day. Each person carried about 30 pounds of equipment. All the members of the party, except for the leader, slept poorly that night. The next morning the young climber felt weak and dizzy and had a severe headache. A snowstorm and moderate winds forced the group to spend that day and night in the hut. During the night the young climber began to moan and thrash about, shouting that he was being attacked by snakes. When aroused, he was irrational, incoordinate, and barely able to stand. He could not walk without assistance. Later in the night he lapsed into a coma. The next day he was carried down on a mule to the road and taken to a nearby hospital. For two days he remained in a coma and then gradually regained consciousness. For the next two weeks he had difficulty in maintaining his balance and could not walk without assistance. He had no memory of the episode, starting with the first day of the climb to the hut. He slowly recovered, but one year later his sense of balance was still slightly impaired.

These acute illnesses occurring in previously healthy, physically fit young people are not unusual, esoteric infectious diseases but rather are common consequences of rapid ascent to high altitude. Acute mountain sickness, high altitude pulmonary edema, and high altitude cerebral edema occur all too frequently and can ruin a vacation, and may even cause death or disability. Each of these conditions can be prevented, recognized, and treated by appropriate methods. Unfortunately, however, many physicians still seem unaware of the prevalence of high altitude medical problems. Acute altitude illness continues to result in disability and death in high mountain regions throughout the world.

This volume is not intended to present a complete review of all the complex physiological adjustments to high altitude. Only the physiological changes that have major clinical relevance are examined.

HIGH ALTITUDE MEDICINE

CHAPTER 1

Physiological Effects of High Altitude

SUMMARY

The major effect of high altitude upon human physiology is a decrease in oxygen pressure and content in the arterial blood. The atmosphere at high altitude contains the same percentage of oxygen, 20.93 percent, as at sea level, but the partial pressure is reduced. It is the partial pressure that drives oxygen from the lungs into the blood. At 18,000 feet (5,850 m) the atmospheric pressure, and therefore the partial pressure of oxygen, is about half that of sea level. At 29,000 feet (9,425 m), it is only about one-third that of sea level. Symptoms of high altitude discomfort usually begin above 8,000 feet (2,600 m) and become more severe the higher the altitude and the more rapid the ascent. Four altitude ranges should be considered where physiological and medical problems may occur: (1) moderate (intermediate) altitude, 5,000-8,000 feet (1,500-2,440 m); (2) high altitude, 8,000-14,000 feet (2,440-4,270 m); (3) very high altitude, 14,000-18,000 feet (4,270-5,490 m); and (4) extreme altitude, 18,000-29,028 feet (5,490-8,848 m). Barometric pressure falls with increasing altitude, but this relationship is not constant: barometric pressure varies at a given altitude with changes in weather, as well as between the equator and the poles. For example, a barometric pressure of 253 mm Hg on the summit of Mount Everest would be only 224 mm Hg at the same altitude in the latitude of Mount McKinley. Weather changes may result in equivalent altitude variations of as much as 1,000 feet (304 m). Small variations in barometric pressure may have important physiological consequences especially at extreme altitudes.

• • •

The most important effect of high altitude upon physiological processes is a decrease in the oxygen pressure and content in the circulating blood. This decrease is directly related to the decrease in barometric pressure. As barometric pressure decreases, the partial pressure of oxygen also decreases, because the percentage of oxygen in the atmosphere at high altitude remains the same as at sea level (see Fig. 1.1). At sea level the oxygen content of the atmosphere is 21 percent and the atmospheric pressure is 760 mm Hg; therefore the partial pressure of inspired oxygen is about 160 mm Hg (760 x .21). If 100 percent oxygen is breathed, the partial pressure of oxygen will be 760 mm Hg and many more molecules of oxygen will enter the blood from the alveoli. At 18,000 feet (5,490 m) the atmospheric pressure is about half that at sea level. The partial pressure of oxygen will also be halved, resulting in a smaller number of molecules of oxygen entering the blood. The same effect can be achieved by breathing a mixture of nitrogen and 10 percent oxygen as shown in the far right of Figure 1.1. The partial pressure of inspired oxygen is moistened

2

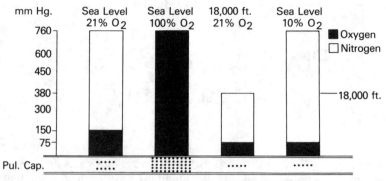

Pressure of O_2 at sea level and 18,000 ft.

Figure 1.1. The effect of barometric pressure and the partial pressure of oxygen under various conditions. The partial pressure refers to the partial pressure of the inspired air. As shown on the far right, breathing a mixture of 10 percent oxygen will have approximately the same effect as breathing air at 18,000 feet (5,490 m). As soon as the air reaches the airways the water vapor pressure of 47 mm displaces oxygen, nitrogen, and carbon dioxide. The oxygen pressure at the alveoli will decrease correspondingly to about 110 mm Hg while breathing air, or to 710 mm while breathing 100 percent oxygen. Dots in the figure indicate the relative number of molecules of oxygen.

by the water vapor in the airways, which reduces the oxygen pressure in the alveoli by about 47 mm Hg. The water vapor pressure is the same at high altitude as at sea level. Since the barometric pressure is lower at high altitude, the effect of water vapor pressure in reducing the oxygen pressure in the inspired air will be greater than at sea level. The decrease in oxygen in the blood at high altitude is compensated for by several physiological mechanisms, the most important of which is an increase in pulmonary ventilation. Pulmonary ventilation does not, however, completely compensate for the lower oxygen pressure, and as a result arterial oxygen tension and content fall as the altitude increases.

Hypoxia and Hypoxemia
In a general sense both hypoxia and anoxia refer to a lack of oxygen. In a more specific sense, hypoxia is defined as a decrease in the *partial pressure* of oxygen in blood or tissues. Altitude hypoxia is related to the decrease in barometric pressure and the resulting decrease in the partial pressure of inspired oxygen. Hypoxemia, a more specific term, refers to a decrease in the oxygen *content* of arterial blood. Hypoxemia occurs at high altitude because arterial blood is not fully saturated with oxygen owing to its low arterial tension. At sea level, hypoxemia with a low oxygen saturation and a low arterial oxygen tension of arterial blood may occur as a result of chronic pulmonary disease, pneumonia, or congenital heart disease. Hypoxemia may also occur in the presence of a normal arterial oxygen tension under unusual conditions, such as carbon monoxide poisoning or methemoglobinemia where the hemoglobin is partially bound to other substances that prevent full saturation with oxygen. In these conditions arterial oxygen tension may be normal, but the arterial oxygen saturation may be markedly decreased.

Altitude hypoxia differs from the more common varieties of hypoxia observed at sea level in patients with pulmonary disease. Altitude hypoxia is associated with hypocapnia, that is, a low arterial carbon dioxide pressure (PCO_2), in contrast to the patient with pulmonary disease at sea level where arterial PCO_2 is frequently normal or elevated. Some medical conditions at sea level are associated with hypoxia and a normal or low arterial PCO_2 including cyanotic congenital heart disease, left ventricular failure, cardiac pulmonary edema, and interstitial pulmonary disease.

The effect of acute hypocapnic hypoxia has been the subject of many studies. In general, obvious symptoms usually do not occur until the arterial PO_2 reaches 40 mm Hg, which occurs at about 18,000 feet (5,500 m). Levels of PO_2 from 60 to 40 mm Hg occur between 8,000 feet (2,500 m) and 10,000 feet (3,030 m), and may result in a mild to a moderate decrease in mental acuity. The relationship between altitude, barometric pressure, partial pressure of oxygen, and blood gases is shown in Table 1.1.

All altitudes in this volume are expressed in feet above sea level (feet) and meters (m). One foot equals .305 meters and one meter equals 3.281 feet. Barometric pressure is expressed as mm Hg. The conversion from meters to feet is summarized in Table 1.2.

Several abbreviations will be employed in this book. PO_2 refers to the partial presssure of oxygen expressed in mm Hg. In some publications the pressure is expressed as Torr units in recognition of Evangelista Torricelli, who invented the mercury barometer. One Torr unit is equivalent to one mm Hg. PCO_2 is the partial pressure of carbon dioxide. PAO_2 and $PACO_2$ refer to the partial pressure of these gases in the alveoli, and PaO_2 and $PaCO_2$ are the partial pressure of these gases in arterial blood. For purposes of simplicity and clarity, the terms alveolar PO_2-PCO_2 and arterial PO_2-PCO_2 will be used instead of PAO_2-$PACO_2$ and PaO_2 and $PaCO_2$. Oxygen saturation of blood is expressed as a percentage, SAO_2.

Table 1.1
Arterial Blood Gas Values at Various Altitudes Up to the
Summit of Mount Everest (mm Hg)

Feet	Meters	BP	PiO_2	PaO_2	$PaCO_2$	SAO_2 %
0	0	760	149	94	41	97
5,000[a]	1,500	630	122	66	39	92
8,000[a]	2,500	564	108	60	37	89
10,000[a]	3,000	523	100	53	36	85
12,000[a]	3,600	483	91	52	35	83
15,000[a]	4,600	412	76	44	32	75
18,000[a]	5,500	379	69	40	29	71
20,000[a]	6,100	349	63	38	21	65
24,000[a]	7,300	280	52	34	16	50
28,028[b]	8,848	253	43	28	7.5	70

SOURCES: [a]Hecht, ref. 11; [b]West et al., ref. 12. In source [b] data from one subject, arterial PCO_2 were obtained by extrapolation from venous samples drawn hours later at a lower altitude.

NOTES: The estimated arterial oxygen saturation is higher at 28,028 feet (8,848 m) than at 24,000 feet (7,300 m) owing to the severe alkalosis and the left shift of the hemoglobin oxygen dissociation curve.

SYMBOLS: BP = barometric pressure mm Hg, PiO_2 = partial pressure of inspired oxygen, PaO_2 = arterial oxygen pressure, $PaCO_2$ = arterial carbon dioxide pressure, SAO_2 % = arterial oxygen saturation.

4

Table 1.2
Conversion of Meters to Feet

meters	feet	meters	feet	meters	feet	meters	feet
3,300	10,827	4,700	15,420	6,100	20,013	7,500	24,607
3,400	11,155	4,800	15,748	6,200	20,342	7,600	24,935
3,500	11,483	4,900	16,076	6,300	20,670	7,700	25,263
3,600	11,811	5,000	16,404	6,400	20,998	7,800	25,591
3,700	12,139	5,100	16,733	6,500	21,326	7,900	25,919
3,800	12,467	5,200	17,061	6,600	21,654	8,000	26,247
3,900	12,795	5,300	17,389	6,700	21,982	8,100	26,575
4,000	13,124	5,400	17,717	6,800	22,310	8,200	26,903
4,100	13,452	5,500	18,045	6,900	22,638	8,300	27,231
4,200	13,780	5,600	18,373	7,000	22,966	8,400	27,560
4,300	14,108	5,700	18,701	7,100	23,294	8,500	27,888
4,400	14,436	5,800	19,029	7,200	23,622	8,600	28,216
4,500	14,764	5,900	19,357	7,300	24,951	8,700	28,544
4,600	15,092	6,000	19,685	7,400	24,279	8,800	28,872

SOURCE: *American Alpine Club Journal* 1989; 31:128.

Aircraft

Cabin pressures in modern jet aircraft are maintained at a level between 5,000 and 6,000 feet (1,525-2,000 m) and rarely may reach the equivalent of 8,000 feet (2,440 m). Even on long transoceanic flights, altitude exposure causes few symptoms in normal healthy subjects, although symptoms do sometimes occur in patients with pulmonary or cardiac disease. Obesity, alcohol, sedative drugs that depress respiration, prolonged immobility, and sleep may cause hypoventilation and intensify the hypoxemia under these conditions. Flights in smaller nonpressurized aircraft may exceed altitudes of 10,000 feet (3,050 m) and oxygen may be available only to the pilot and copilot.

Altitude and Barometric Pressure

For the purposes of discussion it is convenient to define four altitude levels at which medical problems may occur:

1. *Intermediate altitude*—5,000-8,000 feet (1,500-2,440 m). Intermediate altitude is an acceptable term for elevations below 8,000 feet (2,440 m). Significant altitude illness is rare in this altitude range. High altitude pulmonary edema, for example, is virtually unknown among skiers in the Lake Tahoe area of California, where lodges and hotels are located at altitudes of 6,000-7,000 feet (1,830-2,135 m), but it has been observed in nearly all ski areas above 8,000 feet (2,440 m). Patients with cardiac or pulmonary disease may exhibit increased symptoms in this altitude range and some persons may even experience mild symptoms of acute mountain sickness as low as 6,700 feet (2,000 m).[1]

2. *High altitude*—8,000-14,000 feet (2,440- 4,270 m). Most altitude-related medical problems occur between 8,000 feet (2,440 m) and 14,000 feet (4,270 m), because these are the elevations visited by the greatest number of people. Altitudes

exceeding 14,000 feet (4,270 m) are rarely reached by tourists in the United States or Europe.

Altitude illness is largely dependent upon the altitude at which one sleeps and not upon the highest elevation attained for a short period of time.

3. *Very high altitude*—14,000-18,000 feet (4,270-5,490 m). Very high altitudes are commonly encountered by climbers and trekkers in many parts of the world, including South America and the Himalayas. These altitudes are frequent locations for climbing party base camps where climbers may stay for many days or weeks. It is very dangerous to ascend to these altitude levels without gradual acclimatization.

4. *Extreme altitude*—18,000-29,028 feet (5,490-8,848 m). The extreme altitude ranges are only reached by expeditionary mountain climbers, and then only for a short time. Acute medical problems at these altitudes are more frequently related to terrain and weather (falls, avalanches, frostbite, hypothermia) than to the usual altitude medical conditions, since at these altitudes most climbers will have been acclimatized and those susceptible to altitude problems will have descended. Less frequent but more serious medical problems such as cerebral edema and pulmonary embolism may first occur in this altitude range, however, even in well-acclimatized climbers; pulmonary edema and cerebral edema may occur if ascent is rapid or the work load is too great in this altitude range.

A prolonged stay at altitudes above 18,000 feet (5,490 m) results in altitude deterioration rather than continued improvement in acclimatization, and for this reason climbers who are setting up routes and camps up to 27,000 feet (8,235 m) usually return to base camp for several days before moving up rapidly for the summit climbs. Members of the 1960 Himalayan Scientific and Mountaineering Expedition spent more than five months at 19,000 feet (5,795 m) at Mingbo La near Mount Makalu. Although the group tolerated this altitude reasonably well, they all lost weight. Colleagues who joined the group after a five-month acclimatization period appeared to be more fit and active than the men who wintered at 19,000 feet (5,795 m).[2]

Natives who live continuously at very high altitude also probably experience deterioration. Miners who work at the Auconquilcha sulfur mine in Chile at 19,516 feet (5,950 m) prefer to live at 14,235 feet (4,340 m) and travel daily up to the mine to work. Many miners go down to Amincha, 13,776 feet (4,200 m), on weekends. The miners know that living at the mine would result in deterioration.[3]

Barometric Pressure

Barometric presssure falls nearly exponentially with increasing altitude and can be estimated by a knowledge of the altitude and standard tables. The relation of altitude to barometric pressure is shown in Figure 1.2. The upper curve is that calculated from a formula developed by Zuntz when a mean temperature of +15 degrees centigrade and a sea-level pressure of 760 mm Hg are assumed.[4] The lower curve was developed from the internationally adopted altimeter calibration formula. The relationship between barometric pressure and altitude for the Standard Atmosphere has also been described by Haldane and Priestly.[5] It can be seen that on the summit of Mount Everest at 29,028 feet (8,848 m) the barometric pressure would be 269 mm Hg according to the Zuntz formula and 236 mm Hg according to the altimeter scale—a difference equivalent to between 1,000 feet (305 m) and 1,500 feet of altitude (458 m). The actual pressure measured by Dr. Chris Pizzo on the summit of Mount Everest during the American Medical Research Expedition to Everest in

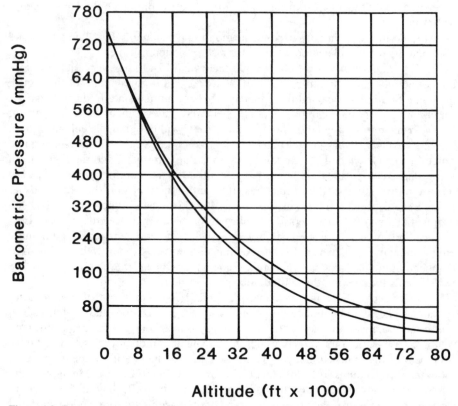

Figure 1.2 Two curves showing relation of barometric pressure to altitude. The upper curve is drawn from the Zuntz formula. The lower curve is the international altitude calibration curve. From West et al., ref. 6.

October 1981 was 253 mm Hg, which was 17 mm higher than that predicted by the international altimeter calibration formula.[6,7,8] At extreme altitudes small variations in barometric pressure may make great difference in climbing ability. Barometric pressure *at the same elevation* is lower at higher latitudes nearer the poles, as in Alaska, than nearer the equator. Therefore, at an elevation of 20,000 feet (6,100 m) in Alaska, for example, the partial pressure of oxygen is lower than at the same elevation near the equator and at the summit of Mount Everest. The barometric pressure of approximately 253 mm would be predicted to be only about 224 mm at the same elevation in the latitude of Mount McKinley. The reason for this phenomenon is that there is a very large mass of heavy cold air in the stratosphere above the equator, as the atmosphere is "piled" up owing to the effect of convection and radiation. This air mass weighs more than the air mass nearer the poles. Thus local barometric pressure at all elevations around the equator is higher, compared with more northern and southern areas nearer the poles.

Barometric pressure will also reflect changes in the weather (Fig.1.3). During the winter of 1960-61 a range of barometric pressure from 372 to 384 mm Hg, equivalent to an altitude variation of 750 feet (230 m), was observed at the Silver Hut at 19,000 feet (5,795 m) in the Everest region.[2] In the Everest area barometric

Barometric Pressures on Mt. Everest

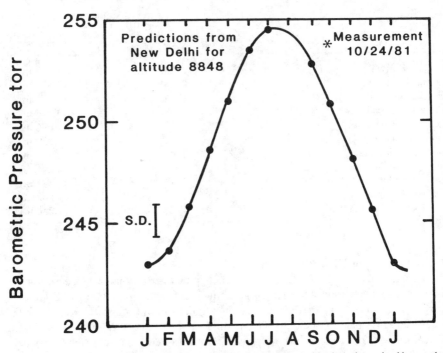

Figure 1.3. Variations in barometric pressure for 29,028 foot (8,848 m) altitude as determined by weather balloons released from New Delhi, India, in 1981. Mean monthly standard deviation as shown by the asterisk indicates the barometric pressure on Mount Everest on October 24, which was higher than normal. From West et al., ref. 6.

pressure during the warm, clear days from May to October was about 10-11 mm higher than in December to February during cold, stormy days. This is one reason that it will be very much more difficult to climb Everest in the winter without supplemental oxygen. At Keystone, Colorado, 9,300 feet (2,840 m), the average change of barometric pressure between good weather and a storm is about 10-20 mm Hg with maximum changes as much as 40 mm Hg. This corresponds to an altitude change of 500-1,000 feet (150-300 m) and a maximum change of about 2,000 feet (610 m).[9] Seasonal changes in barometric pressure are important at higher elevations. In midsummer the barometric pressure is significantly higher on Mount McKinley and may be as much as an equivalent altitude of 3,000 feet (915 m) on the summit.[10] Thus the effect of altitude upon man cannot be predicted simply by the height above sea level. Barometric pressure varies with seasons, location on the earth, weather, and temperature. Against these physical factors the physiological response of the climber must also be considered.

High Altitude Cities

Many cities in the United States and elsewhere in the world are at altitudes where mild or severe altitude effects may occur. Some of these cities are shown in Table 1.3.

Table 1.3
High Altitude Cities of the World

| City | Altitude | |
	(feet)	(meters)
La Paz, Bolivia	12,730	(3,883 m)
Lhasa, Tibet	12,000	(3,660 m)
Cuzco, Peru	11,380	(3,471 m)
Climax, Colorado, U.S.A.	11,190	(3,413 m)
Leadville, Colorado, U.S.A.	10,150	(3,096 m)
Quito, Ecuador	9,343	(2,850 m)
Bogotà, Colombia	8,563	(2,612 m)
Mexico City, Mexico	7,347	(2,241 m)
Denver, Colorado, U.S.A.	5,400	(1,647 m)
Casper, Wyoming, U.S.A.	5,123	(1,562 m)
Salt Lake City, Utah, U.S.A.	4,255	(1,248 m)

Tourist Access to High Mountains

Aircraft, autos, railroads, and cable car facilities permit the easy access of even the most sedentary tourist to many high altitude cities and mountain passes or summits. In Hawaii one can drive from sea level to the summit of Mauna Kea at 13,780 feet (4,200 m) in about one hour. This is the location of six large telescopes making observations at optical and infrared wave lengths. In Peru one can reach Morococha at 14,900 feet (4,540 m) within three hours from Lima by rail or auto. San Cristóbal is a mining town in the central Peruvian Andes, which can be reached via an all year road. The altitude is 15,600 feet (4,758 m). In Europe, trains, cable cars, and téléfériques reach altitudes above 10,000 feet (3,050 m). The Jungfrau Joch in the Swiss Alps at 11,397 feet (3,476 m) is reached by a railroad. The highest point that can be reached by a modern cable car is above Mérida, Venezuela. This car transports tourists from the center of town at 5,400 feet (1,647 m) to 15,800 feet (4,820 m) in 45 minutes. A restaurant, viewpoints, and other facilities are provided at the highest station.

Ski Resorts

In the United States many ski resorts provide access to mountains as high as 10,000 feet (3,050 m) to 14,000 feet (4,270 m). A list of representative U.S. ski resorts and their elevations is shown in Table 1.4. Most of these resorts are in the Rocky Mountains. The highest ski resort in the U.S. is at Breckenridge, Colorado, at 9,630 feet (2,940 m) and the top of the ski run is 12,213 feet (3,725 m). Most ski resorts in Europe are located below 8,000 feet (2,440 m), but summit ridges of 12,000 feet (3,660 m) to 14,000 feet (4,270 m) can be reached by chair lifts and cable cars. In Chile one ski lift starts at 9,230 feet (2,815 m) and reaches to 11,370 feet (3,468 m). At 17,050 feet (5,200 m) in Bolivia there is a rope tow that is reached by road from La Paz at 12,730 feet (3,773 m). In Mexico skiers can stay at the modern Tlacmacas Lodge at 12,950 feet (3,950 m) and ski on the upper slopes of Popocatepetl (summit 17,887 feet/5,456 m), but there are no lift facilities. In 1988-89, it is estimated that 7.7 million skiers visited the top ten ski resorts in Colorado.

Table 1.4
Altitudes of Selected Ski Areas in the United States

	Base (feet)	Top (meters)	Altitude (feet)	(meters)
California				
Mammoth Lakes	9,000	(2,745)	11,053	(3,371)
Squaw Valley	8,200	(2,500)	8,900	(2,715)
June Lake	8,100	(2,470)	10,212	(3,115)
Kirkwood	7,700	(2,350)	9,800	(2,890)
Sugar Bowl	6,883	(2,100)	8,383	(2,557)
Alpine Meadows	6,840	(2,086)	8,637	(2,637)
Heavenly Valley	6,600	(2,015)	10,167	(3,100)
Colorado				
Leadville	10,500	(3,203)	11,700	(3,567)
Loveland Basin	10,500	(3,200)	11,500	(3,508)
Breckenridge	9,630	(2,940)	12,213	(3,725)
Copper Mountain	9,600	(2,928)	11,600	(3,538)
Crested Butte	9,375	(2,860)	11,250	(3,430)
Keystone	9,300	(2,840)	12,450	(3,797)
Telluride	8,735	(2,664)	11,890	(3,626)
Snowmass	8,212	(2,505)	11,808	(3,600)
Arapahoe Basin	8,200	(2,500)	11,500	(3,813)
Vail	8,200	(2,500)	11,250	(3,430)
Aspen	8,000	(2,440)	11,800	(3,600)
Utah				
Park City	8,900	(2,715)	10,000	(3,050)
Alta	8,600	(2,623)	10,550	(3,218)
Idaho				
Sun Valley	5,787	(1,765)	9,150	(2,790)
Wyoming				
Jackson Hole	6,311	(1,925)	10,466	(3,186)
New Mexico				
Santa Fe	10,283	(3,136)	12,100	(3,690)
Sandia Peak	9,650	(3,943)	10,378	(3,165)
Taos	9,207	(2,808)	11,819	(3,605)

Trekkers and Climbers

Organized treks to all parts of the world permit rapid access to very high altitudes. Since ascent is often rapid, the stay at high altitude is often prolonged, and heavy daily physical exertion is usually involved. Severe altitude illness is frequent under these conditions. The limitations of rapid transport and the lack of medical facilities contribute to numerous fatalities.

A popular trek in Nepal reaches its highest altitude at the Everest Base Camp at 17,500 feet (5,340 m). Many participants on this trek climb to the nearby summit of Kala Patar at 18,500 feet (5,640 m). Trekkers who walk from Katmandu, 4,500 feet (1,375 m), have few serious altitude problems because the walk takes two to three weeks, which allows for a gradual ascent and acclimatization. Serious problems, however, occur when trekkers fly to Lukla at 9,200 feet (2,810 m) and begin the walk from this point. In three to four days these trekkers can be above 14,000 feet (4,270 m). One can also fly from Katmandu to the Everest View Hotel at 12,700 feet (3,875 m), a short distance from the trail to the Everest Base Camp.

In Peru many treks cross passes as high as 15,400 feet (4,697 m), and base camps are as high as 14,000 feet (4,270 m). Serious altitude illness is common under these conditions, since these elevations can be reached within two to three days after leaving sea-level cities.

Some well-known mountain peaks are within easy access of major cities where guide services for summit climbs are available. From Mexico City one can climb Popocatepetl by driving two to three hours to the Tlacamas Lodge, 12,950 feet (3,950 m), and starting up the mountain the following morning. In Arequipa, Peru, to climb El Misti, 18,500 feet (5,645 m), one can drive to a roadhead at 12,000 feet (3,660 m) to begin the climb. El Pichincha, 15,728 feet (4,800 m), is on the outskirts of Quito, Ecuador, at 9,134 feet (2,786 m). Mount Fuji, 12,395 feet (3,780 m), in Japan can be climbed in one day by starting at the Fifth Station at 7,800 feet (2,380 m). Few people experience severe mountain sickness on Fuji, because it is possible to reach the summit and return in one day, and that is too short a time for symptoms of mountain sickness to become severe. Commonly climbed mountains are listed in Table 1.5. Popular climbs that require more advanced technical skills are made on Mount McKinley, Alaska; Huascaràn, Peru; Aconcagua, Argentina; Chimborazo, Ecuador; Mount Kenya, Africa; and most Himalayan peaks.

High Altitude Populations

In many parts of the world, populations have resided at high altitude for many generations. In Peru, human bones have been found at 14,000 feet (4,270 m) in the Lauricocha region; radiocarbon tests indicate that they are approximately 9,000 years old. More recently, signs of ancient human habitation have been found as high as 18,000 feet (5,490 m) in the Andes, though it is not known whether these dwellings were permanent or temporary living accommodations or fortifications.

High altitude areas of the world where there are large populations of permanent residents include the Andes of South America, the Caucasus of Eastern Europe, Ethiopia, Tibet, Africa, and the Himalaya. It is estimated that about 38 million people live above 8,000 feet (2,440 m). In Peru the highland population living above 8,000 feet (2,440 m) is estimated to be about 4 million (Table 1.6). About 80,000 Peruvians live in Cerro de Pasco, altitude 14,200 feet (4,330 m), and 6,000 live in the mining town of San Cristóbal 15,600 feet (4,758 m). La Paz, the capital city of Bolivia, is at 12,730 feet (3,883 m) and has a population of approximately one million.

Permanent residents of high altitude regions possess physiological characteristics that clearly are the result of generations of high altitude life. In the past, native highlanders rarely traveled to sea level, but now that modern transport facilities are readily available, many high altitude residents do travel to sea level areas for vary-

Table 1.5
Important Mountain Peaks of the World

Mountain	Location	Altitude	
U.S.A.			
Mount McKinley	Alaska	20,320 ft.	(6,198 m)
Mount Rainier	Washington	14,500 ft.	(4,422 m)
Mount Whitney	California	14,500 ft.	(4,422 m)
Mount Shasta	California	14,200 ft.	(4,362 m)
Pikes Peak	Colorado	14,110 ft.	(4,303 m)
Mauna Kea	Hawaii	13,896 ft.	(4,205 m)
Grand Teton	Wyoming	13,766 ft.	(4,200 m)
Longs Peak	Colorado	13,000 ft.	(3,965 m)
Mount Hood	Oregon	11,000 ft.	(3,355 m)
Mexico - South America			
Aconcagua	Argentina	23,080 ft.	(7,039 m)
Ojos del Salado	Chile	22,580 ft.	(6,887 m)
Huascaràn	Peru	22,334 ft.	(6,812 m)
Chimborazo	Ecuador	20,561 ft.	(6,271 m)
Cotopaxi	Ecuador	19,357 ft.	(5,904 m)
El Misti	Peru	19,100 ft.	(5,826 m)
Pico Orizaba	Mexico	18,700 ft.	(5,704 m)
Popocatepetl	Mexico	17,887 ft.	(5,452 m)
Ixtacihuatl	Mexico	17,343 ft.	(5,286 m)
Europe			
Mont Blanc	France	16,500 ft.	(5,032 m)
Monte Rosa	Switzerland	15,200 ft.	(4,635 m)
Weisshorn	Switzerland	14,800 ft.	(4,505 m)
Matterhorn	Switzerland	14,000 ft.	(4,270 m)
Africa			
Kilimanjaro	Tanzania	19,210 ft.	(5,893 m)
Mount Kenya	Kenya	16,500 ft.	(5,033 m)
Japan			
Mount Fuji	Japan	12,395 ft.	(5,551 m)
New Zealand			
Mount Cook	New Zealand	12,350 ft.	(3,765 m)
Himalayas			
Everest	Tibet-Nepal	29,000 ft.	(8,850 m)
K2	Karakorams	28,240 ft.	(8,610 m)
Kangchenjunga	Sikkim	28,200 ft.	(8,600 m)
Lhotse	Tibet-Nepal	27,900 ft.	(8,500 m)
Makalu	Nepal	27,780 ft.	(8,470 m)
Dhaulagiri	Nepal	26,800 ft.	(8,170 m)
Cho Oyu	Tibet-Nepal	26,750 ft.	(8,155 m)
Nanga Parbat	Karakorams	26,650 ft.	(8,125 m)
Manaslu	Nepal	26,650 ft.	(8,125 m)
Annapurna	Nepal	26,500 ft.	(8,080 m)
Gasherbrum 11 and 1V	Karakorams	26,470 ft.	(8,070 m)
Hidden Peak	Karakorams	26,450 ft.	(8,065 m)
Broad Peak	Karakorams	26,400 ft.	(8,045 m)

Table 1.6
**Estimated Number of Permanent High Altitude Residents and Annual High
Altitude Visitors Worldwide at Altitudes Above 8,000 feet (2,439 m), 1984-1986**

Continent	Country	Permanent residents	Percent total	Visitors	Percent total
Africa	Ethiopia	7,379,000	19	61,000	<1
	Kenya	6,125,000	16	541,000	1
			35		2
Asia	Afghanistan	4,778,000	12	9,000	<1
	Bhutan	426,000	1	2,000	<1
	China-Tibet	1,800,000	5	30,000	<1
	India-Sikkim	?	?	?	?
	India-Kashmir	?	?	?	?
	Nepal	4,798,000	12	181,000	<1
	Russian Commonwealth				
	Tadzhik	1,140,000	3	?	?
	Kirgiz	1,059,000	3	?	?
			36		<1
North America	Colorado	120,000	<1	14,370,000	39
	New Mexico	90,000	<1	5,000,000	14
	Utah	70,000	<1	10,600,000	29
	Wyoming	40,000	<1	4,750,000	13
			1		95
South America	Bolivia	2,443,000	6	127,000	<1
	Chile	1,097,000	3	394,000	<1
	Ecuador	2,902,000	8	350,000	<1
	Peru	4,069,000	11	300,000	<1
			28		3
Total		38,336,000	100%	36,715,000	100%

SOURCES: L Moore. Altitude aggravated illness: Examples from pregnancy and prenatal life. *Ann. Emerg. Med.* 1987; 16:965-73.

ing periods of time. If sufficiently prolonged (1-4 weeks) a sea-level sojourn can result in some loss of acclimatization, and altitude illness may recur upon reascent. High altitude residents may exhibit certain forms of high altitude illness that are dependent upon prolonged hypoxia. These include "chronic mountain sickness" (Monge's disease), "chronic mountain polycythemia," and pulmonary hypertension.

High Altitude Research Stations

High altitude research is carried out in many parts of the world, including China. A partial listing of some of the better known research stations is presented in Table 1.7.

Table 1.7
Important High Altitude Research Stations of the World

Name and location	Altitude
U.S.A.	
Mount Evans, Colorado	14,264 ft. (4,350 m)
Summit Hut, White Mountain, California	14,246 ft. (4,354 m)
Pikes Peak, Colorado	14,110 ft. (4,304 m)
Mount Wrangell, Alaska	14,000 ft. (4,270 m)
Mauna Kea Summit, Hawaii	13,800 ft. (4,209 m)
Barcroft Laboratory, White Mountain, California	12,470 ft. (3,803 m)
Climax, Colorado	11,190 ft. (3,413 m)
Echo Lake Research Station, Colorado	10,700 ft. (3,264 m)
Leadville, Colorado	10,500 ft. (3,203 m)
Crooked Creek, White Mountain, California	10,150 ft. (3,096 m)
Kole Kole, Hawaii	10,020 ft. (3,056 m)
Mauna Kea Observatory, Hawaii	9,800 ft. (2,989 m)
South America	
Cesar Tejos, Chile	20,000 ft. (6,100 m)
Laboratorio Fisica	
Cosmica Chacaltaya, near La Paz, Bolivia	17,060 ft. (5,203 m)
Ticlio, Peru	15,400 ft. (4,700 m)
Institute of Andean Biology, Morococha, Peru	14,900 ft. (4,545 m)
Instituto de Biologia, Mina Aguilar	
de La Altura, Argentina	14,763 ft. (4,503 m)
Cerro de Pasco, Peru	14,200 ft. (4,331 m)
Infernillo, Chile	14,170 ft. (4,322 m)
La Oroya, Peru	12,230 ft. (3,730 m)
University of La Paz, Bolivia	11,800 ft. (3,600 m)
Instituto Geofisico de Huancayo, Peru	10,990 ft. (3,352 m)
Eva Perón, Argentina	10,170 ft. (3,102 m)
Europe	
Capanna Margherita, Monte Rosa, Italy	14,953 ft. (4,559 m)
Observatoire Vallot, Mont Blanc, France	14,281 ft. (4,356 m)
L'Aiguille du Midi, Mont Blanc, France	11,810 ft. (3,602 m)
Laboratorio Testa, Grigia, Val D'Aosta, Italy	11,417 ft. (3,482 m)
Jungfraujoch High Altitude Research Station,	
Berner Oberland, Switzerland	11,397 ft. (3,476 m)
Sonnblick, Austria	10,190 ft. (3,108 m)
Grossglockner, Austria	9,840 ft. (3,000 m)
Cal d'Olen (Instituto Angelo Mosso), Italy	9,512 ft. (2,900 m)
Instituto Angelo Mosso, Monte Rosa, Italy	9,396 ft. (2,866 m)
Obergurgl, Austria	6,560 ft. (2,000 m)
Other areas	
Himalayan Rescue Association, Nepal	14,000 ft. (4,270 m)
Everest View Hotel, Nepal	12,700 ft. (3,874 m)
Mount Fuji, Japan	12,370 ft. (3,773 m)
Gulmarg Laboratory, India	9,900 ft. (3,020 m)
Italian Research Laboratory, Lobuche, Nepal	16,175 ft. (4,930 m)

NOTE: Many altitude stations are being operated elsewhere in the world, including China.

References

1. MONTGOMERY A, MILLS J, and LUCE J. Incidence of acute mountain sickness at intermediate altitude. *JAMA* 1989; 261:732-34.
2. PUGH L. Physiological and medical aspects of the Himalayan Scientific and Mountaineering Expedition. *Brit. Med. J.* 1962; 2:621-27.
3. DILL D. Personal communication.
4. ZUNTZ N, LOEWY A, MULLER F, and CASPARI W. Atmospheric pressure at high altitudes. In *Höhenklima und Bergwanderungen in ihrer Wirkung auf den Menschen.* Berlin: Bong, 1906. Translation of relevant pages in J West, ed., *High altitude physiology.* Stroudsburg, Pa: Hutchinson, Ross, 1981:37-39.
5. HALDANE J, and PRIESTLEY J. *Respiration.* 2d. ed. New Haven, Conn: Yale University Press, 1935:323.
6. WEST J, LAHIRI S, MARET K, PETERS R, JR., and PIZZO C. Barometric pressures at extreme altitudes on Mt. Everest: Physiologic significance. *J. Appl. Physiol.* 1983; 54:1188-94.
7. WEST J. Oxygenless climbs and barometric pressure. *Am. Alpine J.* 1984; 26:126-33.
8. WEST J. Man on the summit of Mount Everest. In J West and S Lahiri, eds., *High altitude and man.* Bethesda, Md. American Physiological Society, 1984: 5-17.
9. NICHOLAS R. Personal communication.
10. MOORE T. The worlds great mountains: Not the height you think. Am. Alpine J. 1968; 16:109-16.
11. HECHT H. A sea level view of altitude problems. *Am. J. Med.* 1971; 50:703-8.
12. WEST J, HACKETT P, MARET K, MILLEDGE J, PETERS J, JR., et al. Pulmonary gas exchange on the summit of Mt. Everest. *J. Appl. Physiol.* 1983; 55:678- 87.

CHAPTER 2

Respiration and Pulmonary Function

SUMMARY

Ascent to high altitude is accompanied by an increase in pulmonary ventilation as a result of the hypoxic stimulus acting primarily via the peripheral chemoreceptors and the respiratory center. Arterial PCO_2 falls and an alkalosis ensues during the first few days of altitude exposure. The alkalosis is partially corrected by renal compensation, but a moderate alkalosis persists. The increase in ventilation also persists; marked increases in ventilation occur during exercise compared with sea-level values at the same degree of exercise.

Several changes in pulmonary function occur upon ascent, including a small decrease in vital capacity, a marked decrease in breath-holding time, and increases in maximum breathing capacity and FEV_1 (forced expired volume in one second). Although resting pulmonary diffusing capacity is unchanged with ascent to high altitude, at very high altitudes exercise is accompanied by an impairment in gas exchange and a decrease in arterial PO_2. The magnitude of the decrease is proportional to the altitude and the amount of exercise with considerable individual variations.

• • •

Peripheral Chemoreceptors

Ascent to high altitude is accompanied by an increase in pulmonary ventilation as a result of the hypoxic stimulus acting primarily via the peripheral chemoreceptors and the respiratory center. This increase in alveolar ventilation constitutes one of the most important physiological adjustments that permits man to function even at extreme altitudes. The increase is dependent upon several integrated control systems.

The carotid body located just above the bifurcation of the common carotid artery is the principal sensing organ for arterial oxygen tension; the aortic bodies have a similar function, but are less important. These organs constitute the peripheral chemoreceptors. The carotid body, though it weighs only 10 mg, has a large blood flow per unit of weight and surface area, which enables it to respond promptly to changes in arterial oxygen; it is sensitive to oxygen partial pressure and not to oxygen content. The carotid body also responds, though only weakly, to changes in carbon dioxide partial pressure.[1]

Central Respiratory Centers

The main sensors for changes in PCO_2 are the central medullary chemoreceptors, usually known as the respiratory center, but actually a pair of centers deep in the medulla, just below the surface of the fourth ventricle and immersed in cerebrospinal fluid. The central chemoreceptors are sensitive to pH changes in the cerebrospinal fluid. Carbon dioxide is rapidly diffusible across the blood brain barrier. As arterial carbon dioxide levels increase, the PCO_2 in the cerebrospinal fluid also increases, and there is a corresponding increase in cerebrospinal fluid hydrogen ion concentration and a decrease in pH. It is this decrease in pH that is sensed by the central chemoreceptors that increase ventilation.

Carbon Dioxide (CO_2)

During acclimatization, the ventilatory response to carbon dioxide is gradually increased so that a greater ventilation occurs with lower levels of carbon dioxide, presumably because of an increased sensitivity to carbon dioxide (Fig. 2.1). The influence of hypoxia on the response to carbon dioxide remains the same as at sea level, so that a fall in arterial PO_2 still increases the response to carbon dioxide. This represents an interaction between arterial carbon dioxide and oxygen tension in controlling respiration. If the respiratory response to CO_2 is measured at several different oxygen tensions, the slope of the response to CO_2 becomes steeper as alveolar PO_2 is lowered (Fig. 2.2). The significance and basis of this increased sensitivity to CO_2 are not known, although exaggerated chemoreceptor discharge is one possibility.[2]

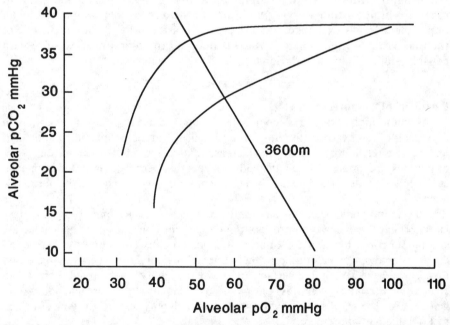

Figure 2.1. Alveolar gas concentrations and altitude. The upper line indicates the arterial PO_2 and PCO_2 in subjects exposed to an increasing simulated altitude in a hypobaric chamber. The lower line is obtained from residents at high altitude and acclimatized mountaineers. The diagonal straight line indicates possible PO_2 and PCO_2 values as a result of ventilation occurring at 12,000 feet (3,600 m). The decrease in arterial PCO_2 reflects the increase in ventilation, which increases sharply below an alveolar PO_2 of about 50 mm. The lower PCO_2 in the acclimatized represents the higher ventilation, which is an important adjustment to high altitude. From Rahn and Otis, ref. 15.

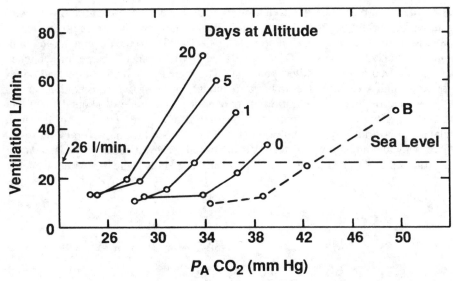

Figure 2.2. The effect of acclimatization upon the ventilatory response to arterial PCO_2 in normal subjects brought to 14,300 feet (4,340 m). Note that during the altitude stay the ventilatory response to arterial PCO_2 is shifted to the left and the response curve becomes steeper, indicating an increased response. The steady-state method was employed. Numbers at the top of each curve indicate the number of days at altitude. Redrawn from Kellogg, ref. 19.

Cerebrospinal Fluid and Respiration

As a result of the hypoxia-driven increase in respiration, both blood and cerebrospinal fluid carbon dioxide fall very nearly together, as one would expect, and this inhibits respiration. However, the body appears to choose between the dangerous effects of increased hypoxia and the less serious consequences of carbon dioxide depletion. Individual differences in ventilatory response result in variable effects of carbon dioxide and oxygen; in some persons carbon dioxide may have greater control, and in others oxygen may dominate.[3]

Severinghaus and others in 1963 presented data suggesting that this cerebrospinal fluid alkalosis is prevented by active transport of bicarbonate ions out of the cerebrospinal fluid, resulting in an increase in acidity and a stimulation of ventilation, which would facilitate acclimatization.[4] This concept was also employed to explain the gradual return to pre-ascent values of ventilation upon descent to sea level after a stay at high altitude.[5] Subsequently, other workers have found that the pH of the lumbar and intracranial cerebrospinal fluid in men at high altitude was more alkaline that at sea level.[6,7] The mechanism of the slow secondary increase in ventilation at high altitude is therefore not clear, but changes in neuromodulators acting on respiratory control neurons may be involved.[8]

Hypoxic Ventilatory Response (HVR)

The increase in ventilation due to hypoxia, or the hypoxic ventilatory reponse (HVR), may also be affected by the arterial PCO_2 because ventilation is inhibited as the PCO_2 falls with the increase in ventilation. To determine the HVR, subjects are exposed over a period of five to ten minutes to decreasing concentrations of oxygen, with arterial oxygen saturation determined usually by an earpiece oximeter. In order to maintain a constant CO_2 stimulus, CO_2 is added to the inspired air to maintain a constant alveolar PCO_2 (Isocapnic HVR).[8,9] Tests can also be performed when CO_2 is allowed to fall (poikilocapnic test). The increase in ventilation usually does not occur until alveolar PO_2 is reduced to about 50 mm Hg, which is equivalent to a 12.5 percent oxygen concentration at sea level or an altitude of about 10,200 feet (3,100 m). The relation of ventilation to arterial PO_2 is hyperbolic, but linear in relation to arterial oxygen saturation (Fig. 2.3). Depending on several conditions there is a wide range of values for HVR in normal sea-level subjects; coefficients of variation range from 23 percent to 73 percent.[9] The HVR decreases with advancing

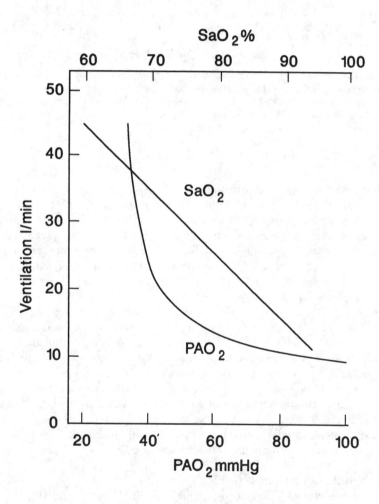

Figure 2.3. Hypoxic ventilatory response (HVR). Note the increase in ventilation as PCO_2 held constant. The relation of ventilation to the arterial oxygen saturation is linear. From Weil et al., ref. 9.

age,[9] and men have a lower HVR than women; also, prolonged hypoxia over many years will result in a low HVR.[10] It is known that chronic mountain sickness is more common in older men who have lived for many years at high altitude. Severe hypoxia may depress the HVR.[11,12,13] There is also some evidence that prolonged training for distance sports may decrease the HVR.[14] A low HVR has been implicated in the occurrence of acute mountain sickness and high altitude pulmonary edema.

There may also be geographical differences in HVR. For example, high altitude natives in South America have a greater blunting of chemosensitivity than do Himalayan natives, and this may be a factor in the higher incidence of chronic mountain sickness in South America. Centuries of acclimatization may have something to do with the apparent beneficial higher hypoxic ventilatory response in the Himalayan natives, which has evolved over the million years that they have lived at high altitude, compared with the 20,000-40,000 years of native residence in the South American Andes.

Respiration at High Altitude

Although there are individual differences in the sensitivity and response of the respiratory control mechanisms, in general ventilation will become substantially increased at about 10,000 feet (3,050 m). A detectable increase may be evident as low as 5,000 feet (1,500 m). The increase occurs primarily in the depth of ventilation, and there is little change in respiratory rate until higher high altitudes are attained (Table 2.1). This is of diagnostic value to the physician because an abnormally high resting respiratory rate may be an early sign of high altitude pulmonary edema or pneumonia. When there is an acute increase in ventilation, arterial PCO_2 falls and the pH rises, and ventilation decreases.[15] For this reason the ventilatory response to hypoxia is less than would have occurred if arterial PCO_2 had not decreased.

Table 2.1
Resting Minute/Volume and Respiratory Rate at
High Altitude in Normal Acclimatized Subjects

Altitude (feet)	Minute/volume liters/min BTPS	Respiratory rate per minute
Sea level	8.85 - 9.1 ± 2.8[a]	12
12,000	9.71	14
18,000	11.06	12
19,000	12.0	19[a]
21,200	13.4	20[a]
22,000	15.31	15[23]
24,400	23.4 ± 3.6[b]	27[b]

SOURCE: Rahn and Otis, ref. 15.

[a]Additional data from Nevison et al., ref. 54.

[b]Additional data from Wagner et al., ref. 27.

Following an acute increase in ventilation at any given altitude there is a further slow increase in ventilation that continues for days, or for weeks, depending on the altitude. Arterial PCO_2 further decreases and arterial PO_2 rises slightly. The increased ventilation persists in the sojourner and is about 20 percent higher than it is in the native resident.[8] For example, at the moderate altitude of 12,500 feet (3,812 m) arterial PCO_2 may fall to 30 mm Hg in the first day, while arterial PO_2 falls less sharply as a result. A mild alkalosis will be present, with a pH of about 7.48. The renal response to the alkalosis is a conservation of hydrogen ions and the excretion of fixed base in the urine to restore the pH of the blood close to, but not quite to the normal value of 7.40. Renal compensation is largely accomplished during the first week of high altitude exposure, and during this time the respiratory center becomes more responsive to carbon dioxide and permits important but not exclusive control of respiration again by carbon dioxide. This process may take one month or more.[9] Ventilatory regulation by carbon dioxide is retained by long-term residents and may be considered an adaptive phenomenon. One of the functional changes in chronic mountain sickness is the loss of this sensitivity to CO_2. Sensitivity to hypoxia, despite individual variations, is usually unchanged or slightly increased in the high altitude sojourner, but is diminished in the high altitude resident. High altitude natives exhibit a higher arterial PCO_2 than that found in acclimatized lowlanders who have a similar arterial PO_2, indicating a relative hypoventilation in the natives.[16]

Compared with sojourners, the high altitude resident exhibits only a small increase in ventilation during acute hypoxia. Native residents also have a slightly lower arterial PO_2 and a higher arterial PCO_2 than do visitors both at rest and during exercise. Furthermore, this relative insensitivity to hypoxia persists in the high altitude native even after long periods of sea-level residence; this does not occur in the sojourner. It appears that one must have been born at high altitude, or must have lived there for many years since before puberty, to develop a persistent insensitivity to hypoxia.[17,18] A valuable historical account of the development of concepts of acclimatization and the control of breathing has been published by Kellogg.[19]

Ventilation at rest is only slightly increased in the visitor, but during exercise it increases more than at sea level. This results in perceptible and even uncomfortable dyspnea on exertion during the first few days at altitude.[20,21,22] The increase in exercise ventilation is associated with increased respiratory work.[23] High altitude natives ventilate less during a similar exercise level than do sojourners (Fig. 2.4).

Exercise and Ventilation

Ventilation measured in the same subjects during graded exercise at sea level and again at high altitude is greater at high altitude for each work level (Figs. 2.4 and 2.5); correcting the high altitude ventilatory volumes for sea-level barometric pressure shows the same volume of gas moved as at sea level (Fig. 2.5). In a later experiment, Grover found that after correction for sea-level pressure the volume ventilated was actually less than at sea level, and he postulated that relative "hypoventilation" occurs at high altitude during exercise.[22] Correcting ventilatory volumes at altitude to sea-level barometric pressure is of questionable value, however, because the respiratory control system and the respiratory muscles sense volumes as they are at high altitude and not as they are reduced to sea-level pressures.

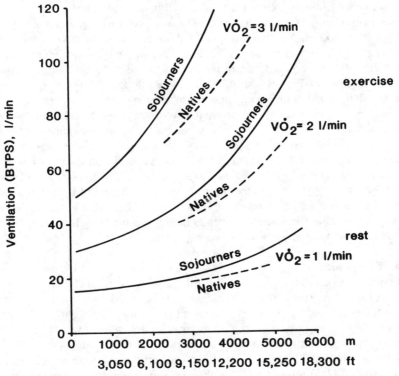

Figure 2.4. Minute ventilation in relation to altitude at rest and during three levels of exercise in high altitude natives and sojourners. Note the very high levels of ventilation approaching maximum voluntary ventilation in sojourners during exercise. From Lenfant and Sullivan, ref. 20.

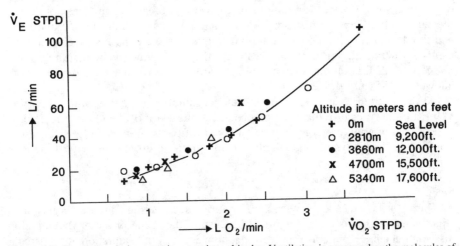

Figure 2.5. Ventilation during exercise at various altitudes. Ventilation is expressed as the molecules of air ventilated (V_E STPD) and is thus independent of altitude and only related to the oxygen consumption. Of course, to achieve this delivery of oxygen the uncorrected ventilation becomes progressively greater. Redrawn from Christensen, ref. 21.

Studies carried out at extreme altitudes by Pugh[24] and West[25] have shown that ventilation during maximum exertion increases in a linear manner up to about 21,000 feet (6,400 m) (170 L/min BTPS). Above this altitude, West predicted a decrease in maximum exercise ventilation. This was not observed in Operation Everest II, where ventilation during maximum exercise did not increase from an equivalent altitude of 16,000 feet (4,870 m) to 20,000 feet (6,100 m).[26] It has been predicted that ventilation during maximum exertion on the summit of Mount Everest may be as low as 60 L/min owing to the marked decrease in maximum exercise.[25] Although the lower air density decreases the work required to move air at altitude, the very high volume and rapid rate demand more muscular effort. For example, at 20,660 feet (6,300 m) on Everest in 1981, the mean volume of air moved by eight subjects during exertion was 207 L/min at 62 breaths per minute, and at 29,000 feet (8,848 m) during Operation Everest II it was 184 L/min at a rate of 65/min. These are exhausting levels of work—simply to move air, which decreases the oxygen available for tissues other than the respiratory muscles. At such levels, the fatigue of diaphragmatic or chest muscles may limit work.

Work of Breathing

No one has measured the work of breathing during exercise at extreme altitudes, but some facts suggest that it may be higher than expected. The lower air density at high altitude does reduce the work of breathing, but the very high ventilatory volumes and respiratory rates still require moving the rib cage at high velocities. During the 1981 American Medical Research Expedition to Mount Everest (AMREE) at an altitude of 20,800 feet (6,300 m), the mean ventilation of eight subjects during exercise at 1,200 kg/min was 207 L/min at a respiratory rate of 62 breaths/min.[7,25] In Operation Everest II at the highest simulated altitude, 29,200 feet (8,848 m), maximum exercise in six subjects required a minute ventilation of 184 L/min.[26] At this level of exercise there was a significant limitation of diffusion in the lung that was highly suggestive of some degree of pulmonary edema.[27] Breathing oxygen during exertion decreases ventilation and the work of breathing but does not restore the sea-level values.[28] Pulmonary edema may be present under these conditions and the decrease in pulmonary compliance due to the edema may figure significantly in increasing the work of breathing: that is, fatigue of the diaphragm and muscles of respiration may perhaps limit ventilatory performance and in that way allow arterial PCO_2 to rise.

At high altitudes the maximum oxygen consumption is decreased in proportion to the altitude. Because there is no decrease in the work of breathing, the oxygen cost of breathing may become a very large part of the total body oxygen consumption, so that less oxygen is available for other muscle groups and vital functions (Figs. 2.6 and 2.7).

Sleep

During sleep at sea level the respiratory drive decreases and arterial oxygen falls slightly, although this is not important because of the shape of the oxyhemoglobin dissociation curve, which is relatively flat above an arterial saturation at 90 percent at sea level. At high altitudes the decrease in arterial oxygen and arterial carbon dioxide is important in facilitating periodic breathing, which results from the pendulum-like shift of respiratory control between peripheral (oxygen) and central (carbon dioxide) centers.

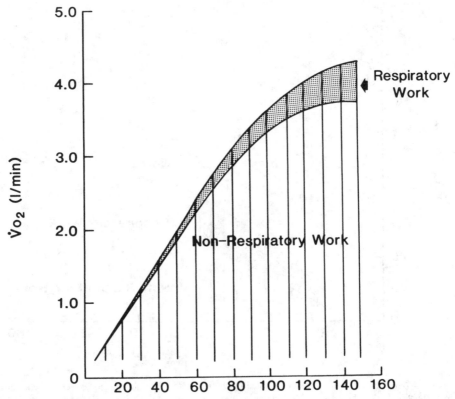

Figure 2.6. The relation between ventilation and oxygen consumption during exercise at sea level. The amount of oxygen consumed by the respiratory muscles is indicated by the shaded area and that consumed by the rest of the body by vertical lines. Note that even during maximum effort only a small percentage of the total oxygen consumption is required to breathe. From Cherniak, ref. 23.

Periodic breathing is commonly observed during sleep, but it may also be observed in the resting, awake state.[28,29] It may occur as low as 8,000 feet (2,440 m), and at very high altitudes it may persist for weeks. The few high altitude natives (Sherpas) studied have not exhibited periodic breathing and have exhibited only nominal decreases in arterial oxygen saturation during sleep.[30] It has been observed that Andean natives, however, do desaturate during sleep.[31]

Pulmonary Function

During the first 12-24 hours at high altitude, vital capacity decreases slightly, reaching a maximum of about 4 percent on the third day; it then returns slowly to normal sea-level values over a period of one to six weeks (Fig. 2.8).[32,33,34,40] The slight decrease is of no clinical significance and is probably due to an increased intrathoracic blood volume in the pulmonary arteries and right heart. A decrease in vital capacity of more than 10 percent is abnormal and in young persons may be a sign of high altitude pulmonary edema. In older persons a greater decrease in vital capacity may occur without clinical evidence of pulmonary edema.[41]

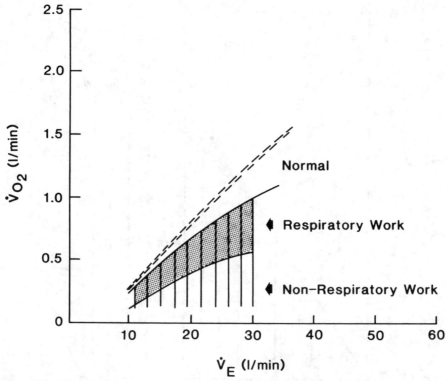

Figure 2.7. The amount of oxygen consumed by the respiratory muscles during exercise in chronic hypoxia at high altitude. Note that the amount of oxygen required for respiration is increased for each workload and the total amount of exercise performed is sharply limited. The amount of oxygen required to breathe is therefore nearly half that of the total oxygen required by the body. From Cherniak, ref. 23.

Breath-holding time is decreased at high altitude (Fig. 2.9).[33,42] Consolazio and his workers recorded a decrease from a mean value of 68.8 seconds at sea level to 25.8 seconds by the sixth day at 14,000 feet (4,270 m) in sixteen normal young men.[33] Maximum breathing capacity is increased at high altitude probably owing to the decreased air density (Fig. 2.10). The maximum breathing capacity in sixteen subjects increased from 182 L/min at sea level to 277 L/min at 14,000 feet (4,270 m); FEV_1 was increased from 85.5 percent to 91.7 percent. (FEV_1 is the percentage of the total vital capacity that can be forcibly expired in one second; normal values are 80-90 percent.) The changes in breath-holding time, maximum breathing capacity, and FEV_1 persisted throughout the 22-day stay at high altitude.[33] Similar findings have been reported by Thomas.[35] Further studies of pulmonary function in Operation Everest II subjects revealed that vital capacity decreased by 14±3 percent over the 40 day stay in the hypobaric chamber. The decrease resolved slowly upon return to sea level over 48 hours (Fig. 2.11.). Chest x-rays recorded immediately upon return to sea level revealed prominence of the main pulmonary artery and a diffuse increase in pulmonary density compatible with interstitial edema. The decrease in vital capacity was probably due to subclinical pulmonary edema and an increase in pulmonary blood volume. Forced expiratory flow (FEF) 25-75 percent increased

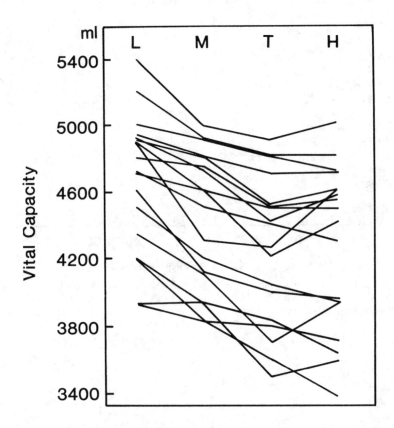

Figure 2.8. Decrease in vital capacity in seventeen normal subjects ascending from L (Lima, sea level) to M (Matucana, 7,836 feet; 2,389 m) and to T (Ticlio, 15,606 feet; 4,758 m), and descending to H (Huancayo, 10,073 feet; 3,271 m). From A Hurtado, ref. 33.

by 82±3 percent due to the decreased air density[36] (Fig. 2.12). In young women exposed to the same altitude, the changes were similar except for a smaller increase in maximum breathing capacity.[37,38,39,40,41,42] Normal standards for expiratory flow velocities at 10,610 feet (3,100 m) have been published.[42,43,44] Higher flow velocities were present in young subjects.

Transient, less striking, changes occur in lung volumes during ascent to high altitude.[32] Residual volume is initially increased and then decreases over five days to level off at about 10 percent above sea-level values. Expiratory reserve volume increases progressively over six days and remains elevated. Functional residual capacity and total lung volume are increased.

In the Andean natives of Peru, prolonged exposure to high altitude has been accompanied by an increase in vital capacity, expiratory reserve, residual volume,

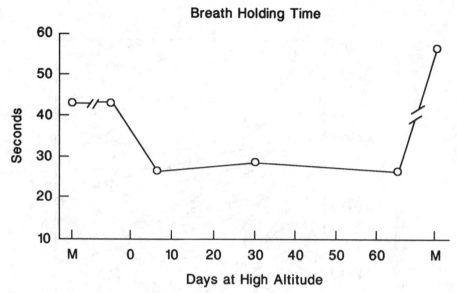

Figure 2.9. Breath-holding time in eight women at 700 feet (228 m) and during a 65-day stay at Pikes Peak, 14,110 feet (4,300 m). Breath-holding time was greater upon return to low altitude than before ascent. Redrawn from Shields et al., ref. 37.

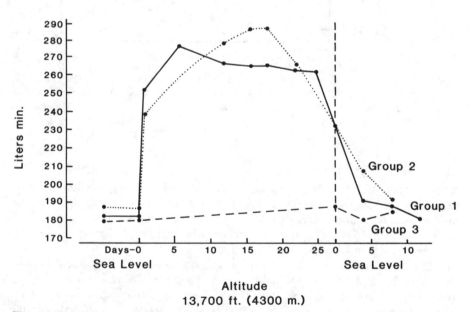

Figure 2.10. Maximum breathing capacity in normal young males at sea level and during exposure to 14,110 feet (4,300 m). Group 1 consisted of eight subjects who made a gradual ascent in two weeks to 14,110 feet (4,300 m). Group 2, also eight subjects, made a rapid ascent to the same level. Group 3 consisted of eight subjects who remained at sea level throughout the study. Redrawn from C. Consolazio et al., ref. 34.

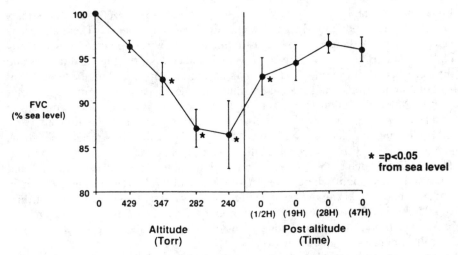

Figure 2.11. Vital capacity in 8 subjects during a 40 day stay in a hypobaric chamber and upon return to low altitude. Barometric presures (Torr) are indicated and the number of hours after leaving the chamber. From Welsh, et al. ref. 36.

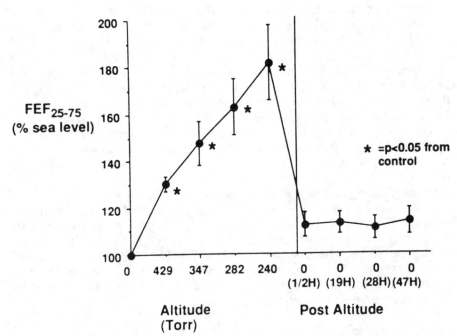

Figure 2.12. Forced expiratory flow (FEF_{25-75}) in 8 subjects during a 40 day stay in a hypobaric chamber and upon return to low altitude. Barometric pressures (Torr) are indicated and the number of hours after leaving the chamber. From Welsh et al, ref. 36.

functional residual capacity, and total lung volume. These changes have been erroneously referred to by Hurtado as a "physiologic emphysema." These characteristics of the native Peruvian do not justify the term emphysema since neither airway obstruction nor disruption of alveolar walls is a feature of the highland natives and the net effect of the volume changes is an increase in total lung volume,[45] but without an accompanying increase in anatomic dead space. The ratio of alveolar ventilation to perfusion (VA/C) throughout the lung is either not significantly changed or possibly is only slightly improved during ascent to high altitude.[46]

In the lung, oxygen tension in the alveoli is higher than in arterial blood. This alveolar-arterial difference is normally 5-10 mm Hg in sea-level subjects at rest. This gradient is due to the anatomic barrier of the alveolar-capillary membrane and a physiological shunt where some mixed venous blood enters the left ventricle. Mixed venous blood can bypass the pulmonary alveoli by two routes: (1) bronchial and Thebesian veins entering the pulmonary veins and left ventricle, and (2) passage of blood through pulmonary alveoli that are closed or poorly ventilated (ventilation perfusion mismatch).

Shortly after ascent there is no change or only a small increase in the resting pulmonary diffusing capacity as measured by the carbon monoxide method in the newcomer to high altitude,[47] but during exercise at high altitude, or under induced hypoxia, the alveolar- arterial oxygen difference in normal subjects increases as a result of ventilation-perfusion mismatching and a limitation of diffusion.[48] Under these conditions postpulmonary and intrapulmonary right-to-left shunting is negligible.

This phenomenon was studied under controlled conditions during Operation Everest II using a multiple inert gas elimination technique.[27] At sea level, ventilation-perfusion inequality was present only during heavy exercise with an oxygen consumption of 3 L/min or more. This inequality became progressive with increasing altitude up to 25,000 feet (7,625 m), where a diffusion limitation was evident at the lightest level of exercise and was detectable in several subjects at rest. The ventilation-perfusion inequality was not reversed by breathing 100 percent oxygen. All the subjects had pulmonary hypertension that became more marked during exercise. In one subject a physiologic shunt equal to 25 percent of the cardiac output was observed at rest, which increased to 50 percent during exercise. The most likely explanation for these abnormalities was a variable degree of interstitial pulmonary edema.[27,49] The possibility of intracardiac shunting via a patent foramen ovale was not excluded.

Haldane's intriguing theory that oxygen secretion by the lung was a factor in acclimatization has not been substantiated, but it is important to note that simultaneous measurements of alveolar and arterial oxygen have not been made in acclimatized subjects above 14,000 feet (4,270 m). Most studies of high altitude natives show an increase in diffusing capacity of about 20-30 percent with an A-a gradient decreasing to about 2 mm Hg,[50,51] owing possibly to a larger internal lung surface, or perhaps to a more complete perfusion of the apices of the lung as a result of the pulmonary hypertension of high altitude.

Postural Hypoxemia

Arterial oxygen saturation at high altitude is lower in the supine position than it is when sitting erect or standing. In ten normal subjects at 12,230 feet (3,730 m) the mean arterial oxygen saturation was 89 percent sitting erect or standing and 84 percent in the supine position (Fig. 2.13). No further decrease occurred in the supine position with the head lower than the feet.[52] Ward and his associates studied seven normal subjects with asymptomatic polycythemia in Denver, Colorado to determine the effect of posture on arterial PO_2. In the sitting position the mean arterial PO_2 was 69.6 mm Hg and in the supine position the mean PO_2 was 54.9 mm Hg. The authors suggested that the difference was probably related to changes in the position of the diaphragm with the resultant decrease in pulmonary volume and it was concluded that postural hypoxemia could result in polycythemia at moderate altitudes.[53] The authors did not exclude the possibility of shunting via a patent foramen ovale.[54]

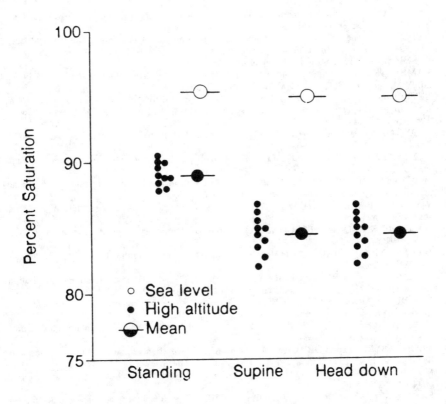

Figure 2.13. Relation of arterial oxygen saturation to posture in ten normal subjects at 12,230 feet (3,730 m). Subjects were studied when standing erect (left), lying supine (middle), and lying supine with the body tilted headward at a 30-degree angle (right). Note the fall in oxygen saturation when supine. From Hultgren, ref. 52.

Sleep hypoxemia may be an additional causative factor. Further studies of this phenomenon are clearly indicated. The observations indicate that when performing blood gas studies at high altitude the position of the subject must be constant and specified, otherwise positional effects will affect the results.

In conclusion, the increase in alveolar ventilation by the ventilatory pump is the most important and rapidly acting adjustment that the body makes to high altitude. Ventilation is precisely adjusted to arterial PO_2 by the glomus cells of the carotid body. After an initial renal adjustment to respiratory alkalosis by excretion of bicarbonate, the control of ventilation is regained by the interaction of carbon dioxide and oxygen. All the other changes in respiratory function that occur—including a more uniform ventilation-perfusion ratio, a decreased alveolar-arterial gradient, and increased diffusing capacity and an increase in vital capacity—are relatively minor.

References

1. MCDONALD D. Peripheral chemoreceptors. In T Hornbein, ed., *Regulation of breathing*. New York: Marcel Dekker, 1981: 105-319.
2. KELLOGG R. The role of CO2 in altitude acclimatization. In D Cunningham and B Lloyd, eds., *The Regulation of human respiration: The proceedings of the J.S. Haldane Centenary Symposium.* Oxford: Blackwell Scientific Publications, 1963: 379-95.
3. LAMBERTSEN C. Chemical control of respiration at rest. In *Medical physiology*, 12th Edition. ed., V Mountcastle. St. Louis: C. V. Mosby, 1968: 713-63.
4. SEVERINGHAUS J, MITCHELL R, RICHARDSON B, and SINGER M. Respiratory control at high altitude suggesting active transport regulation of cerebrospinal fluid pH. *J. Appl. Physiol.* 1963; 18:1155- 66.
5. CRAWFORD R, and SEVERINGHAUS J. CSF pH and ventilatory acclimatization to altitude. *J. Appl. Physiol.* 1978; 45:275-83.
6. DEMPSEY J, FORSTER H, and DoPICO G. Ventilatory acclimatization to moderate hypoxemia in man. *J. Clin. Invest.* 1974; 53:1091-1100.
7. WEISKOPF R, GABEL R, and FENEL V. Alkaline shift in lumbar and intracranial CSF in man after five days at high altitude. *J. Appl. Physiol.* 1976; 41:93.
8. WARD M, MILLEDGE J, and WEST J. *High altitude medicine and physiology*, Philadelphia: University of Pennsylvania Press, 1989: 86-95.
9. WEIL J, BYRNE-QUINN E, SODAL I, et al. Hypoxic ventilatory drive in normal man. *J. Clin. Invest.* 1970; 49:1061-72.
10. WEIL J, BYRNE-QUINN E, SODAL L, et al. Ventilatory control in the athlete. *J. Appl. Physiol.* 1971; 30:91-98.
11. MILLHORN D, ELDRIDGE R, KILEY J, and WALDROP T. Prolonged inhibition of respiration following acute hypoxia in glomectomized cats. *Respir. Physiol.* 1984; 57:331-40.
12. MOORE L, HARRISON G, MCCULLOUGH R, et al. Low acute hypoxic ventilatory response and hypoxic depression in acute altitude sickness. *J. Appl. Physiol.* 1986; 60:1407-12.
13. HACKETT P, ROACH R, SCHOENE R, et al. Abnormal control of ventilation in high altitude pulmonary edema. *J. Appl. Physiol.* 1988; 64:1268-72.
14. KRONENBERG R, and DRAGE C. Attenuation of the ventilatory and heart rate responses to hypoxia and hypercapnia with aging in normal men. *J. Clin. Invest.* 1973; 52:1812-19.
15. RAHN H, and OTIS A. Man's respiratory response during and after acclimatization. *Am. J. Physiol.* 1949; 157:445-62.
16. SANTOLAYA R, LAHIRI S, ALFARO R, and SCHOENE R. Respiratory adaptation in the highest inhabitants and highest Sherpa mountaineers. *Respir. Physiol.* 1989; 77:253-62.
17. SEVERINGHAUS J. Hypoxic respiratory drive and its loss during chronic hypoxia. *Clin. Physiol.* 1972; 2:57-79.
18. WEIL J, BYRNE-QUINN E, SODAL I, FILLEY G, and GROVER B. Acquired attenuation of chemoreceptor function in chronically hypoxic man at high altitude. *J. Clin. Invest.* 1971; 50:186-95.
19. KELLOGG R. Altitude acclimatization. A historical introduction emphasizing the regulation of breathing. *Physiologist* 1968; 11:37-57.
20. LENFANT C, and SULLIVAN K. Adaptation to high altitude. *N. Engl. J. Med.* 1971; 284:1298-1308.

21. CHRISTENSEN E. Sauerstaffaufnahme und Respiraterische Funktionen in grossen Hohen. *Skan. Arch Physiol.* 1937; 76:88-100.
22. GROVER R. Effects of hypoxia on ventilation and cardiac output. *Ann. N.Y. Acad. Sci.* 1975; 6:663- 73.
23. CHERNIAK R. Oxygen cost of breathing as a limiting factor in physical performance. In J Hatcher and D. Jennings, eds., *International symposium on cardiovascular and respiratory effects of hypoxia.* New York: Hafner, 1966: 346-59.
24. PUGH L, GILL M, LAHIRI J, MILLEDGE J, WARD M, and WEST J. Muscular exercise at great altitude. *J. Appl. Physiol.* 1964; 19:431-40.
25. WEST J, BOYER D, GRABER D, et al. Muscular exercise at extreme altitudes on Mount Everest. *J. Appl. Physiol.* 1983; 55:688-98.
26. SUTTON J, REEVES J, WAGNER P, et al. Tolerable limits of hypoxia for the lungs: Oxygen transport. In J Sutton, C Houston, and G Coates, eds., *Hypoxia: The tolerable limits.* Indianapolis: Benchmark Press, 1988: 123-32.
27. WAGNER P, SUTTON J, REEVES J, et al. Operation Everest II: Pulmonary gas exchange during a simulated ascent of Mt. Everest. *J. Appl. Physiol.* 1987; 63:2348-59.
28. MILLEDGE J, and LAHIRI S. Respiratory control in lowlanders and Sherpa highlanders at altitude. *Respir. Physiol.* 1967; 2:310-22.
29. WEIL J, KRYGER H, and SCOGGIN C. Sleep and breathing at high altitude. In C Guilleminault and W Dement, eds., *Sleep apnea syndromes.* New York: A. R. Liss, 1978: 119-23.
30. LAHIRI S, MARET K, SHERPA M, and PETERS M, JR. Sleep and periodic breathing at high altitude: Sherpa natives versus sojourners. In J West and S Lahiri, eds., *High altitude and man.* Bethesda, Md: American Physiological Society, 1984: 73-90.
31. ROACH P. Personal communication.
32. TENNEY S, RAHN H, STROUD R, and MITHOEFER J. Adaptation to high altitude: Changes in lung volumes during the first seven days at Mount Evans, Colorado. *J. Appl. Physiol.* 1953; 5:607-13.
33. HURTADO A. *Aspectos fisicos y patologicos de la vida en las alturas.* Lima, Peru: Imprenta Rimac, 1937.
34. CONSOLAZIO C, JOHNSON H, MATOUSH L, NELSON R, and ISAAC C. Respiratory function in normal young adults at sea level and 4300 meters. *Military Med. Feb.* 1968:96-105.
35. THOMAS P, HARDING R and MILLEDGE J. Peak expiratory flow at altitude. *Thorax* 1990; 45:620-22.
36. WELSH C, WAGNER P, REEVES J, et al. Operation Everest-II. Spirometric and radiographic changes in acclimatized humans at simulated high altitudes. *Am. Rev. Respir. Dis.* 1993; 147:1239-44.
37. SHIELDS J, HANNON J, HARRIS C, and PLITNER W. Effects of altitude acclimatization on pulmonary function in women. *J. Appl. Physiol.* 1968; 25:606-9.
38. HANNON J, SHIELDS J, and HARRIS C. A comparative review of certain responses of men and women to high altitude. In C Helferich, ed., *Proceedings Symposia on Arctic Biology and Medicine VI: The physiology of work in cold and altitude.* Fort Wainwright, Alaska: Arctic Aeromedical Laboratory, 1966.
39. HANNON J. Comparative altitude adaptability of young men and women. In L Folinsbee, J Wagner, J Borgia, B Drinkwater, J Gliner, and J Bedi, eds., *Environmental stress: Individual human adaptations.* New York: Academic Press, 1978: 335-50.
40. HANNON J. High altitude acclimatization in women. In R Goddard, ed., *The effects of altitude on physical performance.* Chicago: Athletic Institute, 1966: 37-44.
41. DILL D, HILLYARD S, and MILLER J. Vital capacity, exercise performance, and blood gases at altitude as related to age. *J. Appl. Physiol.* 1980; 48:6-9.
42. RAHN H, BAHNSON H, MUXWORTHY J, and HAGEN I. Adaptation to high altitude: Changes in breath holding time. *J. Appl. Physiol.* 1953; 6:154-57.
43. KRYGER M, ALDRICH F, REEVES J, and GROVER R. Diagnosis of airflow obstruction at high altitude. *Am. Rev. Resp. Dis.* 1978; 117:1055-58.
44. THOMAS P, HARDING P, and MILLEDGE J. Peak expiratory flow at altitude. *Thorax* 1990; 45:620-22.
45. HURTADO A. Respiratory adaptations in the Indian natives of the Peruvian Andes: Studies at high altitude. *Am. J. Phys. Anthropol.* 1932; 17:137-65.
46. HAAB P, HELD D, ERNST H, and FARHI L. Ventilation- perfusion relationships during high altitude adaptation. *J. Appl. Physiol.* 1969; 26:77-81.
47. KREUZER F, and VAN LOOKEREN C. Resting pulmonary diffusing capacity for CO_2 and O_2 at high altitude. *J. Appl. Physiol.* 1965; 20:519-24.

48. TORRE-BUENO J, WAGNER P, SALTZMAN H, GALE G, and MON R. Diffusion limitation in normal humans during exercise at sea level and simulated altitude. *J. Appl. Physiol.* 1985; 58:989-95.
49. WAGNER P. The lungs during exercise. *News in Physiol. Sci.* 1987; 2:6-10.
50. DeGRAFF A, JR., GROVER R, JOHNSON B, et al. Diffusing capacity of the lung in Caucasians native to 3100 m. *J. Appl. Physiol.* 1970; 29:71-6.
51. REMMERS J, and MITHOEFER J. The carbon monoxide diffusing capacity in permanent residents at high altitude. *Respir. Physiol.* 1969; 6:233.
52. HULTGREN H. Unpublished observation.
53. WARD H, BIGELOW B, and PETTY T. Postural hypoxemia and erythrocytosis. *Am. J. Med.* 1968; 45:880-88.
54. NEVISON T, ROBERTS J, LACKEY W. SCHERMAN R, and AVERILL K. *Himalayan Scientific and Mountaineering Expedition, I.U.S.A.F. High altitude physiologic studies.* Lovelace Foundation, Albuquerque, N. Mex., and School of Aerospace Medicine, TX., 1962:1960-61.

CHAPTER 3

The Systemic Circulation

SUMMARY

Ascent to high altitude is accompanied by stimulation of the systemic circulation by the sympathetic nervous system. This is largely mediated by the effect of hypoxia upon the carotid bodies and consequent central nervous system activation of epinephrine and norepinephrine secretion. Epinephrine activity is transient, but norepinephrine activity and consequent alpha stimulation persist for many days. The major effects are an increase in heart rate, blood pressure, and cardiac contraction velocity. Venoconstriction and an increase in central blood volume also occur. An important result is an increase in cardiac work, which can be estimated by the product of the heart rate and the systolic blood pressure, that is, "the double product." Cardiac function as measured by systolic time intervals, echo-Doppler methods, and invasive studies is normal. Left ventricular volume is decreased. Electrocardiographic changes compatible with pulmonary hypertension and right ventricular hypertrophy occur. Prolonged exposure to high altitude is accompanied by a decrease in sympathetic activity to levels below pre-ascent values. The net effect is a lower cardiac output, a wider arteriovenous oxygen difference, and a lower blood pressure. These changes are present in high altitude residents and may even persist for many days after descent. These features of the systemic circulation may be responsible for the lower prevalence of coronary artery disease and hypertension in high altitude populations.

• • •

Circulatory Changes

Several important circulatory changes occur during acute exposure to high altitude. These include an increase in ventilation, heart rate, cardiac output, and blood pressure as well as changes in regional blood flow by selective vasoconstriction.

Vasoconstriction occurs selectively, involving the muscles, skin, and viscera. Vasodilatation occurs in the coronary circulation. Vasoconstriction does not occur in the cerebral circulation. By these mechanisms blood is diverted to essential organs with a high metabolic rate.[1] Acidosis augments the vasoconstrictive response to hypoxia, but hypocapnic alkalosis, which occurs during the first few days at high altitude, attenuates the response.

Severe hypoxemia (an arterial PO_2 of 40 mm Hg or less) will result in vasodilatation by local effects upon the vascular bed. Responses are greater in the coronary and cerebral vessels and substantially less in limb vessels and renal vessels. Chronic hypoxia attenuates the vasoconstrictor response to acute hypotensive stresses. The response can be reverted to normal by the administration of oxygen.[1]

These initial responses to high altitude are due to hypoxic stimulation of the carotid bodies, which increase sympathetic activity. Animal studies have shown that if the carotid arteries are perfused with hypoxic blood, systemic blood pressure increases, systemic vasoconstriction occurs, myocardial contractile force increases, and the mean velocity of left ventricular circumferential shortening is increased. If only the systemic circulation is perfused by hypoxic blood, these changes do not occur and systemic vascular resistance falls.[2]

Acute Induced Hypoxia in Unacclimatized Subjects

In 31 normal subjects breathing 11.7 percent oxygen in nitrogen at sea level the following changes at rest were observed (see Table 3.1): (1) arterial oxygen saturation fell from 95 to 74 percent, (2) heart rate increased from 75 to 98/min, (3) cardiac output increased from 3.4 to 4.3 L/min/m², (4) mean brachial arterial pressure and systolic pressure did not change significantly, and (5) the double product (heart rate x systolic blood pressure – 100) increased from 950 to 1,200 units.[3] (The double product is an approximate measure of cardiac work.)

The effect of acute hypoxia is even more striking when exercise is performed during hypoxia.[4] In thirteen normal subjects moderate exercise was performed while breathing 11.7 percent oxygen in nitrogen (see Table 3.2). The following changes occurred: (1) arterial oxygen saturation decreased from 98 to 66 percent, (2) heart rate increased from 70 to 126/min, (3) cardiac output increased from 9.1 to 22.2 L/min/m², (4) mean blood pressure increased from 85 to 95 mm Hg, (5) mean systolic blood pressure increased from 119 to 154 mm Hg, (6) the double product increased from 840 to 1,940 units, indicating that cardiac work had more than doubled. Kikuchi and his associates obtained similar results in a study of cardiovascular changes occurring in nine subjects who ascended on different days to four simulated altitudes of 13,000 feet (4,000 m) up to and including 21,300 feet (6,500 m). After 30 minutes of exposure to each altitude, noninvasive measurements were made, including echocardiography.[5] Pertinent changes included: (1) a decrease in left ventricular end systolic dimensions, (2) an increase in contraction velocity, (3) an increase in heart rate and cardiac output, (4) an increase in hematocrit, indicating

Table 3.1
Effect of Acute Hypoxia at Sea Level in 31 Normal Subjects

	Room air	Hypoxia[a]
Heart rate/min	75 (51-100)	98 (70-164)
Brachial mean pressure, mm Hg	96 (63-119)	94 (62-123)
Peripheral resistance (dynes/sec/cm-5)	1,326 (906-2,050)	1,030 (410-2,100)
Cardiac index (L/min/m²)	3.4 (2.1-5.0)	4.3 (1.9-7.5)
Pulmonary artery pressure, mean mm Hg	14 (7-19)	20 (12-36)
Pulmonary arteriolar resistance (dynes/sec/cm-5	102 (32-213)	157 (52-358)
Arterial O_2 saturation, percent	95 (90-99)	74 (57-87)
Brachial systolic pressure, mm Hg	127 (100-144)	123 (96-140)
Double product		
Heart rate x systolic pressure/100	950[a]	1,200

SOURCES: Data from eight subjects studied in the author's laboratory (ref. 3) and by Doyle et al., *Circulation*, 1952; 5:263-70; and Westcott et al., *J. Clin. Invest.* 1951; 30:957-70. Mean values and ranges are shown.

[a] Breathing 11.7 percent oxygen in nitrogen.

Table 3.2
Effect of Acute Hypoxia Upon Exercise at Sea Level in 13 Normal Subjects
(Age 22-34 Years)

	Room air Rest	Room air Exercise	Hypoxia Exercise
Respiratory rate/min	11 (8-16)	15 (8-22)	19 (9-32)
Ventilation, L/min	8.6 (6-10)	16.1 (11-21)	25.8 (18-36)
Heart rate, beats/min	70 (56-97)	97 (80-125)	126 (100-150)
Brachial systolic pressure, mm Hg	119 (92-136)	131 (101-156)	154 (118-180)
Brachial diastolic pressure, mm Hg	68 (56-85)	73 (63-82)	72 (60-91)
Brachial mean pressure, mm Hg	85 (75-100)	92 (82-105)	95 (84-115)
Arterial O_2 saturation, percent	98 (96-99)	98 (96-99)	66 (56-84)
Cardiac output, L/min	9.1 (5.1-15.4)	15.4 (9.2-24.8)	22.2 (14-32)
Cardiac index, L/min/m²	5.1 (2.8-8.6)	8.6 (5.0-14.0)	12.2 (7.8-16.8)
Double product (mean)			
(Heart rate x systolic pressure/100)	840 units	1,270	1,940

SOURCE: Hultgren, ref. 4.

NOTES: Resting data are shown in the left hand column, exercise in room air in the middle column, and exercise while breathing 11.7 percent oxygen in nitrogen in the right-hand column. Supine cycle ergometry exercise was performed at a submaximum level to increase oxygen consumption by approximately 100 percent. Note that when exercise is performed during hypoxia, striking increases in ventilation, heart rate, and cardiac output occur compared with exercise breathing room air. Cardiac work is substantially higher. Mean arterial blood pressure is not significantly changed, indicating a fall in systemic peripheral resistance. Arterial oxygen saturation is lower than when breathing the same low oxygen mixture at rest (66 percent vs 74 percent). Mean values and ranges are shown.

a decrease in plasma volume, and (5) an increase in epinephrine levels at the highest altitude. Systemic blood pressure (6) did not change significantly. These data indicate that acute hypobaric hypoxia resulted in enhanced myocardial contractility, probably mediated by chemoreceptor stimulation of epinephrine release. Cardiac work was clearly increased. There was no evidence of left ventricular dysfunction.

The effect of acute hypoxia upon the circulation and coronary blood flow in calves has been studied by Manohar and his associates.[6] Hypoxia was produced by breathing a mixture of 14 percent oxygen in nitrogen, which lowered arterial oxygen tension to 48 mm Hg. Aortic systolic, diastolic, and mean pressure rose. The heart rate increased, hence the double product increased. Left ventricular myocardial blood flow increased from 1.10 to 175 ml/min/gm, a 60 percent increase (see Table 3.3).

Acute Hypoxia in Acclimatized Natives

Continued residence at high altitude modifies the circulatory response to acute hypoxia. This was studied by the administration of 11.7 percent oxygen in nitrogen upon the circulation in acclimatized high altitude natives at 12,230 feet (3,730 m). This is a severe stimulus (inspired PO_2 = 64 mm Hg) and corresponds to an altitude of approximately 22,000 feet (6,710 m). The resting arterial oxygen saturation decreased from 89 to 59 percent. Systemic arterial mean pressure decreased from 92

Table 3.3
Cardiovascular Responses of Calves at Sea Level and High Altitude to Acute Hypoxia

	Sea level			High altitude		
	Room air	Acute hypoxia	Percent change	Room air	Acute hypoxia	Percent change
Heart rate/min	90 ± 5	141 ± 14	+57%	102 ± 4	127 ± 8	+20%
Cardiac output ml/min/Kg	113 ± 14	123 ± 17	+ 9	141 ± 15	108 ± 10	-23
Art. PO_2 mm Hg	90 ± 1	48 ± 1		91 ± 1	48 ± 1	
Art. PCO_2 mm Hg	39 ± .4	32 ± .7		38 ± .7	35 ± .5	
PA_m mm Hg	34 ± 3	43 ± 4	+26	73 ± 9	98 ± 10	+29
SBP mm Hg	137 ± 3	144 ± 7	+ 5	116 ± 5	121 ± 9	+4.5
Double product	123 ± 5	203 ± 11	+65	118 ± 4	1.54 ± 7	+30
LV cor. flow ml/min/Kg	1.11 ± .06	1.75 ± .31	+58	.98 ± .8	1.05 ± 0.11	+ 7
RVEDP mm Hg	7 ± 1	8 ± 1	+14	17 ± 2	24 ± 2	+40
Per. Vasc. R. units	104 ± 08	120 ± 10	+15	70 ± 9	98 ± 10	+40

SOURCE: Manohar et al., ref. 6.

NOTES: High altitude calves were exposed to an altitude equivalent to 11,500 feet (3,500 m) in a hypobaric chamber for 53 days. Acute hypoxia was produced by breathing 14 percent oxygen in nitrogen.

to 85 mm Hg, and systemic arterial resistance decreased from 945 to 849 dynes/sec/cm^{-5}. The effect of posture upon this severe degree of hypoxia is shown in Figure 3.1. In the supine position there was an insignificant change in blood pressure during hypoxia. When the study was repeated with the subject sitting erect, there was a significant drop in blood pressure. The usual response to acute hypoxia in normal subjects at sea level consists of an increase in cardiac output and blood pressure; this response is greatly diminished in high altitude residents. In 32 high altitude natives, 11 percent oxygen was administered at 12,400 feet (3,782 m) for fifteen minutes while hemodynamic variables were measured. Arterial saturation decreased from 88 percent (PaO_2 59 mm Hg) to 59 percent (PaO_2 30 mm Hg). Mean pulmonary artery pressure rose from 23 to 43 mm Hg and pulmonary artery wedge pressure fell from 8 to 6 mm Hg. A significant finding was a decrease in stroke volume from 89 to 69 ml with only a slight increase in cardiac output, from 4.0 to 4.3 L/min. Heart rate increased from 72 to 100/min. Mean arterial pressure decreased from 90 to 81 mm Hg, and peripheral resistance decreased from 1,120 to 944 dynes/sec/ cm^{-5}.[7,8] A diminished response of the sympathetic nervous system to acute hypoxia seems evident and has been observed by others as a result of chronic exposure to high altitude.[1,9-11]

Heart Rate

Upon ascent to high altitude the heart rate increases over sea level values both at rest and during exercise (Figs. 3.2, 3.3, 3.4 and Table 3.4). The increase is usually first apparent above 10,000 feet (3,050 m). The heart rate is higher in women com-

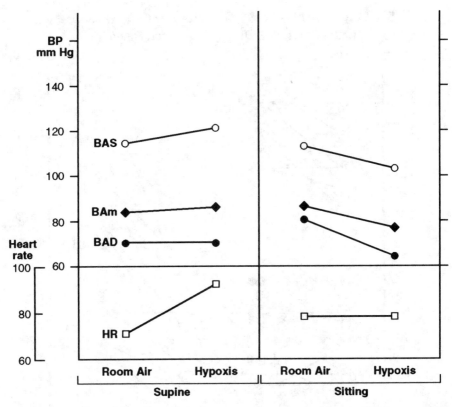

Figure 3.1. Effect of acute hypoxia and posture upon heart rate and blood pressure in eight normal high altitude residents at 12,230 feet (3,730 m). Ten percent oxygen was administered for ten minutes. Mean arterial oxygen saturation was 67 percent. Note fall in systemic blood pressure with unchanged heart rate response in the sitting position. The fall in blood pressure could be due to deficient reflex sympathetic vasoconstriction. BAS = brachial arterial systolic pressure; BAM = brachial arterial mean pressure; BAD = brachial arterial diastolic pressure; HR = heart rate. From Hultgren, unpublished observations and ref. 7.

pared to men.[33] The increase in heart rate is accompanied by an increase in blood pressure (Fig. 3.2). The tachycardia is related to increased sympathetic activity, which stimutates beta receptors in the heart. A rise in the level of plasma and urinary catecholamines accompanies this response.[12] The tachycardia is abolished by beta blockade.[13] Although beta blockade reduces the heart rate during exercise, cardiac output is maintained by an increase in stroke volume.[14] A few persons will exhibit a relative bradycardia upon ascent to high altitude. After five to seven days the heart rate decreases, but under conditions of more severe hypoxia at high altitude, such as in high altitude pulmonary edema, a tachycardia occurs that is roughly proportional to the degree of hypoxia; the respiratory rate is also increased. This latter change is of diagnostic value in the detection of the initial stages of high altitude pulmonary edema, where resting heart rates and respiratory rates are increased.

For the same level of exercise the heart rate is higher at high altitude than at sea level. This holds true for both newcomers to high altitude and high altitude residents (Fig. 3.4). During exercise at high altitude the heart rate that can be attained during

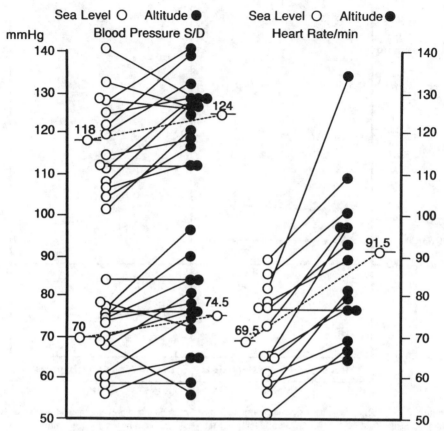

Figure 3.2. Effect of ascent from sea level to 12,470 feet (3,803 m) upon resting blood pressure and heart rate in thirteen normal subjects age 13-54 years. Measurements were made 48 hours after arrival from sea level. From Hultgren, unpublished observations.

maximum exercise decreases in proportion to the altitude (Fig. 3.5). For example, in one study the heart rate at sea level in normal young subjects was 192/min at a maximum work load of 1,500-1,800 kg m/min (13.4- 15.7 METS). At 21,000 feet (6,400 m) the heart rate was 146/min at a maximum work load of 900-1,050 kg m/min (7.7-9.0 METS). At 24,000 feet (7,440 m) the heart rate of two subjects was 135/min at a maximum work load of only 600 kg m/min (5.1 METS).[15] On the summit of Mount Everest the heart rate of one climber was 110/min at rest and 120/min during exercise; at sea level, the same subject's heart rate was 58/min at rest and 190/ min during maximum exercise.[16] Additional data on exercise heart rates at various altitudes were provided by Operation Everest II, where seven normal subjects underwent a simulated ascent of Mount Everest over a 40-day period in a hypobaric chamber (Fig. 3.5).[17] At sea level the maximum heart rate was 177/min, compared with 124/min at 29,000 feet (8,845 m). At that highest altitude, the maximum heart rate was achieved after 30 seconds of exercise, but within two minutes a decrease of six beats per minute had occurred. This was not observed during exercise at lower altitudes.

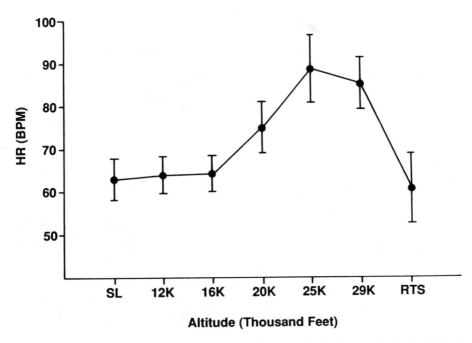

Figure 3.3. Resting heart rates in six young men exposed to a progressive increase in simulated altitude in a hypobaric chamber over a 40-day period. The slow increase in heart rate is due to the gradual ascent profile. Mean values and one standard deviation are shown. From Malconian et al., ref. 45.

Cardiac Output

Acute hypoxia results in an increase in cardiac output due to sympathetic stimulation. This effect is evident upon ascent to high altitude, where the cardiac output is increased by approximately 20 percent for the first few days after arrival. The increased output is evident both at rest and during moderate exercise. The maximum cardiac output that can be attained is less than at sea level, however.[18,19]

One important circulatory change that appears after five to ten days at high altitude is a decrease in the cardiac output at rest and during exercise. Alexander and his associates studied normal subjects who performed graded supine cycle ergometer exercise at four levels of effort at sea level and then repeated the same exercise protocol ten days after arrival at 10,150 feet (3,100 m).[20] Cardiac output was measured by the Fick method. For each level of exercise the stroke volume and cardiac output at high altitude were approximately 16 percent below sea level values (Fig. 3.6). Coronary blood flow during exercise was also decreased, but the decrease was proportional to the decrease in left ventricular work.[21] The lower cardiac output during exercise is more marked in sojourners than in high altitude native residents.[22] Wolfel and his associates, who measured cardiac output at rest and during exercise in seven men at sea level and after 21 days at 14,110 feet (4,300 m), found that cardiac output at rest and during a similar level of exercise decreased by 25 percent.[23] Even at moderate altitudes a decrease in cardiac output and stroke volume after several days of acclimatization has been observed. Sime and his workers obtained similar results in eight subjects brought from sea level to 7,800 feet (2,380 m). After five days the cardiac index was reduced by 20 percent and by 15 percent

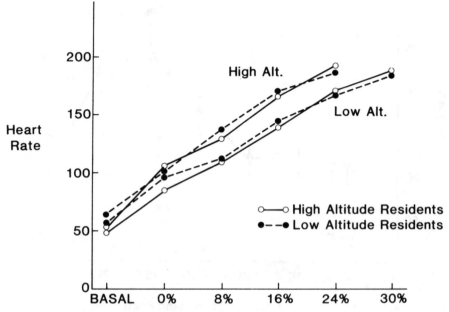

Figure 3.4. Heart rate response to treadmill exercise at a constant speed of 3.0 miles per hour with a progressive increase in grade. Five sea level residents were compared with five high altitude residents native to 10,150 feet (3,100 m). Exercise was performed by both groups of subjects at sea level and within 48 hours of arrival at high altitude. From Alexander et al., ref. 20.

Table 3.4
Resting Heart Rates at Various Altitudes in Normal Acclimatized Sea-Level Dwellers Exposed for Periods of 20 Days to Several Months

Altitude		Number of subjects	Altitude Heart rate/min range		Sea level Heart rate/min range	
Feet	Meters		Mean	SD	Mean	SD
10,170[a]	3,100	10	69	SD ± 11	71	± 11
12,700[b]	3,874	10	77	SD ± 14	64	SD ± 8
14,100[c]	4,300	5	76	SD ± 4	62	SD ± 4
17,500[d]	5,400	12	70	SD ± 9	59	SD ± 10
18,532[e]	5,650	11	90	SD ± 12	67	SD ± 11
19,000[f]	5,470	9	83	68 - 110		
20,000[g]	6,100	6	86	59 - 102	64 ± 4	SD ± 4
20,500[d]	6,300	12	78	SD ± 12	59	SD ± 10
21,200[f]	6,440	5	82	64 - 101		
25,000[g]	7,620	5	95	58 - 118	64 ± 4	SD ± 4
29,000[g]	8,800	4	99	80 - 118	64 ± 4	SD ± 4

SOURCES: [a]Hultgren et al, ref. 8; [b]Hultgren, ref. 4; [c]Wolfel et al., ref. 23; [d]Karliner et al., ref. 16; [e]Hirata et al., ref. 37; [f]T Nevison et al., *1960-61 Himalayan Scientific and Mountaineering Expedition, I.U.S.A.F. High altitude physiologic studies,* Lovelace Foundation, Albuquerque, N.Mex.; [g]Reeves et al, ref. 17.

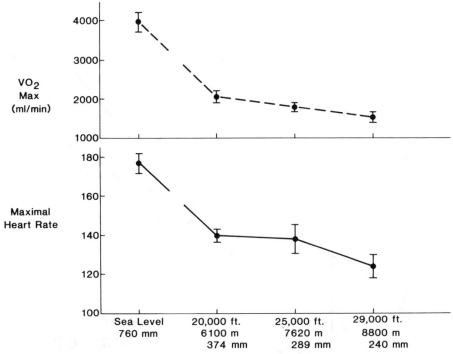

Figure 3.5. Maximum heart rate in seven normal young men who spent 40 days in a hypobaric chamber with a slow simulated ascent to 29,000 feet (8,800 m) (Operation Everest II). The decrease in maximum heart rate parallels the decrease in maximum O_2 consumption shown above. From Reeves et al., ref. 17.

during exercise. Resting heart rate was unchanged, but the heart rate during maximum exercise decreased from 165/min to 156/min.[24]

The arm to tongue circulation time is prolonged at high altitude.[25,26] This may be a reflection of the decrease in cardiac output (Table 3.2). The resting cardiac output of high altitude natives is lower than that of sea level dwellers (Table 3.5). When high altitude natives descend to sea level their cardiac output remains lower than that of sea-level subjects at rest and during similar levels of exercise for several days (Fig. 3.7).[27]

Left Ventricular Function

The decreased cardiac output associated with prolonged exposure to high altitude raises the possibility that chronic hypoxia results in an impairment of left ventricular function. Studies of the effect of altitude upon left ventricular function have employed three methods:

Systolic time intervals. This method requires a carotid pulse tracing, a phonocardiogram, and simultaneous electrocardiogram. The pre-ejection period (PEP) is measured from the onset of the QRS complex of the electrocardiogram to the onset of the rise of the carotid pulse. The left ventricular ejection time (LVET) is measured from the onset of the rise of the carotid pulse to the initial component of the second heart sound. The ratio of the PEP/LVET is normally 34-37 percent ± 5 percent. A low stroke volume and abnormal left ventricular function, as seen in

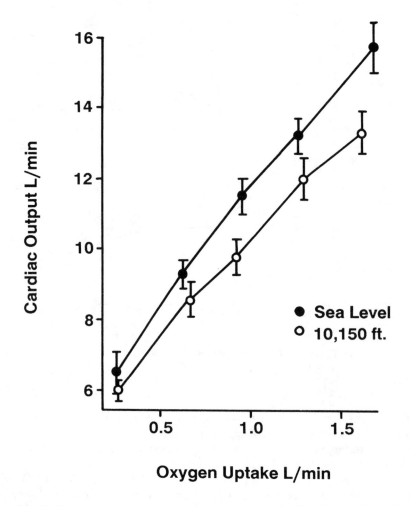

Figure 3.6. Cardiac output response to submaximum supine exercise. Each point indicates the mean value for eight subjects studied first at sea level (solid dots) and again after ten days at 10,150 feet (3,100 m) (open circles). Vertical bars indicate standard error of the mean (SEM). At each work load, cardiac output is less at high altitude, the decrease being as great as two liters per minute at an oxygen uptake of 1.61 per minute. Exercise at the same work load was performed at sea level and altitude. From Alexander et al., ref. 20.

severe coronary disease, result in an increase in the PEP/LVET ratio. Ratios as high as 60 percent have been reported in some patients. The abnormally high values are due to an increased duration of the PEP and a shortening of the ET. Other factors that will prolong the PEP/LVET ratio include a decrease in blood volume, a decrease in stroke volume, a decrease in left ventricular volume, and changes in loading conditions. The use of systolic time intervals in evaluating changes in cardiac function

Table 3.5
Systemic Circulation at Rest in 30 High Altitude Residents at
12,470 feet (3,803 m) and 16 Normal Sea-Level Subjects

	Hultgren		Sime	
	High altitude residents	Sea-level normals	Morococha residents	Lima two years
Number of subjects	30	16	11	11
Age in years	30	25	20.6	22.6
Body surface area, m^2	1.65	1.71	1.54	1.54
Hematocrit, percent	54	44	55.4	41.9
Arterial saturation, percent	85	95	78.5	97.3
Ventilation, L/min/m^2	8.79	6.26	5.24	4.80
O$_2$ consumption, ml/min/m^2	154	132	158	161
A-V difference, ml/100 ml	5.0	3.8	4.22	3.63
Cardiac index, L/min/m^2	3.4	3.6	3.83	4.32
Heart rate	73	77	77	59

NOTES: Hultgren's data (ref. 7) are compared with data from Sime (ref. 27) on 11 high altitude residents at Morococha, in Peru, 14,900 feet (4,500 m), who were studied after two years' residence at Lima, sea level. Cardiac output is lower and A-V difference is greater at high altitude compared with sea level in both the United States residents and Peruvians.

is most accurate when measurements are made in the same subject under standard conditions.[28]

Echocardiograms. Both M mode and two dimensional echocardiograms provide valuable information regarding LV function, including left ventricular-left atrial volumes, ejection fraction, ratio of peak systolic pressure to end systolic volume, contraction velocity, and the mean normalized systolic ejection rate.

Left ventricular diastolic pressure. Measurement of the pulmonary artery wedge pressure via a catheter inserted into a peripheral vein permits an accurate estimation of left ventricular filling pressure. Normally this pressure does not exceed 6 mm Hg at rest and rises to less than 12 mm during exercise. Higher pressures are usually associated with left ventricular dysfunction.

Systolic Time Intervals

Early studies of normal subjects at sea level and during the first four days at 12,000 feet (3,660 m) indicated a prolongation of the PEP interval and a shortening of the LVET with a resulting increase in the PEP/ LVET ratio.[29] These results were interpreted as evidence of left ventricular dysfunction,[29] but further studies showed that this interpretation was erroneous. Fowles and Hultgren, working with ten normal subjects at 12,470 feet (3,803 m), carried out systolic time interval studies that included measurements of cardiac dimensions and other indices of left ventricular function using echocardiography.[30] The pre-ejection period/left ventricular ejection time ratio increased by 16 percent (Fig. 3.8). Echocardiographic dimensions, however, decreased at high altitude with left atrial and left ventricular diameters reduced by 10 to 12 percent (Fig. 3.9). The percent of fractional shortening and mean normalized velocity of circumferential fiber shortening remained normal.

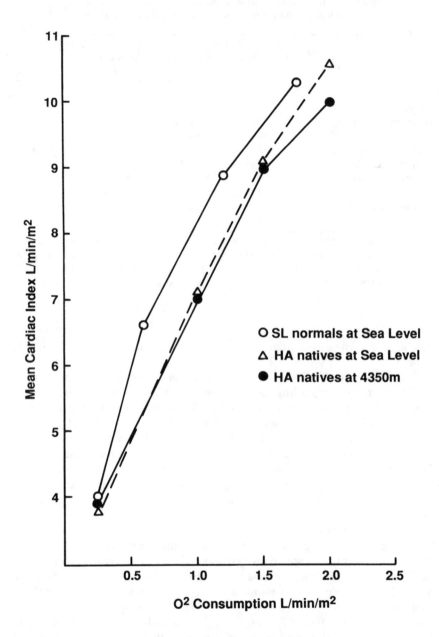

Figure 3.7. Cardiac output during graded cycle ergometer exercise. The open circles represent four normal sea level subjects studied at sea level. Open triangles represent eight high altitude natives living at 14,355 feet (4,350 m) studied at sea level 8-13 days after descent. Solid circles represent eight high altitude natives studied at 14,355 feet (4,350 m) before descent. From Vogel et al., ref. 19.

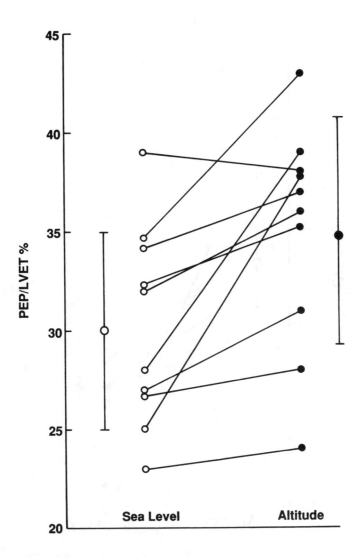

Figure 3.8. Changes in the ratio of the pre-ejection period/left ventricular ejection time (PEP/LVET) following ascent from sea level to 12,470 feet (3,803 m). The mean value of 30.1 percent at sea level increased to 34.9 percent at altitude (p=0.01). These changes were accompanied by a decrease in left ventricular dimensions, as shown in Table 3.2. From Fowles and Hultgren, ref. 30.

Isovolumetric contraction time was shorter at high altitude, suggesting increased contractility (see Table 3.6).

In subjects living for six weeks at 17,600 feet (5,350 m), the same authors found PEP/LVET ratios to be prolonged to a similar degree, and left ventricular dimensions were also decreased. These results indicate that the reduction in stroke volume and the decrease in left ventricular dimensions are not a transient phenomenon but

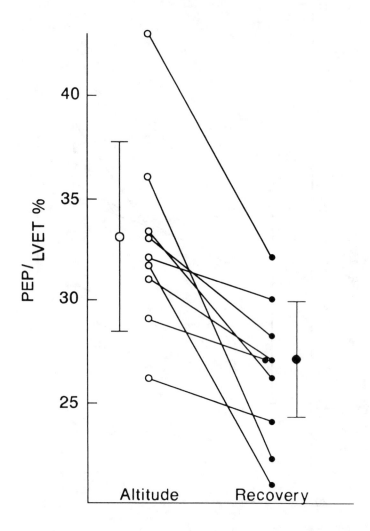

Figure 3.9. Change in duration of the pre-ejection period/left ventricular ejection time (PEP/LVET) after descent from several weeks of high altitude exposure. For each subject, open circles represent the immediate postdescent, or altitude, condition, and solid circles the values after three days of recovery at low altitude. The larger circles represent the mean value for altitude and recovery and the vertical lines the standard deviation. The change in PEP/LVET was statistically significant ($p < 0.005$). Subjects were living for six weeks at 17,500 feet (5,260 m). These data indicate that the prolongation of the PEP/LVET ratio persists for several weeks at high altitude but returns to normal within three days after descent. From Fowles and Hultgren, ref. 30.

Table 3.6
The Effect of Acute Exposure of 10 Normal Subjects to 12,470 Feet (3,803 M) on Cardiac Function Determined by Systolic Time Intervals and Echocardiography

	Sea level Sea level	High Altitude High altitude	Percent of change	p Value
Heart rate, beats/min	64 ± 8	77 ± 14	+20	0.01
PEP/LVET	0.301 ± 0.050	0.349 ± 0.057	+16	0.01
LVICT, m/sec	39 ± 10	29 ± 9	-26	0.01
LA, mm	36 ± 2.9	32 ± 3.4	-11	0.001
LVID$_{ed}$ mm	50 ± 5.9	45 ± 3.3	-10	0.005
% FS	38 ± 7.1	39 ± 5.0	+2.6	NS
Vcf, circ/sec	1.09 ± 0.27	1.14 ± 0.19	+4.6	NS

SOURCE: Fowles and Hultgren, ref. 30.

NOTES: Studies were performed at sea level and 48 hours after arrival at high altitude. The results indicate that with the prolongation of the PEP/ LVET ratio there is a decrease in the end-diastolic diameter of the LV and no change in LV function—that is, percent FS and Vcf are essentially unchanged. All measurements are expressed as mean ± standard deviation. The p values were determined by paired t tests. % FS = percent fractional shortening; LA = left atrial diameter; LVICT = left ventricular isovolumic contraction time; NS = not significant; PEP/LVET = ratio of pre-ejection time/left ejection time; Vcf = velocity of circumferential shortening.

may persist for weeks. Within three days of returning to sea level these measurements returned to normal (Fig. 3.10). Similar results were obtained by Grover, who studied eleven subjects daily after ascent to 10,300 feet (3,096 m). Mean left ventricular end-diastolic echocardiographic dimensions fell after six to eight days with a 20 percent decrease in plasma volume as reflected by a rise in hematocrit (Fig. 3.11). The PEP/LVET ratio was increased 24 and 48 hours after arrival. All indices of contractility were unchanged at rest and slightly enhanced during exercise.[31] On the basis of these studies, we can say that the altitude associated increase in the PEP/LVET ratio does not indicate a decrease in left ventricular function but rather is associated with a smaller left ventricular volume and probably a decrease in plasma volume.

It is of interest that Graybiel and his workers demonstrated a decrease in heart size as determined by serial roentgenograms in four normal subjects exposed to simulated high altitude in a hypobaric chamber for one month with a gradual ascent to 22,500 feet (6,863 m).[32]

Blood Volume and Systolic Time Intervals

Plasma volume decreases with ascent to high altitude. This is a consistent response in both men and women.[33] Kelm and his associates studied the relationship between plasma volume and the PEP/LVET ratio in an experiment in which eleven healthy subjects followed a regimen of seven days of dietary salt restriction, which reduced plasma volume. The PEP/LVET ratio was measured at rest and during isometric handgrip exercise (three minutes of 50 percent maximum force); the subjects were then given a saline infusion to restore plasma volume to the control level. The PEP/LVET ratio was 33.3 percent (rest) and 35.5 percent (exercise) before the saline infusion and 28.1 percent (rest) and 30.6 percent (handgrip)

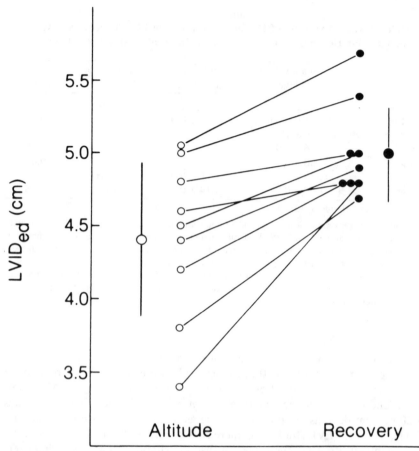

Figure 3.10. Change in left ventricular minor-axis dimension at end-diastole (LVID$_{ed}$) after descent from chronic altitude exposure. The open circles represent each subject's measurement in the immediate postdescent, or altitude, condition, and the solid circles the values after three days of recovery at low altitude. The larger circles indicate the mean values for altitude and recovery and the vertical lines the standard deviation. The change in left ventricular dimension was statistically significant ($p<0.005$). From Fowles and Hultgren, ref. 30.

after the infusion. The decrease in plasma volume by dietary salt restriction thus prolonged the PEP/LVET ratio at rest and during exercise with a decrease toward normal values when plasma volume was restored.[34] In normal subjects at sea level the administration of furosemide results in a decrease in plasma volume and a similar increase in the pre-ejection period/left ventricular ejection fraction ratio. Buch and his associates reported similar effects of pre-load reduction upon systolic time intervals.[35]

Echocardiography In Operation Everest II

Echocardiographic studies were made by Suarez at sea level and simulated altitudes of 15,000 feet (4,755 m), 18,000 feet (5,490 m), 20,000 feet (6,168 m), 25,000 feet (7.625 m), and 29,000 feet (8,845 m) in eight normal subjects. In all

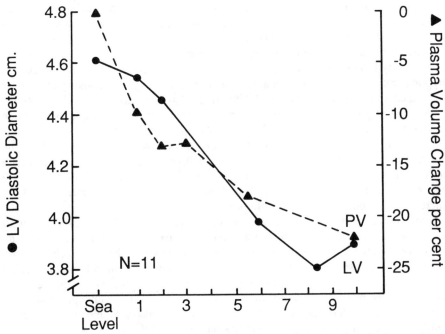

Figure 3.11. Decrease in left ventricular and diastolic diameter and plasma volume in eleven subjects during a nine day stay at high altitude (13,120 feet). These data suggest that the decrease in left ventricular volume is probably a result of the decrease in total blood volume. From Grover et al., ref. 18.

subjects, during ascent to 25,000 feet (7,625 m) resting left ventricular end-diastolic, end-systolic, and stroke volumes progressively decreased with mean reductions of 21 percent, 40 percent, and 14 percent, respectively. During moderate exercise, reductions of 23 percent, 43 percent, and 14 percent, respectively, occurred, compared with sea-level exercise. Indices of left ventricular function, including ejection fraction, ratio of peak systolic pressure to end systolic volume, and mean normalized systolic ejection rate at rest remained normal.[36] The results are similar to those obtained by Fowles and Alexander.[30,31] Hirata and his colleagues recently performed 2D echocardiography on eleven climbers at 16,465 feet (5,020 m) and at 18,532 feet (5,650 m). The results confirmed previous studies. Cardiac function remained normal, left ventricular volumes decreased, ejection fraction, rate of circumferential shortening, and fractional shortening all increased. Septal motion was abnormal. Of interest is the observation that left ventricular posterolateral wall motion was increased, apparently to compensate for the abnormal septal motion.[37] These data are compatible with maintenance of normal cardiac function even during exercise at extreme altitudes.

Left Ventricular Filling Pressure
No direct measurements of left ventricular filling pressure in man via the left atrium or left ventricle have been made at high altitude under conditions of severe induced hypoxia at rest or during exercise. Several investigators have, however, measured pulmonary artery wedge (PAW) pressure under these conditions. These

studies have demonstrated normal PAW pressures at rest and during exercise.[38] Even in the presence of severe high altitude pulmonary edema and marked hypoxemia at 12,400 feet (3,782 m), PAW pressure has been shown to remain normal.[39]

Additional information regarding left ventricular function at extreme altitudes is provided by Reeves and his associates from Operation Everest II. Five subjects in a hypobaric chamber were studied at rest and during erect cycle ergometry exercise at simulated altitudes of 20,000 feet (6,100 m), 25,000 feet (7,620 m), and 29,000 feet (8,845 m). Right atrial pressures were not elevated during exercise at any altitude and in fact were lower than sea level values. Pulmonary artery wedge pressures were not elevated at rest or during exercise at any of the three altitudes. The relation between stroke volume and right and left ventricular filling pressure at each altitude and level of exercise was normal, indicating no impairment of right or left ventricular function. Also, oxygen breathing reversed the hypoxemia but did not increase heart rate, suggesting that hypoxia was not depressing the heart rate. Stroke volume was decreased but cardiac output was maintained by an increase in heart rate. The decrease in stroke volume was commensurate with the decrease in filling pressures and the decrease in left ventricular dimensions as shown by echocardiography.[17] These results clearly indicate that cardiac rate and pump functions during maximum exercise are not impaired by extreme, chronic hypoxemia. Since blood volume measurements were not made, however, some of the changes observed, such as decreased left ventricular dimensions, filling pressures and stroke volume, could have resulted from a decreased plasma volume.[36,38]

Plasma Volume and Cardiac Output

The decrease in plasma volume that occurs during ascent to high altitude may be one of the mechanisms involved in the lower cardiac output during exercise (Fig. 3.11). An argument against this concept is the observation that dextran infusions that restore blood volume and filling pressures to normal sea level values have not improved the stroke volume during exercise.[40,41] These studies were limited to a few subjects, however, and further research is needed to settle this point. It is possible that chronic hypoxia sets the central control mechanism at a lower cardiac output. Wolfel suggested that a decrease in plasma volume could not explain the decrease in resting and exercise cardiac output observed in seven normal subjects who spent 21 days at 14,110 feet (4,300 m), since at 21 days an increase in red cell mass had restored the blood volume to the pre-ascent level, yet cardiac output was still low.[23]

The Electrocardiogram

Resting ECG's. Several studies have been made of the resting electrocardiogram at high altitude.[42,43,44] Recordings made on members of the American Research expedition to Mount Everest (AMREE) at altitudes of 17,500 feet (5,338 m), 20,500 feet (6,253 m), and 26,200 feet (4,000 m) revealed the expected increase in resting heart rate with increasing altitude, a rightward shift of the QRS axis, and an increase in the amplitude of the P wave in lead 2. At extreme altitude, three subjects developed right ventricular conduction defects and three others developed deep S waves in the precordial leads.[16] More controlled observations were made in seven normal subjects in a hypobaric chamber during a 40-day simulated ascent of Mount Everest to 29,000 feet (8,845 m). Several significant changes occurred: (1) increase in P wave amplitude in inferior leads (2,3, and V) F, (2) negative displacement of P waves in leads V_1-V_2, (3) increasing depth of S waves in V_6, (4) inversion of T waves in V_1, and (5) shift of the frontal plane axis to the right. No conduction defects or arrhythmias were observed. The above changes were related to the altitude attained, with the most striking changes being present at the highest altitudes (Fig. 3.12). The changes were similar to those observed on Mount Everest and are compatible with an increase in right ventricular pressure and pulmonary hypertension. The ECG's reverted to normal with descent to sea level.[45,46]

Exercise ECG's. Heavy exercise can be performed at extreme altitudes without evidence of myocardial ischemia. Symptom-limited upright cycle ergometry exercise tests were performed during OEII at four altitude levels. Maximum heart rates during exercise varied from 98/min to 160/min. Cardiac arrhythmias were not present at rest, but ventricular premature beats occurred in four subjects during exercise. The arrhythmias were benign and no sustained or repetitive beats were observed. Even under maximum effort at extreme altitudes, there were no ST-T wave changes that might indicate myocardial ischemia. Minor repolarization abnormalities occurred following exercise and consisted of slight QT prolongation or prominent U waves, which could have been related to exertional alkalosis.[45] No ischemic changes occurred during sleep.[46] These results indicate that, despite the low arterial PO_2 and maximum effort, myocardial ischemia does not occur at extreme altitudes, and they support other observations that under these conditions left ventricular function is normal.

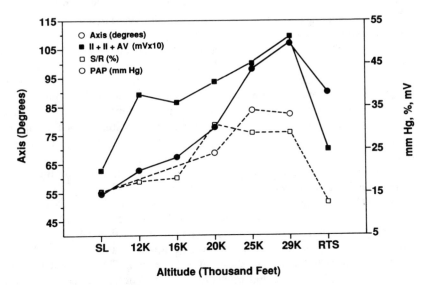

Figure 3.12. ECG changes and mean pulmonary artery pressure in seven normal subjects subjected to a progressive increase in altitude in a hypobaric chamber (Operation Everest II). The frontal plane axis (solid circles) becomes more inferiorly directed (right axis deviation), the height of the P waves in leads II, III and AV become taller, and the S waves in the left precordial leads become deeper as altitude and mean pulmonary artery pressure increase. The changes begin to reverse 24 hours after return to sea level. From Malconian et al., ref. 45.

Blood Pressure

Acute exposure to high altitude is frequently accompanied by a modest rise in blood pressure for the first few weeks. In thirteen normal subjects brought from sea level to 12,470 feet (3,803 m) and studied two days after arrival systolic and diastolic blood pressures rose as well as heart rates (Fig. 3.2). Kamat observed a rise in resting blood pressure in 31 of 32 subjects who ascended to an altitude between 11,500 feet and 13,000 feet (3,506 m-3,963 m).[47] The elevated pressure persisted for the three weeks at altitude and returned to normal after descent. Vogel and his associates observed a rise in mean arterial pressure in four sea level residents brought to 14,355 feet (4,350 m). The mean arterial pressure rose from 100 mm Hg to approximately 128 mm Hg two days after arrival and persisted for ten days. The resting heart rate rose from 68/min to approximately 92/min on day 2, but the rate decreased to 78/min on day 10.[19] Eight high altitude natives brought from 14,355 feet (4,350 m) to sea level exhibited a decrease in mean blood pressure from 113 to 103 mm Hg eight to thirteen days after descent. Heart rate slowed slightly from 64 to 58/min. Blood pressure was higher during exercise in both groups at high altitude than at sea level. Wolfel and his associates observed a rise in systemic blood pressure in eleven subjects who spent three weeks at 14,110 feet (4,300 m). Propranolol given to six subjects blunted the blood pressure rise. The authors concluded that sympathetic stimulation was one of the etiologic factors.[23] Other studies have shown that the rise in resting blood pressure is accompanied by an elevation of systolic, diastolic, and mean blood pressure during submaximum exercise (Fig. 3.13).[18,20,48] Prolonged residence at high altitude is associated with a low systemic blood pressure (Fig. 3.14): natives of the Peruvian Andes, for example, have lower blood pressures than do their counterparts living at sea level.[49,50] Systolic pressure is affected more than diastolic pressure. For reasons not yet explained, although the usual rise in systolic pressure seen in normal sea level subjects with advancing age does not occur in high altitude Peruvian natives, it does occur in Tibetans, who live at even higher altitudes.[51]

The effect of residence at high altitude upon blood pressure has also been studied in the United States. Appleton measured the blood pressure in 2,872 high school students living at 4,000 feet (1,220 m), 6,000 feet (1,830 m), and over 7,700 feet (2,350 m). Mean systolic blood pressure at the highest altitude was 119 mm Hg compared with 124 mm Hg in students living at 4,000 feet (1,220 m). There was no significant difference in diastolic pressure.[52]

In persons born at sea level who move to high altitude and live there for several years, there is a decrease in systolic blood pressure and a small decrease in diastolic pressure.[53,54] This finding is based on yearly examinations of 100 men who were born at sea level and resided at elevations between 12,400 feet (3,782 m) and 14,000 feet (4,270 m) for periods of two to fifteen years (mean duration 8.4 years), continuing during that time to follow their sea level occupations and dietary and social habits. The results of the study are shown in Figure 3.15. The mechanism of the effect of high altitude upon blood pressure in man is not clear. Hemodynamic studies suggest that systemic peripheral resistance is not decreased, but cardiac output is moderately depressed.[8,38]

Animal studies also have shown a decrease in blood pressure associated with chronic hypoxia. Restrained monkeys brought to 12,470 feet (3,803 m) for four weeks demonstrated an initial rise in aortic blood pressure persisting for three

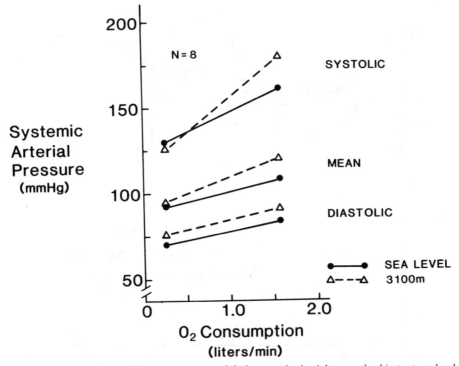

Figure 3.13. Systemic arterial pressure at rest and during exercise in eight normal subjects at sea level and after ten days at 10,150 feet (3,100 m). Both systolic and diastolic pressures are elevated during exercise at high altitude compared with sea level by about 18 and 4 mm Hg, respectively. Similar exercise performed on the first day of altitude exposure gave results similar to those at sea level. From Alexander et al., ref. 20.

weeks, and then a decrease to lower than normal control levels. This decrease persisted for two weeks after return to sea level. The animals were studied for four weeks at sea level before ascent and for four weeks after descent.[55]

Venous Tone

A decrease in venous compliance and an increase in venous tone occur during acute hypoxia and exposure to high altitude.[56] This is probably due to the increase in sympathetic nervous system activity that accompanies ascent, and it may be a compensatory response to the decrease in plasma volume.

Reflex Vasoconstriction

Although reflex vasoconstriction is a common response to acute altitude exposure, experimental evidence indicates that in subjects with chronic hypoxemia reflex vasoconstriction may be impaired. Lower body negative pressure is a test of the function of the sympathetic nervous system in maintaining blood pressure. This maneuver pools blood in the legs, and the normal response is an increase in heart rate and vasoconstriction, which prevents a fall in blood pressure. Lower body negative pressure applied to hypoxemic patients results in a fall in arterial pressure,

54

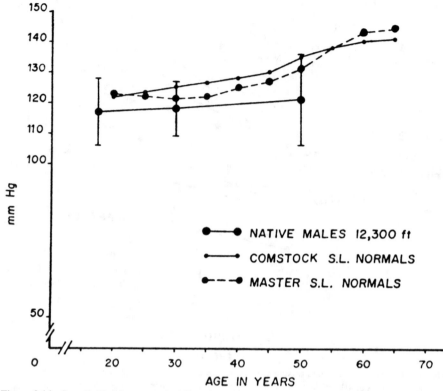

Figure 3.14. Systolic blood pressure in 150 male natives living at an altitude of 12,400 feet (3,757 m) in the Peruvian Andes. Sea-level values are indicated as obtained by Comstock[a] and Master[b]. Brackets indicate one standard deviation.

[a] G. Comstock. An epidemiologic study of blood pressure levels in a biracial community in the southern United States. *Am. J. Hyg.* 1957; 65:271-315.

[b] A. Master. The normal blood pressure range and its clinical implications. *JAMA* 1950; 143:1464-70.

slight constriction of forearm vessels, and only a small increase in heart rate. When oxygen is administered the fall in arterial pressure is prevented by vasoconstriction and heart rate increases normally (see Fig. 3.16).[1,9]

Impaired reflex vasoconstriction in high altitude residents is also evident by an abnormal response to the Valsalva maneuver.[8] During and after the release of a twelve-second Valsalva maneuver the increase and subsequent decrease in heart rate as well as the blood pressure overshoot are less than are seen in normal subjects at sea level (Fig. 3.17). Similar alterations in the response to a Valsalva maneuver are seen in patients with ideopathic orthostatic hypotension due to adrenergic sympathetic insufficiency.[57] Diminished sympathetic responses due to hypoxia have been demonstrated in animals. Maher and his workers have shown that in dogs under conditions of chronic hypoxia the heart rate response to an infusion of isoproterenol is attenuated.[10] The decreased responsiveness may be due in part to an increase in the activity in the effect of O-methyltransferase, an enzyme that inactivates catecholamines.[11] Voelkel and his workers have shown that in rats under conditions of chronic hypoxia the density of beta adrenergic receptors in the left ventricle is

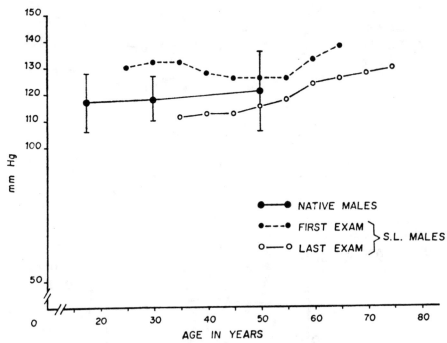

Figure 3.15. Systolic blood pressure of white men born at sea level who moved to high altitude, 12,000-14,000 feet (3,782-4,270 m). The first measurement of blood pressure was recorded within the first two to four days of high altitude residence. The last measurement of blood pressure was recorded from two to fifteen years later (mean interval approximately 8.4 years). These data indicate that prolonged residence at high altitude results in a decrease in systolic blood pressure, but the rise with advancing age still occurs. From Marticorena et al., ref. 53, and Hultgren, ref. 54.

decreased.[58] These observations have practical clinical applications, since under conditions of severe hypoxia, shock may occur more easily and may be more severe as a result of impaired vasoconstriction.

Distribution of Blood Volume and Blood Flow

Ascent to high altitude results in several changes in regional circulatory beds that tend to distribute blood flow and blood volume to central vascular beds.[1] Constriction of the veins of the forearm in normal subjects following ascent to 14,000 feet (4,270 m) has been demonstrated by plethysmography.[56,59] Hypoxia with normocapnia had no effect upon the forearm veins, but hypoxia with hypocapnia resulted in venous constriction. The cutaneous circulation is also affected by high altitude, as manifested by a decrease in blood flow to the hand. The effect is evident only when the skin temperature is zero degrees centigrade or above. If one considers hand blood flow to represent the cutaneous circulation, Durand estimates that ascent to high altitude will decrease the cutaneous blood volume by approximately 250 ml.[59,60] Roy and his workers demonstrated significant increases in pulmonary blood volume in soldiers returning to high altitude.[61] An increase in pulmonary blood volume would explain the modest decrease in vital capacity that occurs upon ascent to high altitude. Jaeger and his workers demonstrated an increase

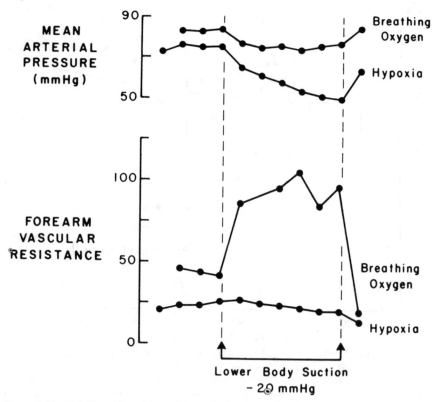

Figure 3.16. Inhibiting effect of hypoxia on reflex vasoconstriction. During hypoxia and lower body negative pressure, a marked fall in blood pressure occurs and vascular resistance does not rise. With oxygen breathing, vascular resistances rise normally, preventing the fall in blood pressure. From Heistad and Abboud, ref. 1.

in intrathoracic fluid volume in men at high altitude, which may also be a manifestation of a shift of blood from the periphery to the lungs.[62] Part of the shift of blood to the lungs could be due to peripheral vasoconstriction. Vogel and his workers evaluated regional blood flow distribution during simulated acute high altitude exposure in man, dogs and rabbits.[63] They observed an increase in cardiac output and a rise in systemic blood pressure that were probably related to cardiac inotropic and chronotropic sympathetic stimulation. They also noted an increased venous return with an increase in central blood volume. Regional blood flow changes included a relative decrease in renal and splanchnic blood flow with blood flow being diverted to heart and brain.

In the dog, and probably in man, this diversion of blood flow does not interfere with normal renal, hepatic, and intestinal function.[63] Renal blood flow is maintained in native residents at altitudes of 12,300-14,900 feet (3,752-4,545 m), but renal plasma flow is reduced and filtration rate is slightly reduced, and as a result the filtration fraction is increased.[64] The renal plasma flow is lowest in patients with chronic mountain sickness. Renal oxygen uptake is normal.[65]

These studies indicate that at high altitude blood shifts from the peripheral, splanchnic, and renal vascular beds to the lungs. This phenomenon could play a role

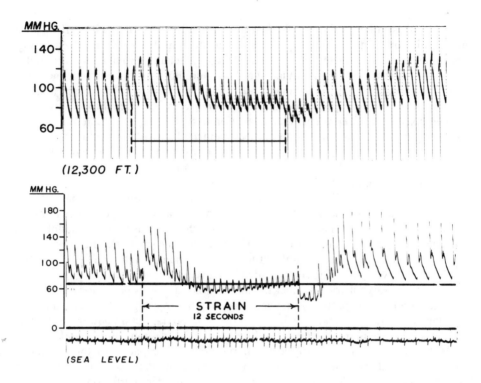

MM HG.

140—
100—
60—

(12,300 FT.)

MM HG.

180—
140—
100—
60—

STRAIN
12 SECONDS

0—

(SEA LEVEL)

Figure 3.17. Brachial arterial pressure and heart rate response to a twelve-second Valsalva maneuver in a high altitude native (above) and a normal sea level subject (below). Note the increased heart rate in the normal subject during the strain and the reflex slowing of the rate during the overshoot. Only minimal changes in heart rate occur in the high altitude native, indicating a decrease in autonomic function.[57] The blood pressure response in the native is also abnormal and approaches a "square wave" response. From Hultgren et al., ref. 8.

in increasing pulmonary artery pressure and facilitating the development of pulmonary edema.

Coronary Circulation

The coronary circulation in the high altitude resident has attracted considerable attention owing to the low prevalence of coronary artery disease and myocardial infarction in the native Andean Indian population. Grover and colleagues have shown that after ten days of residence at 10,150 feet (3,100 m) normal subjects had a lower coronary blood flow than they had at sea level. The decrease in flow was proportional to the decrease in left ventricular work, since the cardiac output at rest and during exercise was decreased.[21] Coronary flow appears to be adequate in newcomers to high altitude, as evidenced by the absence of ST depression during maximum exercise of normal subjects at 25,000 feet (7,625 m) in a hypobaric chamber described earlier in this chapter.[45]

Moret studied coronary blood flow and myocardial metabolism in Andean residents at 12,140 feet (3,700 m) and 14,200 feet (4,330 m) and compared the results with similar studies performed at sea level.[66] Coronary blood flow and myocardial oxygen consumption were lower at high altitude than at sea level. Substrates usually extracted by the heart (glucose, lactate, pyruvate, and free fatty acids) were the same at high altitude and there were no signs of anaerobic metabolism. The cardiac output and estimated left ventricular work were decreased at high altitude. The authors speculated that the decrease in coronary blood flow and oxygen consumption represented an adaptation to high altitude. A more reasonable explanation is that cardiac output and left ventricular work are reduced at high altitude, and since the oxygen-carrying capacity of the blood is increased by the increase in hemoglobin, less coronary blood flow is required to deliver the necessary oxygen for cardiac work.

Arias-Stella and Topilsky carried out a postmortem study of the coronary circulation in ten hearts from subjects who had been born and who spent their lives at 14,200 feet (4,330 m). An acrylic resin injection technique was used. The number of branches of the main coronary trunk was increased and the small peripheral branches were more numerous in the high altitude hearts than in hearts from sea level residents that were used for comparison.[67] Valdivia has found that in guinea pigs maintained in a hypobaric chamber the number of capillaries per myocardial fiber was increased.[68] This probably indicates that capillary recruitment rather than new capillary formation occurs in response to tissue hypoxia, but an additional factor may be a decrease in muscle mass resulting from a decrease in cardiac work.

Hultgren and Miller measured the maximum flow capacity of the coronary circulation in 7 dogs living at 14,200 feet (4,330 m) in the Peruvian Andes and in 37 control dogs from sea level by the technique of postmortem perfusion,[69] a method that has been used by previous workers to measure the flow capacity of the renal and coronary arterial circulation in human kidneys and hearts.[70,71] In the experiment, fresh dog hearts obtained at autopsy were refrigerated for 24 hours until rigor had disappeared. Small, thin-walled cannulae were placed in the orifices of the coronary arteries via the aorta, and the arterial bed was perfused from a pressure reservoir at mean pressures of 60-140 mm Hg at 20 mm Hg increments. Flow was recorded in ml/min at each perfusion pressure. After each study the wall of the left ventricle was dissected free from the septum, and the fat and vessels were removed to obtain the weight of the left ventricular myocardium. Total myocardial weight was estimated to be 70 percent of the heart weight to allow for nonmyocardial tissues. Flow rates of seven dog hearts from high altitude at five levels of mean pressure showed similar linear increases in flows to those seen in sea level controls (Fig. 3.18). Further data are presented in Table 3.7. Flow rates expressed as ml/min/gm of myocardium at a mean pressure of 100 mm were 3.0 ml in the high altitude hearts compared with 2.5 ml in the sea level hearts. These values are comparable to those reported by Dock in human hearts, which exhibited a flow rate of 2.1-3.5 ml/min under similar experimental conditions.[71] Flow rates per 100 grams of left ventricle were 532 ml/min for high altitude hearts and 513 ml/min for sea level dogs. Although this difference is not significant ($p > 0.75$), the slightly greater flow in the high altitude hearts could be due to the moderate right ventricle hypertrophy of high altitude. This degree of hypertrophy increases total heart weight by approximately 10 percent.[72] Murphy and Lynch have shown by postmortem injection studies an increase in the size of the coronary vascular bed to the right ventricle in patients with moderate right ventricular hypertrophy due to pulmonary disease.[73]

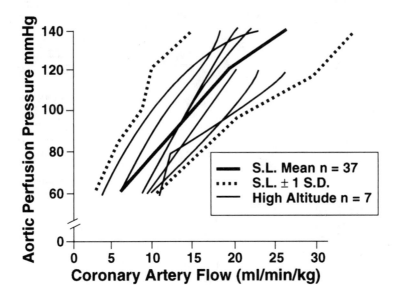

Figure 3.18. Maximal coronary flow capacity determined by post-morten kerosene perfusion in seven high altitude dogs and 37 sea level dogs. From Hultgren et al., ref. 69.

Similar results were obtained in Manohar's experiment with calves exposed to a simulated altitude of 11,500 feet (3,500 m) for 53 days.[6] Maximum coronary flow was measured by radionuclide-labeled microspheres, and it was found that maximum left ventricular coronary blood flow was the same in the high altitude calves as in the sea level calves; blood flow to the right ventricle, however, was greater than that in the sea level calves: 1.65 ml/min/gm as compared with 0.47 ml/min/gm. Right ventricular weight was greatly increased owing to severe pulmonary hypertension in the high altitude calves, and the weight of the left ventricle had decreased slightly. These data indicate that the functional cross-sectional area of the right ventricular coronary bed increases in proportion to the increase in right ventricular mass. The functional cross-sectional area of the left ventricular coronary bed was not increased. Actually, there appeared to have been a slight decrease in left ventricular mass and a corresponding decrease in maximum left ventricular flow. These studies are compatible with the physiological studies of Grover and Moret, who found no increase in coronary blood flow in normal subjects at high altitude.[21,66]

In summary, these studies all support the concept that at high altitude left ventricular work is not substantially increased and may actually be slightly decreased. Right ventricular work is clearly increased, as evidenced by right ventricular hypertrophy and an increase in the functional cross-sectional area of the right ventricular coronary bed. These results do not conflict with the study of Arias-Stella, who showed that hearts of high altitude residents had more branches of the main coronary arteries and more peripheral ramifications than did hearts of sea

Table 3.7
Maximum Flow Capacity of the Coronary Circulation in Dogs
at High Altitude and Sea Level

		Sea level (n = 37)	Altitude (14,200 ft) (n = 13)
Body wt. kg	mean	18 kg	13 kg
	range	8 - 42	6.5 - 18
Heart wt. gms	mean	143 gms	86 gms
	range	64 - 322	61 - 129
LV wt. gms	mean	51 gms	41 gms
	range	19 - 322	22 - 49
Total flow, ml/min			
at 100 mg Hg = Hg		251 ml	179 ml
Flow/100 gms LV mean			
at 100 mm Hg513 ml		532 ml	
Flow per minute per			
gram of myocardium[a]			
at 100 mg Hg mean pressure		2.5 ml	3.0 ml
Heart wt/body wt		143/18	86/13
		8.0 gms/kg	6.6 gms/kg
Flow per min per kg			
body wt at 100 mm Hg		14.0 ml	13.8 ml

SOURCE: Hultgren et al., ref. 69.

NOTES: Maximum flow capacity was determined by postmorten kerosene perfusion. The flow per minute corrected for heart weight or body weight is essentially similar in both groups of dogs; the slightly higher flow per minute per gram of myocardium and per 100 grams of left ventricle in the high altitude animals does not approach statistical significance ($p=.08$).

[a] Weight of myocardium assumed to be 70 percent of total heart weight.

level residents. Increased vascularization does not necessarily indicate an increased flow but rather may be an adaptation to hypoxemia.

The effect of altitude upon the systemic circulation is bimodal. With *acute* exposure to altitude, sympathetic stimulation increases heart rate, blood pressure, contraction velocity, and cardiac output for the first few days. Subsequently, with chronic exposure to altitude, cardiac output at rest and during exercise decreases and remains lower than pre-ascent levels. Even high altitude residents exhibit a lower cardiac output than do their sea level counterparts. Circulatory responses to sympathetic stimulation are diminished. Over years of exposure, systemic blood pressure is decreased; cardiac work remains low. Whether these factors are responsible for the low incidence of coronary disease and systemic hypertension in high altitude residents remains speculative.

References

1. HEISTAD D, and ABBOUD F. Circulatory adjustments to hypoxia. Dickinson W. Richards Lecture. *Circulation* 1980; 61:463-70.
2. KAHLER R, GOLDBLATT L, and BRAUNWALD E. The effects of acute hypoxia on the systemic venous and arterial systems and on myocardial contractile force. *J. Clin. Invest.* 1962; 41:1553-63.
3. HULTGREN H. Circulatory responses to acute hypoxia in normal subjects at sea level. To be published.
4. HULTGREN H. Circulatory responses to acute hypoxia in high altitude residents at altitude. To be published.
5. KIKUCHI K, ASANO K, and TAKAHASHI H. Cardiovascular responses at supine rest under acute hypobaric hypoxia. In *High altitude medical science*, ed, G Ueda, S Kusama, and N Voelkel. Matsumoto, Japan: Shinshu University, 1988: 45-50.
6. MANOHAR M, PARKS C, BUSH M, and BISCARD G. Transmural coronary vasodilator reserve and flow distribution in unanesthetized calves sojourning at 3,500 m. *J. Surg. Res.* 1985; 39:499-509.
7. HULTGREN H, JANIS B, MARTICORENA E, and MILLER H. Diminished cardiovascular response to acute hypoxia at high altitude. *Circulation* 1967; 36; suppl. 2:146. (Abstract).
8. HULTGREN H, KELLY J, and MILLER H. Pulmonary circulation in acclimatized man at high altitude. *J. Appl. Physiol.* 1965; 20:233-38.
9. HEISTAD D, ABBOUD F, MARK A, and SCHMID P. Impaired reflex vasoconstriction in chronically hypoxemic patients. *J. Clin. Invest.* 1972; 51:331-37.
10. MAHER J, DENNISTON J, WOLFE D, et al. Cardiovascular responsiveness to B-adrenergic stimulation and blockage in chronic hypoxia. *Am. J. Physiol.* 1975; 228:447-81.
11. MAHER J, DENNISTON J, WOLFE D, and CYMERMAN A. Mechanism of the attenuated cardiac response to B-adrenergic stimulation in chronic hypoxia. *J. Appl. Physiol.* 1978; 44:647-51.
12. DOWNING S. Automonic influences on cardiac function in systemic hypoxia. In *International symposium on the cardiovascular and respiratory effects of hypoxia*, ed. J Hatcher and D Jennings. New York: Hafner, 1966: 208-30.
13. RICHARDSON D, KONTOS H, RAPER A, and PATTERSON J, JR. Modification by beta-adrenergic blockage of the circulatory responses to acute hypoxia in man. *J. Clin. Invest.* 1965; 46:77-85.
14. REEVES J, MOORE L, WOLFEL E, et al. Activation of the sympatho-adrenal system at high altitude. In *High altitude medicine*, ed G Ueda, J Reeves, and M Sekiguchi. Matsumoto, Japan: Shinshu University, 1992: 10-23.
15. PUGH L. Physiological and medical aspects of the Himalayan Scientific and Mountaineering Expedition. *Brit. Med. J.* 1962; 2:621-27.
16. KARLINER J, SARNQUIST F, GRABER D, et al. The electrocardiogram at extreme altitude: Experience on Mt. Everest. *Am. Heart J.* 1985; 109: 505-13.
17. REEVES J, GROVES B, SUTTON J, et al. Operation Everest II: Preservation of cardiac function at extreme altitude. *J. Appl. Physiol.* 1987; 63:531- 39.
18. GROVER R, WEIL J, and REEVES J. Cardiovascular adaptation to exercise at high altitude. In *Exercise and sport sciences review*, ed. K Pandolf. New York: Macmillan, 1986: 269-302.
19. VOGEL A, HARTLEY H, CRUZ J, and HOGAN R. Cardiac output during exercise in sea level residents at sea level and high altitude. *J. Appl. Physiol.* 1974; 36:169-72.
20. ALEXANDER J, HARTLEY H, MODELSKI M, and GROVER R. Reduction of stroke volume during exercise in man following ascent to 3,100 m altitude. *J. Appl. Physiol.* 1967; 23:849-58.
21. GROVER R, LUFSCHANOWSKI R, and ALEXANDER J. Decreased coronary blood flow in men following ascent to high altitude. In *Hypoxia, high altitude, and the heart*. Adv. Cardiol 5. Basel: S. Karger, 1970: 72-79.
22. PUGH L. Cardiac output in muscular exercise at 19,000 ft. (5,800 m). *J. Appl. Physiol.* 1964; 19:441-47.
23. WOLFEL E, SELLAND M, MAZZEO R, and REEVES J. Sympathetic hypertension at 4,300 m is related to sympathoadrenal activity. *J. Appl. Physiol.* 1994; 76:1643-50.
24. SIME F, PENALOZA D, RUIZ L, et al. Hypoxemia, pulmonary hypertension, and low cardiac output in newcomers at low altitude. *J. Appl. Physiol.* 1971; 36:561-65.
25. RAMIREZ A, MARTICORENA E, GAMBOA R, and DIAZ C. El tiempo circulatorio en la altura y a nivel del mar. *Arch. Inst. Biol. Andina* 1970; 3:106-11.
26. MONGE C, CAZORLA G, WHITTEMBURG J, et al. A description of the circulatory dynamics in the heart and lungs of people at sea level and at high altitude by means of the dye dilution technique. *Acta Physiol. Lat. Am.* 1955; 5:189-210.

27. SIME F, PENALOZA D, and RUIZ L. Bradycardia, increased cardiac output, and reversal of pulmonary hypertension in altitude natives living at sea level. *Brit. Heart J.* 1971; 33:647-57.
28. LIST W, GRAVENSTEIN J, and SPODICK D, eds. *Systolic time intervals.* Berlin: Springer-Verlag, 1980.
29. BALASUBRAMANIAN K, MATHEW O, TIWARI S, et al. Alterations in left ventricular function in normal man on exposure to high altitude. *Circulation* 1978; 57:1180-85.
30. FOWLES R, and HULTGREN H. Left ventricular function at high altitude examined by systolic time intervals and M-mode echocardiography. *Am. J. Cardiol.* 1982; 52:862-66.
31. ALEXANDER J, and GROVER R. Mechanism of reduced cardiac stroke volume at high altitude. *Clin. Cardiol.* 1983; 6:301-3.
32. GRAYBIEL A, PATTERSON J, and HOUSTON C. The changes in heart size in man during partial acclimatization to simulated high altitudes. *Circulation* 1950; 1: 991-99.
33. HANNON J, SHIELDS J, and HARRIS C. A comparative review of certain responses of men and women to high altiutde. In *Proceedings of the Symposia on Arctic Biology and Medicine, VI: The physiology of work in cold and altitude,* ed. C. Helffereich. Fort Wainwright, Alaska: Arctic Aeromedical Laboratory, 1966.
34. KELM M. GRIEB E, SCHWIDDESSEN V, et al. Influence of acute volume loading on the systolic time intervals during isometric handgrip in normal subjects. Unpublished Ms.
35. BUCH J, EGEBLAD H, HANSEN P, et al. Correlation between changes in systolic time intervals and left ventricular end-diastolic diameter after preload reduction. *Brit. Heart J.* 1980; 44:668-71.
36. SUAREZ J, ALEXANDER J, and HOUSTON C. Enhanced left ventricular systolic performance at high altitude during Operation Everest II. *Am. J. Cardiol.* 1987; 60:137-42.
37. HIRATA K, BAN T, JINNOUCHI Y, and KUBO S. Echocardiographic assessment of left ventricular function and wall motion at high altitude in normal subjects. *Am. J. Cardiol.* 1991; 68:1692-97.
38. HULTGREN H, and GROVER R. Circulatory adaptation to high altitude. *Ann. Rev. Med.* 1968; 19:119-52.
39. HULTGREN H, LOPEZ C, LUNDBERG E, and MILLER H. Physiologic studies of pulmonary edema at high altitude. *Circulation* 1964; 29:393-408.
40. GROVER R. Pulmonary circulation in animals and man at high altitude. *Ann. N.Y. Acad. Sci.* 1965; 127: 632-39.
41. HARTLEY H. Effects of high altitude environment on the cardiovascular system of man. *JAMA* 1971; 215: 241-44.
42. DAS B, TEWARI S, PARASHAR S, et al. Electrocardiographic changes at high altitude. *Indian Heart J.* 1983; 35:30-33.
43. JACKSON F, and DAVIES H. The electrocardiogram of the mountaineer at high altitude. *Brit. Heart J.* 1960; 22:671-85.
44. MILLEDGE J. Electrocardiographic changes at high altitude. *Brit. Heart J.* 1963; 25:291-98.
45. MALCONIAN M, ROCK P, HULTGREN H, et al. The electrocardiogram at rest and during a simulated ascent of Mt. Everest (Operation Everest II). *Am. J. Cardiol.* 1990; 65:1475-80.
46. MALCONIAN M, HULTGREN H, NITTA M, et al. The sleep electrocardiogram at extreme altitudes (Operation Everest II). *Am. J. Cardiol.* 1990; 65:1014-20.
47. KAMAT S, and BANERJI B. Study of cardiopulmonary function on exposure to high altitude: Acute acclimatization to an altitude of 3,500 ft. to 4,500 ft. *Am. Rev. Resp. Dis.* 1972; 106:404-13.
48. STENBERG I, EKBLOM J, and MESSIN R. Hemodynamic response to work at simulated altitude, 4,000 m. *J. Appl. Physiol.* 1966; 21:1589-94.
49. MARTICORENA E, SEVERINO J, and CHAVEZ A. Presión arterial sistemica en el nativo de altura. *Arch. Inst. Biol. Andina* 1967; 2:18-26.
50. ZAPATA B, and MARTICORENA E. Presión arterial systemica en el individuo senil de altura. *Arch. Inst. Biol. Andina.* 1968; 2:220-28.
51. SEHGAL A, KRISHAM I, MALHOTRA R, and GUPTA M. Observations on the blood pressure of Tibetans. *Circulation* 1968; 37:36-44.
52. APPLETON F. Possible influence of altitude upon blood pressure. *Circulation* 1967; 36, suppl. 2: 55. Abstract.
53. MARTICORENA E, RUIZ L, SEVERINO J, et al. Systemic blood pressure in white men born at sea level; changes after long residence at high altitudes. *Am. J. Cardiol.* 1969; 23:364-68.
54. HULTGREN H. Reduction of systemic arterial blood pressure at high altitude. *Adv. Cardiol.* (Basel) 1970; 5:49-55.
55. INGE W. Effects of high altitude on pulmonary and systemic blood pressures in unanesthetized monkeys. M.S. thesis, University of California, Berkeley, 1965.
56. WEIL J, BATTOCK D, GROVER R, and CHIDSEY C. Venoconstriction in man upon ascent to high altitude: Studies on potential mechanisms. *Fed. Proc.* 1969; 28:1160-63.

57. EWING D. Practical bedside investigation of diabetic autonomic failure. In *Autonomic failure: A textbook of clinical disorders of the autonomic nervous system,* ed. R. Bannister, London: Oxford University Press, 1983: 372-76.

58. VOELKEL N, HEGSTRAND N, et al. Effects of hypoxia on density of B-adrenergic receptors. *J. Appl. Physiol.* 1981; 50:363-66.

59. DURAND J, and MARTINEAUD J. Resistance and capacitance vessels of the skin in permanent and temporary residents at high altitude. In *High altitude physiology: Cardiac and respiratory aspects,* ed. R Porter and J Knight. Edinburgh: Churchill, Livingston, 1971: 159-86.

60. DURAND J, VERPILLAT J, PRADEL M, and MARTINEAUD J. Influence of altitude on the cutaneous circulation of residents and newcomers. *Fed. Proc.* 1969; 28:1124-28.

61. ROY S, GULERIA J, KHANNA J, et al. Immediate circulatory response to high altitude hypoxia in man. *Nature* 1969; 217:1177-78.

62. JAEGER J, SYLVESTER J, and CYMERMAN A. Evidence of increased intrathoracic fluid volume in man at high altitude. *J. Appl. Physiol.* 1979; 47:670-76.

63. VOGEL J, PULVER R, and BURTON T. Regional blood flow distribution during simulated high altitude exposure. *Fed. Proc.* 1969; 28:1155-59.

64. MONGE C, LOZANO R, MARCHENA J, et al. Kidney function in the high altitude native. *Fed. Proc.* 1969; 28:1199-1203.

65. CONSOLAZIO C, NELSON R, MATOUSH L, and HANSEN J. Energy metabolism at high altitude (3,475 m). *J. Appl. Physiol.* 1966; 21:1732-40.

66. MORET J. Coronary blood flow and myocardial metabolism in man at high altiutde. In *High altitude physiology: Cardiac and respiratory aspects,* ed. R Porter and J Knight. Edinburgh: Churchill, Livingston, 1971: 131-48.

67. ARIAS-STELLA J, and TOPILSKY M. Anatomy of the coronary circulation at high altitude. In *High altitude physiology,* ed. R Porter and J Knight: 149-57.

68. VALDIVIA E. Total capillary bed of the myocardium in chronic hypoxia. *Fed. Proc.* 1962; 21:221. Abstract.

69. HULTGREN H, MILLER H, and HARDING J. Maximum coronary flow capacity in dogs living at high altitude. In *Hypoxia: The adaptations,* ed. J Sutton, G Coates, and J Remmers. Toronto: B.C. Decker, 1990; 278. Abstract.

70. COX A, and DOCK W. The maximal flow capacity of the renal arterial bed in man. *J. Exper. Med.* 1941; 74:167-76.

71. DOCK W. The capacity of the coronary bed in cardiac hypertrophy. *J. Exper. Med.* 1941; 74: 177-85.

72. HULTGREN H, MARTICORENA E, and MILLER H. Right ventricular hypertrophy in animals at high altitude. *J. Appl. Physiol.* 1963; 18:913-18.

73. MURPHY M, and LYNCH W. A comparison of the size of the arterial vascular bed to the right ventricular mass in patients with chronic obstructive pulmonary disease. *Am. Heart J.* 1979; 98: 453-58.

CHAPTER 4

Pulmonary Circulation

SUMMARY

The pulmonary circulation at sea level serves largely as a passive conduit to permit optimal gas exchange. Local decreases in ventilation, as in airway obstruction or pneumonia, evoke local vasoconstriction to minimize hypoxemia. Exposure to high altitude is associated with a generalized pulmonary arteriolar constriction and a prompt, modest rise in pulmonary artery pressure. Part of the pressure elevation is related to the increased cardiac output during the first few days at high altitude. The rise in pressure is proportional to the altitude and the alveolar PO_2. Left ventricular filling pressure is not elevated. Hypoxic pulmonary arteriolar constriction is a calcium-dependent phenomenon. High altitude natives exhibit an altitude-related pulmonary hypertension with considerable individual variation. Exercise and acute hypoxia will further increase the pressure; oxygen and descent will lower the pressure. An anatomical increase in resistance owing to medial hypertrophy is also present, since the elevated resistance decreases only slowly with descent to sea level. Pulmonary hypertension results in a moderate degree of anatomical hypertrophy of the free wall of the right ventricle. It is of interest that such hypertrophy is present in nearly all animal species studied at high altitude. Right ventricular hypertrophy is also evident in the electrocardiogram of high altitude residents, more commonly in children than in adults. Pulmonary hypertension of high altitude has important physiological consequences such as in the genesis of high altitude pulmonary edema, possible limitation of physical exercise, and other implications not yet understood.

$\bullet \ \bullet \ \bullet$

Acute Exposure

Acute exposure to high altitude results in an increase in pulmonary artery pressure owing primarily to a hypoxia-mediated increase in pulmonary arteriolar (precapillary) resistance. Left ventricular filling pressure, which is usually estimated by the pulmonary artery wedge pressure (PAW), remains normal. Only a minor part of the initial pressure rise is related to the elevated cardiac output, since pulmonary artery pressure remains elevated after ten days, at which time cardiac output has decreased. The rise in pulmonary artery pressure occurs in the presence of the initial alkalosis of high altitude and a decrease in plasma volume, both of which would tend to minimize the pressure rise. The rise in pressure is usually modest, increasing from the sea-level normal mean value of 14 mm ± 3 mm to approximately 21 mm Hg at 10,150 feet (3,100 m).[1,2,3] The pressure elevation is prompt and is proportional to the altitude attained. Pulmonary artery pressure will become elevated in newcomers to even modest altitudes. Eight sea-level athletes brought to 7,800 feet (2,380 m) exhibited a rise of mean pulmonary artery pressure from 11 to 13 mm Hg after five days. Mean pulmonary artery pressure after exercise was 21 mm Hg at sea level and 28 mm Hg at altitude.[4] Calculated pulmonary arteriolar resistance may increase to several times sea-level values. During exercise, the pulmonary artery pressure rises, owing primarily to an increase in cardiac output with little change in resistance.[1,5]

Recent studies of the pulmonary circulation have been made on eight subjects who made a simulated ascent to 29,000 feet (8,790 m) in a hypobaric chamber over a 40-day period as part of the project Operation Everest II.[6] In this experiment, cardiac catheterization studies were performed using a Swan-Ganz thermodilution, balloon-tipped catheter to measure cardiac output, pulmonary artery wedge pressure, and pulmonary artery pressure. The subjects were tested both at rest and during maximum upright cycle exercise at altitudes equivalent to 20,000 feet (6,200 m), 25,000 feet (7,700 m), and 29,000 feet (8,790 m) as well as at sea level. When the altitude studies were performed the subjects had spent from 18 to 33 days in the chamber undergoing a gradual ascent, so some degree of acclimatization had occurred. The pressures depicted in Figure 4.1 represent the differences between the mean pulmonary artery pressures and the pulmonary artery wedge pressures and therefore reflect pulmonary arteriolar (precapillary) resistance. The pressures both at rest and during exercise at 20,000 feet (6,200 m) are higher than those reported from other studies done at lower altitudes.[5] Even higher pressures were recorded at 25,000 feet (7,000 m) and 29,000 feet (8,790 m). It is of interest that although oxygen promptly restored pulmonary artery pressure toward sea level values, this did not occur above 25,000 feet (7,700 m), where the pulmonary artery pressure had reached a plateau and was not affected by oxygen. At 29,000 feet (8,790) the resting and exercise pressures were similar to those at 25,000 feet (7,700 m). The reason for

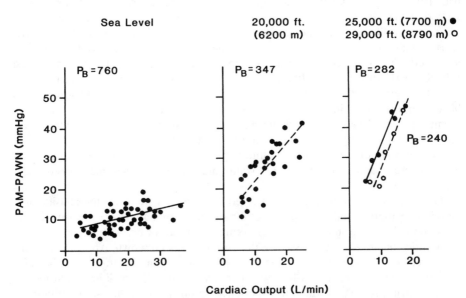

Figure 4.1. Gradient between mean pulmonary artery pressure and wedge pressure and thermodilution cardiac output during cycle ergometer exercise at sea level and at three simulated altitudes. Open circles are data from 240 mm barometric pressure. PA=pulmonary artery; PAW=pulmonary artery wedge pressure; P_B=barometric pressure. Data from Groves et al., ref. 6.

Table 4.1

Hemodynamics at Rest and During Maximum Erect Cycle Ergometer Exercise in Normal Subjects at Sea Level and at Three Simulated Altitudes in a Hypobaric Chamber

	Sea level PB 760		20,000 ft. (6,100 m) PB 347		25,000 ft. (7,625 m) PB 282		29,000 ft. (8,450 m) PB 240	
	Rest	Exercise	Rest	Exercise	Rest	Exercise	Rest	Exercise
RA mean mm Hg	2.6	9.4	0.5	4.5	0	5.3	1.5	4.7
PAP mean mm Hg	15	33	24	41	34	54	33	48
PAW mean mm Hg	7	21	7	9	7	5	8	7
PAP-PAW, gradient (mm)	8	12	17	32	27	49	21	41
C.O., L/min	6.7	30	6.2	25	6.3	15	6.1	15
Arterial O_2, sat. %	97	96	76	61	68	59	58	49
Arterial PO_2, mm	99	94	41	32	37	32	30	27
Pul. V. resistance	96	40	216	128	344	240	240	224
BA mm Hg	96	120	96	109	90	115	90	108

SOURCE: Groves et al., ref. 6.

ABBREVIATIONS: RA=right atrium; PAP=pulmonary artery pressure; PAW=pulmonary artery wedge pressure; CO=cardiac output; Pul. V.=pulmonary vascular (precapillary); PB=barometric pressure; BA=brachial arterial mean pressure. Pulmonary vascular resistance in dynes sec. cm.$^{-5}$.

the apparent lack of further rise of pulmonary pressure during exercise above 25,000 feet (7,700 m) is unknown. One possible explanation may be that the cardiac output had also reached a plateau and did not increase to a higher level. During exercise at 29,000 feet (8,790 m) the mean arterial PO_2 was 27 mm Hg with an arterial oxygen saturation of 49 percent. (The results are summarized in Table 4.1 and Figure 4.1.) During maximum exercise at sea level the pulmonary artery wedge pressure increased but not during the altitude studies. Other studies from Operation Everest II have clearly shown that pulmonary artery wedge pressure at rest and during exercise at extreme altitudes is not elevated but is slightly decreased. (These results have been discussed in Chapter 3 on systemic circulation.) The lack of a rise in pulmonary artery wedge pressure during exercise at simulated altitudes in the Operation Everest II study is more consistent with previous hemodynamic studies of patients at high altitude with high altitude pulmonary edema[7] and normal subjects during exercise and indicates that left ventricular function is well maintained under these conditions.[8]

One important finding that has emerged from several studies is the considerable individual variation in the magnitude of the rise in pulmonary artery pressure during acute hypoxia. Some subjects exhibit striking elevations of pressure, whereas others show little change.[9-12] The reason for this difference is unknown. Are some persons "hyperreactors" who have more intense hypoxic arteriolar constriction? It has also been postulated that some sea-level dwellers have unusually thick arteriolar medial walls, which might cause them to experience an unusually high rise in pulmonary artery pressure during acute altitude hypoxia.[13] This concept is supported by a study made of the coatimundi, a raccoon-like animal of Mexico and Central and South America, which lacks pulmonary collateral ventilation and has thick-walled pulmonary arteries. The response of the coatimundi's pulmonary artery pressure to hypoxia is greater than that of other mammals except the pig and cow. At an arterial PO_2 of 44 mm Hg the coatimundi's mean pulmonary artery pressure rose to 50 mm Hg despite an alkalosis of pH 7.56. Cardiac output did not increase.[14]

Subjects with a history of high altitude pulmonary edema will exhibit a greater rise than normal subjects in pulmonary artery pressure and resistance at high altitude.[15] Pulmonary artery pressure will increase when sea-level subjects are made hypoxic by breathing a low oxygen mixture.[16] The increase in pressure in these subjects is due largely to an increase in cardiac output with only a modest increase in resistance. Continued exposure to high altitude leads to an initial progressive rise in pulmonary artery pressure over the first year with little further rise thereafter. High altitude residents have higher pulmonary artery pressures than newcomers.[17]

Pulmonary Vasoconstriction

In 1946 Von Euler and Liljestrand showed in a study of the cat that breathing 10 percent oxygen resulted in a rise in pulmonary artery pressure without a change in left atrial pressure.[18] These observations led to numerous studies to elucidate the mechanism of hypoxic pulmonary vasoconstriction. Most of these studies indicated that alveolar hypoxia was the primary stimulus and that desaturation of systemic arterial blood had no pressor effect. Further research has indicated that desaturation of pulmonary artery blood probably has some vasoconstrictive effect in the presence of alveolar hypoxia or during exercise.[19] The major stimulus, however, is alveolar hypoxia.[20,21] Hypoxic pulmonary vasoconstriction exists to a variable degree in all mammalian species. Three general mechanisms by which hypoxia could result in vasoconstriction have been suggested by McMurty and Raffestin: (1) a direct excitatory effect upon pulmonary arteriolar smooth muscle; (2) a release of a chemical mediator from extravascular lung tissue, for example, mast cells, neuroepithelial bodies, autonomic nerve endings, or possibly vascular endothelium; (3) an inhibition of the activity of a continuously acting vasodilator.[22] The last hypothesis is based upon three lines of evidence that deserve comment.

1. Hypoxic vasoconstriction is dependent upon the influx of extracellular calcium into the smooth muscle fibers of the pulmonary arterioles. For example, hypoxic vasoconstriction in a perfused rat lung is rapidly reversed by a return to normoxic ventilation or by the injection of verapamil, which blocks the influx of calcium into the cells.

2. Inhibition of glycolysis by hypoxia increases the pressor sensitivity to hypoxia by a decrease in mitochondrial oxidative phosphorylation with a resultant inhibition of potassium ion (K+) conductance.

3. Inhibitors of K+ conductance allow hypoxic contractions in isolated smooth muscle, and this may be a valid model for pulmonary hypoxic vasoconstriction.[22] Oxygen then may be a pulmonary arteriolar dilator, and hypoxia represents a deficiency of this vasodilator.

Mechanisms of hypoxic pulmonary vasoconstriction have been reviewed by Voelkel and his associates.[23] They reaffirm the following general concepts: (1) the precapillary arterioles are the major focus of vasoconstriction; (2) hypoxic vasoconstriction is observed in denervated lungs; (3) vasoconstriction is calcium dependent; (4) the major stimulus to vasoconstriction is alveolar hypoxia.

It is evident that the mechanism of hypoxic pulmonary vasoconstriction is a very complex question and the exact mechanisms have yet to be defined. One important clinical implication of these studies, however, relates to the fact that calcium channel-blocking drugs lower the elevated pulmonary vascular resistance, and may prove useful in the treatment of some patients with primary pulmonary hypertension.[24] In particular, nifedipine has recently been reported to relieve symptoms of high altitude pulmonary edema.[25,26] Drugs that act as pulmonary vasodilators and have been used in the treatment of primary pulmonary hypertension at sea level, but for the most part not at high altitude, are listed in Table 4.2 Nitric oxide, an endothelium derived relaxing factor synthesized locally in the pulmonary circulation, has been shown to reduce pulmonary artery pressure in patients with high altitude pulmonary edema.[27]

High Altitude Natives

Hurtado in 1932 was the first to suggest that pulmonary hypertension might be present in the high altitude native.[28] He based his suggestion on the autopsy finding

Table 4.2
Pulmonary Vasodilator Drugs That Have Been Used in the Treatment of Primary Pulmonary Hypertension

Alpha-adrenoceptor antagonists
    Phentolamine
    Phenoxybenzamine
    Prazosin
Beta-adrenoceptor agonists
    Isoproterenol
    Terbutaline
Direct acting vasodilators
    Diazoxide
    Hydralazine
    Nitroprusside
    Isosorbide dinitrate
    Nitroglycerin
Calcium-influx blockers
    Verapamil
    Nifedipine
    Dilitiazam
Inhibitors of angiotensin
Converting enzyme (captopril)
Prostaglandins and cyclo-oxygenase inhibitors
Prostaglandin I_2 (prostacyclin)
Indomethacin
Anticholinergics (acetylcholine)
Serotonergic blockers (ketanserin)
Oxygen
Tolazoline-stimulates H_2 receptors
Nitric oxide

SOURCES: McGoon and Vliestra 1984, ref. 25. and Vender 1994, ref.55.

NOTES: With the exception of oxygen, acetylcholine, and isoproterenol, none of these drugs has been investigated in high altitude man.

of dilated central pulmonary arteries and thickened arteriolar walls in a native resident of Morococha, a mining center at 14,900 feet (4,540 m), northeast of Lima, Peru. In 1956, Rotta, also working in Peru, performed the first cardiac catheterization studies of high altitude natives.[16] He found that residents of Morococha had a mean pulmonary artery pressure of 28 mm Hg, compared with 12 mm Hg in residents of Lima. From the numerous studies that have since been made of pulmonary circulation of high altitude residents, several observations are of clinical and physiological significance.

1. *Geographical variations.* High altitude residents exhibit an elevation of pulmonary artery pressure that is roughly proportional to the altitude (Fig. 4.2 and Table 4.3).[29,30,31] In the United States the mean pulmonary pressure is increased in residents who live above 6,600 feet (2,000 m): residents of Denver, Colorado, for example, at 5,400 feet (1,635 m) have a mean pressure of 15 ± 3 mm Hg. In South America, on the other hand, there seems to be no elevation in pulmonary artery

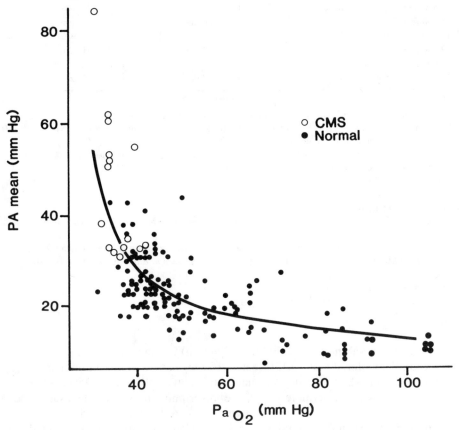

Figure 4.2. Relation of mean pulmonary artery pressure to arterial oxygen tension in residents of Mexico and South America. The line of best fit excluding chronic mountain sickness (CMS) patients results in the equation $Y = 8 + \frac{397}{x-22}$ where Y = PA pressure and X=PaO_2.

CMS patients lie on an extension of the normal curve. From Reeves and Grover, ref. 34.

Table 4.3
Mean Pulmonary Pressures (PAm) in Children and Adults from Various Altitudes

Altitude	Location	Number in study	Age	PAm	RANGE	Source of data
		Children (<14 years of age)				
Sea level	United States	25	6-14	13.5±3		Weir[a]
7,300 feet (2,230 m)	Mexico City	21	11-14	15		Vogel[b] & Michelli[c]
14,200 feet (4,330 m)	Peru	25	6-14	28	18-62	Sime[d]
14,200 feet (4,330 m)	Peru	7	1- 5	45	28-70	Sime[d]
		Adults (>14 years of age)				
Sea level	United States	39	20-31	13±4		Weir[a]
Sea level	United States	26	15-44	14	11-17	Hultgren[e]
Sea level	India	44	27± 5	12.8±4		Viswanathan[f]
Sea level	Peru	25	17-20	12±2	9-17	Penaloza[g]
5,250 feet (1,600 m)	Denver, Colorado	9	12-45	16		Vogel[b]
10,150 feet (3,100 m)	Leadville, Colorado	28	13-17	25	11-45	Vogel[b]
11,500 feet (3,500 m)	Bolivia	19	16-44	27±6		Escourrou[h]
11,800 feet (3,600 m)	Bolivia	11	adults	23±1		Antezana[i]
13,000 feet (3,965 m)	Tibet	22	adults	28±8		Grover[j]
12,300 feet (3,750 m)	Peru	26	18-49	22	14-31	Hultgren[e]
14,900 feet (4,540 m)	Peru	38	17-34	28	13-62	Penaloza[g]
14,900 feet (4,540 m)	Peru	33	adults	27	13-56	Cruz[k]

SOURCES:

[a]E Weir and J Reeves. *Pulmonary hypertension.* Mount Kisko, N.Y.: Futura, 1984.

[b]J Vogel, W Weaver, R Rose, et al. Pulmonary hypertension on exertion in normal men living at 10,150 ft. (Leadville, Colorado). *Medicina thoracalis* 1962; 19:461-77.

[c]Michelli A, Villacis P, de la Mora P, and Alvarez V. Observaciones sobre los valores hemodynamicos y respiratias obtemas en sujetos normales. *Arch. Inst. Cardiol. Mex.* 1960; 30:507-11.

[d]Sime et al., ref. 33

[e]Hultgren et al., ref. 36.

[f]Viswanathan et al., ref. 12.

[g]D Penaloza, F Sime, N Banchero, et al. Pulmonary hypertension in healthy men born and living at high altitudes. *Am. J. Cardiol.* 1963; 11:150-57.

[h]P Escourrou, P Calmon, J. Chastang, et al. Pulmonary pressure and blood gases of Andean residents of el. 4800 m.: Effect of 100% O_2 inhalation. In *Abstracts of the Second Banff International Hypoxia Symposium,* 1984.

[i]Antezena et al., ref. 29.

[j]R Grover. Personal communication.

[k]Cruz et al., ref. 31.

pressure until an altitude of 11,500 feet (3,500 m) is attained. Adolescent residents of Leadville, Colorado, at 10,150 feet (3,100 m) have a higher pulmonary artery pressure (25 mm Hg) than do Peruvian natives at 12,400 feet (3,750 m) (23 mm Hg). Tibetan men, furthermore, may have lower pulmonary artery pressures and a lower pulmonary artery pressure response to acute hypoxia than do residents of North or South America at similar altitudes.[32] However, variations in reported pulmonary artery pressures must be interpreted with caution, because of differences in the zero reference point from which pressures are measured. In adults some workers still use 10 cm from the table top in the supine position—a point that corresponds to the mid-chest in most adults whose chest anteroposterior diameter is about 20 cm.

Obviously this is inappropriate in a child. Some workers use a point 5 cm below the sternum, which would also be inappropriate for a child or for someone with a large anteroposterial chest diameter. This would give a lower value for the PA mean pressure by about 5-10 mm Hg in a large man with an anteropostero chest diameter of 30 cm. The preferred reference point for persons of varying size and age is the midpoint of anteroposterior chest diameter.

2. *Effects of age.* Except for higher pressures in children up to the age of five years, no relationship appears to exist between the pulmonary artery pressure and age.[33,34] In experiments on isolated, perfused ferret lungs, hypoxia elicited more pulmonary vasoconstriction in four-month-old animals than in seven-month-old animals.[35] In adults pulmonary artery pressure is not related to age (Fig. 4.3). There does not appear to be any clear relationship between hematocrit and pulmonary artery pressure despite impressive variations of the hematocrit in high altitude natives.[36,37]

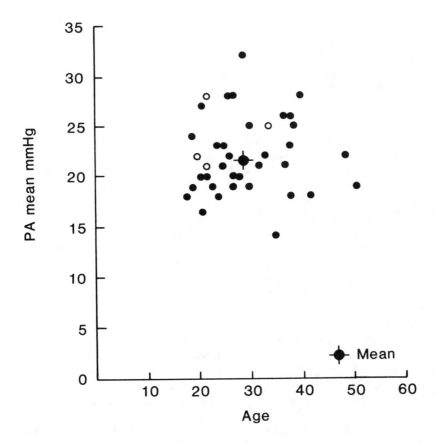

Figure 4.3. Relationship between age and pulmonary artery mean pressure in natives of the Peruvian Andes at 12,230 feet (3,730 m) and 14,200 feet (4,330 m). In subjects above the age of eighteen there is no relation between age and pulmonary artery mean pressure. Open circles are values from Rotta et al, ref. 16; closed circles are values from Hultgren et al., ref. 36.

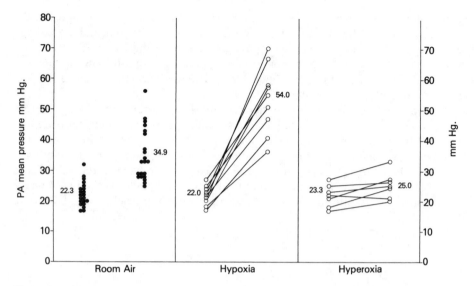

Figure 4.4. Response of mean pulmonary artery pressure to supine exercise in Peruvian natives at 12,230 feet (3,730 m) breathing room air, while breathing 11.7 percent oxygen in nitrogen, and while breathing 100 percent oxygen. Supine cycle ergometer exercise of equal levels was performed during each period. From Hultgren and Miller, ref. 48.

3. *Pulmonary vascular resistance.* The elevated pulmonary artery pressure in high altitude residents is due primarily to an increase in pulmonary arteriolar resistance, which is approximately double the sea-level value. Part of the increased resistance is probably anatomical, and related to an increase in the thickness of the muscular media relative to the lumen of the pulmonary arterioles.[38] This concept is supported by histologic studies, and also by the observation that the administration of 100 percent oxygen lowers both the pressure and resistance, although not completely to sea level values.[39] High altitude natives who go to sea level exhibit a fall in pressure and resistance, but they attain normal levels only after a period of two years, and then a residual abnormality persists: exercise and acute hypoxia still result in an abnormal rise in pulmonary artery pressure, although the resting pressure is within normal limits.[40] At high altitude the wall of the main pulmonary artery and its major branches is thick, and the increased thickness of the muscular media and elastic tissue reflect the presence of chronic pulmonary hypertension.[41,42]

4. *Exercise.* During exercise the high altitude Peruvian native exhibits a marked increase in pulmonary artery pressure (Fig. 4.4). For example, residents of Morococha, at 14,900 feet (4,540 m), had a mean pulmonary artery pressure at rest of 29 mm Hg, which rose to 60 mm Hg during exercise (range 32 to 115 mm Hg).[43,44] The rise in pressure was due primarily to the increase in cardiac output, since pulmonary arteriolar resistance did not change. When the same level of exercise was performed under conditions of added hypoxia (by breathing a low oxygen mixture) the rise in pulmonary artery pressure was found to be almost twice as much as the pressure that occurs while breathing ambient air. The reason for the difference is a hypoxic rise in pulmonary arteriolar resistance, which is approximately

Table 4.4
Effect of Exercise in High Altitude Natives at 12,230 feet (3,730 m)

	Rest Room air	Exercise Room air	Exercise Hypoxia	Exercise 100% O_2
Number of subjects	23	23	9	9
Hematocrit, percent	56.5 (50-67)	57.5 (52-68)	58 (53-69)	57.5 (52-68)
Arterial O_2 saturation, %	86 (80-92)	85 (77-93)	55 (51-60)	99 (98-100)
Cardiac index, L/min/m^2	4.6	7.5	6.2	5.5
Heart rate beats/min	71 (54-89)	97 (80-140)	148 (132-178)	103 (85-134)
PA pressure; mean mm Hg	22 (17-32)	35 (25-56)	54 (36-70)	25 (20-33)
PA wedge pressure, mean mm Hg	6.5 (4-11)	6.7 (1-12)	5.6 (3-10)	6.8 (5-11)
Pulmonary arteriolar resistance dynes, sec/cm^{-5}	220	172	435	169
BA mean pressure, mm Hg	97 (85-104)	111 (98-126)	109 (100-133)	112 (109-115)
BA systolic pressure, mm Hg	124 (111-148)	140 (121-160)	147 (107-170)	155 (130-175)

SOURCES: Groves et al., ref. 6, and Hultgren and Miller, ref. 48.

NOTES: Supine cycle ergometer exercise was performed while the subjects were breathing room air, a low oxygen mixture, and 100 percent oxygen. Note the rise in pulmonary artery pressure with exercise, a normal wedge pressure, and a fall in pulmonary vascular resistance. Exercise during acute hypoxia was accompanied by a rise in pulmonary resistance but wedge pressure did not increase; 100 percent oxygen prevented the rise in pulmonary artery pressure unlike the results of studies performed in the hypobaric chamber (OE II). PA=pulmonary artery; BA=brachial artery.

doubled (Table 4.4). When the same subjects were given 100 percent oxygen during exercise, no significant rise in pulmonary artery pressure occurred. This could explain, in part, the beneficial effect of oxygen breathing in climbers at extreme altitudes.

5. *Acute hypoxia.* Acute hypoxia produced by breathing 10-12 percent oxygen in nitrogen at sea-level causes a modest rise in pulmonary artery pressure in sea level dwellers (Table 4.5, Fig. 4.5).[10,11,12] Acute hypoxia in the high altitude native results in a more striking rise in pulmonary artery pressure and resistance,[9,44] the magnitude of the rise depending upon the altitude and the degree of hypoxia. There is also considerable individual variation in the response. In one normal native of high altitude at 12,300 feet (3,750 m), hypoxia sufficient to produce an arterial oxygen saturation of 59 percent resulted in a mean pulmonary artery pressure of 62 mm Hg. The response time of the pulmonary circulation to acute hypoxia and hyperoxia is rapid (see Fig. 4.6).

6. *Clinical implications.* The clinical implications of these studies are important. At high altitude any condition that results in increased hypoxia such as high altitude pulmonary edema, pneumonia, acute respiratory insufficiency due to pulmonary disease, or hypoventilation as in sleep hypoxia will be accompanied by a rise in pulmonary artery pressure.

The role of severe hypoxic pulmonary hypertension in reducing and limiting cardiac output at high altitude is a significant possibility, but clear experimental evidence is lacking. In primary pulmonary hypertension at sea level, resting cardiac

Table 4.5
Effect of Acute Hypoxia at Rest in High Altitude Native Residents Studied
at 12,230 feet (3,730 m) and Normal Subjects Studied at Sea Level

| | High altitude | | Sea Level | |
	Room air	Hypoxia	Room air	Hypoxia
Number of subjects	31	31	26	26
Hematocrit	56.1		41.5	
Arterial O_2 saturation, %	89 (81-96)	59 (41-7)	95 (90-99)	74 (57-87)
Cardiac index, L/min/m^2	3.88	4.14	3.37	4.26
Heart rate, beats/min	74 (55-100)	99 (60-140)	75 (52-100)	98 (70-164)
PA pressure; mean mm Hg	21 (13-32)	44.5 (23-87)	14 (7-19)	20 (12-36)
PA wedge pressure mean, mm Hg	7.3 (1-13)	6 (1-11)	6.7 (3-13)	6.7 (2-12)
Pulmonary arteriolar resistance dynes/sec cm^{-5}	178 (81-408)	409 (100-671)	102 (32-213)	157 (52-358)
BA mean pressure, mm Hg	92 (76-116)	85 (59-144)	96 (63-119)	93.5 (62-123)
BA systolic pressure, mm Hg	123 (105-152)	119 (92-184)	127 (105-160)	123 (105-159)

SOURCES: Sea level data from Doyle et al., ref. 10; Wescott et al., ref. 11; and from the author's laboratory (eight subjects). High altitude data from Hultgren, ref. 9.

NOTES: Hypoxia was produced by breathing a mixture of 11.7 percent oxygen in nitrogen at both sea level and altitude. The degree of hypoxia produced at altitude was more severe than at sea level (arterial oxygen saturation 59 percent vs 74 percent). Pulmonary artery pressure and pulmonary vascular resistance increase markedly at high altitude but only slightly at sea level. Pulmonary artery wedge pressures remained normal.

output is frequently reduced and cardiac output may increase only modestly or not at all during exercise. The pulmonary circulation thus acts as a restriction to forward blood flow in a manner similar to that of a stenotic mitral valve. Indirect evidence of the effect of pulmonary hypertension in limiting cardiac output at high altitude comes from isolated experiences. Manohar and his colleagues studied severe hypoxic pulmonary hypertension in calves exposed to 11,480 feet (3,500 m). When these calves were taken to sea level, they had a mean pulmonary artery pressure of 73 mm Hg ± 9 and a cardiac output of 141 ± 15 ml/min/kg. When they were subjected to acute hypoxia the pulmonary artery pressure rose to 98 mm Hg ± 10 with a fall in cardiac output to 108 ± 10 ml/min/kg.[45] In Peru, one human patient with high altitude pulmonary edema had a mean pulmonary artery pressure of 71 mm Hg and a cardiac index of 2.6 L/min/m^2. While he was breathing 100 percent oxygen, the pulmonary artery pressure fell to 57 mm Hg and the cardiac index rose to 3.8 L/min/m^2.[7] This observation indicates that increasing the degree of hypoxic pulmonary hypertension will be accompanied by a decrease in cardiac output, and a decrease in pulmonary hypertension may result in an increase in cardiac output. Right ventricular failure did not occur with either of these studies: the right atrial pressure remained normal.

Zonal Distribution of Blood Flow

Owing to the effect of gravity, in the erect position the apical portion of the lungs receives less blood flow than the basal zone. Normally, about 17 percent of the cardiac output perfuses the right upper zone in the sitting position, compared

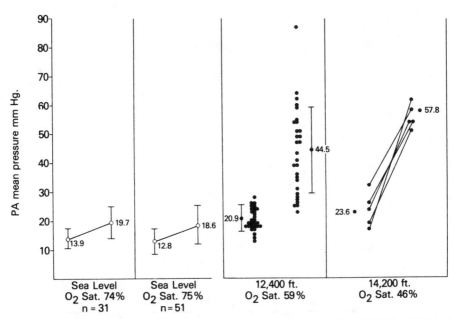

Figure 4.5. Response of the pulmonary artery mean pressure to acute hypoxia at 12,230 feet (3,730 m) and 14,200 feet (4,330 m) in native Peruvian highlanders living at these altitudes. Hypoxia was induced by breathing 11 percent oxygen in nitrogen. The rise in pressure is greater at 14,200 feet (4,330 m). The most rapid rise occurs during the first two minutes of hypoxia. Note that one subject at the lower elevation had an unusually marked rise in pressure. From Hultgren, ref. 9.

with a flow of 26 percent in recumbency. It has been speculated that an advantage of pulmonary hypertension at high altitude is better perfusion of the apical zones of the lung. However, isotope studies performed in Bolivian highlanders at 12,200 feet (3,600 m) have shown a flow distribution of cardiac output to the upper zone of the lungs that is almost identical to that found in lowlanders, despite a pulmonary artery mean pressure that is 7.7 mm Hg higher in the highlanders.[29]

Right Ventricular Hypertrophy

Right ventricular hypertrophy due to pulmonary hypertension has been demonstrated in high altitude natives by various methods. Kerwin employed chest roentgenograms to determine the heart size of 273 normal Peruvian highlanders living between 10,000 and 15,000 feet (3,050 and 4,575 m) in the Andes.[46] Compared with published normal values of sea level residents, the transverse cardiac diameter was increased 11.5 percent + 7.1 (S.D.) and the frontal area was increased 16.3 percent + 14.4. The increase in size is probably due to an increase in right ventricular volume as well as to right ventricular hypertrophy. Heart size did not increase with advancing age. In the newborn native, the relative weight of the free wall of the right ventricle was found to be the same as in infants born at sea level, but postnatal right ventricular hypertrophy occurred rapidly, so that by the age of three months the right ventricular weight exceeded sea level values (Figs. 4.7 and 4.8). By three months the maximum degree of hypertrophy had occurred, and this seems to have persisted throughout adult life.[47] The weight of the free wall of the

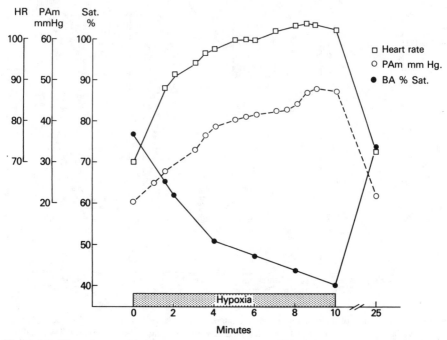

Figure 4.6. The response of pulmonary artery mean pressure (PAm), heart rate, and arterial oxygen saturation (BA% sat.) to acute hypoxia in a 30-year-old high altitude native at 12,230 feet (3,730 m). Upon the cessation of hypoxia the subject returned to room air breathing. Data from Hultgren, ref. 9.

right ventricle expressed as a percent of the total heart weight (RV/T ratio) is approximately 32 percent at 12,300 feet (3,750 m) compared with 24 percent in sea-level subjects and represents a 50 percent increase in right ventricular weight. This is only a moderate degree of hypertrophy and is comparable to that found at sea level in patients with chronic pulmonary disease.[48] In congenital heart disease with associated pulmonary hypertension in sea-level patients right ventricular weight may be increased as much as 300 percent. The degree of right ventricular hypertrophy at high altitude is related to the level of altitude, the pulmonary artery pressure, and the degree of daily physical activity. The weight of the left ventricular free wall and septum have been found to be normal when related to body surface area. The total heart weight/body weight ratio is also normal. Increased right ventricular diameter in 56 percent of 43 men living at 13,000 feet (3,965 m) in Peru has been reported by Carrillo.[49] The increased right ventricular diameter was more common in the elderly and in subjects with a hematocrit greater than 60 percent.

Animal Studies

Right ventricular hypertrophy of a similar degree to that of human high altitude residents has been found in other animal species living at high altitude, including cattle, rabbits, lambs, pigs, cats, horses, guinea pigs, dogs, llamas, and viscachos (Fig. 4.9).[50] Young steers develop marked pulmonary hypertension when brought to high altitude.[45] When taken to 12,700 feet (3,900 m), steers have developed a three-

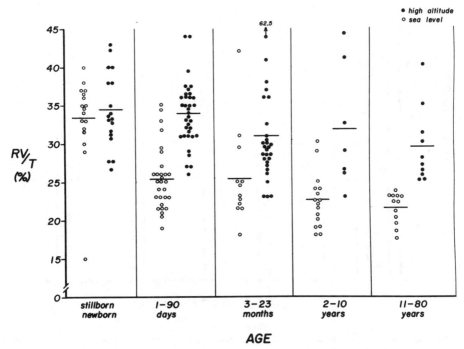

Figure 4.7. Ratio of the weight of the right ventricle to the total heart weight (RV/T%) in various age groups in sea level residents and native highlanders at 12,400 feet (3,730 m). Note the nearly equal RV/T% ratio at birth, but between one and 90 days relative right ventricle hypertrophy persists in the highlanders, with little significant change in the ratio thereafter. During this time relative right ventricular weight in the sea-level children is decreased. Relative right ventricular hypertrophy is higher in children at both elevations from 1-90 days than thereafter. From Hultgren and Miller, ref. 47.

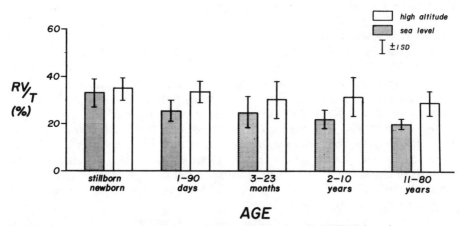

Figure 4.8. Relative weight of the right ventricle expressed as the ratio RV/T(%) in various age groups at sea level and high altitude, 12,230 feet (3,730 m). The brackets represent one standard deviation. The relative weight of the right ventricle becomes greater at about three months of age, with little change thereafter. Data from Hultgren and Miller, ref. 47.

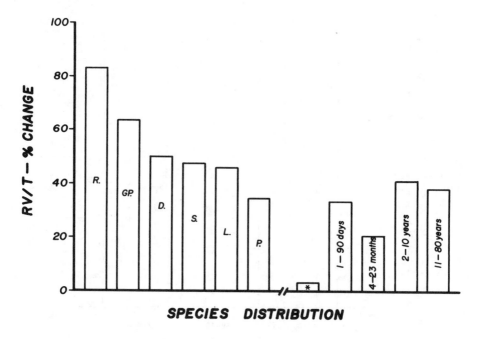

Figure 4.9. Comparison of the degree of right ventricular hypertrophy expressed as a percentage increase over sea level values in six adult animal species and human beings at high altitude. R=rabbits; GP=guinea pigs; D=dogs; S=sheep; L=lambs; P=pigs; *=stillborn and newborn human beings. All animal species had right ventricular hypertrophy. Data from Hultgren et al., ref. 50.

fold rise in pulmonary artery pressure. Some animals exhibit marked variability in the pressure rise, and some develop right ventricular failure (brisket disease).[51]

The Electrocardiogram

The electrocardiogram reflects the presence of right ventricular hypertrophy in the high altitude native. If one employs as a single criteria of right ventricular hypertrophy an R/S ratio of >50 percent in lead V_1 or V_2, approximately 20 percent of adults living at 12,300 feet (3,750 m) will have electrocardiographic evidence of right ventricular hypertrophy. The prevalence of right ventricular hypertrophy patterns is higher in children than in adults, despite the fact that the degree of anatomical hypertrophy is similar.[52,53,54] There is no exact correlation between the resting pulmonary artery pressure and the electrocardiogram in the relatively few subjects studied, nor is there any correlation between the hematocrit and the electrocardiogram. Descent to sea level results in a reversal of the pattern of right ventricular hypertrophy to normal.

My associates and I have recorded electrocardiograms in children and adults residing at 12,230 feet (3,730 m), 14,200 feet (4,330 m), and 15,600 feet (4,758 m) in Peru (see Table 4.6, Figs. 4.10 and 4.11).[53] The prevalence of right ventricular hypertrophy patterns in adults was similar at all three altitudes, but at 15,600 feet

Table 4.6
Electrocardiographic Evidence of Right Ventricular Hypertrophy in 64 Adults
(Age 18-51) and 62 Children (Age 5-14 Years) at Three Levels of High Altitude in Peru

Altitude	Number of subjects	A QRS >110 degrees (percent)	R/S V_1 >1.0 (percent)	R/S V_{5-6} <1.0 (percent)	RVH* (percent)
12,230 feet	A28	32%	25%	11%	18%
(3,373 m)	C20	22	32	9	20
14,200 feet	A15	36	27	20	20
(4,330 m)	C22	32	29	18	29
15,600 feet	A15	38	14	38	29
(4,760 m)	C20	74	55	30	60
TOTALS	A58	35	22	22	22
	C62	40	37	19	31

SOURCE: Toole et al., ref. 53.
ABBREVIATIONS: A=adult; C=children; AQRS=frontal plane QRS axis; R/S-V_1=ratio of R wave to S wave in V_1; R/S-V_{5-6}=ratio of R wave to S wave in V_5-V_6; RVH=right ventricular hypertrophy.
*Two or more criteria.

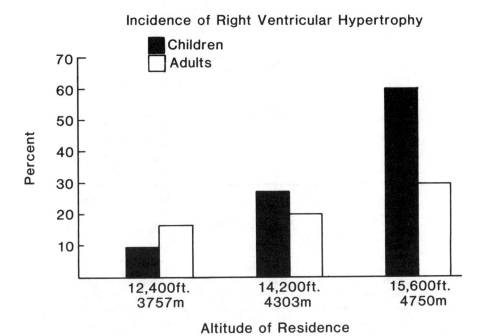

Figure 4.10. Prevalence of signs of right ventricular hypertrophy in the electrocardiogram of children and adults, living at three altitude levels in the Peruvian Andes. Criteria for right ventricular hypertrophy: two of the following three abnormalities: (1) frontal plane QRS axis >110 degrees; (2) R/S ratio in V, >100 percent; (3) R/S ratio in V5-6 <100 percent. Data from Toole et al., ref. 53.

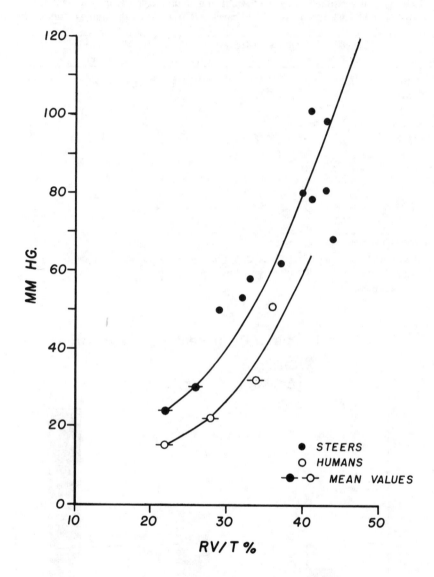

Figure 4.11. Relation between the ratio of the weight of the right ventricle to the total heart weight (RV/T ratio) and mean pulmonary artery pressure in human beings and steers. Human pressure data at sea level and high altitude are reported elsewhere (ref. 36). The two higher values in human subjects are derived from hemodynamic studies in patients with emphysema and dissection of the heart, in six cases of emphysema. The RV/T range from 30-40 percent in human beings is related to a substantially lower PA pressure than in steers, which exhibit higher PA pressures and a greater degree of RV hypertrophy. Data on steers obtained from Grover et al., ref. 51.

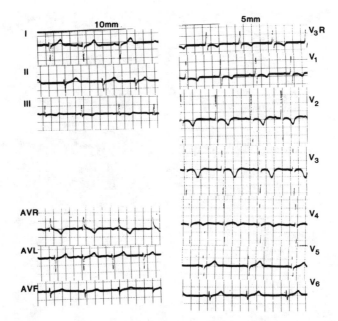

Figure 4.12. Electrocardiogram of a healthy eleven-year-old boy living at 15,600 feet (4,758 m) in the Peruvian Andes, showing a classic pattern of right ventricular hypertrophy. At this altitude, about 60 percent of children will have similar electrocardiograms.

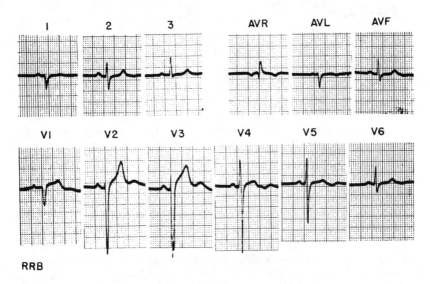

Figure 4.13. Electrocardiogram of a 28-year-old office worker living at 15,000 feet (4,575 m). The hematocrit was 75 percent. The chest film is shown in Figure 4.13. Although there is marked right axis deviation (+150 degrees), the precordial leads do not suggest right ventricular hypertrophy but are instead more compatible with an increased lung volume. Precordial leads were recorded one and two intercostal spaces lower than the above leads and revealed no significant difference in the QRS complexes from the above record. The systemic blood pressure was normal.

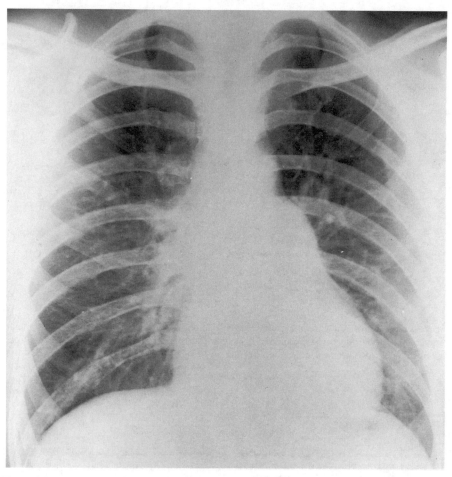

Figure 4.14. Chest film of a 28-year-old office worker who lived and worked at a mining facility at 15,000 feet (4,550 m) in the Peruvian Andes. His hematocrit was 75 percent. He was asymptomatic. Prominence of the main pulmonary artery and rounding of the cardiac apex compatible with pulmonary hypertension and right ventricular hypertrophy are a common finding in chest roentgenograms of high altitude natives.

(4,758 m) right ventricular hypertrophy patterns were substantially more common in children (60 percent versus 29 percent in adults). The reason for the lower prevalence of right ventricular hypertrophy patterns in adults is not clear, although it may be that adults have a greater chest volume in relation to body size than children. Hurtado in 1932 reported that high altitude natives had an increased chest circumference, increased pulmonary artery pressure, larger lateral chest diameters, and increased estimated chest volumes compared with sea-level adults.[28] Thus, the chest contour may modify the electrocardiogram just as the chest contour of pulmonary emphysema may modify the electrocardiogram at sea level (Figs. 4.12, 4.13, 4.14).

References

1. KRONENBERG R, SAFAR P, LEE J, et al. Pulmonary artery pressure and alveolar gas exchange in man during acclimatization to 12,400 feet (3,780 m). *J. Clin. Invest.* 1971; 50:827-37.

2. ALEXANDER J, HARTLEY L, MODELSKI M, and GROVER R. Reduction of stroke volume during exercise in man following ascent to 10,150 ft., (3,100 m) altitude. *J. Appl. Physiol.* 1967; 23:849-58.

3. REEVES J, and GROVER R. Approach to the patient with pulmonary hypertension. In *Pulmonary hypertension*, ed. E Weir and J Reeves. Mount Kisko, N.Y.: Futura, 1984: 1-44.

4. SIME F, PENALOZA D, RUIZ L, et al. Hypoxemia, pulmonary hypertension, and low cardiac output in newcomers at low altitude. *J. Appl. Physiol.* 1974; 36:561-65.

5. VOGEL J, GOSS J, MORI M, and BRAMMEL H. Pulmonary circulation in normal man with acute exposure to high altitude 14,260 feet (4,630 m). *Circulation* 1956; 34, Suppl. 3:233. Abstract.

6. GROVES B, REEVES J, SUTTON J, et al. Operation Everest II: Elevated high-altitude pulmonary resistance unresponsive to oxygen. *J. Appl. Physiol.* 1987; 63:521-30.

7. HULTGREN H, LOPEZ C, LUNDBERG E, and MILLER H. Physiologic studies of pulmonary edema at high altitude. *Circulation* 1964; 29:393-408.

8. REEVES J, GROVES B, SUTTON J, et al. Operation Everest II: Preservation of cardiac function at extreme altitude. *J. Appl. Physiol.* 1987; 63:531-39.

9. HULTGREN H. The pulmonary circulation in high altitude residents during exercise: The effects of acute hypoxia and 100 percent oxygen breathing. (MS. in preparation.)

10. DOYLE J, WILSON J, and WARREN J. The pulmonary vascular responses to short term hypoxia in human subjects. *Circulation* 1952; 5:263-70.

11. WESCOTT R, FOWLER N, SCOTT R, et al. Anoxia and human pulmonary vascular resistance. *J. Clin. Invest.* 1951; 30:957-70.

12. VISWANATHAN R, JAIN S, SUBRAMANIAN T, et al. Pulmonary edema of high altitude II: Clinical, aerohemodynamic, and biochemical studies of a group with a history of pulmonary edema at high altitude. *Am. Rev. Resp. Dis.* 1969; 100:334-41.

13. WAGENVOORT C, and WAGENVOORT N. Hypoxic pulmonary vascular lesions in man at high altitude and in patients with chronic respiratory disease. *Pathologia e Microbiologia* 1973; 39:276-82.

14. HANSON W, BOGGS D, KAY M, et al. Collateral ventilation and pulmonary arterial smooth muscle in the coati. *J. Appl. Physiol.* 1993; 74:2219-24.

15. HULTGREN H, GROVER R, and HARTLEY L. Abnormal circulatory responses to high altitude in subjects with a previous history of high altitude pulmonary edema. *Circulation* 1971; 44:759-70.

16. ROTTA A, CANEPA A, HURTADO A, et al. Pulmonary circulation at sea level and at high altitude. *J. Appl. Physiol.* 1956; 9:328-36.

17. GROVER R, OKIN J, and OVERY H. Natural history of pulmonary hypertension in normal adult residents of high altitude. *Circulation* 1965; 32, Suppl. 2: 102. Abstract.

18. EULER V, and LILJESTRAND G. Observations on the pulmonary arterial pressure in the cat. *Acta Physiol. Scand.* 1946; 12:301-20.

19. LOCKHART A, ZELTER M, MENSCH-DECHENE J, et al. Pressure flow volume relationships in pulmonary circulation of normal highlanders. *J. Appl. Physiol.* 1976; 41:449-56.

20. MARSHALL C, and MARSHALL B. Site and sensitivity of hypoxia pulmonary vasoconstriction. *J. Appl. Physiol.* 1983; 55:711-16.

21. HUGHES J, and RUBIN L. Relation between mixed venous oxygen tension and pulmonary vascular tone during normoxic, hyperoxic, and hypoxic ventilation in dogs. *Am. J. Cardiol.* 1984; 54:1118-23.

22. MCMURTY I, and RAFFESTIN B. Potential mechanisms of hypoxic pulmonary vasoconstriction. In *The pulmonary circulation in health and disease*, ed. J Will, C Dawson, K Weir, and C Buckner, New York: Academic Press, 1987, 455-68.

23. VOELKEL N, MCDONNELL T, CHANG S, et al. Mechanisms of hypoxic vasoconstriction. In *High altitude medical science*, eds. G Ueda, S Kusama, and N Voelkel. Shinsu University, Matsumoto, Japan: 1988, 13-28.

24. McGOON M, and VLIESTRA R. Vasodilator therapy for primary pulmonary hypertension. *Mayo Clin. Proc.* 1984; 59:672-77.

25. OELZ O. A case of high-altitude pulmonary edema treated with Nifedipine. *JAMA* 1987; 257:780.

26. HACKETT P, GREEN E, ROACH R, et al. Nifedipine and hydralazine for treatment of high altitude pulmonary edema. In *Hypoxia: The Adaptations*, ed. J Sutton, G Coates, and J Remmers. Philadelphia: B.C. Decker, 1990: 221. Abstract.

27. SCHERRER U, UOLLENWEIDER L, DELABAYS A, et al. Inhaled nitric oxide for high altitude pulmonary edema. *N. Engl. J. Med.* 1996; 334:624-9.
28. HURTADO A. Respiratory adaptations in the Indian natives of the Peruvian Andes. Studies at high altitude. *Am. J. Phys. Anthropol.* 1932; 17:137-65.
29. ANTEZANA G, BARRAGAN L, COUDERT J, et al. The pulmonary circulation of high altitude natives. In *High altitude physiology and medicine*, ed. W Brendel and R Zink. New York: Springer Verlag, 1982.
30. KHOURY G, and HAWES C. Primary pulmonary hypertension in children living at high altitude. *J. Pediatr.* 1963; 62:177-85.
31. CRUZ J, BANCHERO N, SIME F, et al. Correlation between pulmonary artery pressure and level of altitude. *Dis. of the Chest.* 1964; 46:446-51.
32. GROVES B, SUTTON J, DROMA T, et al. Absence of hypoxic pulmonary hypertension in normal Tibetans at 3,658 m. In *Hypoxia and mountain medicine*, ed. J Sutton, G Coates, and C Houston. Burlington, VT: Queen City Printers, 1992: 304. Abstract.
33. SIME F, BANCHERO N, PENALOZA D, et al. Pulmonary hypertension in children born and living at high altitudes. *Am. J. Cardiol.* 1963; 11:143-49.
34. REEVES J, and GROVER R. High-altitude pulmonary hypertension and pulmonary edema. In P Yu and J Goodwin, eds., *Progress in Cardiology*, Philadelphia: Lea & Febiger, 1975: 99-118.
35. GREGORY T, CHAPLEAU M, SUMMER W, and LEVITSKY M. The effects of aging on hypoxic pulmonary vasoconstriction. *The Physiologist* 1984; 27:263. Abstract.
36. HULTGREN H, KELLY J, and MILLER H. Pulmonary circulation in acclimatized man at high altitude. *J. Appl. Physiol.* 1965; 20:233-38.
37. DAVIDSON W, JR., FEE E, and M NAGILL E. Influence of aging on pulmonary hemodynamics in a population free of coronary disease. *Clin. Res.* 1988; 36:271A. Abstract.
38. ARIAS-STELLA J, and SALDANA M. The terminal portion of the pulmonary arterial tree in people native to high altitude. *Circulation* 1963; 28:915-25.
39. HULTGREN H, KELLY J, and MILLER H. Effect of oxygen upon pulmonary circulation in acclimatized man at high altitude. *J. Appl. Physiol.* 1965; 20:239-43.
40. SIME F, PENALOZA D, and RUIZ D. Bradycardia, increased cardiac output, and reversal of pulmonary hypertension in altitude natives living at sea level. *Brit. Heart J.* 1971; 33:647-57.
41. SALDANA M, and ARIAS-STELLA J. Studies on the structure of the pulmonary trunk II: The evolution of the elastic configuration of the pulmonary trunk in people native to high altitudes. *Circulation* 1963; 27:1094-1100.
42. SALDANA M, and ARIAS-STELLA J. Studies on the structure of the pulmonary trunk III: The thickness of the media of the pulmonary trunk and ascending aorta in the high altitude native. *Circulation* 1963; 27:1101.
43. BANCHERO N, SIME F, PENALOZA D, et al. Pulmonary artery pressure, cardiac output, and arterial oxygen saturation during exercise at high altitude and at sea level. *Circulation* 1966; 33:249-62.
44. GROVER R. Hypoxia and pulmonary hypertension at high altitude. *Ann. N.Y. Acad. Sci.* 1965; 127: 632-39.
45. MANOHAR M, PARKS C, BUSCH M, and BISGARD G. Transmural coronary vasodilator reserve and flow distribution in unanesthetized calves sojourning at 11,550 ft. (3,500 m). *J. Surg. Research* 1985; 39: 499-509.
46. KERWIN A. Observation on the heart size of natives living at high altitudes. *Am. Heart J.* 1944; 28:69-80.
47. HULTGREN H, and MILLER H. Human heart weight at high altitude. *Circulation* 1967; 35:207-18.
48. HULTGREN H, and MILLER H. Right ventricular hypertrophy at high altitude. *Ann. N.Y. Acad. Sci.* 1965; 127:627-31.
49. CARRILLO A, BRYCE A, AMAT Y LEON F, et. al. M-mode echocardiography in healthy men born and living at high altitude. *J. Am. Coll. Cardiol.* 1983; 1:592. Abstract.
50. HULTGREN H, MARTICORENA E, and MILLER H. Right ventricular hypertrophy in animals at high altitude. *J. Appl. Physiol.* 1963; 18:913-18.
51. GROVER R, REEVES J, WILL D, and BLOUNT S, JR. Pulmonary vasoconstriction in steers at high altitude. *J. Appl. Physiol.* 1963; 18:567-74.
52. PENALOZA D, GAMBOA R, MARTICORENA E, et al. The influence of high altitudes on the electrical activity of the heart: Electrocardiographic and vectorcardiographic observations in adolescence and adulthood. *Am. Heart J.* 1961; 61:101-15.

53. TOOLE J, HULTGREN H, and KELLEY J. The electrocardiogram at high altitude. *Clin. Res.* 1962; 10:74. Abstract.
54. ROTTA A, and LOPEZ A. Electrocardiographic patterns in man at high altitude. *Circulation* 1959; 19:719- 28.

CHAPTER 5

Blood and Plasma Volume

Part I: Red Cells-Hemoglobin

SUMMARY
The hypoxemia of high altitude causes the kidneys to release erythropoietin, which stimulates red cell production. The result is a slow increase in red cell mass, which plateaus in three to twelve months. Iron absorption increases three to four fold, and reticulocytes increase. The hemoglobin and hematocrit of high altitude residents are increased roughly in proportion to both the arterial oxygen saturation and the altitude. Above 10,000 feet (3,250 m) hemoglobin is roughly related to altitude in a linear fashion. Considerable individual variation exists in hematocrit. At an altitude of 14,200 feet (4,615 m) hematocrits in healthy persons may vary from 50 to 70 percent. Other factors that influence the hematocrit include diet, level of activity, fluid balance, age, and occupation. Descent to sea level results in an abrupt decrease or cessation of red cell production with a decrease in iron absorption and reticulocytes. A steady state is reached after three to six months.

Although thrombotic episodes in various vascular beds are not uncommon at high altitude, especially in sojourners, attempts to relate high altitude exposure in normal subjects to various coagulation factors have not been productive. In certain high altitude illnesses, however, such as high altitude pulmonary edema, decreases in platelet counts and a rise in fibrinopeptide A suggest the presence of enhanced fibrin formation and intravascular thrombosis. Coagulation abnormalities have also been reported in calves with the development of brisket disease upon ascent to high altitude.

• • •

Red Cell Volume

In 1891 Viault[1] demonstrated the presence of an increased hemoglobin concentration in the blood of animals living in Morococha, Peru (altitude 14,900 feet/4,545 m). Subsequently other workers found that polycythemia was common in high altitude residents, and roughly related to the altitude, and that the hematocrit returned to normal upon descent to sea level.[2,3,4]

Ascent to High Altitude

Red cell production increases upon ascent to high altitude owing to an increased secretion of erythropoietin; the erythropoietin activity is proportional to the degree of hypoxia, and the increased secretion is evident within a few hours of ascent.[4,5,6] This initial increase in erythropoietin in plasma and urine subsides after a few days, but levels remain higher than normal throughout the stay at high altitude. In about one year after ascent, red cell production reaches its maximum, usually around 30 percent higher than at sea level.[5,6,7] The life span of the red cell is normal and equilibrium is maintained by increased red cell destruction.[6,8] The magnitude of the rise in erythropoietin activity is related to altitude up to extreme altitudes, where hypoxic depression of the bone marrow may decrease the rate of red cell production.[9] Reynafarje and his associates studied ten normal sea level subjects who were taken to Morococha at 14,900 feet (4,545 m) and remained there for one year.[7] From 16 to 20 days at Morococha three subjects increased their hemoglobin from 13.7 gms percent to 17.1 gms and their hematocrit increased from 44.2 percent to 53.3 percent. The red cell mass continued to increase for eight months, when it reached a plateau. During the first two months, as the red cell mass increased, the plasma volume decreased by an equal volume; at eight months the total blood volume was higher than at sea level but was not greater than that found in natives of high altitude (Fig. 5.1). The increased red cell production was accompanied by an increase in reticulocytes and erythroprotoporhyrins; iron absorption also was greatly increased. Women who may be iron-deficient and persons on an iron-deficient diet will exhibit a smaller increase in red cell mass. Increases in red cell mass also occur in high altitude climbers (Fig. 5.2). In nineteen acclimatized members of the American Medical Research Expedition to Everest the mean hemoglobin at 20,700 feet (6,314 m) was 18.8 gms percent ± 1.4, and the mean hematocrit was 53 percent ± 5.0 (Fig. 5.3). There was no relation between hematocrit and climbing performance or the degree of acclimatization.[10]

High Altitude Natives

In high altitude residents the red cell mass is increased in proportion to the altitude of habitation and their arterial oxygen tension. The critical arterial oxygen tension at which red cell mass starts to increase is a PO_2 of 70 mm Hg, which is equivalent to an altitude of about 5,000 feet (1,525 m) (Fig. 5.4). Red cell mass, however, is increased in a linear relation to arterial oxygen saturation. The increase begins when the arterial oxygen tension falls below the level where arterial oxygen

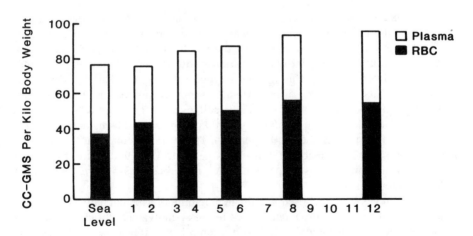

Figure 5.1. Mean values of red cell and plasma volumes in ten male subjects, who were taken from sea level to Morococha, Peru, 14,900 feet (4,540 m), where they lived continuously for one year. Red cell mass and total blood volume are increased, but there is no change in plasma volume at one year. Plasma volume is decreased during the first two months. From Reynafarje, ref. 6.

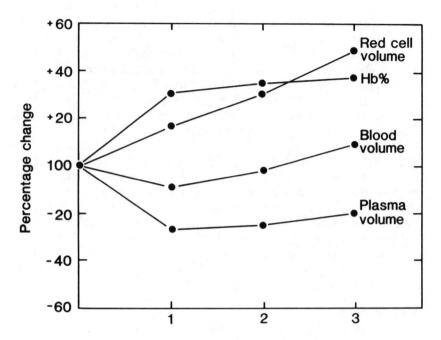

Figure 5.2. Mean changes in hemoglobin, red cell volumes, plasma volume and total blood volume in four subjects during an eight month Himalayan expedition. (1) After 18 weeks between 13,000 feet (4,000 m) and 19,000 feet (5,800 m). (2) After 3 to 6 weeks at 19,000 feet. (3) After 9 to 14 weeks at 19,000 feet or above 19,000 feet. Red cell volume progressively increases. Plasma volume is decreased. From Pugh, ref. 9.

saturation begins a sharp decrease.[11] This implies that red cell production, and presumably erythropoietin production also, are more dependent on oxygen saturation, and therefore on oxygen delivery to the tissues, than on oxygen tension. At any level of high altitude, wide individual variations in hematocrit may be found that cannot be related to the resting arterial oxygen saturation.[12] This indicates that factors other than the degree of hypoxia affect red cell production. Regional and probably genetic variations occur in red cell mass at equivalent altitudes. In Leadville, Colorado (altitude 10,150 feet/ 3,100 m), the normal hematocrit range for adults is 46 to 58 percent (mean 50.2 percent). The average hematocrit for Peruvian natives living at 12,230 feet (3,730 m) is 54 percent. At 14,900 feet (4,545 m) in Peru the mean hematocrit is 60 percent.[3,4] As the red cell mass increases, plasma volume decreases slightly.

Recent studies have proposed that the hemoglobin of Tibetan natives is considerably lower than that of Peruvian natives living at equivalent altitudes. Beall and associates measured hemoglobin levels in a sample of 270 healthy adult Tibetans (ages 20-79) living at 10,800-12,500 feet (3,294-3,813 m) in Nepal. Mean hemoglobin levels were 16.1 gms/100 ml in adult males, and 98 percent of the adult males had hemoglobin levels within two standard deviations of a sea level reference population mean. In comparison with studies from the Peruvian Andes it was concluded that high altitude Himalayan natives have hemoglobin levels one to two

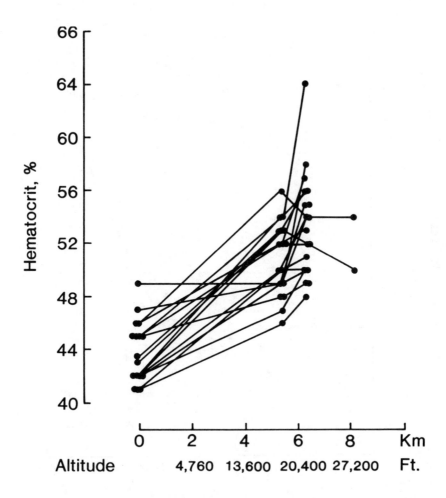

Figure 5.3. Hematocrits at various altitudes in normal male subjects (ages 26-52 years) who were members of the American Medical Research Expedition to Mount Everest in 1982. From Winslow et al., ref. 10.

grams lower than those of Andean natives living at the same altitude.[13] These results must be interpreted with caution, however, since only hemoglobin was measured, samples were transported considerably distances for analysis, and nutritional factors were not excluded. Indeed, Sherpas may not be representative of permanent high altitude residents because they move frequently from high to low altitudes. Studies of a small number of Sherpas by the American Medical Research Expedition to Everest did not confirm Beall's observations.[14] Residents of the Pamir Mountains in Tadzhikistan living at 11,800 feet (3,600 m) have a mean hemoglobin of 18.5 gms and a mean hematocrit of 61.0 percent, which is comparable to the values observed at equivalent altitudes in Peru.[15] The normal hemoglobin value for male residents of La Oroya, Peru, altitude 12,230 feet (3,730 m), is 15.9 gm/100 ml range-14.1 - 17.7 gms. This value is similar to that reported by Beall. Hemoglobin values in relation

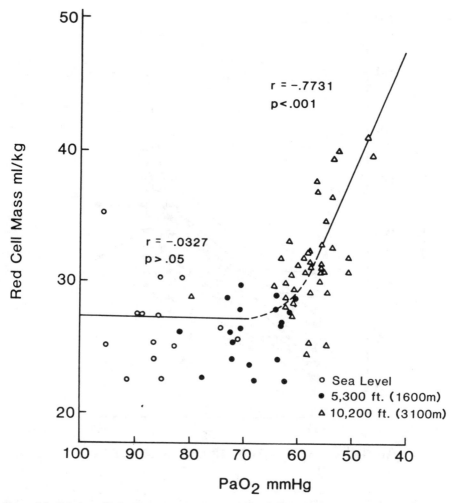

Figure 5.4. Relation of red cell mass to arterial PO₂ at various altitudes. Note the sharp increase in red cell mass at an arterial PO₂ of 70 mm, which corresponds to an altitude of approximately 5,000 feet (1,500 m). From Weil et al., ref. 11.

to the altitude in the South American Andes are shown in Figure 5.5. Monge has pointed out that the hemoglobin levels in rural Peruvian Quechua Indians and rural Nepalese are on the same regression line relating altitude to hemoglobin, indicating that the hemoglobin responses to altitude are similar in these two populations. Urban dwellers in Peru have a higher hemoglobin than do rural dwellers. Hematocrit values are also similar in rural dwelling Nepalese and Quechuas.[16]

Winslow and his associates studied 29 Chilean males living at 12,134 feet (3,700 m) and 30 Sherpas living in Nepal at the same altitude. The hematocrit of the Chilean Indians was slightly higher than that of the Sherpas: 52.2 ± 4.6 percent versus 48.4 ± 4.5 percent, respectively, p <0.003. There was a similar but lesser difference in hemoglobin concentrations, and the red cell counts were similar.[17]

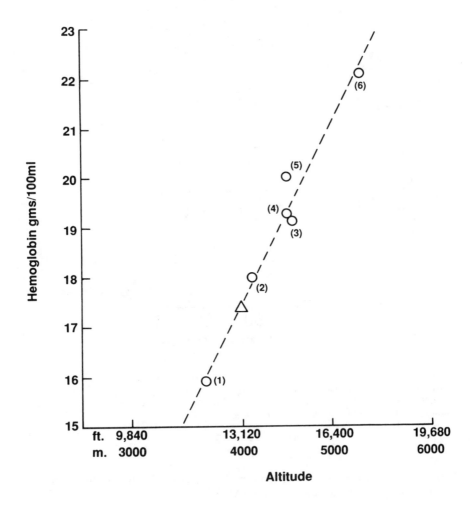

Figure 5.5. Hemoglobin in relation to altitude in the South American Andes. Numbers indicate source references below. Triangle refers to studies in Bolivian highlanders. From Beall et al., ref. 13.

SOURCES:

1. Normal blood values from Chulec General Hospital La Oroya, Peru, altitude 12,230 feet (3,750 m), 475 males, aged 20-60 years.
2,3 Monge C. Natural acclimatization to high altitudes: Clinical conditions. In *Life at high altitudes*. Pan-American Health Organization, 1966. Data from 3.138 miners without silicosis between 13,200 feet (4,000 m) and 14,500 feet (4,400 m) and 3,138 miners living above 14,500 feet (4,400 m).
4. Hurtado A. Some physiologic and clinical aspects of life at high altitude. In *Aging of the Lung (10th Hahnemann Symposium)*, ed. L Cander and J Mayer. New York: Grune and Stratton, 1964: 257. Data from 83 natives living at 14,900 feet (4,540 m) in the Peruvian Andes (Morococha).
5. Hurtado A. In *Handbook of physiology; adaptation to the environment*, ed. D Dill, E Adolph and C Wilber. Washington, DC: American Physiological Society, 1900; Sect. 4:843.
6. Dill D, Talbot J and Consolazio W. Blood physiochemical system XII: Man at high altitude. *J. Biol. Chem.* 1937; 118:649-66.

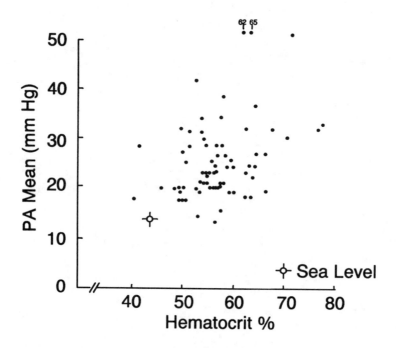

Figure 5.6. Hematocrit and mean resting pulmonary artery pressure at 12,230 feet (3,730 m) and 14,200 feet (4,303 m) in high altitude residents in Peru. o = normal sea level pressure. Only a very crude relationship is evident. From Hultgren, unpublished data.

Several unknown variables other than the hematopoietic response to altitude may have been responsible, as pointed out by Monge.[16]

Polycythemia

There is considerable individual variation in the hemoglobin levels of high altitude residents even in the same age groups living at similar altitudes and carrying out similar levels of daily physical activity (Fig. 5.6). In Peru, hemoglobin values in two different mining populations living at the same altitude may be significantly different without any obvious explanation. For example, the mean hemoglobin in residents of Ticlio, at 15,090 feet (4,600 m), is 18.5 gms, whereas residents of San Antonio at the same altitude have a mean hemoglobin of 21.5 gms.[16-19] In 526 healthy men in La Paz, Bolivia, altitude 12,730 feet (3,883 m), the mean hemoglobin was 18.8 gms/dl ± 1.4 gms.[20] Very high hematocrits exceeding 70 percent may occasionally be seen in apparently asymptomatic individuals without evidence of cardiac or pulmonary disease. An example was described by Santolaya and his associates.[21] A 34 year-old miner who had lived in the Aucanquilcha mining area in Chile, 19,156 feet (5,950 m), for eight years was found to have a hematocrit of 75 percent compared with an average value of 59 percent in five other miners living in

Table 5.1

Systemic Oxygen Transport in 22 Sea level Residents and
High Altitude Natives at Rest and During Exercise

	Rest		Exercise	
	Sea level (350 feet)	14,900 feet	Sea level (350 feet)	14,900 feet
Hgb gms %	14.8	19.4	15.4	20.1
O_2 cap. ml/L	198	259	208	269
Art O_2 Sat, %	95.7	78.4	94.9	69.4
Art O_2 Content, ml/L	190	202	197	186
O_2 uptake ml/min/m^2	153	161	719	779
Cardiac index 1/min/m^2	3.97	3.97	6.83	7.70
Systemic O_2 transport ml/min/-m^2	756	803	1,350	1,430

SOURCE: Data from Banchero et al., ref. 24.

the same area. He did not complain about his health nor were his physical activities limited. His arterial PO_2 was 32 mm Hg and his PCO_2 was 31 mm Hg. This condition has been defined as chronic high altitude polycythemia or excessive polycythemia of high altitude and should not be confused with symptomatic chronic mountain sickness. Chronic high altitude polycythemia has been observed at 10,150 feet (3,100 m) in the Rocky Mountains, where one group of nine asymptomatic subjects had a mean hematocrit of 59 percent ± 1.9.[22]

Oxygen Transport

An important effect of the increase in red cell mass is the resultant increase in oxygen-carrying capacity, which allows oxygen delivery to the tissues to occur without an obligatory increase in cardiac output and cardiac work.[23] Banchero and his workers measured the cardiac output and oxygen transport in 22 normal subjects at sea level and in 35 high altitude natives living at 14,900 feet (4,545 m). Studies were carried out at rest and during equivalent amounts of supine, cycle ergometer exercise. At rest and during exercise, oxygen transport was maintained at high altitude with essentially the same cardiac output that was measured at sea level (Table 5.1).[24] Anemia at high altitude has an adverse effect on physical performance. Anemic men in La Paz, Bolivia, altitude 12,730 feet (3,883 m), had an estimated VO_{2max} that was 21 percent lower than that of non-anemic men.[20]

Oxygen transport is maintained by an increase in cardiac output when the hemoglobin content decreases. A marked compensatory increase in cardiac output occurs when the hemoglobin content falls below 7 gms percent.[25] An example of this adaptation is illustrated by a case report from Alaska in which a 23 year-old schoolteacher who was climbing alone on Mount McKinley developed severe intestinal bleeding and weakness at 17,700 feet (5,400 m). After two days of bleeding, she was able to climb down 700 feet, where she made camp. Several days later, after spending a total of 16 days at 17,000 feet (5,185 m), she was evacuated by helicopter. She was weak, but able to walk. Her sensorium was clear. Her heart rate was 88/min, blood pressure 100/30 mm Hg, red cell count 1.36 million, hemoglobin 3.8 gms/100 ml, and hematocrit 12.7 percent. A chest x-ray was normal and revealed no definite cardiac enlargement or pulmonary edema, but a duodenal ulcer was demonstrated by barium x-ray. After several transfusions the patient recovered completely.[26] It is remarkable that this patient was able to survive for such a long period at a very high altitude with such a marked decrease in the oxygen carrying capacity of her blood. An increase in cardiac output maintained appropriate tissue oxygen delivery without the development of cardiac failure or pulmonary edema. These observations indicate that the contribution of polycythemia to acclimatization at high altitude is probably small and even a low red cell volume can be compensated for by an increase in cardiac output.

Age and Red Cell Mass

Wittenbury and Monge reported that hematocrits in natives living at 14,900 feet (4,545 m) exhibit a progressive increase up to 34 years.[27] Further studies have shown a slow increase in hemoglobin up to 50 years in high altitude residents. The increase was approximately from 18.3 gms at 20-29 years to 19.2 gms at 50 years. Sea level control populations did not exhibit any change in hemoglobin with age. Vital capacity decreased more with advancing age at high altitude than at sea level. The hypoxic ventilatory responses decreases with age, but studies have not been done in high altitude dwellers.[17] The prevalence of hemoglobin levels ≥21.3 gms in healthy high altitude Peruvian miners age 40-49 years is 18.8 percent; the prevalence increases with age, and at 60-69 years the prevalence is 33.7 percent.[19] Collier and Chiodi studied subjects living at Mina Aquilar in Argentina at 14,800 feet (4,515 m). Their data indicated no relation between age and red cell count, hematocrit, or hemoglobin.[28] The difference in these results may be related to differences in the populations studied.

Table 5.2
Normal Blood Values in Residents at Morococha and Lima, Peru

| | Morococha | | Lima | |
	Number of residents	Blood Values	Number of residents	Blood Values
Hemoglobin	83	20.10±00.22	250	15.64± 0.05
Red cells, mill/cu mm	83	06.44±00.09	250	05.11±00.02
Hematocrit, percent	83	59.50±00.68	250	46.60±00.15
Mean corpuscular, vol cu micr	83	92.80±00.77	250	91.20±00.30
Mean corpuscular Hgb micr gm	83	31.50±00.31	250	30.90±00.11
Mean corpuscular Hgb conc percent	83	33.90±00.15	250	33.80±00.08
Mean corpuscular diameter, micr.	32	07.74±00.01	130	07.48±00.01
Reticulocytes, percent	83	01.00±00.07	250	00.40±00.02
Bilirubin total, mg/100 ml	57	01.28±00.13	250	00.76±00.03
Platelets, 1000/cu mm	41	419.0±22.47	80	406.0±14.98
Leucocytes 100/cu mm	72	07.04±00.19	140	06.68±00.10

SOURCE: Hurtado, refs. 2 and 31.

Blood Viscosity

Blood viscosity is increased at high altitude, but its effect upon the circulation in man has not been clearly demonstrated. Reducing red cell mass by removing blood and infusing an equivalent amount of plasma or plasma substitute does not increase physical working capacity at high altitude.[29] An exception may be in patients with chronic mountain sickness.[30] Despite variations in hematocrit from 40 to 75 percent, there is no correlation between hematocrit and mean pulmonary artery pressure in high altitude residents in Peru (Fig. 5.6).

Red cell indices in high altitude natives are normal.[31,32] The number of white blood cells and platelets is normal. The increased red cell production is reflected by an increase in reticulocytes to a value of about one percent and the increased red cell destruction by an elevation of total serum bilirubin to about 1.28 mg/100 ml.[29,33] The slight increase in serum bilirubin reflects destruction of the larger red cell mass. Normal hematologic values for high altitude residents and sea level subjects are shown in Table 5.2. Ascent to extreme altitudes (above 18,500 feet/ 5,643 m) results in an increase in mean corpuscular hemoglobin concentration.[10]

Descent

Descent to sea level by high altitude residents is accompanied by a marked decrease in red cell production with the maximum decrease attained about three to five weeks after descent. Erythropoietin levels become undetectable. The red cell mass progressively decreases so that after two months it may be lower than that of sea level dwellers. Red cell life span remains normal.[6] Plasma volume increases, so that total blood volume remains essentially unchanged or decreases slightly after several months.[5,34] Upon descent, the decrease in red cell production is reflected by a decrease in reticulocytes and iron utilization. Iron absorption decreases.[35] These changes are slowly restored to normal values after three to six months.[6,7]

Leucocytes

Ascent to high altitude does not affect the number or distribution of white cells. An early report indicated that at high altitude the number and percentage of lymphocytes is increased.[36] I have found no confirmation of this observation. Normal values for residents of La Oroya, Peru, 12,400 feet (3,782 m) do not indicate an increased percentage of lymphocytes compared to sea level values.

Hemoglobin

Hemoglobin is a large protein molecule consisting of four polypeptide subunits, each of which is linked to an iron containing prosthetic group, *heme*. Oxygen binds reversibly to the iron atom, and each hemoglobin molecule can bind four molecules of oxygen. About 97 percent of the oxygen in the blood is physically bound to hemoglobin and about 3 percent is dissolved in the plasma.

Variant hemoglobins. There are many mutant hemoglobins in man, which occur in about 0.5 percent of all human beings; however few of these are clinically important. Sickle cell anemia and the sickle cell trait result from the presence of S-hemoglobin. This hemoglobin has a slightly unusual molecular configuration, which can result in changes of the shape of the red cell as a result of various stimuli. Hypoxemia will induce changes in the shape of the cells (sickling), and the abnormal cells may clump into masses occluding vessels and capillaries (see Chapter 26 "Sickle Cell Disease").

Another unusual variant hemoglobin is known as the Andrew Minneapolis form. This type of hemoglobin results in a left shift of the oxygen dissociation curve and thus may be of advantage to a person at high altitude. To test this hypothesis, two subjects with this form of hemoglobin were transported to 10,200 feet (3,100 m) with two unaffected siblings as controls. The affected subjects experienced a lesser increase in heart rate, a lesser increase in erythropoietin, and no decrease in VO_{2max} compared with the control subjects. The p50 was 17.1 mm Hg in the affected subjects and 27.0 mm Hg in the controls. The authors suggested that a left-shifted oxygen dissociation curve confers a degree of preadaptation to high altitude.[37]

F Hemoglobin

Newborn infants have a high percentage of F (fetal) hemoglobin, which, because it has a high affinity for oxygen, enables the fetus to extract oxygen rapidly through the placenta from the mother's blood. The oxygen dissociation curve is thus shifted to the left of the adult hemoglobin curve. After birth the curve moves to about 7 mm to the right of the adult curve, thus providing a greater facility for oxygen release in the tissues. Since this coincides with the physiological anemia of the postnatal period, the shift in the curve compensates for what would otherwise require a 50 percent increase in blood flow.[38] Many animals living at high altitude have high levels of F hemoglobin.

Coagulation Factors

For several reasons, considerable attention has been given to studies of coagulation factors in the blood of sojourners and residents of high altitude. (1) Venous thrombosis and pulmonary embolism have occurred in high altitude climbers. (2) Small thrombi have been found in the pulmonary arterioles and capillaries of

Table 5.3
Blood Coagulation Factors at High Altitude

Researcher	Conditions of Study	Results	
Marticorena 1968 (ref. 41)	10 subjects brought to 14,200 feet (4,600 m)	Whole blood Coagulation time	↓
Garvey 1968, 1969 (refs. 39,40)	Monkeys at 17,500 feet (5,338 m) for 28 days in a hypobaric chamber (data from animals with hematocrits ≥ 65%	Prothrombin time	↑
		Partial thromboplastin time	→
		Fibrinogen	↑
		Euglobulin lysis time	→
		Split product activity	↑
Hultgren 1970 (ref. 49)	7 subjects brought to 12,470 feet (3,803 m)	Platelets	→
		Fibrinogen	→
		Quick time	→
		Thrombin time	→
		PTT	→
		AHG	→
		Coagulation time	→
		Fibrin split products	→
		Euglobulin clot lysis	→
		Hematocrit	

Table 5.3 continues on the next page

Table 5.3 (cont.)
Blood Coagulation Factors at High Altitude

Researcher	Conditions of Study	Results	
Genton 1970 (ref. 43)	4 calves brought to 14,100 feet (4,300 m) for 10 days Pulmonary hypertension developed	Decrease in platelet count (600,000 to 200,000)	↓
		Platelet adhesiveness	↑
		Platelet survival	↓
		Fibrinogen survival	↓
		Partial thromboplastin time	↓
		Prothrombin time	↑
Singh 1972 (ref. 42)	38 soldiers - residents for 2 years at 12,000-18,000 feet (3,660-5,550 m).	Plasma fibrinogen	↑
		Fibrinolytic activity	↑
		Platelet adhesiveness	↑
		Platelet factor III	↑
	A. 6 who developed pulmonary hypertension	Factor V	↑
		Factor VIII	↑
		Prothrombin time	0
		Platelet count	0
	B. 32 who did not develop p.h.	Plasma fibrinogen	↑
		Fibrinolytic activity	↑
Coates & Gray 1982 (ref. 45)	16 subjects exposed to 20,000 feet (6,100 m) in a hypobaric chamber 2 hours	Protamine paracoagulation test	→
		Platelet count - a drop of 10% for 3 days after decompression	↓
Gray 1975 (ref. 46)	2 subjects exposed to 9,800 feet (3,000 m) and	Platelet counts decreased 7 and 25%	↓
	7 subjects exposed to 12,470 feet (3,778m) 24 hours	Platelet accumulation in lungs	→
Maher 1976 (ref. 47)	8 subjects brought to 14,436 feet (4,400 m) in a hypobaric chamber	Mean partial Thromboplastin time *	↓
		Fibrinogen *	↓
		Factor VIII *	
		Fibrin degradation products	3/7
		Platelet aggregation	→
		2/3 diphosphoglycerate	↑
		Platelet count	→
		Factor III availability	→
		Membrane lipid	→
		Peroxidase formation	→
		Prothrombin time	→
		Thrombin time	→
Andrew 1987 (ref. 48)	5 subjects exposed to 25,000 feet (7,625 m) in a hypobaric chamber for 40 days	14 coagulation factors rest	→
		Factor VIII exercise	↑

patients with high altitude pulmonary edema and chronic mountain sickness and may be a contributing factor in the pathogenesis of these syndromes. (3) Cerebral venous thrombosis has been observed in cases of high altitude cerebral edema. (4) The marked polycythemia of Peruvian high altitude residents suggests an increased tendency to develop thrombosis comparable to that seen at sea level in patients with polycythemia vera. (5) Exposure to high altitude has been reported to result in changes in blood factors, which may give indirect evidence of an increased tendency to intravascular thromboses particularly in the pulmonary circulation. The results of nine studies are summarized in Table 5.3.

Garvey reported autopsy studies and coagulation abnormalities in rhesus monkeys exposed to a simulated altitude of 17,500 feet (5,300 m) for 28 days in a hypobaric chamber. Hemorrhages and thromboses were found in the brain and lungs. Coagulation studies were compatible with accelerated intravascular coagulation, including marked decreases in Factors VIII and IX and modest decreases in Factors V and XI. Fibrin degradation products were present in the serum. The coagulation abnormalities improved with heparin therapy. It was concluded that the coagulopathy was due to the increased viscosity of the blood in the microcirculation. The hematocrit varied from 58 to 80 percent.[39,40]

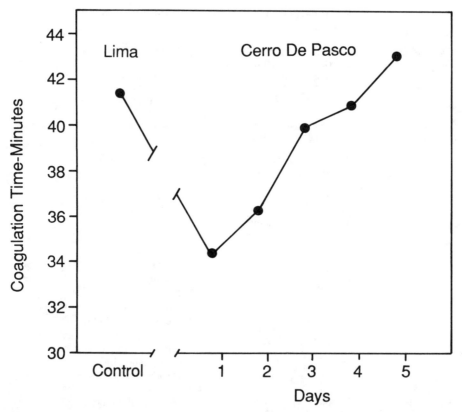

Figure 5.7. Whole blood coagulation time in silconized tubes in ten normal subjects brought from sea level to 14,200 feet (4,330 m). From Marticorena, ref. 41.

Marticorena in 1968 reported a decrease in whole blood coagulation times from 42 seconds to 34 seconds in ten subjects brought from sea level to 14,200 feet (4,330 m) (Fig. 5.7). The maximum decrease occurred on the first day after arrival, and there was a return to normal values by the fifth day.[41] Singh studied 38 Indian soldiers who had lived for two years between 12,000 feet (3,660 m) and 18,000 feet (5,490 m).[42] In six men who developed pulmonary hypertension, increases were observed in plasma fibrinogen, fibrinolytic activity, platelet adhesiveness, Factor III, Factor V, and Factor VIII. In the 32 soldiers who did not develop pulmonary hypertension, the only increases seen were in plasma fibrinogen and fibrinolytic activity. Platelet adhesiveness was increased.

Genton and his associates also found changes in coagulation factors in acute pulmonary hypertension induced in four calves that were taken from 5,400 feet (1,647 m) to 14,110 feet (4,300 m) and kept there for ten days.[43] Pulmonary artery pressure increased from 40 mm Hg to 90 mm Hg (mean). The hematocrit increased by 25 percent. Ten coagulation factors were studied. Positive findings included a fall in platelet count from 600,000 to 200,000, an increase in platelet adhesiveness by 143 percent, and a 63 percent decrease in platelet survival. Fibrinogen survival decreased by 35 percent, partial thromboplastin time decreased by 53 percent, and prothrombin time increased by 50 percent. The authors concluded that these changes were compatible with a moderate consumption coagulopathy related to the development of pulmonary hypertension. There was no evidence, however, of platelet accumulation in the lungs, and lung biopsies showed no evidence of thrombosis.

Bärtsch and his associates studied coagulation factors in 66 climbers at 14,810 feet (4,557 m). Twenty-five were clinically well, 24 had mild acute mountain sickness (AMS), 13 had severe AMS, and 4 had high altitude pulmonary edema.[44] Coagulation times, euglobulin lysis time, and fibrin fragment E were normal in all groups without significant changes; however, fibrinopeptide A (FPA), a molecular marker of in vivo fibrin formation, was elevated in patients with pulmonary edema to 4.2 ng/ml ± 2.7 (p<0.0001) compared with other groups that had mean values between 1.6 ± 0.4 and 1.8 ± 0.7 ng/ml.

Coates studied seven subjects exposed to 12,470 feet (3,800 m) for 24 hours and found no evidence of platelet sequestration in the lungs.[45] Gray, in an earlier study, observed a slight decrease in platelet counts in subjects exposed to high altitude.[46] Other studies of coagulation factors in human subjects exposed to high altitude for variable periods of time have yielded essentially negative results.[47,48] Some studies have shown changes that might suggest intravascular thromboses, but results are not consistent and are hardly convincing.[47,48,49]

In 27 patients with high altitude pulmonary edema (HAPE) studied in Japan by Kobayashi and his associates, platelet counts were decreased and prothrombin time was slightly prolonged upon admission to hospital with a return toward normal values upon recovery.[50] Bärtsch and his associates examined blood coagulation factors during altitude exposure to 14,764 feet (4,500 m) and in patients with HAPE. Ascent to high altitude does not result in activation of coagulation factors in normal subjects nor in subjects who were susceptible to HAPE. In the majority of cases of HAPE there was evidence of in vivo fibrin generation which subsides rapidly with oxygen treatment at low altitude. It was concluded that these changes in coagulation factors were a consequence of clinical HAPE and not a causative factor.[51] One may conclude from these studies that exposure of normal subjects to high altitude is not accompanied by any consistent abnormality in blood factors that might suggest an increased tendency to intravascular thrombosis. It may be more informative to study patients who have acute altitude illness syndromes.

In permanent residents of high altitude, despite the presence of a high hematocrit, an increased tendency to intravascular thrombosis does not seem to be present. This is in accord with the medical experience of several hospitals in the Peruvian Andes, where postoperative pulmonary embolism is rare.[52] A possible mechanism is a relative deficiency of plasma coagulation properties, since the plasma constitutes a smaller percentage of the total blood volume.

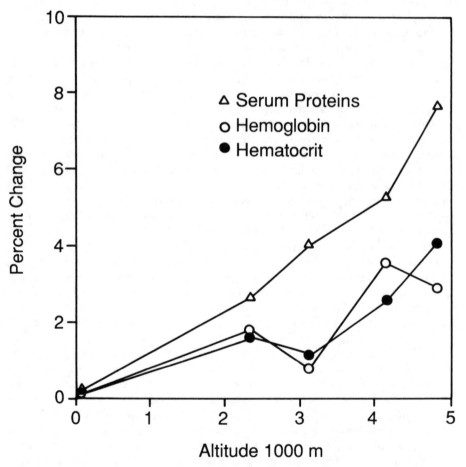

Figure 5.8. Increase in mean levels of serum proteins, hematocrit, and hemoglobin (HB) observed within the first three hours after arrival at the altitudes of 7,840 feet (2,390 m), 10,300 feet (3,140 m), 13,660 feet (4,165 m), and 15,860 feet (4,835 m). These changes are compatible with a decrease in plasma volume roughly related to the altitude attained. From Hurtado, ref. 2.

Part II: Plasma Volume

SUMMARY

Ascent to high altitude results in a prompt decrease in plasma volume. The decrease in plasma volume is substantial and results in a 10 to 15 percent decrease in total blood volume. There is also an associated increase in serum proteins, hemoglobin, and hematocrit. Changes in hemoglobin and hematocrit provide a simple method of estimating acute changes in plasma volume. The decrease in plasma volume may persist at high altitude for up to 60 days. Blood volume is high in afternoon hours and is moderately increased following prolonged exercise. The decrease in plasma volume at high altitude offers little adaptive advantage in terms of an increased hematocrit, but it may impair exercise capacity and cause orthostatic hypotension, and it may also exacerbate hypotension resulting from volume depleting diuretics.

• • •

Grawitz in 1895 first observed that altitude exposure results in a decrease in plasma volume.[53] Since then, many other workers have confirmed and extended his observations.[54,55,56] Plasma volume decreases rapidly, and there is a corresponding increase in hematocrit, hemoglobin, and serum proteins (Fig. 5.8). The mean decrease in plasma volume amounts to 20 to 30 percent, or the equivalent of between 500 and 600 ml, with marked individual variations. About half the decrease occurs within the first 24 hours, but the decrease continues over a period of about 30 days and remains at the lower level for several months (Fig. 5.9). The decrease appears to be more prominent in men than in women, as indicated by the increase in hematocrit (Fig. 5.10).[57,58] On expeditionary climbs the decrease in plasma volume reaches a maximum at eighteen weeks, after which there is a modest increase, prob-

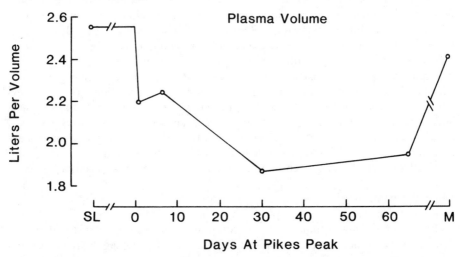

Figure 5.9. Effect of altitude exposure on the plasma volume of eight young women brought from sea level to Pikes Peak at 14,100 feet (4,260 m) as reported by Hannon et al., ref. 57. Values on the ordinate are expressed in liters. SL on the abscissa refers to low altitude measurements made in Missouri.

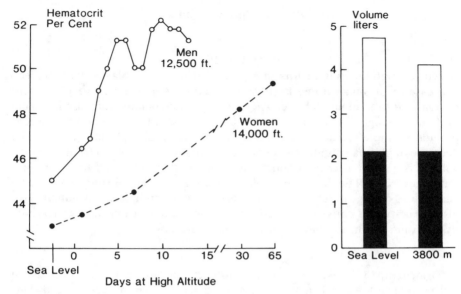

Figure 5.10. Increase in hematocrit following ascent to high altitude. The increase is greater in the four men than in the eight women. As shown in the right-hand panel the increase in hematocrit from 45 to 52 percent represents a 25 percent decrease in plasma volume. From Grover et al, ref. 58.

ably as a result of continuous heavy physical activity.[56] The decrease in plasma volume upon ascent to high altitude is slower in older men but at five to six days the magnitude of the decrease is the same as in younger men.[59]

The stimulus is hypoxia. Acute hypoxia will result in similar changes occurring within a few minutes (Fig. 5.11). Decreases in plasma volume have also been reported in rabbits, rats, and other animals brought to high altitude.[4] Earlier studies of soldiers on Pikes Peak, 14,110 feet (4,300 m), indicated that intracellular fluid volumes were increased while total body water was unchanged or even slightly elevated. Extracellular fluid was not changed.[54] More recent studies by Hoyt and his associates indicated that a ten-day exposure in a hypobaric chamber to an equivalent simulated altitude resulted in a significant decrease in total body water, intracellular water, and plasma volume, but without any significant change in extracellular fluid.[60] Since extracellular fluid did not change, the decrease in plasma volume cannot be due to a decrease in fluid intake or dehydration but rather must have been the result of a fluid shift from the vascular compartment. This hypothesis does not exclude the effect of excessive fluid loss, blunted thirst, and inadequate fluid intake at high altitude, which may result in a decrease in a total body water, extracellular fluid, hemoconcentration, and a further decrease in plasma volume.

Diurnal Variation

A slight diurnal variation in plasma volume has been reported at high altitude with a lower plasma volume in the morning upon awakening, as estimated by a hematocrit that is about 4 percent higher (Fig. 5.12).[61] This change may be due to a greater degree of arterial desaturation during sleep, since plasma volume changes occur rapidly with increasing hypoxia.[62] The nocturnal decrease in plasma volume

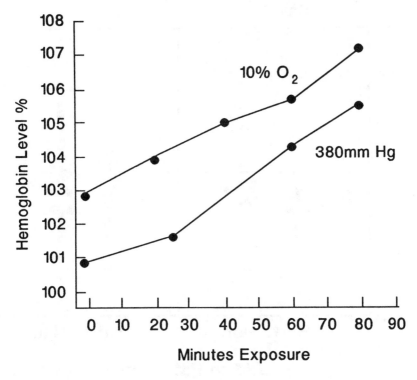

Figure 5.11. Effects of reduced atmospheric pressure and reduced oxygen tension at sea level atmospheric pressure on blood hemoglobin level of human subjects. These changes probably reflect hemoconcentration from a decrease in plasma volume. Values on the ordinate are expressed in percent as determined by the Gower-Haldane method. Drawn from data included in the report of Gregg, Lutz, and Schneider, ref. 62.

may explain the fact that symptoms of acute mountain sickness, including headache, dizziness, weakness, orthostasis, and fatigue, are frequently most severe early in the day, soon after arising.

Exercise

Supine cycle ergometer exercise of short duration in normal subjects has resulted in a rise in hematocrit of approximately 2.5 to 4.5 percent.[63] The hematocrit returns to the pre-exercise level within a few minutes. Similar changes occurred in acclimatized high altitude residents, although the magnitude of the decrease in hematocrit was slightly less (Fig. 5.13). An increase in hemoglobin was observed after exhausting treadmill exercise at Morococha, Peru, (14,900 feet/4,545 m), in normal newcomers to high altitude and high altitude natives. The mean increase in hemoglobin was 3.7 percent.[4,32] Upright treadmill exercise is usually accompanied by a smaller change in hematocrit than upright or supine cycle ergometer exercise.[63] These changes are of little clinical importance, however, aside from showing that

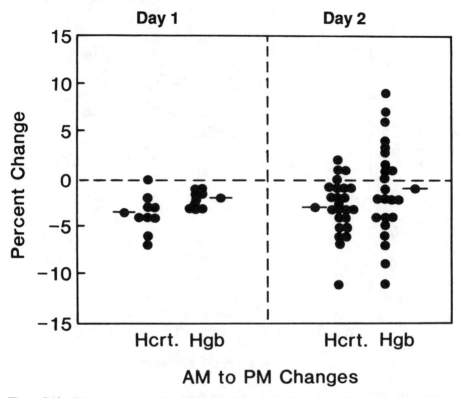

Figure 5.12. Change in hematocrit and hemoglobin from 7:00 a.m. to 5:00 p.m. in nine subjects at 12,470 feet (3,800 m). The decreases in hematocrit and hemoglobin indicate that plasma volume is lowest in the morning. From Hultgren et al, ref. 61, and unpublished observations.

when experimental studies are made of supine exercise appropriate corrections must be made for changes in hematocrit and hemoglobin in calculating arterial oxygen saturation and the hemoglobin-oxygen content. Changes in hematocrit and hemoglobin are frequently used to estimate changes in plasma volume, but they provide only an approximate estimate during acute alterations of volume. The method depends upon a constant number of circulating red cells and a constant red cell volume. Changes in plasma osmolality may change the red cell volume, since red cells act as osmometers, but only during periods of dehydration or extended exercise duration (>two hours) does the plasma osmolality change sufficiently to affect red cell size.[64] It should be noted that changes in the hematocrit are not truly reflective of changes in plasma volume if red cell mass is constant. Changes in hematocrit are always less than changes in plasma volume. For example, an increase in hematocrit of 3 percent indicates a decrease in plasma volume of 11.4 percent. Van Beaumont has developed an equation and a nomogram reflecting changes in hemoglobin, hematocrit, and plasma volume.[65] Upright exercise of longer duration, such as climbing for several hours, has resulted in a decrease in hematocrit of about 4 percent, which returned to the pre-exercise level in two to four hours. Older subjects experienced a smaller change in hematocrit. Pugh observed a small but

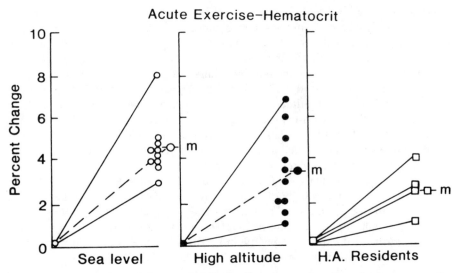

Figure 5.13. Percent change in hematocrit following five minutes of moderate (oxygen consumption doubled) supine exercise. Studies were performed in ten normal subjects at sea level and were repeated 48 hours after exposure to 12,470 feet (3,800 m) altitude. The right panel shows the effect of similar exercise in four acclimatized high altitude residents at 12,470 feet (3,800 m). From Hultgren et al, ref. 61, and unpublished observations.

significant fall in hematocrit of 2.1 percent in six subjects after a 28-mile walk.[66] Williams and his workers studied the effect of seven consecutive days of strenuous hill walking in five subjects.[67] By the fifth day there had been a fall in hematocrit to a maximum of 11 percent. The change was not due to red cell destruction. Sodium and water retention occurred. Calculations indicated that by day 5 plasma volume had increased 22 percent, interstitial fluid volume had increased 17 percent, and intracellular volume had decreased 8 percent. Facial or ankle edema was present in all subjects by the fifth day. Similar results were obtained in six subjects walking seven hours a day for five days at 10,200 feet (3,110 m). All subjects had leg edema as measured by an increase in lower leg volume.[68] The proposed mechanism was an activation of the renin-aldosterone system.[69] Another possibility that remains to be investigated is a decrease in the secretion of the atrial naturetic factor with resulting sodium and water retention. Facial edema has been described in Japanese mountain guides after arrival at high altitude.[70] Further studies of blood volume changes during high altitude exposure are clearly needed to determine whether or not women exhibit different changes than men, whether elderly subjects exhibit only slight changes, and what role atrial naturetic hormones play in blood volume changes.

Total Blood Volume

Although it is well accepted that ascent to high altitude is associated with a prompt decrease in plasma volume, less information is available regarding changes in plasma volume and red cell volume over a long period of time. This problem has been addressed by Wolfel, who studied seven normal subjects at sea level and after 21 days of residence at 14,110 feet (4,300 m).[71] Blood and plasma volumes were determined at sea level and after 18 days at high altitude. Total blood volume did not significantly change from the sea level value to 18 days. This was attributed to an increase in red cell volume. At sea level the mean plasma volume of the subjects was 3,505 ml, the red cell volume was 2,399 ml, and the hematocrit was 41.2 percent. After 18 days at altitude the plasma volume had decreased to 2,869 ml, the red cell volume had increased to 2,877 ml, and the hematocrit was 50.2 percent. Thus the total blood volume at altitude was 5,732 ml, which was similar to the sea level value of 5,896 ml. These observations suggest that the decrease in cardiac output in these subjects could not be explained by a decrease in blood volume. In this study blood volume was not measured upon arrival at altitude, but it was assumed that the usual decrease in plasma volume had occurred.

The decrease in plasma volume upon ascent to high altitude is probably due not to splenic release of red cells but rather to a movement of fluid out of the vascular bed. The resulting slight rise in hematocrit and hemoglobin offers little value in terms of acclimatization; the decrease in total blood volume, however, may result in some impairment of exercise capacity and postural hypotension, and it may be a factor in the mechanism of syncope of high altitude.

References

1. VIAULT F. On the large increase in the number of red cells in the blood of the inhabitants of the high plateaus of South America. In *High altitude physiology*, ed. J West. Stroudsberg, PA: Hutchinson Ross, 1981; 333-34.
2. HURTADO A. Studies at high altitude. Blood observations on the Indian natives of the Peruvian Andes. *J. Appl. Physiol.* 1932; 100:487-505.
3. HURTADO A, MERINO C, and DELGADO E. Influence of anoxemia on the hemopoetic activity. *Arch. Int. Med.* 1945; 75:284-322.
4. REYNAFARJE C. Hematologic changes during rest and physical activity in man at high altitude. In *The physiologic effects of high altitude*, ed. W Weihe. New York: Macmillan, 1964; 73-85.
5. REYNAFARJE C, RAMOS J, FAURA J, and VILLAVICENCIO. Humoral control of erythropetic activity in man during and after altitude exposure. *Proc. Soc. Exp. Biol. Med.* 1964; 116:649.
6. REYNAFARJE C, LOZANO R, and VALDIUIESO J. The polycythemia of high altitudes: Iron metabolism and related aspects. *Blood* 1959; 14:433-55.
7. FAURA J, RAMOS J, REYNAFARJE J, et al. Effect of altitude on erythropoiesis. *Blood* 1969; 33:668-76.
8. BERLIN N, REYNAFARJE C, and LAWRENCE J. Red cell life span in the polycythemia of high altitude. *J. Appl. Physiol.* 1954; 7:271-72.
9. PUGH L. Physiological and medical aspects of the Himalayan Scientific and Mountaineering Expedition, 1960-61. *Brit. Med. J.* 1962; 2:621-27.
10. WINSLOW R, SAMAJA M, and WEST J. Red cell function at extreme altitude on Mount Everest. *J. Appl. Physiol.* 1984; 56:109-16.
11. WEIL J, JAMIESON G, BROWN D, and GROVER R. The red cell mass-arterial oxygen relationship in normal man. *J. Clin. Invest.* 1968; 47:1627-39.
12. MONGE C. Natural acclimatization to high altitudes clinical conditions. In *Life at high altitudes*, ed. A Hurtado. Washington, D.C.: World Health Organization, 1966:47.
13. BEALL C, STROHL K, and BRITTENHAM G. Reappraisal of Andean high altitude erythrocytes from a Himalayan perspective. *Seminars in Respir. Med.* 1983; 5:195-201.
14. *Everest-The testing place*, ed. J West. New York: McGraw-Hill, 1985:85.
15. MIRRAKHIMOV M. Biological and physiological characteristics of the high altitude natives of Tien Shan and the Pamis. In *The biology of high altitude peoples*, ed. P Baker. International Biological Programme No. 14. Cambridge: Cambridge University Press, 1978; 299-315.
16. MONGE C, BONAVIA D, LEON-VELARDE F, and ARREGUI A. High altitude populations in Nepal and the Andes. In *Hypoxia: The adaptation*, ed. J Sutton, G Coates, and J Remmers. Toronto: B. C. Decker, 1990.

17. WINSLOW R, CHAPMAN K, GIBSON C, et al. Different hematologic responses to hypoxia in Sherpas and Quechuas. *J. Appl. Physiol.* 1989; 66:2561-69.
18. KRONENBERG R, and DRAGE C. Attenuation of the ventilatory and heart rate responses to hypoxia and hypercapnia with aging in normal men. *J. Clin. Invest.* 1973; 52:1812-19.
19. MONGE C, LEON-VELARDE F, and ARREGUI A. Increasing prevalence of excessive erythrocytosis with age among healthy high altitude miners. *N. Engl. J. Med.* 1989; 321;1271. Correspondence.
20. TUFTS D, HAAS J, BEARD J, and SPIELVOGEL H. Distribution of hemoglobin and functional consequences of anemia in adult males at high altitude. *Am. J. Clin. Nutr.* 1985; 42:1-11.
21. SANTOLAYA R, LAHIRI S, ALFARO R. and SCHOENE F. Respiratory adaptation in the highest inhabitants and highest Sherpa mountaineers. *Resp. Physiol.* 1989; 77:253-62.
22. KRYGER M, MCCULLOUGH R, COLLINS D, et al. Treatment of excessive polycythemia of high altitude with respiratory stimulant drugs. *Am. Rev. Resp. Dis.* 1978; 117:455-64.
23. LENFANT C, and SULLIVAN K. Adaptation to high altitude. *N. Engl. J. Med.* 1971; 284:1298-1308.
24. BANCHERO H, SIME F, PENALOZA D, et al. Pulmonary pressure, cardiac output, and arterial oxygen saturation during exercise at high altitude and at sea level. *Circulation* 1966; 33:249-62.
25. VARAT M, ADOLPH R, and FOWLER N. Cardiovascular effect of anemia. *Am. Heart J.* 1972; 83:415-26.
26. WILSON R. Anemia at high altitude. *Alaska Med.* 1977; 19:49-52.
27. WHITTENBURY J, and MONGE C. High altitude, hematocrit, and age. *Nature* 1972; 238:278-79.
28. COLLIER C, and CHIODI H. Age and high altitude polycythemia. *J. Clin. Res.* 1981; 29:99A.
29. SARNQUIST F, SCHOENE R, HACKETT P, and TOWNES B. Hemodilution of polycythemic mountaineers: Effects on exercise and mental function. *Aviat. Space Environ. Med.* 1986; 57:313-17.
30. WINSLOW R, MONGE C, BROWN H, et al. The effect of hemodilution on oxygen transport in high altitude polycythemia. *J. Appl. Physiol.* 1985; 59:1495- 1502.
31. HURTADO A. Some physiologic and clinical aspects of life at high altitude. In *Aging of the lung*, 10th Hahneman Symposium, ed. L Cander and J Mayer. New York: Grune and Stratton, 1965.
32. HURTADO A, et al. *Mechanisms of natural acclimatization 56-1.* Air University School of Aviation Medicine, USAF, Randolph AFB, Texas 1956.
33. SIRI W, VAN DYKE D, WINCHELL H, et al. Early erythropoietin, blood, and physiologic responses to severe hypoxia in man. *J. Appl. Physiol.* 1966; 21:73-80.
34. REYNAFARJE C, LOZENO R, and VALDIVIA J. The polycythemia of high altitudes: Iron metabolism and related aspects. *Blood* 1959; 14:433-55.
35. REYNAFARJE C, and RAMOS J. The influence of altitude changes on the intestinal iron absorption. *J. Lab. and Clin. Med.* 1961; 57:848-55.
36. STAINES M, JAMES T and ROSENBERG C. Lymphocyte increase and altitude. *Arch. Int. Med.* 1914; 14:376-82.
37. HEBBEL R, EATON J, KRONENBERG R, et al. Adaptation to altitude in subjects with a high hemoglobin oxygen affinity. *J. Clin. Invest.* 1978; 62:593-600.
38. BARTELS H, HILPERT P, and RIEGEL K. Die O2 transportfunktion des blutes während der ersten Lebensmonate von Menschen, Ziegen und Schafen. *Arch. Ges. Physiol.* 1960; 271:160-72.
39. GARVEY M, DENNIS L, and CONRAD M. The coagulopathy of hypobaric induced polycythemia and its reversal with heparin. *Clin. Res.* 1968; 370.
40. GARVEY M, DENNIS L, HILDEBRANDT P, and CONRAD M. Hypobaric erythraemia: pathology and coagulation studies. *Brit. J. Haematol.* 1969; 17:275-82.
41. MARTICORENA E. Tiempo de coagulacíon de sangria y prueba de Rumpel-Leede en la hipoxia aguda por ascensíon a les grandes altura. Thesis, Universidad Peruana "Cayetano Heredia," Lima, Peru, 1968.
42. SINGH I, and CHOHAN I. Blood coagulation changes at high altitude predisposing to pulmonary hypertension. *Brit. Heart J.* 1972; 34:611-17.
43. GENTON E, ROSS A, TAKEDA Y, and VOGEL J. Alterations in blood coagulation at high altitude. In *Advanced cardiology, Vol. 5.* New York; S Karger, 1970; 32.
44. BÄRTSCH P, WABER U, HAEBERLI A, et al. Enhanced fibrin formation in high altitude pulmonary edema. *J. Appl. Physiol.* 1987; 63:752-57.
45. COATES G, GRAY G, NAHMIAS C, POWLES A, and SUTTON P, JR. Platelet survival and sequestration in the lung at altitude. In W Brendel and R Zink, eds., *High altitude physiology and medicine.* New York: Springer Verlag, 1982: 179-82.
46. GRAY G, et al. Effect of altitude exposure on platelets. *J. Appl. Physiol.* 1975; 39:648-51.

47. MAHER J, LEVINE P, and CYMERMAN. Human coagulation abnormalities during acute exposure to hypoxia. *J. Appl. Physiol.* 1976; 41:702-7.
48. ANDREW M, BRODOVICH O, and SUTTON J. Operation Everest II: Coagulation system during prolonged decompression to 282 Torr. *J. Appl. Physiol.* 1987; 63:1262-67.
49. HULTGREN H, LUKIS G, STONE E, and BILISOLY J. Effect of high altitude and exercise on blood coagulation factors. *Clin. Res.* 1970; 18:114. Abstract.
50. KOBAYASHI T, KOYAMA S, KUBO K, et al. Clinical features of high altitude pulmonary edema in Japan. *Chest* 1987; 92:814-21.
51. BÄRTSCH P, HAEBERLI N, NANCER A, et al. High altitude pulmonary edema: Blood coagulation. In *Hypoxia and Molecular Medicine*. J Sutton, G Coates, and C Houston, eds, Vt: Queen City Printers, 1993: 252-58.
52. MARTICORENA E. Personal communication.
53. GRAWITZ E. Ueber die Einwerkung des hohen klimas auf die Zusammensetzung des Bluts. *Klin. Wochenschr.* 1895; 34:740-44.
54. HANNON J, CHINN K, and SHIELDS J. Effects of acute high altitude exposure on body fluids. *Fed. Proc.* 1969; 28:1178-84.
55. ASMUSSEN E, and CONSOLAZIO C. The circulation in rest and work on Mount Evans (4,300 m). *Am. J. Physiol.* 1941; 12:555-63.
56. PUGH L. Blood volume and haemoglobin concentration at altitudes above 18,000 feet (5,500 m). *J. Physiol* (London) 1964; 170:344-54.
57. HANNON J, SHIELDS J, and HARRIS C. Effects of altitude acclimatization on blood composition of women. *J. Appl. Physiol.* 1969; 26:540-47.
58. GROVER R, WEIL J, and REEVES J. Cardiovascular adaptation to exercise at high altitude. In *Exercise and sport sciences reviews*, vol. 14, ed. K Pandolf. New York: Macmillan, 1966.
59. JUNG R, DILL D, HORTON R, et al. Effects of age on plasma aldosterone levels and hemoconcentration at altitude. *J. Appl. Physiol.* 1971; 31:593-97.
60. HOYT R, DURKOT M, KAMIMORI D, et al. Chronic altitude exposure (4,300 m) decreases intracellular and total body water in humans. *Proceedings, Seventh International Hypoxia Symposium, 1991.* Abstract.
61. HULTGREN H, BILISOLY J, FAILS H, et al. Plasma volume changes during acute exposure to high altitude. *Clin. Res.* 1973; 21:224. Abstract.
62. GREGG H, LUTZ B, and SCHEIDER E. The changes in the content of hemoglobin and erythrocytes of the blood in man during short exposures to low oxygen. *Am. J. Physiol.* 1919; 50:216-27.
63. SENAY L, JR., ROGERS G, and JOOSTE P. Changes in blood plasma during progressive treadmill and cycle exercise. *J. Appl. Physiol.* 1980; 49:59-65.
64. GREENLEAF J, CONVERTINO V, and MANGSETH G. Plasma volume during stress in man: Osmolality and red cell volume. *J. Appl. Physiol.* 1979; 47:1031-38.
65. VAN BEUMONT W. Evaluation of hemoconcentration from hematocrit measurements. *J. Appl. Physiol.* 1972; 32:712-13.
66. PUGH L. Blood volume changes in outdoor exercise of 8-10 hour duration. *J. Physiol.* 1969; 200:345-51.
67. WILLIAMS E, WARD M, MILLEDGE J, et al. Effect of the exercise of seven consecutive days hill-walking on fluid homeostasis. *Clin. Sci.* 1979; 56:305-16.
68. WITHEY W, MILLEDGE J, WILLIAMS B, et al. Fluid and electrolyte homeostasis during prolonged exercise at altitude. *J. Appl. Physiol.* 1983; 55:409-12.
69. MILLEDGE J, CATLEY E, WILLIAMS B, et al. The effect of prolonged exercise at altitude on the resin-aldosterone system. *J. Appl. Physiol.* 1983; 55:413-18.
70. SUMIYOSHI K, SUMIYOSHI M, OTANI N, et al. Changes in blood elements and the circulatory system in climbing. *Japanese Cir. J.* 1964; 28:661-68.
71. WOLFEL E, GROVES B, BROOKS G, et al. Oxygen transport during steady-state submaximal exercise in chronic hypoxia. *J. Appl. Physiol.* 1991; 70:1129- 36.

CHAPTER 6

The Central Nervous System

SUMMARY

The central nervous system has a high demand for oxygen and is therefore physiologically vulnerable to even modest degrees of hypoxia. Because the cerebral cortex is more vulnerable to hypoxia than the lower centers, the earliest abnormalities due to hypoxia involve higher cortical functions. An important adjustment is an increase in cerebral blood flow mediated by hypoxia upon ascent to high altitude. Hypocapnic vasoconstriction lessens the hypoxic increase in flow during altitude exposure. Many different measurable functions of the central nervous system are impaired at various altitudes. Night vision may be impaired as low as 5,000 feet (1,525 m); other visual functions, such as critical flicker fusion frequency, visual acuity, central visual acuity, visual search, and target tracking, are first impaired between 8,000 feet (2,400 m) and 14,000 feet (4,270 m). At higher altitudes, code tasks, conceptual reasoning, memory, learning rate, verbal expression, and mood changes may also be impaired. Some of these altitude-induced abnormalities may persist after descent, including visual memory, verbal expression, and finger tap-ping ability. In twelve climbers (AMREE) who spent several weeks between 18,000 feet (5,490 m) and 23,000 feet (7,010 m) only finger tapping ability remained impaired at one year. Despite numerous exposures to extreme altitudes and severe hypoxic episodes related to high altitude pulmonary edema in some expedition climbers, there is so far no evidence of permanent impairment of intellectual or other functions of the central nervous system, although further more sensitive studies may reveal some residual impairment.

• • •

The effect of hypoxia of high altitude upon the central nervous system is dependent upon multiple factors. These include: (1) the degree of hypoxia, or altitude, (2) rate of ascent, (3) duration of exposure, (4) respiratory and circulatory response to hypoxia and hypocapnia, (5) prior acclimatization, (6) abnormal conditions such as sleep apnea or pulmonary disease, and (7) individual susceptibility.

The brain uses oxygen at a rate of about 3 ml/100 gm/min. A 1500 gram brain thus requires about 45 ml/ min of oxygen, or about 20 percent of the body's resting oxygen consumption. The brain consumes primarily oxygen and glucose. Brain hypoxia results in decreased glucose utilization and aerobic metabolism with production of lactic acid instead of carbon dioxide and water. As energy stores are depleted, membrane function is impaired, with loss of intracellular potassium, calcium, and brain creatine kinase with resulting neurotransmitter failure.[1,2,3]

Cerebral Blood Flow

Isocapnic Hypoxia. Hypoxia dilates cerebral blood vessels, thus causing an increased flow of blood when the carbon dioxide tension is maintained at a constant level.[4,5] The vasodilatation may be due to a direct effect of hypoxia upon the cerebral vessels, an increase in lactate, and a decrease in pH, or to the release of adenosine, which occurs within a few seconds of the onset of hypoxia and rapidly dilates cerebral vessels.[6] The increase in flow is related to the degree of hypoxia: as long as hypoxia continues, the flow increases, and it will increase sharply when the arterial PO_2 falls below about 60 mm Hg (Fig 6.1). Hypoxia results in an increase in cerebral blood flow to all regions of the brain, with blood flow to the gray matter increasing more than blood flow to the white matter. Normally only about 50 percent of cerebral capillaries at any one time are perfused, but during severe hypoxia about 90 percent are perfused.[4]

Measurements of cerebral blood flow at high altitude by Severinghaus and his associates revealed a 24 percent increase in flow within six to twelve hours; the flow diminished to a 13 percent increase after three to five days. Oxygen breathing reduced the flow to normal values. It is estimated that if the arterial PCO_2 had not decreased, cerebral blood flow would have increased by 60 percent.[7]

Hypocapnic Hypoxia. Hypocapnia has a powerful vasoconstrictive effect upon the cerebral circulation. A reduction in arterial PCO_2 decreases blood flow in an almost linear manner, as shown in Figure 6.2. A decrease in arterial PCO_2 to about 15 mm Hg will decrease blood flow by about 40 percent.[7,8,9] With severe degrees of hypocapnia cerebral blood flow may decrease despite a hypoxic stimulus.

The role of carbon dioxide tension in hypoxia is illustrated by the experiments of Davis and his associates.[10] They studied the time, averaged frequency content of the thirteen lead EEG in occipital and frontal regions in normal subjects during controlled hypoxia. Arterial PCO_2 was controlled, and it fell at a rate related to the subject's oxygen consumption. When PCO_2 was held above the resting arterial level,

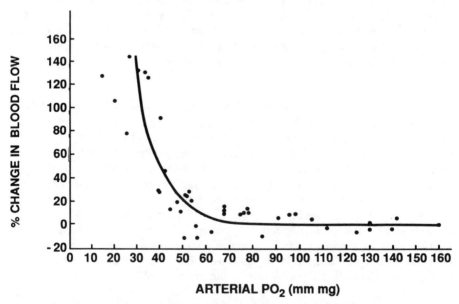

Figure 6.1. Interrelationships between blood oxygen tensions and cerebral blood flow, under normocapnic conditions. Under hypocapnic conditions such as at high altitude the increase in blood flow will be less. From Payne and Hill, ref. 19.

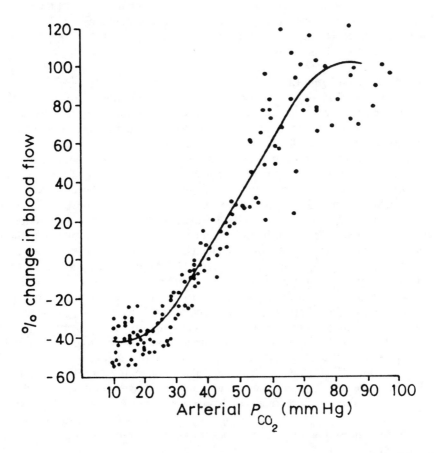

Figure 6.2. Effect of changes of arterial PCO_2 on cerebral cortical blood flow in anesthetized dogs. The zero reference line is at the normal arterial PCO_2 of 40 mm Hg. The blood pressure was normal. From Harper and Glass, ref. 9.

there were no EEG changes even when the arterial oxygen saturation fell to 60 percent. When the PCO_2 was at or below resting levels, EEG changes always occurred, indicating increased amplitude and diffuse theta activity. Amplitude changes were greater in the fronto-temporal regions than in the occipital area and occurred at oxygen saturations as high as 88 percent. There was an inverse relation between PCO_2 and the oxygen saturation necessary to invoke EEC changes. These results indicate that severe levels of arterial desaturation can occur with no detectable cerebral dysfunction if hypocapnia is prevented.

From the foregoing data it is clear that during the first few days at high altitude two opposing factors are constantly active: one is hypoxia with its effect upon cerebral function and its capacity to increase cerebral blood flow; the other is hypocapnia, which reduces cerebral blood flow with consequent effects upon cerebral function. The symptoms of acute mountain sickness may be due in part to these opposing stimuli. Some of the symptoms of acute mountain sickness may also be related to the alkalosis and thus resemble symptoms of the hyperventilation syndrome at sea level. Hypoxia, by its increase in cerebral blood flow, may result in headache and retinal hemorrhages.

Effects of Hypoxia Upon the CNS

General Effects. About 40 percent of the brain consists of neuronal cells that have a high energy requirement in order to carry out their functions of maintenance of cellular membrane integrity, electrical depolarization, and release of neurotransmitters. Acute hypoxia results initially in an impairment of electrical activity, gross congnitive dysfunction, and coma. This may be present for several hours, and there may be recovery of function upon re-oxygenation. Finally, cell membrane integrity is lost, brain oxygen consumption falls, and irreversible damage occurs. Neuronal cells, probably because of their higher oxygen consumption, are more susceptible to hypoxia than are glial or vascular cells. Further hypoxia results in a depletion of energy stores, loss of membrane integrity and consequent loss of cellular potassium, cellular edema with an influx of sodium, an increase in intracranial pressure, petechial hemorrhages, and areas of brain infarction.[11,12,13] Myers has suggested that the occurrence, degree, and distribution of hypoxic brain injury may be determined by lactic acid accumulation in brain tissue. An increase in the concentration of lactic acid may result in altered cell membrane structure and function.[3]

Visual impairment. Common types of visual impairment may begin as low as 5,000-8,000 feet (1,525-2,400 m). The impairment may involve night vision, light sensitivity, critical flicker fusion frequency, visual acuity, and central visual field vision.[14,15] Above 17,000 feet (5,185 m), visual target tracking decreases abruptly.[16]

Blindness. Because vision is one of the functions of the central nervous system that is most sensitive to impairment by hypoxia, it is not surprising that episodes of blindness have been described in high altitude climbers. Loss of vision due to central nervous system hypoxia may occur as cortical blindness or as a result of vascular spasm.

Cortical blindness results from the effects of severe hypoxia upon the visual cortex. Hackett described six cases of cortical blindness occurring at 14,000 feet (4,300 m) in sojourners.[17] All episodes were transient, varying from 20 minutes to 24 hours with intermittent periods of normal vision. Blindness was bilateral; in three cases there was some light perception. No macular hemorrhages or papilledema were seen. Pupils reacted to light. All cases responded within minutes to breathing oxygen and 5 percent carbon dioxide, and/or descent. In some instances decreases or dimming of vision occurred without complete loss of vision. Upon recovery no visual defects remained. None of the patients had an abnormal degree of hypoxia from the altitude, nor did any have high altitude pulmonary edema or severe mountain sickness. Cortical blindness also occurs in carbon monoxide poisoning; presumably as a consequence of brain hypoxia.

Houston reported instances of blindness that suggest vascular spasm as a possible etiology.[18] Such episodes may represent migraine equivalents, since the onset was sudden, brief, and often associated with scintillating scotomata, and in these cases there also was a common history of migraine attacks at sea level.

Code tasks and conceptual reasoning. Several tests of mental function are employed in studies of hypoxia. Code tasks consists of translating scrambled letters

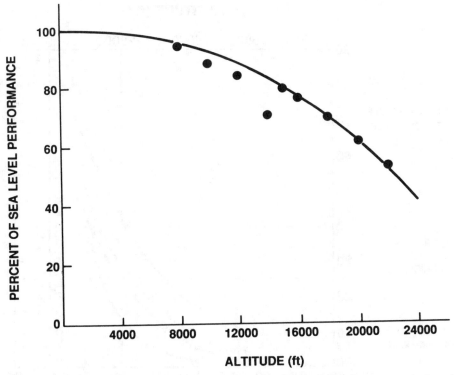

Figure 6.3. The short-term effect of rapid altitude change in a hypobaric chamber upon a paired-word association task. From McFarland, ref. 15.

to words or converting a message into a coded one, using a simple transfer code. Conceptual reasoning tests require drawing parallels or conclusions from a short statement or a parable. A slow decrease in code tasks begins at 10,000 feet (3,050 m) with a more rapid decrement above 16,000 feet (4,880 m). At 12,000 feet (3,660 m) conceptual reasoning ability declines, and the decline becomes more rapid after 14,000 feet (4,270 m).[16]

Memory. Memory tests, including a paired-word association test, show a decrement beginning at 8,000 feet (2,440 m), with a more rapid decline above 12,000 feet (3,660 m) (Fig. 6.3).[16] The degree of impairment in the performance of four mental tests in relation to oxygen saturation and altitude is shown in Figure 6.4.

Cognitive performance. Studies of cognitive performance generally employ several tasks, including the Tower task, addition, map compass, and computer interaction. The Tower task requires the ability to visualize anticipated movements of puzzle blocks, to foresee the consequences of block movements under consideration, and to relate intended actions to consequences learned previously. Such skills require analysis, logical reasoning, and the ability to relate current information to prior experiences. The mental processes involved are similar to those required for a person assembling components on a mechanical guidance system, engine carburetor, or other mechanical assembly. Addition consists of adding a series of numbers appearing on the computer screen. Map compass requires association of direction

114

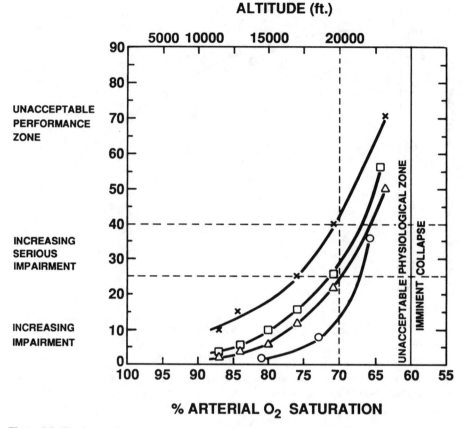

Figure 6.4. The degree of impairment in performance of four mental tests in relation to oxygen level and short-term exposure to a simulated altitude in a hypobaric chamber. Tests are: X Memory, □ Computation, △ Decision making, O Alertness. from McFarland, ref. 15.

and degree relationships and the ability to calculate distance or a new grid coordinate. Computer interaction evaluates a person's global transactions with a computer system. Information is entered into the calculator and one of six sequential operations is performed. Cognitive performance was studied in seven subjects who participated in a simulated ascent of Mount Everest in a hypobaric chamber (Operation Everest II). Performance was determined repeatedly with the addition, computer interaction, map, compass, and Tower tasks from 15,000 feet (4,500 m) to 25,000 feet (7,600 m). The results are shown in Fig. 6.5. Performance declined linearly with altitudes above 15,000 feet (4,500 m)—noticeable mainly in a slower rate of performance rather than in an increased number of errors. All four tasks deteriorated comparably at altitude. Two and a half days after descent the performances were similar to those at 25,000 feet (7,600 m). Ten mood factors were also evaluated; only four of these showed significant changes with altitude. This indicates that the selection of cognitive tasks resulted in performance measures with a greater sensitivity to altitude than those that evaluated mood.[16]

In summary, three general zones of central nervous system impairment at high altitude have been recognized:

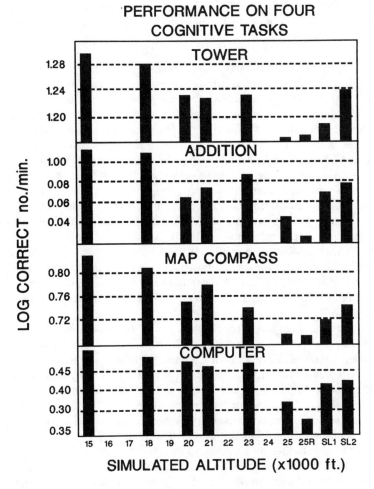

Figure 6.5. Performance on four cognitive tasks at simulated altitudes in a hypobaric chamber.

The Tower Task requires the ability to visualize anticipated movements of puzzle blocks, foresee the consequences of block movements under consideration and to relate intended actions to consequences learned previously. Such skills require analysis, logical reasoning and ability to relate current information to prior experiences. The mental processes involved are similar to those required for a person assembling components on a mechanical guidance system, engine carburetor or other mechanical assembly.

Addition consists of adding a series of numbers appearing on the computer screen.

Computer interaction evaluates a person's global transactions with a computer system. Information is entered into the calculator and one of six sequential operations is performed.

Note marked decrement at 25,000 feet (7,625 m) with a rapid return the first two days at sea level (SL2). From Kennedy et al., ref. 16.

1. 5,000-12,000 feet (1,525-3,660 m). Arterial oxygen saturation 95-85 percent. Minimal sensory impairment may be evident.
2. 12,000-16,000 feet (3,660-4,880 m). Arterial oxygen saturation 85-75 percent. Minimal mental impairment is present.

3. 16,000-22,000 feet (4,880-6,710 m). Arterial oxygen saturation less than 55 percent. Central nervous system depression, impairment of motor function, and syncope may occur.

Most of these observations have been obtained from studies in normal subjects in hypobaric chambers, usually with a rapid rate of ascent and short periods of hypoxia.[19,20] The conditions under which the central nervous system is studied should be carefully defined in terms of the degree of hypoxia, the rapidity of ascent, and the duration of exposure, including the presence and degree of acclimatization. For example, rapid exposure over a ten-minute period to a simulated altitude of 30,000 feet (9,150 m) will result in the onset of unconsciousness in 90-100 seconds.[21] The gradual exposure of normal subjects to 28,000 feet (8,485 m) in a hypobaric chamber over 40 days results in only modest changes in mental function.[16]

Several studies have been made under field conditions at high altitude. Studies at 15,400 feet (4,700 m) in Chile by McFarland revealed impairment of simple and complex psychological functions in normal subjects brought to that altitude by train or car. Tests included arithmetical tests, writing ability, appearance and disappearance time of after-images following exposure to bright light, memory, perseverances, auditory threshold, and understanding of words. Impairment of function was slight below 17,589 feet (5,330 m), and it was even less evident following acclimatization.[22-25]

Sharma measured psychomotor efficiency in 27 Indian troops brought to 13,200 feet (4,000 m) for periods of time up to four years.[26,27] Eye-hand coordination decreased over the first 10 months of exposure and then, within 24 months, recovered to approximately half that of the sea level value. This study may show the beneficial effect of acclimatization and its time course, although it is possible that the improvement was due in part to learning how to perform the test more efficiently.

Gill and his associates have described decreased mental efficiency in card sorting during acclimatization at an altitude of 19,000 feet (5,800 m).[28] They found that accuracy was only attained by spending more time and more effort in concentration. Similar results were obtained by Cahoon at 15,000 feet (4,600 m).[29]

During the 1981 American Medical Research Expedition to Everest psychometric tests were carried out at sea level, at 17,820 feet (5,400 m), and at 21,000 feet (6,300 m). Tests were repeated after descent and one year later. Finger tapping speed decreased significantly during the high altitude stay: the mean rapid tapping values for the right (dominant) hand were 53.7 (sea level) and at 17,820 feet (5,400 m), 50.8 at 21,000 feet (6,300 m), 48.1 in subjects returning to 21,000 feet (6,300 m) from 26,400 feet (8,000 m), and 45.4 immediately after the expedition.[29,30,31] Persistence of intellectual impairment was noted in some members of the expedition. These included learning rate, memory, and the expression of verbal material. The defects were present three days after descent to Katmandu, but not one year later. A bilateral reduction in motor speed persisted in some subjects for one year.

Recently, Townes and Hornbein and their associates reported neuropsychological and physiological studies on 41 subjects who had been subjected to altitudes of more than 17,600 feet (5,488 m) for many days.[30] Studies were made before ascent and from one to 30 days after descent. Several abnormalities were noted, including a decline in visual and verbal long-term memory and poor performance on the aphasia screening test. These impairments were not present one year later. Of interest is that a higher ventilatory response to hypoxia correlated with a reduction in verbal learning and poor long-term verbal memory after descent. The authors concluded that persons with a more vigorous response to hypoxia had more residual neuro-behavioral impairment, possibly because the decrease in cerebral blood flow resulting from their more severe hypocapnia more than offset their increase in arterial oxygen saturation.

Mental Performance at High Altitude: Practical Aspects

Many persons at high altitude must do work requiring a high level of mental acuity and concentration—such as astronomers, altitude research workers, employees in high altitude mines, construction workers, and climbers. The studies reviewed in this chapter indicate several general suggestions to maintain efficient mental performance.

Mental tasks can usually be reliably performed if a longer time is taken for the work. Work should be reviewed carefully after each task has been done to detect errors or omissions. This can best be done by working with an assistant who reviews the work as each task is completed. The use of a checklist and an assistant is helpful if the work requires a succession of several steps, such as recording a 12-lead ECG machine or operating a pressure recorder apparatus. The author once recorded 12-lead electrocardiograms in a group of school children at 15,400 feet (4,700 m) after having driven up from a lower altitude that morning. Since a limited time was available, the work had to be completed quickly, and there were several steps involved, including an explanation of the procedure, placing electrodes on proper limbs and on the precordium, and recording each lead with the proper switch activated. Working alone resulted in frequent errors. When an assistant developed a checklist and reminded me of each correct step, no errors occurred.

Frequent rest breaks as well as a shorter working day or a siesta hour will result in improved performance. Sleep deprivation owing to frequent nocturnal awakenings may play a role in diminished performance. Performance is usually most impaired on the first and second day of altitude exposure. After that there is a steady improvement in performance, and for this reason two or three days of rest and acclimatization before carrying out important tasks may be a good solution.[29]

The ability to work after ascent to high altitude has been investigated in astronomers and workers at the telescopes on Mauna Kea on the island of Hawaii, where six telescopes are located at an altitude of 13,776 feet (4,200 m). Three groups of people work on the mountain. Shift workers stay at the summit to maintain and service the telescopes. They usually spend three weeks on the summit and one week at sea level. Astronomers stay at living quarters located at Pohaku 9,020 feet (2,751 m). They work with the telescopes at night and sleep during the day at their quarters. Protocols and data evaluations are carried out at this level and no changes are made at the telescope level. Carry-around oxygen bottles and oxygen masks are available at the summit but rarely used. Anyone who feels ill is given oxygen and brought down to Pohaku and if necessary taken to sea level. For safety reasons nobody is permitted to drive down at night. Commuters live at sea level but drive trucks and buses up to the telescopes to deliver equipment and personnel. They are urged to acclimatize at Pohaku but this precaution is not always observed. Above this level the drivers are advised to use oxygen via a plastic face mask at a flow rate of two liters per minute, but this is not always followed.[32]

Eighty percent of the shift workers have some symptoms of AMS on the first day or two at the telescopes. Headache is the most disabling symptom and some workers must use oxygen and descend to Pohaku. After five days only 40 percent of the workers had symptoms. Arterial PO_2 values for these workers on the first day were 41 mm Hg (33-57 mm Hg).[33] Psychometric tests on shift workers showed some deterioration on the first day of arrival, but after five days scores on the digit-span-backward test had returned to sea level values. It was concluded that although immediate ascent to operate high technology equipment may be accompanied by slight deterioration of higher cerebral functions, adequate motivation and familiarity with the procedures to be followed can overcome such problems.[33,34] Serious mountain illness was rare. Over a two-year period, only three workers required oxygen and descent. One had pulmonary edema, one had cerebral edema, and one had severe acute mountain sickness. The number of persons at risk is not known.[33]

Few studies have been done on commercial aircraft flights. Denison has shown that at a pressure equivalent to 8,000 feet (2,440 m) subjects are slower to learn complex mental tasks. Even at an altitude of 5,000 feet (1,525 m) eight subjects were slower to learn complex tasks than a matched group breathing an enriched oxygen mixture.[34]

Psychological and Psychiatric Problems at Very High or Extreme Altitudes

In climbing expeditions at very high or extreme altitudes the following effects on mental function have been reported by Ward[35] and Houston[36]: uncontrolled emotional outbursts, depression, euphoria and mood swings, irritability and explosive behavior, delirium, fixation of ideas, and activation of underlying psychosis and hallucinations. Hallucinations at extreme altitude have been described by many climbers. A common hallucination is that of a "phantom companion", that is, the illusion that an additional person is following the climber. Visual hallucinations consisting of pulsating kite-like objects in space have been described.[37] Two survivors of a tragic climb of Aconcagua, 23,080 feet (7,039 m) reported that on reaching the summit they saw highway equipment, dead mules, skiers, and trees, and heard voices of an Argentine mountain patrol that was never, in fact, near the summit.[38] Houston reported hallucinations experienced by a physician at 14,000 feet (4,270 m). The physician heard voices talking to him and saw people walking nearby. He realized they were hallucinations and descended. A few years later, at a higher elevation, he had more severe hallucinations, became violent, and had to be restrained.[39] Such symptoms may represent cerebral edema and are an indication for prompt descent or oxygen therapy. Greene has reported his observations on mental and psychological changes occurring during the early British Everest expeditions.[40]

Acute Severe Hypoxia

Acute severe hypoxia may occur at very high and extreme altitudes under several circumstances. Acclimatized climbers using oxygen may experience a sudden loss of their oxygen supply. Hornbein removed his oxygen mask on the summit on Everest and while climbing noted a gradual dimming of vision, which regressed during rest.[41] It should be noted that Hornbein and Unsoeld spent the night close to the summit of Everest. This is one of the highest bivouacs in history and the longest stay at that altitude without oxygen. Sudden, heavy exertion may markedly decrease arterial oxygen saturation. Syncope may also occur at rest. In Operation Everest II, two subjects were removed from the chamber after experiencing a transient loss of consciousness while sitting or standing at 25,000 feet (7,625 m).[42] I have seen one healthy 32-year-old runner who had episodes of syncope while carrying a pack between 18,000 feet (5,490 m) and 20,000 feet (6,100 m) on Mount Everest. Upon return to sea level no abnormalities were noted after complete studies, including a treadmill test and ambulatory monitoring. In high altitude pulmonary edema a very marked degree of hypoxemia may be present, and this is probably responsible for loss of consciousness in this illness.[43]

Normal subjects abruptly exposed to extreme altitude will rapidly lose consciousness. Velasquez exposed unacclimatized subjects to a stimulated altitude of 30,000 feet (9,150 m) in a hypobaric chamber by removing their oxygen masks. The subjects lost consciousness in 90-100 seconds. Loss of consciousness was preceded by only moderate hyperventilation.[21] Luft and Noell carried out similar studies by rapid decompression (explosive decompression) in a chamber with an oxy-gen atmosphere.[44] Chamber pressure was reduced from 200 mm Hg to 68 mm Hg in 0.2 seconds, and hypoxic exposures ranged in duration from 6 to 8 seconds. The initial response of the subjects was a complete cessation of all muscular movements and a freezing of facial expression, with eye fixation. Posture was maintained during this phase, which lasted only one or two seconds. This was followed by a sudden loss of consciousness, as the body weakened and the head fell forward and there were convulsive muscular movements. After chamber pressure was returned to the previous level, the subjects recovered slowly from the postural paralysis and did not resume the former erect position until they regained consciousness. Recovery was complete within 15-20 seconds, and there were no apparent residual effects. During the final few seconds of hypoxia the electroencephalogram revealed a flat line, but brain waves returned to normal within 14 seconds of a return to the control pressure. The observation that cessation of rhythmic respiratory movements developed during the test is interesting. Subjective sensations included an initial urge to breathe, a general darkening of the visual field, and amnesia. Such severe degrees of hypoxia are, of course, rarely seen in field situations except perhaps when an oxygen mask is removed at an extreme altitude.

Episodes of hypoxia severe enough to result in unconsciousness rarely result in brain damage if the duration is short and the cerebral circulation is maintained. Glaisher and Coxwell in 1862 ascended in a balloon to an estimated altitude of 29,000 feet (8,766 m). Glaisher became unconscious, and when Coxwell tried to vent the gas from the balloon he found that his arms and hands were paralyzed, so he released the gas by pulling a cord with his teeth. The balloon landed safely and they both recovered and walked several miles to the nearest village "without inconvenience."[45] Another historic episode occurred in 1875, when the balloon Zenith ascended to above 25,000 feet (7,625 m). Tissandier was able to vent the hydrogen and the balloon descended, but his two companions were dead upon reaching the ground.[46]

A more contemporary episode of severe hypoxia with complete recovery is illustrated by the experience of Neils Bohr, the famous atomic physicist. During World War II after Denmark had been invaded by the Germans, Bohr was encouraged by the German high command to continue his research, which had relevance to the development of an atomic bomb. In September 1943, Bohr received warnings that he might be arrested by the Germans, and with the help of the Danish resistance he escaped to Sweden. The British then invited Bohr to come to England to continue his research. Bohr accepted, and after careful planning a British Mosquito reconnaissance bomber landed at the Stockholm airport, completely unarmed to comply with Swedish neutrality. The only place for the passenger was a specially prepared empty bomb bay. Bohr was put in a flying suit and instructed how to use the oxygen equipment, since the aircraft was not pressurized. To avoid the Luftwaffe the aircraft flew at a very high altitude. Bohr had difficulty fitting on his helmet and face mask, which were equipped with earphones, and during the flight he did not hear the pilot instructing him to turn on his oxygen. When they landed in Scotland, Bohr appeared lifeless and the pilot feared that he had succumbed from hypoxia, his brain and knowledge being forever lost to the world. Accounts vary as to Bohr's condition upon landing. Some state that he had probably been unconscious throughout most of the flight but regained consciousness before landing; other reports say that he was unconscious upon landing and was presumed to be dead only to recover after several days in a hospital. None of the accounts state the altitude of exposure, but it may be estimated to have been about 30,000 feet (9,150 m), and the duration of the flight above 15,000 feet (4,575 m) was about four hours. Despite this severe hypoxic injury, Bohr recovered fully and suffered no sequelae, as evidenced by the valuable role he played in atomic research for the Allies and later as director of the Danish Atomic Energy Commission for fifteen years after the war ended.[47]

Another case, also dating from World War II and described by Olson, is that of a twenty-year-old crew member on a bombing mission who became disconnected from his oxygen supply at 25,000 feet (7,625 m). Before he was discovered, he had been without oxygen for 39 minutes at 20,000-25,000 feet (6,100-7,625 m) and for 16 minutes at 12,000-20,000 feet (3,660-6,100 m). Upon landing, he was unconscious, with absent reflexes, bilateral Babinskies, and absent corneal reflexes. For the first eleven hours he was in a complete vegetative state, incontinent, with occasional spastic, uncontrolled bodily motions. He gradually improved and was discharged on the eighteenth day. Although he had no memory of the three days before the episodes or the three days after, he had no persistent neurological, intellectual, or personality defects. Hypothermia may have played a role in his survival, since his electrically heated flight suit had been disconnected, and when he was found there was ice in his nose and mouth.[48]

A similar recent episode involved a young man who stowed away in the wheel-housing of a Boeing 747 aircraft and spent over four hours at an altitude above 25,000 feet (7,625 m). He survived without residual neurological deficiencies. In this case, too, hypothermia may have provided some protection from hypoxia.[49] Gray described 22 patients who had experienced episodes of hypoxia as a result of various medical conditions, with arterial PO_2 values below 21 mm Hg. The lowest PO_2 was 7.5 mm Hg with a mixed venous PO_2 of 2.0 mm Hg. The mean duration of the hypoxic episodes was 40 minutes. During hypoxia 5 patients remained alert, 7 were somnolent, and 7 were comatose; 2 of the comatose patients had decerebrate rigidity and both recovered. Of interest is that only 12 of the 22 patients experienced a long-term recovery without residual effect.[50]

Permanent Effects of Exposure to Extreme Altitude

One recurrent speculation has been that repeated or prolonged exposure to extreme altitude might result in permanent loss of cerebral cells with a consequent decrease in intellectual capacity or persistent neurological deficits.[51] This concept has been disputed effectively by several authors, who have pointed out the high intellectual achievement of persons who have been exposed repeatedly for long periods of time above 25,000 feet (7,625 m).[36,37,38] This view is also supported by a systematic study by Clark et al. of 22 acclimatized mountaineers who spent 26.6 ± 19 nights above 17,500 feet (5,334 m) at a mean altitude of 22,203 feet (6,767 m).[52] Before ascent and after descent, the mountaineers were given a battery of tests—including the Wechsler Adult Intelligence Seals, the Holstead Reitan Battery, and ten other tests—and they were also asked to assess their own functioning. A control group of 29 subjects of a similar age was tested over the same time period but did not go to altitude. After descent, no evidence of intellectual impairment was found in any of the 22 subjects; in fact, the post-descent scores were improved, no doubt because of learning effects. Similar results were obtained in the control subjects. Cavaletti and his associates studied seven climbers who had ascended to a summit of 23,350 feet (7,075 m) without oxygen. Simple tests of memory, language fluency, and ideomotor apraxia at base camp, 17,160 feet (5,200 m), after the climb and 75 days later revealed minor deficits that were not statistically significant.[53] Twenty Polish climbers who had returned from high altitude were studied by Ryn.[54] He reported that four of the climbers had residual abnormalities, which consisted of permanent focal neurologic symptoms. Eight had abnormal EEG patterns or gave impaired performance on the Bender Gastalt test. The significance of these results can be questioned, because all the impaired climbers had been immobilized by a storm for long periods without water or food and had suffered serious damage, and these conditions might have been partly responsible rather than hypoxia alone.

Cognitive impairment after repeated exposure to extreme altitude was evaluated in eight world-class climbers who had attained summits exceeding 28,050 feet (8,500 m) without oxygen by Regard et al.[55] Control subjects were of similar age, education, sex, and experience as the climbers, but they climbed only to moderate altitudes. The studies were two to ten and a half months after exposure. Five of the climbers had mild impairments in concentration, short-term memory, and ability to shift concepts and control errors, but there were no defects in perception or other cognitive activities. The pattern of impairment suggested malfunctioning of bifronto-temporo-limbic structures. Although it was concluded that extreme altitude exposure can cause mild, persistent cognitive impairment, there was no further testing after one to two years, and therefore it is not known whether the impairment was permanent. Repeat testing might well have shown improvement.

A recent study by Capdevila and Rodriguez reported the presence of cortical atrophy detected by MRI scans in ten (38 percent) of 26 climbers exposed for long periods of time to altitudes exceeding 22,960 feet (7,000 m). Scans were recorded 26 days and 36 months after return to sea level. None of the climbers had used oxygen. Similar studies in 21 control sea level subjects revealed no abnormalities. Nearly all climbers had symptoms at altitude including headache, insomnia, anorexia and irritability. Eleven (42 percent) had ataxia. At sea level amnesia, confusion and emotional disturbances occurred in some of the climbers. These are unusual findings and should be confirmed by additional studies. It should be pointed out that all the climbers had been previously exposed to altitudes as high as 22,960 feet (7,000 m) and MRI studies were not done prior to the final ascent.[56]

In summary, there is really no compelling evidence that repeated or even prolonged exposure to extreme altitude results in permanent impairment of intellectual or mental functioning. Although impairment in some test performances may be present as long as one year after exposure, the abnormalities are mild and may be of doubtful practical significance.

I am not aware of any case reports of mountaineers who have spent prolonged periods at extreme altitudes where permanent neurological or mental defects have occurred. (An exception is one person who had a cerebrovascular accident.) On the contrary, one cannot but be impressed by the high level of intellectual functioning and productivity of the many mountaineers who have been repeatedly exposed to extreme altitudes—not simply professional climbers but attorneys, writers, professors, researchers, physicians, and corporation executives. Unfortunately, we have only anecdotal data for such climbers. Studies have been talked of but not carried out, and the question may never be resolved, since with advancing age other factors affecting mental performance may be present to confuse the issue.

References

1. LASSEN N. The brain: cerebral blood flow in hypoxia. In *Hypoxia: Man at altitude*, ed. J Sutton, N Jones and C Houston. New York: Thieme Stratton, 1982; 9-13.
2. GIBSON G. Hypoxia. In *Cerebral energy metabolism and metabolic encephalopathy*, ed. D McCandless. New York: Plenum Press, 1985.
3. MYERS R. A unitary theory of causation of anoxic and hypoxic brain pathology. *Adv. Neurol.* 1979; 26:195-217.
4. EDELMAN N, SANTIAGO T, and NEUBAUER J. Hypoxia and brain blood flow. In J West and S Lahiri, eds., *High altitude and man*. Bethesda, MD: American Physiological Society, 1984: 101-13.
5. BORGSTROM L, JOHANNSON H, and SEISJO B. The relationship between arterial PO_2 and cerebral blood flow in hypoxia. *Acta Physiol. Scand.* 1975; 93:423-32.
6. WINN G, RUBIO R, and BERNE R. The role of adenosine in the regulation of cerebral blood flow. *J. Cerebral Blood Flow and Metab.* 1981; 1:239-44. Editorial.
7. SEVERINGHAUS J, CHIODI H, EGER E, et al. Cerebral blood flow in man at high altitude: Role of cerebrospinal fluid pH in normalization of flow in chronic hypocapnia. *Circulation Res.* 1966; 19:274-82.
8. LAMBERTSEN D. Therapeutic gases: oxygen and carbon 3, dioxide and helium. In *Drill's Pharmacology in medicine*, ed. J Di Palma, New York: McGraw-Hill, 1965.
9. HARPER A, and GLASS H. Effect of alterations in the arterial carbon dioxide tension on the blood flow through the cerebral cortex at normal and low arterial blood pressures. *Neurol. Neurosurg. Psychiat.* 1965; 28:449-52.
10. DAVIS C, REBUCK A, UPTON M, et al. Quantified electroencephalographic changes during controlled hypoxia. *Clin. Res.* 1900; 00:1069. Abstract.
11. HORNBEIN T. Hypoxia and the brain. In *The Lung Scientific Foundations*, ed. R Crystal, J West, et al. New York: Raven Press, 1991:1535-41.
12. BRIERLEY J. In *Greenfield's neuropathology*, ed. W Blackwood and J Corsellis. London: Edward Arnold, 1976:43-85.
13. GIBSON G, PULSINELLI W, BLASS J, and DUFFY T. Brain dysfunction in mild to moderate hypoxia. *Am. J. Med.* 1981; 70:1247-54.
14. McFARLAND R, and EVANS J. Alterations in dark adaptation under reduced oxygen tensions. *Am. J. Physiol.* 1939; 127:37-50.
15. McFARLAND R. Review of experimental findings in sensory and mental function. In *Biomedical problems of high terrestrial elevations*, ed. A Hegnauer, Natick, Mass: U.S. Army Research Institute of Environmental Medicine. 1969:250-65.
16. KENNEDY R, DUNLAP W, BANDERET L, et al. Cognitive performance deficits in a simulated climb of Mount Everest: Operation Everest II. *Aviat. Space Environ. Med.* 1989; 60:99-104.

17. HACKETT P, HOLLINGSHEAD K, ROACH P, et al. Cortical blindness in high altitude climbers and trekkers: A report of 6 cases. In *Hypoxia and Cold*, ed. J Sutton, C Houston, and G Coates. New York: Praeger, 1987: 536. Abstract.

18. HOUSTON C. Transient visual disturbances at high altitude. In *Hypoxia and Cold*, ed. J Sutton, C Houston, and G Coates. New York: Praeger, 1987: 536. Abstract.

19. PAYNE J, HILL D., eds. Oxygen measurements. In *McDowell's blood and tissues*. London: Churchill, 1966: 205-19.

20. MALMO R, FINAN J. A comparative study of eight tests in the decompression chamber. *Am. J. Psychol.* 1944; 57:389-405.

21. VELASQUEZ T. Tolerance to acute anoxia in high altitude natives. *J. Appl. Physiol.* 1959; 14:357-62.

22. McFARLAND R. Psychophysiological studies at high altitude in the Andes and the effects of rapid ascents by aeroplane and train. *Compar. Psych.* 1937; 23:191-225.

23. McFARLAND R. Psychophysiological studies at high altitude in the Andes, II: Sensory and motor responses during acclimatization. *Compar. Psych.* 1937; 23:227-58.

24. McFARLAND R. Psychophysiological studies at high altitude in the Andes, III: Mental and psychosomatic responses during gradual adapation. *Compar. Psych.* 1938; 24:147-88.

25. McFARLAND R. Psychophysiological studies at high altitude in the Andes, IV: Sensory and circulatory responses of the Andean residents at 17,500 ft. *Compar. Psych.* 1938; 24:189-220.

26. SHARMA V, MALHOTRA M, and BASKARVAN A. Variations in psychomotor efficiency during prolonged stay at high altitude. *Ergonomics* 1975; 18:511-16.

27. SHARMA V and MALHOTRA M. Ethnic variations in psychomotor psychological performance under altitude stress. *Aviat. Space Environ. Med.* 1976; 47:248-51.

28. GILL M, POULTON E, CARPENTER A, et al. Falling efficiency at sorting cards during acclimatization at 19,000 feet. *Nature* 1964; 203:436.

29. CAHOON R. Simple decision making at high altitude. *Ergonomics* 1972; 15:157-64.

30. TOWNES B. HORNBEIN T, SCHOENE R, et al. Human cerebral function at extreme altitude. In *High altitude and man*. ed. J West and S Kahiri, Bethesda, MD: American Physiological Society, 1984:31-36.

31. HORNBEIN T, TOWNES B, SCHOENE R, et al. The cost to the central nervous system of climbing to extreme altitude. *N. Engl. J. Med.* 1989; 321:1714-19.

32. FORSTER P. *Work at high altitude: A clinical and physiological study at the United Kingdom Infrared Telescope*, Mauna Kea, Hawaii. Edinburgh Royal Observatory, Occasional Reports, 1983.

33. HEATH D, and WILLIAMS D. *High altitude medicine and pathology*. London: Butterworth's, 1989: 288-94.

34. DENISON D, LEDWITH F, and POULTON E. Complex reaction times at simulated cabin altitudes of 5,000 feet and 8,000 feet. *Aerospace Med.* 1966; 57:1010-13.

35. WARD M. *Mountain medicine*. London: Crosby, Lockwood, Staples. 1975: Chap. 28.

36. HOUSTON C. Personal communication.

37. SMYTHE F. The second assault. In *Everest*. London: Hodder and Stoughton, 1933: 164.

38. LINDLEY R. Secrets of killer mountain. *Sunday Times* (London), June 22, 1975.

39. HOUSTON C. *Going higher*. Boston: Little, Brown, 1987: 173.

40. GREEN R. Mental performance in chronic anoxia. *Brit. Med. J.* 1957; May 4: 1028-31.

41. HORNBEIN T. Everest without oxygen. In *Hypoxia, exercise, and altitude*. ed. J Sutton, C Houston, and N Jones. New York: A.R. Liss, 1983: 409-13.

42. HOUSTON C, SUTTON J, CYMERMAN A, and REEVES J. Operation Everest II: Man at extreme altitude. *J. Appl. Physiol.* 1987; 63:877-82.

43. HULTGREN H, and WILSON R. Blood gas abnormalities and optimum therapy in high altitude pulmonary edema. *Clin. Res.* 1981; 29:99A.

44. LUFT U, and NOELL W. The manfestations of sudden brief anoxia in man. *J. Appl. Physiol.* 1956; 8:444-54.

45. GLAISHER J, FLAMMARION C, DEFONVIELLE E, and TISSANDIER G. Ascents from Wolverhampton. In J. Glaisher, ed., *Travels in the air*. Philadelphia: Lippincott, 1871.

46. TISSANDIER G, Le voyage à grande hauteur du ballon, "le Zenith", *Nature* (Paris) 1875; 3:337-44.

47. MOORE R. *Niels Bohr: The man, his science, and the world they changed*. New York: Knopf, 1966: 308-9.

48. WARD R, and OLSON O. Report of a case of severe anoxia with recovery. *J. Aviat. Med.* 1943; 14:360-65.

49. PAJARES J, and MERAYO F. Unique clinical case both of hypoxia and hypothermia studied in a 18 year old aerial stowaway on a flight from Havana to Madrid. *Aerospace Med.* 1970; 41:1416.

124

50. GRAY F, and HORNER G. Survival following extreme hypoxia. *JAMA* 1970; 211:1875
51. WEST J. Do climbs to extreme altitude cause brain damage? *Lancet* 1986; 2:387-88.
52. CLARK C, HEATON R, and WIENMS A. Neurophychological functioning after prolonged high altitude exposure in mountaineering. *Aviat. Space Environ. Med.* 1983; 54:202-7.
53. CAVALETTI G, MORONI R, GARAUAGLIA P, and TREDICI G. Brain damage after high altitude climbs without oxygen. *Lancet* 1987; 1:101.
54. RYN Z. Psychopathology in alpinism. *Acta. Med. Pol.* 1971; 12:453-67.
55. REGARD M, OELZ O. BRUGGER P, and LANDIS T. Persistent cognitive impairment in climbers after repeated exposure to extreme altitude. *Neurology* 1989; 39:210-12.
56. CAPDEVILA, and RODRIGUEZ FA. Cortical atrophy and other brain magnetic resonance imaging (MRI) changes after extremely high altitude climbs without oxygen. *Int. J. Sports Med.* 1993; 14:232-34.

CHAPTER 7

Endocrine Systems

SUMMARY

Exposure to high altitude has some significant effects upon several endocrine systems, with some clinical consequences. The ACTH stimulation of the adrenal cortex results in a rise in 17 hydroxy corticosteroids and cortisol, which remain elevated for one to four weeks before returning to sea-level values. Increased activity of the sympathetic nervous system is accompanied by an increased release of norepinephrine and, epinephrine. Heart rate, blood pressure, myocardial contraction velocity, and venoconstriction all increase, and carbohydrate and lactate metabolism are affected. After several days or weeks at high altitude the enhanced sympathetic activity subsides, and there is usually a down regulation of activity which persists. Recent studies have indicated that exercise in recent arrivals at high altitude results in an increase in renin, aldosterone, ADH, and ANF. The increase is more marked in persons who subsequently develop acute mountain sickness, and the increase is frequently accompanied by sodium and water retention with systemic edema. It is possible that the diuretic effect of ANF is overcome by the combined effect of aldosterone and ADH.

Thyroid function appears to be increased during exposure to high altitude, with a peak activity in about nine to ten days and a return to pre-ascent levels by the third week. Animals subjected to severe hypoxia have demonstrated a decrease in thyroid function. Iodine deficiency is the principal cause of endemic goiter in mountainous areas of the world. As many as 30-40 percent of high altitude villagers may have visible thyroid enlargement. Thyroid extract given daily will result in a decrease in the size of goiters and may prevent cretinism if started in infancy.

• • •

There is abundant evidence that the physiological stress of hypoxia and high altitude exposure stimulates the adrenal cortex via an increase in ACTH secretion. Major effects are evident within 24 hours, and then there is a gradual restoration to normal levels of these substances after several days of exposure.[1] The secretion of 17 hydroxy corticosteroids (17-OHCS), as estimated by 24-hour urinary excretion, increases rapidly during the first few days at altitude and then returns to sea-level values in one to four weeks.[2-5] An increase in plasma cortisol also occurs.[6,7] Bärtsch and his associates reported an exercise-induced increase in ACTH and cortisol levels in subjects brought to 14,950 feet (4,559 m).[8]

At 17,000 feet (5,185 m) the level of free 17-OHCS in plasma may remain elevated for as long as five weeks; at lower altitudes a return toward sea-level values begins after three days. The effect of a prolonged stay at extreme altitude was studied by Siri.[9] In climbers staying at 17,800 feet (5,429 m) and 21,500 feet (6,558 m) urine values of 17-OHCS were similar to normal sea-level values. The response to ACTH was normal. Eosinophils in the peripheral blood decreased. Similar results were obtained by Mordes.[10] The changes in glucocorticoids are probably due to an increase in cortisol secretion and not to a transient augmentation of cortisol metabolism.[11] The process is initiated by hypoxia, but nonspecific stress may be an additional factor. The increase in steroids at high altitude may not be maximal, since ACTH administration results in a further rise in steroids.[12] In rats, hypoxia results in an increase in adrenal weight and a depletion of ascorbic acid, lipids, and cholesterol. This was observed by Gosney, who exposed rats to a simulated altitude of 18,000 feet (5,500 m) for 28 days. Adrenal weight increased, and there was also an increase in the weight of both cortex and medulla. Histologic changes in the cortex were consistent with increased adrenocortical activity.[13,14]

Sympathetic Nervous System

Ascent to high altitude is accompanied by an increase in activity of the sympathetic nervous system as evidenced by a release of epinephrine and norepinephrine. Dopamine may also be involved, although its significance during high altitude exposure is unknown.

Norepinephrine. Norepinephrine is released mainly at nerve endings in the tissues innervated by the adrenergic nervous system. Pace and his colleagues were the first to show that high altitude exposure was accompanied by an increase in urinary norepinephrine excretion during a fourteen-day sojourn at 12,500 feet (3,800 m). Epinephrine was not increased.[15] Cunningham reported similar findings in subjects at 15,000 feet (4,775 m).[16] Bärtsch reported an increase in norepinephrine levels during exercise in normal subjects exposed to 14,950 feet (4,559 m).[8] Surks and his colleagues studied five subjects before, during, and after an eight-day exposure to 14,100 feet (4,300 m); mean norepinephrine excretion rose progressively, reaching maximum values on the fifth and seventh day of exposure while mean epinephrine excretion remained unchanged (Fig. 7.1).[1] Increased plasma levels of norepinephrine are accompanied by an increase in urinary excretion of metabolites such as vanilmandelic acid. Exercise will also increase norepinephrine levels.[16]

Epinephrine. Early research did not show an increase in plasma epinephrine levels during high altitude exposure, and subsequent studies gave contradictory results,[17] but recent experiments have indicated that epinephrine output is increased at high altitude, especially when the altitude exposure is rapid or is associated with other stresses.[18] For example, Hoon found a prompt rise in urinary catecholamines in 29 subjects with acute mountain sickness at an altitude of 12,000 feet (3,660 m). In 18 subjects who remained well, there was an insignificant rise in catecholamines, and excretion levels were normal throughout the stay.[19]

Tamura studied the catecholamine response of normal subjects to two hours at a simulated altitude of 18,300 feet (6,000 m) in a hypobaric chamber.[20] In repeat exposures that were performed on three successive days, plasma epinephrine and plasma norepinephrine increased for the first two days but fell on the third day owing to pretreatment with dexamethasone. These studies indicate that adrenocortical stimulation by hypoxia accelerates epinephrine production with an increase in blood epinephrine levels. Repeat exposures attenuate the responses.

Epinephrine is released mainly from the adrenal medulla in response to the stress of hypoxia. The increased output of epinephrine occurs during the first few hours of

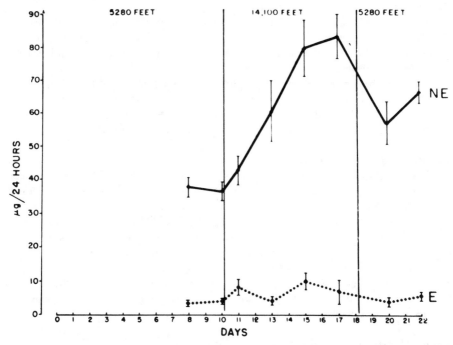

Figure 7.1. Daily urinary excretion of epinephrine (E) and norepinephrine (NE) during acute high altitude exposure. Each point represents the mean ± S.E. for five subjects. Altitude exposure consisted of an eight-day stay at 14,110 feet (4,300 m). From Surks et al., ref. 2.

exposure. Adrenal medullary hyperplasia occurs in rats subjected to a simulated high altitude.[13,21] The mechanism by which hypoxia exerts its effect appears to be by central neural hypoxia. A decrease in plasma volume has also been speculated as a cause. Other studies, however, have indicated that an increase in sympathetic activity, as manifested by systemic venoconstriction, precedes the fall in plasma volume.[22]

The circulatory effects of catecholamines during ascent to high altitude are well known. Major effects are: (1) increased heart rate, cardiac output, and myocardial contraction velocity; (2) increased systolic blood pressure, muscle blood flow, and splanchnic blood flow; and (3) decreased cutaneous blood flow. Norepinephrine is associated with lesser cardiac effects but with increases in systolic and diastolic blood pressure and systemic peripheral resistance.[23,24]

The metabolic effects of the catecholamines consist of an increase in oxygen consumption, blood sugar, and blood lactic acid and changes in carbohydrate metabolism including glycogenolysis. Metabolic effects of high altitude exposure have been recently investigated by Brooks and his associates, who concluded that sympathetic adrenergic responses appear to be important in regulating the metabolic response to high altitude.[25] Epinephrine also seems to increase muscle lactate production and the appearance rate of lactate and muscle glycogenolysis. This study reported a surprisingly close correlation between the mean lactate appearance rate and arterial epinephrine levels both at rest and during exercise, with an R value of 0.99.

Decrease in Catecholamine Effect

After several days or weeks of exposure to an altitude above 9,840 feet (3,000 m) there is evidence of a decrease in the effects of the sympathetic nervous system, especially upon the circulation. This is evident in the decrease in heart rate in relation to the plasma level of norepinephrine during exercise.[18] The effect does not appear to be a result of increased parasympathetic activity. Several investigators have shown that there is a decreased circulatory response to an infusion of isoproterenol.[18,26,27] Voelkel found that hypoxia results in a decrease in the density of cardiac ß-adrenergic receptors, which could explain these responses.[28]

The Parasympathetic System

Few studies have been performed on the response of the parasympathetic nervous system at high altitude. Immediately after arrival at high altitude a sinus bradycardia may be present in some subjects at rest and during exercise (Table 7.1).[29] Atropine in five subjects at high altitude increased the maximum heart rate, suggesting a parasympathetic effect. Atropine in normoxia did not increase the maximum heart rate.[30] Zhuang compared exercise heart rates in native Tibetans and acclimatized Han newcomers to >11,800 feet (3,600 m). The Han Chinese had higher maximum exercise heart rates. Atropine increased heart rates in the Tibetans but decreased the heart rate in the Chinese, suggesting a greater parasympathetic activity in the Tibetans.[31]

Renin-Aldosterone-Angiotensin

Renin is released from the cells of the juxtaglomerular apparatus in the kidney in response to several stimuli, including hypoxia and exercise.[32] Renin release may be stimulated by the sympathetic nervous system and circulating catecholamines. Renin acts by converting angiotensinogen to angiotensin I. Though both these substances are biologically inert, angiotensin I is converted to the physiologically potent angiotensin II by the angiotensin converting enzyme. Angiotensin II is a strong vasoconstrictor and also acts on the adrenals to release aldosterone, which in turn acts on the distal renal tubules to retain sodium. The system can be affected by several conditions pertinent to high altitude exposure.

Table 7.1
Effect of Ascent from Sea Level to 12,230 feet (3,730 m) in Two Normal Subjects Upon Resting Heart Rate and Heart Rate Response to Moderate Exercise

Location	Heart rate			
	Resting		Exercise	
	H.H.	W.S.	H.H.	W.S.
Lima	68	82	63	90
4 hours after arrival at La Oroya	63	60	65	60
3 days after arrival at La Oroya	76	84	94	80

SOURCE: Hultgren and Spickard, ref. 29.

NOTES: Relative bradycardia is evident four hours after arrival, with a higher heart rate three days later. Exercise consisted of 50 step ups to an eighteen-inch-high chair seat.

1. *Acute Hypoxia.* Acute exposure to high altitude results in a decrease in aldosterone secretion.[33,34,35] This is accompanied by a rise in the sodium/potassium ratio in saliva, an increase in total body potassium, a rise in serum potassium and a decrease in aldosterone secretion in the urine.[36,37,38] Although acute hypoxia increases plasma renin, the angiotensin converting enzyme is decreased and plasma aldosterone falls. The mechanism by which the angiotensin converting enzyme is decreased is unknown,[38] but a possible explanation may lie in the increase in central blood volume that occurs with ascent to high altitude. Peripheral venous constriction, a decrease in the cutaneous circulation, and a decrease in splanchnic and renal blood flow will increase central blood volume, including pulmonary blood volume. These effects may stimulate volume receptors and in so doing, decrease angiotensin converting enzyme and aldosterone production. Kotchen has suggested that the increase in renin at high altitude is due to an increase in sympathetic nervous system activity, since propranolol, a beta blocker, prevents the rise.[39] Bouissou and his colleagues could not support this hypothesis. They employed the beta blocker pindolol in twelve subjects at 14,268 feet (4,350 m) and studied its effect on renin and aldosterone during exercise. Pindolol suppressed the rise in renin but did not further reduce aldosterone levels. The results suggested that the suppressive effect of hypoxia upon the renin-aldosterone systems was not mediated via ß-adrenoceptors.[40]

2. *Exercise at Low and High Altitude.* Daily exercise consisting of seven hours of hill walking per day for five days at sea level results in a rise in plasma renin and a rise in aldosterone, but without any change in the angiotensin converting enzyme, which thus facilitates the rise in aldosterone. The effect of the rise in aldosterone results in sodium retention, modest water retention, expansion of the extracellular space, and an increase in plasma volume associated with a fall in hematocrit (Fig. 7.2). Experimental subjects exhibited edema manifested by an increase in leg volume after several days of exercise.[38,41]

When similar exercise is carried out at an altitude of 10,000 feet (3,050 m) the rise in plasma renin is about eight times higher than at sea level (Fig. 7.3). Despite this greater rise in renin levels, aldosterone levels do not increase more than what has been observed at sea level. The angiotensin converting enzyme is lowered at high altitude in contrast to sea level; this accounts for the blunted aldosterone response (Fig. 7.4).

3. *Long-term Altitude Exposure.* At 14,625 feet (4,500 m) resting plasma renin is initially elevated but returns to lower levels within ten days. Serum aldosterone levels decrease and then slowly return to sea-level values. The angiotensin converting enzyme also decreases and then slowly returns to sea-level values.

Exercise studies were made in seven subjects on the American Medical Research Expedition to Mount Everest who were exposed to 20,500 feet (6,300 m) for six weeks.[38] Plasma renin levels rose, as in previous exercise studies at high altitude, but aldosterone levels rose even less than at lower altitudes. Thus, several weeks at this altitude appeared to have substantially diminished the response of aldosterone to an elevation of plasma renin.

Milledge and his colleagues, who carried out these important studies, have suggested several practical implications of their results. Sodium and water retention, with varying degrees of systemic edema during prolonged exercise at sea level, is probably due to increased aldosterone secretion, since the angiotensin converting

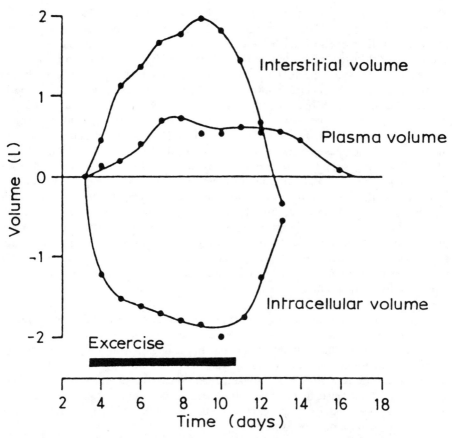

Figure 7.2. Calculated changes in body fluid volumes during several days of hill walking at sea level. Sodium and water retention occurred, along with a modest increase in plasma volume. These changes are frequently accompanied by systemic edema both at sea level and at high altitude. From Williams, ref. 36.

enzyme is not decreased. Despite substantially higher levels of plasma renin during high altitude climbing, the rise in plasma aldosterone is substantially less than at sea level, and sodium and water retention with systemic edema rare under these conditions. The decrease in converting enzyme by hypoxia is probably an important responsible factor. If the decrease is of a lesser magnitude, fluid retention may occur, with a greater tendency to develop acute mountain sickness, pulmonary edema, or cerebral edema.[36,42] High levels of angiotensin II may also be a factor in the rise in systemic blood pressure seen in some subjects during acute exposure to high altitude.[43]

Atrial Natriuretic Factor (ANF)

The role of the atrial natiuretic factor (ANF) in fluid balance and blood volume changes at high altitude remains to be determined. The factor ANF is a peptide secreted primarily by specific granules in specialized cells known as cardiocytes. The greatest concentration of these cells is in the right atrium. A rise in right atrial pressure or volume will cause the release of ANF peptides, which results in

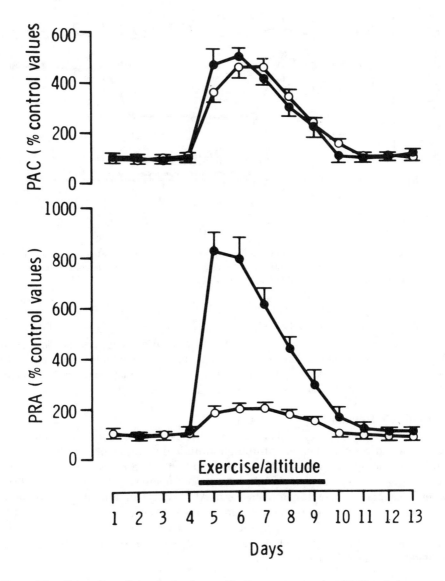

Figure 7.3. Comparison of changes in plasma aldosterone concentration (PAC) and plasma renin activity (PRA) in six normal subjects during exercise at 10,100 feet (3,100 m), compared with exercise at sea level (open circles). Mean values ± S.E. Note that despite the much greater rise in plasma renin activity at high altitude plasma aldosterone is not elevated to higher levels than at sea level. Exercise consisted of five days of hill walking for seven hours daily. From Milledge et al., ref. 37.

an increase in urine volume and a decrease in systolic and diastolic pressures. An important function of ANF is its vasorelaxing effect on the renal arteries and arterioles with a marked increase in glomerular filtration rate and filtration fraction. This results in an increased excreted fraction of filtered sodium as well as increased

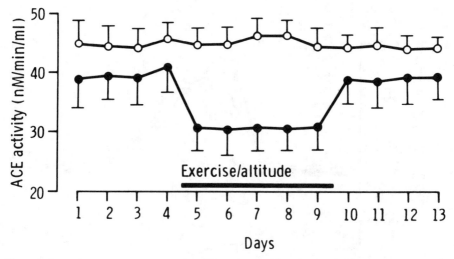

Figure 7.4. Angiotensin converting enzyme from six subjects performing daily exercise at sea level (top) and at high altitude (bottom). Note that a decrease in the enzyme occurs at high altitude but not under the same conditions at sea level. From Milledge et al., ref. 37.

potassium excretion.[44] Milledge and his associates reported that day-long hill-walking exercise is associated with an elevated level of ANF that persists for several days after exercise is discontinued but then subsides, at which time previously elevated aldosterone levels are decreased. They concluded that the unopposed effect of ANF resulted in the diuresis that followed the exercise.[45,46]

Antidiuretic Hormone

The occurrence of a diuresis or an antidiuresis as well as episodes of sodium retention and edema upon ascent to high altitude directed many investigators to study antidiuretic hormone (ADH) activity and hypoxia. Studies were made of the effects of acute hypoxia, high altitude, and exercise upon ADH levels. None of these stimuli resulted in a significant increase in ADH. Claybaugh found a decrease in ADH with mild acute hypoxia (13.9 percent inspired oxygen for 20 minutes) but not with severe hypoxia (11.1 percent oxygen).[33] Hackett found normal levels in trekkers at 14,100 feet (4,300 m) but elevated levels in two patients with high altitude pulmonary edema.[47]

Hormonal Interactions

The role that renin, aldosterone, atrial natiuretic factor, and antidiuretic hormone have in the occurrence of acute mountain sickness has been studied extensively by Bärtsch and his associates.[8] Eight subjects with a prior history of AMS were compared with nine subjects who had never experienced AMS. Ascent to 14,950 feet (4,559 m) in two days was followed by 30 minutes of exercise on a cycle ergome-ter. During the three-day altitude stay, nine subjects developed AMS while eight did not. Two of the subjects with severe AMS received medical treatment and withdrew from the study. Plasma levels of all four hormones were higher during exercise than at rest at both low and high altitudes and were significantly higher in those who developed AMS than in those who remained well. Norepinephrine, ACTH, and cortisol levels were also higher during exercise in those who developed AMS (Fig.7.5). The subjects who developed AMS had a more severe degree of hypoxemia then those who remained well. The authors speculated that sodium and fluid retention was largely due to the increase in aldosterone and antidiuretic hor-

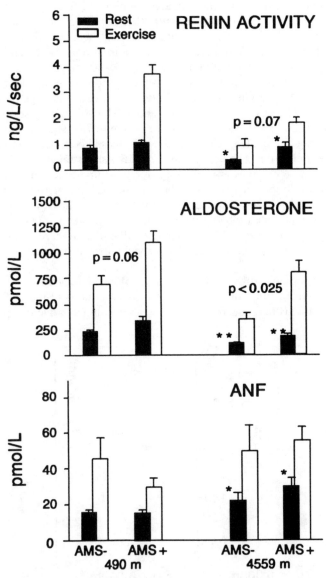

Figure 7.5. Plasma levels at rest and during exercise of renin activity, aldosterone, and atrial natriuretic factor (ANF) in eight subjects without acute mountain sickness (AMS) and nine subjects with acute mountain sickness at 14,950 feet (4,559 m). P values compare exercise-induced increase between groups. *p<0.01, **p<0.005 compared with low altitude values. Redrawn from Bärtsch et al., ref. 8.

mone and that the effect of these two hormones overcame any effect of the atrial natiuretic factor. This is an important study showing significant results in a small number of subjects, and it confirms previous results obtained by these workers.[48]

Thyroid

Thyroid function in man is increased during exposure to high altitude, with a peak rise at nine to ten days and a return to normal levels by the third week. Surks found elevated levels of thyroxine-binding globulin and free T_4 (thyroxine) during the first two weeks at 14,100 feet (4,300 m).[49,50] Dragan reported a rise in the uptake of triiodothyronine by red cells in sojourners at 6,400 feet (1,950 m).[51] A peak was reached by the tenth day, and there was a return to normal by the end of the third week. Moncloa transported ten young men to 14,100 feet (4,300 m) and studied thyroid function for fourteen days. The 24-hour thyroidal I^{131} uptake rose from 34 percent to 51 percent. The basal metabolic rate was not changed.[52] Studies by AMREE indicated a rise in serum T_3, T_4, and TSH levels during several weeks of exposure to 20,500 feet (6,300 m) as shown in Figure 7.6. The fact that T_3 concentrations were not as elevated as T_4 suggests a decreased peripheral conversion of T_4 to T_3.[53] Other field studies and one chamber study made similar observations.[54,55,56]

Although these changes are probably of little importance in terms of human performance or illness at high altitude, the mechanism of the changes is still unexplained. Several factors, including an increase in ventilation, heart rate, and sympathetic stimulation, probably increase the basal metabolic rate slightly during the first few days at altitude.[57,58] It is also possible that an increase in sympathetic stimulation due to hypoxia is part of the mechanism of the increase in thyroid function.

Studies in animals subjected to severe prolonged hypoxia have indicated a decrease in thyroid function. Connors and his associates found in hypoxic rats an elevation of TSH but a decrease in T_3 and T_4, presumably due to a primary defi-

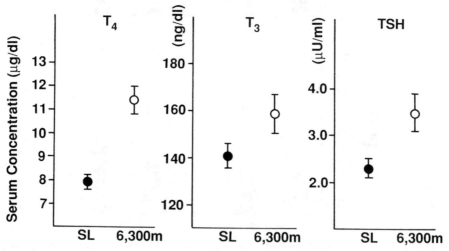

Figure 7.6. Mean fasting serum concentrations of thyroxine (T4), triiodothyronine (T3), and thyroid-stimulating hormone (TSH) at sea level (SL; n=17) and 20,660 feet (6,300 m) (n=13). Vertical lines ± SEM. From Blume, ref. 53.

ciency of thyroid secretion.[59] Martin and his workers studied the histology of the thyroid gland of hypoxic rats and concluded that the changes indicated a direct depressant effect of hypoxia upon the thyroid gland.[60] The simulated altitude was 24,570 feet (7,560 m). Gosney, on the other hand, concluded from his experimental work that hypoxia in rats resulted in a primary inhibition of the hypothalamic-pituitary axis with a decrease in TSH.[14] His studies were conducted at a simulated altitude of 18,000 feet (5,500 m). The decrease in thyroid function was not due to iodine deficiency. Other explanations to be considered are a reduced requirement for thyroxine in peripheral tissues, an altered responsiveness to TSH by the thyroid, or a direct depressant effect of hypoxia upon the thyroid.[49,51,52] The degree of hypoxia in these animal experiments was severe—18,000-24,570 feet (5,500-7,560 m)—and under these conditions there is considerable weight loss, greater than that observed in human studies. It is possible that weight loss may also play a role in the decrease in thyroid function.

In animals, the decrease in thyroid function may also have systemic effects. Fregley and Otis exposed rats to 13 percent oxygen for twelve weeks and observed a protective effect against experimentally induced renal hypertension during the altitude exposure.[61] They suggested that a depression of thyroid function was a possible mechanism of the antihypertensive effect.

Iodine deficiency is the principal cause of endemic goiter in mountainous and glaciated areas of the world owing to the low iodine content of soil. The lack of iodine results in an inadequate formation of thyroid hormone and an increased output of TSH from the pituitary.[62] Johannes studied a village at 9,800 feet (3,000 m) in the Himalayas for evidence of goiter. In 296 villagers enlargement of the thyroid gland was present in 43 percent of females and 7 percent of males. There was no one who could be clinically diagnosed as having endemic cretinism.[63] Surveys of hypothyroidism in Nepal have been reported by Worth and Shah.[64] Above 9,000 feet (2,745 m) 45 to 64 percent of the people had goiter, mostly grade I (palpable but not visible). The percentage of people with visible goiters is smaller but highly variable between villages being as high as 70 percent in some areas. Cretinism is rare. Mental retardation was not systematically evaluated but diagnosed only when apparent during a routine physical examination. In people with visible goiters mental retardation varied between 2 and 6 per 1,000 persons examined.

Ward reported a 32-percent prevalence of goiter in the general high altitude population at Dhan Kuta in Nepal.[65] Some of the goiters were huge and resulted in gross disfigurement. In this case, surgical treatment and administration of radioiodine were not feasible methods of management, but treatment with thyroid extract offered a practical method. Thyroid extract in a dose of 60 mg daily increasing to a total daily dose of 300 mg daily over a five-week period resulted in a marked decrease in the size of the goiters in six weeks. (Thyroid tablets which are less expensive than synthetic thyroid L-thyroxine are now a preferable preparation.) Recent studies of myxedematous cretinism in Zaire have shown that iodine supplements can result in a biochemically euthyroid state in younger children with cretinism, but only rarely in older children.[66] In eight rural Andean villages over 10,000 feet (3,050 m) 54 percent of the population in some villages had goiters and evidence of cretinism was present in 10 percent.[67]

136

References

1. SURKS M. Endocrine adaptations to high altitude exposure. In *Biomedical problems of high terrestrial elevations*, ed. A Hegnauer. Natick, Mass.: U.S. Army Research Institute of Environmental Medicine, 1969: 186-203.
2. SURKS M, BECKWITT H, and CHIDSEY C. Changes in plasma thyroxine concentration and metabolism, catecholamine exertion, and basal oxygen consumption in man during acute exposure to high altitude. *J. Clin. Endocrinol. and Metab.* 1967; 27:789-99.
3. HALHUBER M, and GABL F. 17-OHCS excretion and blood eosinophils at an altitude of 2,000 m. In W Weihe, ed., *The physiologic effects of high altitude* New York: MacMillan, 1964: 131-40.
4. MacKINNON P, MONK-JONES M, and FOTHERBY K. A study of various indices of adrenocortical activity during 23 days at high altitude. *J. Endocrinol.* 1963; 26:555-56.
5. MONCLOA F, DONAYRE J, SOBREVILLA L, and GUERRA-GARCIA R. Endocrine studies at high altitude: I. Adrenal cortical function in sea level natives exposed to high altitudes (4300 m) for two weeks. *J. Clin. Endocrinol. and Metab* 1965; 25:1640-42.
6. FRAYSER R, RENNIE I, GRAY G, and HOUSTON C. Hormonal and electrolyte response to exposure to 17,500 ft. *J. Appl. Physiol.* 1975; 38:636-42.
7. SUTTON J, VIOL G, GRAY G, et al. Renin, aldosterone, electrolyte, and cortisol responses to hypoxic decompression. *J. Appl. Physiol.* 1977; 43:421-24.
8. BÄRTSCH P, MAGGIORINI M, SCHOBERSBERGER W, et al. Enhanced exercise-induced rise of aldosterone and vasopressin preceding mountain sickness. *J. Appl. Physiol.* 1991; 71:136-43.
9. SIRI W, CLEVELAND A, and BLANCHE P. Adrenal gland activity in Mount Everest climbers. *Fed. Proc.* 1969; 28:1251-56.
10. MORDES J, BLUME F, BOYER S, et al. High altitude pituitary-thyroid dysfunction on Mount Everest. *N. Engl. J. Med.* 1983; 308:1135-38.
11. KLEIN K. Discussion of paper by Halhuber and Gabl. In W. Weihe, ed., *The physiologic effects of high altitude*. New York: Macmillan, 1964:136.
12. MONCLOA F, BETCHA L, VELASCO I, and GOÑEZ C. ACTH stimulation and dexamethasone inhibition in newcomers to high altitude. *Proc. Soc. Exp. Biol. and Med.* 1966; 122:1029-31.
13. GOSNEY J. Adrenal corticomedullary hyperplasia in hypobaric hypoxia. *J. Pathol.* 1985; 146:59.
14. GOSNEY J. Histopathology of the endocrine glands in hypoxia. In *Aspects of hypoxia*, ed. D. Heath. Liverpool: Liverpool University Press, 1986:132.
15. PACE N, GRISWOLD R, and GRUNBAUM B. Increase in urinary norepinephrine excretion during 14 days sojourn at 3,800 m elevation. *Fed. Proc.* 1964; 23:521. Abstract.
16. CUNNINGHAM W, BECKER E, and KREUZER F. Catecholamines in plasma and urine at high altitude. *J. Appl. Physiol.* 1965; 20:607-10.
17. MYLES W, and DUCKER A. The excretion of catecholamines in rats during acute and chronic exposure to altitude. *Can. J. Physiol. Pharmacol.* 1971; 49:721-26.
18. RICHALET J, The heart and adrenergic system in hypoxia. In *Hypoxia: The adaptations*, ed. J Sutton, J Coates, and J Remmers. Toronto: B.C. Decker, 1990:231-40.
19. HOON R, SHARMA S, BALASUBRAMANIAN Y, and CHADHA K. Urinary catecholamine excretion in induction to high altitude (3658 m) by air and road. *Am. J. Physiol.* 1977; 42:728-30.
20. TAMURA Y, MIYAMOTO N, KANDA K, et al. Catecholamine response to altitude exposure in man. In *High altitude medical science*, ed. G. Ueda, S Kusama, and N Voelkel, Matsumoto, Japan: Shinshu University, 1988:144-48.
21. KLAIN G. Acute high altitude stress and enzyme activities in the rat adrenal medulla. *Endocrinology* 1972; 91:1447-49.
22. WEIL J, BATTOCK D, GROVER R, and CHIDSEY C. Venoconstriction in man upon ascent to high altitude: Studies on potential mechanisms. *Fed. Proc.* 1969; 28:1160-64.
23. DOWNING S. Autonomic influences on cardiac function in systemic hypoxia. In *International symposium on the cardiovascular and respiratory effects of hypoxia*, ed. J Hatcher and D Jennings. New York: Hafner, 1966:208-31.
24. HEISTAD D, and ABBOUD F. Circulatory adjustments to hypoxia. Dickinson W. Richard Lecture. *Circulation* 1980; 61:463-70.
25. BROOKS G, BUTTERFIELD G, WOLFE R, et al. Decreased reliance on lactate during exercise after acclimatization to 4300 m. *J. Appl. Physiol.* 1991; 71:333-41.
26. MAHER J, DENNESTON J, et al. Cardiovascular responses to ß-adrenergic stimulation and blockade in chronic hypoxia. *Am. J. Physiol.* 1975; 228:447-81.
27. ANTEZANA A, RICHALET J, ANTEZANA G, and KACIMI R. Response to isoproterenol in high altitude residents. In *Hypoxia and Mountain Medicine*, ed. J Sutton, G Coates and C Houston. Burlington VT. Queen City Printers Inc. 1992:297. Abstract.

28. VOELKEL N, HEGSTRAND N, et al. Effects of hypoxia on density of ß-adrenergic receptors. *J. Appl. Physiol.* 1981; 50:363-66.

29. HULTGREN H, and SPICKARD W. Medical experiences in Peru. *Stanford Med. Bull.* 1960; 18:76-95.

30. HARTLEY L, VOGEL J, and CRUZ J. Reduction of maximal exercise heart rate at altitude and its reversal with atropine. *J. Appl. Physiol.* 1974; 36:362-65.

31. ZHUANG J, DROMA J, SUTTON J, et al. Sympathetic and parasympathetic influences during exercise in Tibetan and Han ("Chinese") residents of Lhasa (3658 m). In *Hypoxia and Mountain Medicine*, ed. J Sutton, G Coates and C Houston. Burlington VT. Queen City Printers Inc. 1992:297. Abstract.

32. AYRES P, HUNTER R, WILLIAMS E, and RUNDO J. Aldosterone excretion and potassium retention in subjects living at high altitude. *Nature* 1961; 191:78-80.

33. CLAYBAUGH J, HANSEN J, and WOZNIAK D. Response to antidiuretic hormone to acute exposure to mild and severe hypoxia. *J. Endocrinol.* 1978; 77:157-60.

34. KEYNES R, SMITH G, STATER H, et al. Renin and aldosterone at high altitude in man. *J. Endocrinol.* 1982; 92:131-40.

35. MAHER J, JONES L, HARTLEY L, et al. Aldosterone dynamics during graded exercise at sea level and high altitude. *J. Appl. Physiol.* 1975; 39:18-22.

36. WILLIAMS E. Electrolyte regulation during the adaptation of humans to life at high altitudes. *Proc. Royal Soc.* 1966; 165:266-80.

37. MILLEDGE J, CATLEY E, WILLIAMS W, et al. Effect of prolonged exercise at altitude on the renin-aldosterone system. *J. Appl. Physiol.* 1983; 55:413-18.

38. MILLEDGE J. Renin-aldosterone system. In J West and S Lahiri, eds., *High altitude and man.* Bethesda, Md.: American Physiological Society, 1984:47-57.

39. KOTCHEN T, HARTLEY L, RICE T, et al. Renin, norepinephrine, and epinephrine response to graded exercise. *J. Appl. Physiol.* 1971; 31:178-84.

40. BOUISSOU P, RICHALET F, GALEN M, et al. Effect of adrenoceptor blockade on renin-aldosterone and a-ANF during exercise at altitude. *J. Appl. Physiol.* 1989; 67:141-46.

41. WILLIAMS E, WARD M, MILLEDGE J, et al. Effect of the exercise of seven consecutive days of hill-walking on fluid homeostasis. *Clin. Sci.* 1979; 56:305-16.

42. SINGH I, KHANNA P, SRIVASTAVA M, et al. Acute mountain sickness. *N. Engl. J. Med.* 1969; 280:175-218.

43. KAMET S, and BANERJI B. Study of cardiopulmonary function on exposure to high altitude. *Am. Rev. Resp. Dis.* 1972; 10(C):404-13.

44. deBOLD A. Atrial naturetic factor: A hormone produced by the heart. *Science* 1985; 230:767-70.

45. MILLEDGE J, BEELEY J, McARTHUR S, and MORICE A. Atrial naturetic peptide, altitude, and acute mountain sickness. *Clin. Sci.* 1989; 77:509-14.

46. MILLEDGE J, McARTHUR S, MORICE A, et al. Atrial natriuretic peptide and exercise-induced fluid retention in man. *J. Wilderness Med* 1991; 2:94-101.

47. HACKETT P, FORSLING M, MILLEDGE J, and RENNIE D. Release of vasopressin in man at altitude. *Horm. Metab. Res.* 1978; 10:571.

48. BÄRTSCH P, SHAW M, FRANCIOLLI M, et al. Atrial natriuretic peptide in acute mountain sickness. *J. Appl. Physiol.* 1988; 65:1929-37.

49. SURKS M. Elevated PBI, free thyroxine, and plasma protein concentration in man at high altitude. *J. Appl. Physiol.* 1966; 21:1185-90.

50. SURKS M. Effect of thyrotropin on thyroidal iodine metabolism during hypoxia. *Am. J. Physiol.* 1969; 216:436-39.

51. DRAGAN I, and POP T. Researches concerning the thyroid function during effort at medium altitude. *J. Sports Med. and Physiol. Fitness* 1969; 9:162-64.

52. MONCLOA F, GUERRA-GARCIA R, SUBASTE C, et al. Endocrine studies at high altitude. I. Thyroid function in sea level natives exposed for two weeks to an altitude of 4,300 meters. *J. Clin. Endocrinol. and Metab.* 1966; 26:1237-39.

53. BLUME D. Metabolic and endocrine changes at altitude, In J West and S Lahiri, eds., *High altitude and man.* Bethesda, Md.: American Physiological Society, 1984:37-45.

54. RASTOGI G, MALHOTRA M, SRIVASTAVA M, et al. Study of the pituitary-thyroid functions at high altitude in man. *J. Clin. Endocrinol. and Metab.* 1977; 44:447-52.

55. STOCK M, CHAPMAN C, STIRLING J, and CAMPBELL I. Effects of exercise, altitude, and food on blood hormone and metabolite levels. *J. Appl. Physiol. Respir. Environ. Exercise Physiol.* 1978; 45:345-49.

56. KOTCHEN T, MOUGHEY A, HOGAN A, et al. Thyroid responses to simulated high altitude. *J. Appl. Physiol.* 1973; 34:165-68.

57. GROVER R. Basal oxygen uptake of man at high altitude. *J. Appl. Physiol.* 1963; 18:909-12.
58. HUANG S, ALEXANDER J, GROVER R, et al. Increased metabolism contributes to increased resting ventilation at high altitude. *Resp. Physiol.* 1981; 57:377-85.
59. CONNORS J, and MARTIN L. Altitude-induced changes in plasma thyroxine, 3, 5, 3_1-triiodothyronine, and thyrotropin in rats. *J. Appl. Physiol. Respirat. Environ. Exercise Physiol.* 1982; 53:313-15.
60. MARTIN L, WESTENBERGER G, and BULLARD R. Thyroidal changes in the rat during acclimatization to simulated high altitude. *Am. J. Physiol.* 1971; 221:1057-63.
61. FREGLEY M, and OTIS A. Effect of chronic exposure to hypoxia on blood pressure and thyroid function of hypertensive rats. In W Weihe, ed., *The physiologic effects of high altitude.* New York: Macmillan, 1964:141-52.
62. McCARRISON R. Observations on endemic cretinism in the Chitral and Gilgit valleys. *Lancet* 1908; 2:1275-80.
63. JOHANNES K, FLEMING W, LELE A, et al. Endemic goiter among isolated villagers in the Warman Valley, Kashmir. *Clin. Res.* 1989; 37:315A.
64. Nepal Health Survey. Worth R and Shah N. Honolulu University of Hawaii Press 1969:49-57.
65. WARD J. The medical treatment of large group III goiters with thyroid extract. *Brit. J. Surg.* 1970; 57:587-88.
66. VANDERPAS J, RIVERA-VANDERPAS T, BOURDOUX P, et al. Reversibility of severe hypothyroidism with supplementary iodine in patients with endemic cretinism. *N. Engl. J. Med* 1986; 315:791-95.
67. FIERRO-BENITEZ R, WILSON P, DeGROTT L, and RAMIREZ I. Endemic goiter and endemic cretinism in the Andean region. *N. Engl. J. Med.* 1969; 280:296-300.

CHAPTER 8

Nutrition and Metabolism

SUMMARY
Ascent to very high and extreme altitudes is accompanied by a progressive weight loss that may amount to as much as 20 percent of total body weight. Anorexia and a decreased caloric intake are the most important causes, although a decrease in water intake and possibly some degree of intestinal malabsorption may be involved. The principal source of weight loss is body fat, but muscle atrophy has also been demonstrated. Total daily caloric requirements may be less than at sea level, since physical working capacity is limited by hypoxia. During the first week of altitude exposure basal metabolism is increased but is only slightly higher than at sea level thereafter. A high carbohydrate diet offers several physiological advantages at high altitude, but individual food preferences and palatability are more important than an arbitrary pre-planned diet. There is no need for a high intake of vitamins and supplemental substances. Minimizing weight loss by eating beyond normal satiety will diminish weight loss and may improve climbing performance.

• • •

Body Weight and Composition

Rapid ascent to high altitude is accompanied by anorexia, a decrease in caloric intake, a decreased water intake with a resultant decrease in urine output, and weight loss (Fig. 8.1). Continued high altitude exposure is accompanied by progressive weight loss largely due to a decreased caloric intake.[1-10] At moderate altitudes weight loss ceases after several weeks, but at extreme altitudes weight loss may be continuous throughout the period of exposure. The decreased caloric intake is primarily related to anorexia.[9]

Body fat is the principal source of weight loss, although some muscle atrophy may also occur. Team members of the American Research Expedition to Mount Everest (AMREE) lost an average of 1.9 kg of body weight during the 250 km 23-day march to base camp at 17,800 feet (5,400 m). Nearly 75 percent of the loss was attributed to a decrease in body fat. During exposure to altitudes above 17,800 feet (5,400 m), over a 26-day period weight loss was further increased to 4.0 kg per man.[6] Similar results were reported by Harvey et al., who studied seventeen members of a Himalayan trekking party. During ascent, all subjects lost body fat but there was little change in lean body mass. During the descent march to sea level further loss of body fat occurred with a slight loss of lean tissue mass as well.[7] A weight loss of 0.45 to 1.36 kg a week at 18,810 feet (5,790 m) was experienced by members of the Silver Hut expedition. Some weight gain occurred on descent to 12,870 feet (3,960 m). Total weight losses by the end of the expedition were 6.4 to 9.0 kg.[9] Dietary intakes for three Himalayan expeditions are summarized in Table 8.1. The dietary intake of protein was low and carbohydrates consituted about 60 percent of the diet. Fluid intake did not exceed three liters per day.[8]

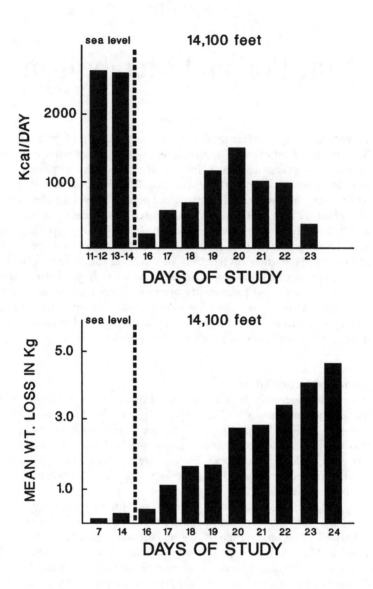

Figure 8.1. A. Mean caloric intake of ten male subjects before and during nine days at 14,100 feet (4,300 m), given a liquid diet of constant composition. **B.** Mean weight loss in kilograms for the ten subjects, who were maintained on a liquid diet at sea level and at high altitude. From Whitten and Janoski, ref. 27.

During Operation Everest II, consisting of a 40-day period of simulated slow ascent in a hypobaric chamber to 25,000 feet (7,620 m), six normal subjects lost weight amounting to an average of 7.6 kg (range 4.2- 12.0 kg), or 9 percent of

Table 8.1
Dietary and Fluid Intake from Three Himalayan Expeditions

Expedition(Percent of diet)	Protein	Fat	Carbohydrate	Total (liters)	Fluid
		K cal			
Cho Oyo 1952[a]					
5,758 m-7,818 m[b]	5	20	75	3,960	2-3
Everest 1953[a]					
5,454 m[c]	9	45	46	3,786	2-3
6,212 m-6,424 m[b]	8	43	49	3,869	2-3
6,667 m[d]	6	15	80	3,208	2-3
Everest 1981[e]					
6,300 m[b]	15	34	51[e,f]	2,224	—

SOURCE: Lickteig, ref. 8

NOTES: The 80 percent carbohydrate intake was used for the Everest assault. The expedition leader, Sir Edmund Hillary, and Tensing Norgay spent most of the night before the successful summit climb making tea at the (27,900 foot/8,454 m) camp. To each cup of tea they added milk and three to four dessert spoons of sugar. Their solid food included sardines and wheat biscuits.

[a] Cho Oyo 1952 and Everest 1953 figures adapted from Pugh.
[b] Climbing
[c] Base camp
[d] Assault on peak
[e] Everest 1981 figures adapted from Boyer and Blume.
[f] Mean daily intake during 3-day studies; highest carbohydrate consumption reached 63 percent of dietary intake.

initial body weight. The loss of body fat was less than the decrease in lean tissue mass and accounted for only 33 percent of the decrease in weight. Arm and leg circumferences were lessened, indicating a decrease in muscle mass.[10] Needle biopsies revealed a 25 percent decrease in the cross-sectional area of muscle fibers with no change in mitochondrial volume or capillary to fiber ratio. CT scans of muscles of the thighs and upper arms revealed a 13-15 percent decrease in muscle area.[11] Although the six subjects were protected from the elements of cold, wind, and low humidity and were offered a palatable, balanced diet with a wide choice of foods, they still lost weight. Caloric intake decreased by an average of 43 percent, and by 63 percent in one person. Above 23,000 feet (7,010 m) the amount of exercise performed daily decreased. There was no evidence of a preference for a high carbohydrate diet; a diminished appetite appeared to be the main reason for the low caloric intake and weight loss. Absorption studies were not done. These results differ from those obtained on expeditions where more fat loss occurred, perhaps owing to the fact that greater amounts of exercise were performed during the expeditionary studies than in the chamber, which may have resulted in a greater negative energy balance.

Additional data are available from a detailed study of seven normal subjects at sea level and after 21 days at 14,100 feet (4,304 m) on Pikes Peak. The subjects were given a carefully controlled liquid diet, and they performed regulated exercise daily. Weight loss occurred despite an apparent adequate energy intake, although the rate of weight loss was less compared with other similar studies. Energy intake to maintain body weight was 3,118 ± 300 Kcal/day. Energy expended during strenuous activity was 37 percent less than at sea level. Weight loss of 2.2 kg was primarily due to a decrease in lean body mass of about 2.8 percent (2.07 kg); only 0.2 kg of body fat was lost. With an increase in caloric intake four of seven subjects exhibited less weight loss.[12]

A prolonged stay at extreme altitude results in muscle wasting. Following an expedition on Lhotse Shar, 27,545 feet (8,398 m), seven expedition members were found to have a reduction in muscle fiber diameter (determined by biopsies of the vastus lateralis).[13] The change was small (75.8-70.5 cm) but statistically significant and it implied a calculated decrease of muscle mass by about 10 to 15 percent. Computer tomography of the thigh indicated a decrease of muscle mass of about 12 percent, which was compatible with the microscopic observations. Biochemical studies suggested a 34 percent decrease in muscle protein.

Gastrointestinal Function

Although the weight loss at high altitude is due largely to anorexia and a deficient caloric intake, several studies have suggested that a decrease in intestinal absorption may also be a causative factor. Rats transported to 14,100 feet (4,300 m) for 26 days exhibited a decrease in body weight and fat with an increase in fecal nitrogen excretion, suggesting a decrease in protein digestion and absorption.[14,15] It was also concluded that carbohydrate and fat absorption was impaired. Boyer and Blume studied fecal fat excretion in 72-hour stool samples on AMREE in three subjects at sea level and at 20,500 feet (6,300 m). The average fat intake at sea level was 161 gm/day with 79 percent absorption; at high altitude the average intake was 79 gm/day with 41 percent absorption.[6,16] The usual normal value for fecal fat is less than 6 grams per day on a 70-100 gram fat diet, which represents 94 percent net absorption. The fecal fat contents of 26 gm/day at sea level and 45 gm/day at high altitude reported by Boyer and Blume are thus higher than usual values but show a considerable standard error. The discrepancy may be due to the methods used in fat determination, or it perhaps indicates mild fat malabsorption occurring at sea level with a greater degree of malabsorption at high altitude. Xylose absorption, which is a measure of the absorbing capacity of the small intestine, was estimated by urinary excretion of oral xylose. A 24 percent decrease in absorption occurred at high altitude. The decrease was thought to be due either to pancreatic deficiency or to hypoxia of the wall of the small intestine.[6] The values of xylose excretion are all within the normal range, however, even though the data suggest a slight reduction at high altitude. If 25 grams of xylose had been administered instead of 5 grams the differences might have been more striking. In such studies serum samples should be analyzed for xylose to eliminate the possibility that a decrease in renal function was the cause of a decrease in urinary secretion.[17]

If fat malabsorption does occur at high altitude it is more likely due to a decrease in mucosal absorption than to pancreatic insufficiency, since pancreatic insufficiency must be severe—that is, a 90 percent reduction in function—before fat absorption is impaired. Mucosal function could be affected by hypoxia or by a reduction in splenic blood flow. Milledge evaluated the effect of hypoxemia upon xylose absorption in sixteen patients with varying degrees of arterial desaturation due to congenital heart disease or chronic lung disease.[18] Xylose absorption was decreased in proportion to the degree of arterial desaturation, which varied between 58 and 78 percent. In nine patients hypoxemia was relieved by oxygen administration or corrective surgery. Xylose absorption was increased in each patient by 11 percent (mean), which was statistically significant (Fig. 8.2). It was postulated that a low tissue oxygen tension impairs xylose absorption.

In the study of seven subjects on Pikes Peak, fecal losses of protein and short chain fatty acids showed no significant changes. It was concluded that no abnormalities of gastrointestinal function could be detected.[11] Rai and his associates studied troops at altitudes of 11,500 feet (3,500 m), 12,540 feet (3,800 m), and 15,400 feet (4,700 m). Fat utilization was 96 percent, 96 percent, and 97 percent on dietary intakes of 128 gms, 168 gms, and 198 gms of fat per day, respectively. Even at 15,400 feet (4,700 m) the digestibility was 98 percent on a large fat intake of 232 gms per day. No ketones were present in urine samples and no diarrhea was observed.[19] Chesler and his workers found no malabsorption of xylose in eleven subjects at 15,900 feet (4,846 m).[20] In another study, Sridharan and his associates

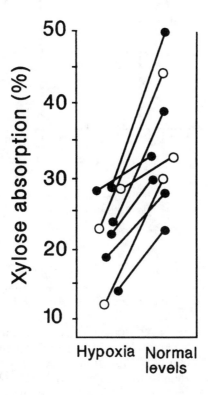

Figure 8.2. Results of xylose absorption tests before and after relief of hypoxia in patients with cyanotic heart disease. Each pair of symbols joined by a line represents one patient. Solid circles represent cyanotic heart disease; open circles represent respiratory disease. Increase in absorption significant (p = <0.001) on paired t-test. Normal values for xylose absorption by the method employed are 23-48 percent (mean 35 percent ± 6 percent). From Milledge, ref. 18.

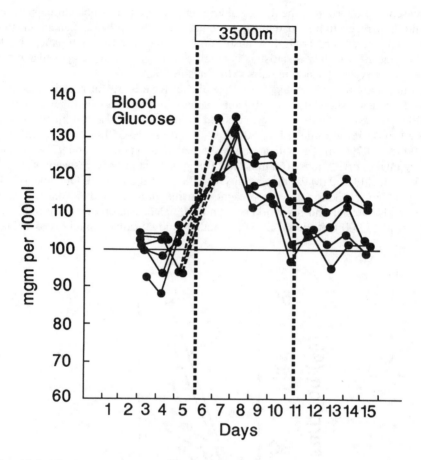

Figure 8.3. Blood glucose concentrations in five normal male subjects at sea level and after being airlifted to 11,400 feet (3,500 m). Redrawn from Williams, ref. 24.

found no change in xylose excretion in ten sea-level residents who were brought to 11,500 feet (3,500 m) for 22 days.[21] The food intake of the subjects was reduced at high altitude but there was no change in the efficiency of food utilization; thus there appears to be no evidence of malabsorption of fat up to 15,400 feet (4,700 m).

Imray and his workers investigated isotopic fat absorption in fifteen climbers at sea level and at 18,000 feet (5,500 m). No evidence for impaired fat absorption was found and pancreatic and small bowel functions were normal. The authors concluded that weight loss at extreme altitude is primarily metabolic in origin, which can be best countered by an increased caloric intake with no special avoidance of fats.[22] Kayser and his colleagues studied dietary protein digestion in six subjects who spent 21 days at 18,000 feet (5,000 m). The average decrease in body weight was 3 percent. No evidence of protein malabsorption was found.[23] In view of these studies, it seems unlikely that high altitude weight loss is due to impaired gastrointestinal function.

Miscellaneous Metabolic Functions

Fasting blood glucose levels at first increase upon ascent to high altitude, probably, in part, because of increased activity of the sympathetic nervous system. Williams observed an increase in blood glucose levels in five men who were air-lifted to 11,400 feet (3,500 m). Elevated levels were present for five to six days after ascent, but after acclimatization there was a decrease to 8 to 10 percent below sea-level control values (Fig. 8.3).[24] Another study of ten men on a controlled liquid diet at sea-level and at 14,100 feet (4,300 m) showed that normal fasting blood glucose levels were maintained and that glucose tolerance curves were normal.[3] Similar results were obtained in Operation Everest II: at simulated altitudes of 22,000 feet (6,710 m) and 25,000 feet (7,625 m) fasting blood glucose levels were not increased over sea-level control values, and glucose tolerance curves were also similar.[10] Different results were obtained on Mount Everest by Blume, who reported a flattening of the glucose tolerance curve in acclimatized subjects compared with sea-level control values. A decrease in glucose absorption was the suggested mechanism.[16] Other possibilities such as weight loss could be responsible. Amtruba reported a decrease in fasting blood sugar with severe weight loss; the observations were made in six obese subjects who experienced a 10 percent weight loss in 40 days while on a 420 calorie diet.[25] Fasting blood sugar decreased from 162 mm/M/L to 69 mg. mmol/L.

During exercise at high altitude, plasma glucose, plasma insulin, and serum growth hormone show similar responses to sea-level exercise values. Hypoglycemia during exercise at high altitude is not severe and cannot be considered a limitation to climbing performance.[26] Plasma glucose levels are lower in high altitude residents and acclimatized visitors to high altitude (Fig. 8.4).

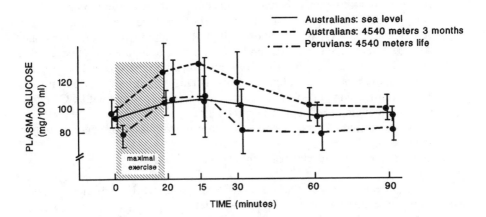

Figure 8.4. Plasma glucose response to maximum exercise (1) at sea level in sea-level dwellers, (2) at 14,900 feet (4,540 m) in sea-level dwellers after three months of acclimatization to altitude, (3) at the same altitude in high altitude dwellers. Plasma glucose levels are lower in the high altitude residents and the acclimatized visitors. From Sutton, ref. 26.

Serum free fatty acids are increased during prolonged stay at 14,000 feet (4,270 m).[25,27] Serum triglycerides are elevated only after the sixth day; serum cholesterol is not changed. Similar results were obtained in Operation Everest II: at 22,000 feet (6,710 m) and 25,000 feet (7,625 m) triglycerides and free fatty acids increased, and there was a modest decrease in total cholesterol and HDL-C.[10] The rise in free fatty acids is attributed to the increased sympathetic stimulation and increased steroid output that accompanied acute altitude exposure.

Hepatic Function

So far, there have been only a few studies of the effect of acute high altitude exposure on hepatic function. Berendsohn in 1962 evaluated hepatic function in 30 men who were born and still lived at an altitude of 14,900 feet (4,545 m) and compared the results with a control sea-level group.[28] The total bilirubin level was increased in the high altitude men, the increase being due to an elevation of the indirect rather than the direct bilirubin. These findings do not necessarily indicate hepatic dysfunction but rather may be related to the polycythemia and increased red cell production that occur at high altitude. Serum proteins were normal in both groups, but serum globulin was increased in the altitude subjects, who also exhibited an increase in inorganic phosphorus and alkaline phosphatase activity. Flocculation tests and transaminase activity were normal. Clinical observations in the Peruvian highlands suggest that hepatic function is normal in both sojourners and residents; for example, the dose of warfarin used for anticoagulation is essentially the same at 14,200 feet (4,330 m) as that used at sea level, that is, 7.5 mg/day.[29] Patients with viral hepatitis, however, appear to have a more fulminant course and a higher mortality at high altitude than at sea level. Animal studies have shown little effect of moderate to severe hypoxia upon hepatic function.

Dietary Composition

High carbohydrate diets have some advantages at high altitude, including:

1. Increased work tolerance, better mental acuity and fewer symptoms.[2]
2. A longer delay to the onset of syncope during acute, severe hypoxia.[30,31]
3. A higher arterial PO_2 as a result of the high R.Q., although this effect is small. At 19,000 feet (5,800 m) a switch from a pure fat to a pure carbohydrate diet would increase arterial PO_2 by only 8 mm, owing to the higher CO_2 production when carbohydrate is burned. This increases ventilation. High fat diets have been recommended in obstructive pulmonary disease with CO_2 retention as a method of reducing CO_2 production.
4. Increased altitude tolerance and a decrease in symptoms of acute mountain sickness.[32,33,34]
5. Greater capacity to produce anaerobic energy.

It has also been suggested that fat metabolism is relatively inefficient because more energy is required to convert fat to body fuel.[35]

Consolazio and his workers demonstrated that a high carbohydrate diet begun eight days before ascent and continued for twelve days at 14,000 feet (4,300 m) not only reduced the clinical symptoms of mountain sickness but also improved physical performance compared with control subjects who consumed a diet with a normal distribution of nutrients.[2] In this experiment a liquid diet was used, consisting of 68 percent of the K cal in carbohydrate and 20 percent in fat. Ten subjects received the high carbohydrate diet and five a normal diet. The group receiving the high carbohydrate diet had significantly fewer symptoms, and the symptoms were of shorter duration than in the subjects on the normal diet. Treadmill walking time to exhaustion was more than doubled in the high carbohydrate diet group compared with the normal diet group (9.6 minutes versus 4.6 minutes). Exercise consisted of walking on a treadmill at 3.4 mph at an 8 percent grade carrying a 20 kg pack.

Other reports of the effect of high carbohydrate diets in reducing the symptoms of acute mountain sickness have been published.[32,33] Astrand and Bergstrom reported that the maximum work time for cross-country skiers was substantially improved on a diet high in carbohydrates, as compared with a normal diet or a diet high in protein and low in carbohydrates.[36] These studies suggest that a high carbohydrate diet is preferable to standard diets during exposure to high altitude. For ascent to altitudes of 7,000-10,000 feet (2,135-3,050 m) for recreational skiing, trekking, or climbing, where meals are obtained in a restaurant, food choices for a high carbohydrate diet are indicated in Table 8.2.

Food preferences of climbers are an important factor in determining the composition of dietary intake.[37,38] Pugh reported that a high fat diet was poorly tolerated on Mount Everest.[39,40] Similar observations were made by the American Everest expeditions,[41,42] and reports from other high altitude expeditions have indicated a voluntary shift from fat and protein to carbohydrates.[6,43] The subjects in Operation Everest II experienced no increased preference for carbohydrates up to 29,000 feet (8,848 m).[10] Rai, however, observed that Indian troops at 15,400 feet (4,700 m) actually preferred a high fat diet.[19]

Freeze-dried foods, although they offer the convenience of reduced weight and bulk as well as rapid cooking time, have been reported to be tasteless and unsatisfying at high altitude.[37,38] Experiences on Mount Everest have indicated that fresh food, bought in the local market, is more palatable and less costly than specially prepared freeze-dried food.[39,40] Sample menus for more aggressive high altitude climbing are shown in Tables 8.2, 8.3, and 8.4. A publication that contains several additional menus for high altitude expeditions is *The Expedition Cookbook*, by Carolyn Gunn.

During approach marches and at base camp most expeditions report that locally obtained foods are highly desirable and of course save the weight, cost, and labor of carrying food. In Nepal along the trek to the Everest base camp a wide variety of fresh vegetables is available including potatoes, lentils, winter crops, and rice; eggs, mutton, chickens, and some fruits. An excellent review of nutrition for high altitude and mountain sports has been published by Lickteig.[8]

Caloric Requirements

Despite the availability of a variety of well selected foods including specialty items catering to individual preferences, caloric intake is reduced at high altitude. On Cho Oyu in 1972 the daily energy intake was 3,200 calories between 19,000 feet (5,800 m) and 22,000 feet (6,710 m), compared with 4,200 calories during the approach march.[40] The energy intake on the Silver Hut expedition (1960-61) at 19,000 feet (5,800 m) was estimated (from diary entries) to be between 3,000-3,200 K cal per day.[9] Above 23,000 feet (7,015 m) on Mount Everest in 1953 the caloric

Table 8.2
Traveler/Restaurant Choices, Moderate Altitude

Meal	Fluids—ad lib	Snack foods
Breakfast		
125 ml (1/2 C) orange juice	250 m (1 C) tea	1/2 banana
15 g (3/4 C) corn flakes	5 g (1 tsp) sugar	
10 g (2 tsp) sugar	500 ml (2 C) water	
250 ml (1 C) skim milk		
1 slice toast		
5 g (1 tsp) margarine		
5 g (1 tsp) jelly		
Lunch		
125 ml (1/2 C) chicken noodle soup	500 ml (2 C) lemonade	1 med apple
6 crackers	250 ml (1 C) water	
113 g (1/2 C) cottage cheese		
120 g (1/2 C) gelatin salad		
120 g (1/2 C) peach halves		
Dinner		
90 g (3 oz) broiled fish	250 ml (1 C) tea	
120 g (1/2 C) parslied potatoes	5 g (1 tsp) sugar	
90 g (1/2 C) mixed vegetables	500 ml (2 C) water	
96 g (1/2 C) sherbet		

Resume normal patterns after 36 to 48 hours.

General Hints
Minimum exercise
No alcohol; increase other fluids
2 to 3 liters of water; drink frequently
Eat foods with higher fluid content
Increase carbohydrates; complex carbohydrates preferred
Eat light meals; smaller amounts
Avoid fried foods
Easy Activity, 1,500 Calories
75% carbohydrate
12% fat
13% protein
2-1/2 liters fluid

SOURCE: Lickteig, ref. 8.

NOTES: Sample diet for altitudes of 8,000 feet to 10,000 feet (2,440 m-3,050 m), where restaurant food is available. Lighter foods should be selected and the percentage of carbohydrates and fluids increased. Light, satisfying foods include soups, crackers, gelatin, turkey, chicken, fish, eggs, canned fruits, breads, cereals, skim milk, sherbet, mashed potatoes, rice, noodles, vanilla wafers, and plain cookies. Baked or broiled foods are preferred to fried foods because frying increases the total dietary fat. Usually the nauseated traveler will shun fried or fatty foods. Fluid consumption should be increased by frequent intake of tea and other mild liquids. This diet can reduce the symptoms of acute mountain sickness during the first three or four days at altitude.

intake was calculated to be only 1,500 calories.[39,40] In a 1982 Everest expedition the average daily intake was 3,000-4,000 calories, and even on this diet the average weight loss was 16 percent. The following year a higher caloric intake was attained

Table 8.3
Sample Diet for More Aggressive,
Active Physical Activity at Higher Altitudes

Meal	Fluids—ad lib	Snack foods
Breakfast		
120 g (1/2 C) applesauce	500 ml (2 C)	8 fig cookies
1 pkg oatmeal/10 g (2 tsp) sugar	milk cocoa	
250 ml (1 C) skim milk	250 ml (1 C) tea	
1 sl bread	5 g (1 tsp) sugar	
5 g (1 tsp) margarine	500 ml (2 C) water	
5 g (1 tsp) jelly		
Lunch		
1 granola bar	500 ml (2 C) lemonade	50 g (1/2 C)
100 g (1 C) banana chips	250 ml (1 C) water	dried fruit
73 g (1/2 C) raisins	250 ml (1 C) tea	
	5 g (1 tsp) sugar	
	250 ml (1 C) eggnog	
Dinner		
250 ml (1 C) vegetable soup	375 ml (1-1/2 C) hot-	hard candies
200 g (1 C) macaroni and cheese	spiced cider mix	
1 pita bread	500 ml (2 C) hot	
125 g (1/2 C) fruit cocktail	flavored gelatin	
	500 ml (2 C) water	

Gradually increase calories as activity increases.

General Hints
Plan one-pot meals that cook in 15 minutes
3 to 5 liters of water per day; drink frequently
It takes 15 to 20 minutes to melt snow to water
It takes 10 to 15 minutes to boil water
Drastic increase of carbohydrate intake
Moderate Climbing, 3,500 Calories
4.4 kg (2 lb) dry food per person
75% carbohydrate
15% fat
10% protein
4 liters fluid
Heavy Climbing, 5,000 Calories
5 kg (2-1/4 lg) dry food per person
5 liters of fluid

SOURCE: Liekteig, ref. 8.

with a resulting weight loss of only 5 percent. For four members of the 1981 American Research Expedition to Mount Everest the caloric intake at 20,666 feet (6,300 m) was 2,224 ± 36 K cal/day, compared with 2,976 + 278 K cal/day at sea level. The average weight loss above 17,800 feet (5,400 m) was 4.0 kg or about 5.4 percent.[6] The energy expenditure of Indian soldiers between 9,000 feet (2,740 m) and 15,000 feet (4,570 m) was 4,200 K cal/day, compared with 3,200 K cal/day at sea level. The soldiers at high altitude were engaged in moderately heavy activity such as road building and ditch digging; sea-level activity was not described.[19] The mean

Table 8.4
Sample Food List for Climbing Parties Providing 3,000 Calories per day with 109 grams of Protein and 86 grams of Fat

	12 man-days actual consumption	Grams	Calories	Daily Protein	Fat	Comment
*Meats, freeze-fried	6 pkg.	19	45	246	30	12	Can be replaced
*Minute Rice	13 oz.	13	31	118	2	—	
Dried low-fat milk	12 pkg.	41	98	370	35	5	
*Dried potato flakes	12 pkg.	12	28	102	2	—	
Instant oatmeal	20 pkg.	22	52	203	7	3	
*Sugar	3 lbs.	48	113	435	—	—	
Cooking oil (e.g. Mazola)	1/2 pt.	8	19	168	—	19	Can be increased
*Oatmeal cookies	3 pkg.	42	100	450	6	15	
Bread	1 loaf	16	38	110	4	1	
Bacon bars	2 pkg.	6	14	85	4	7	
Flavorings	1 pkg.	1-1/2	4	—	—	—	
*Salted nuts	11 oz.	11	26	145	4	12	
*Dried fruit	13 oz.	13	31	103	1	—	e.g. apricot nuggets
Instant tomato juice drink	2 pkg.	4-1/2	2	—	—	—	
Onion soup	1 pkg.	1	2	—	—	—	
*Instant coffee	2 oz.	2	5	—	—		
Powdered cocoa	12 pkg.	12	28	100	5		
*Raisins	12 oz.	12	28	81	—	—	
*Cheese	1 lb.	16	38	152	9	12	
Powered fruit drink	10 pkg.	2	5	2	—	—	
Pepper, salt		2	5	—	—	—	
TOTALS Per man-day		26.7	760	3,000	109	86	

SOURCES: T Jukes, Nutrition for mountaineers. *Proceedings*, Mountain Medicine Symposium, Yosemite, 1975: 21-26.

NOTES: If a higher caloric intake is required, carbohydrates can be increased by adding more sugar, cookies, rice, potatoes, and oatmeal. Instead of freeze-dried meats, other protein sources such as dried beef and tinned meats are recommended. The above menu is an example of that used on an early Everest expedition. Present food processing has added many items not available in earlier years.

*Repackaged in polyethylene bags

caloric intake of climbers on three Himalayan expeditions was 3,410 K cal (range 2,224-3,960) (Table 8.1). The caloric intake of sixteen members of a climb on Mount Kilimanjaro, 18,200 feet (5,551 m) varied from 683 to 2,853 K cal/day with the lower intake at the higher altitudes.

The mean caloric intake of six subjects who completed a six-week simulated ascent in a hypobaric chamber (OE II) to 25,000 feet (7,625 m) decreased from 3,136 K cal/day to 1,789 K cal/day during the final week of the study, despite the availability of a diet selected to satisfy individual food preferences. The mean weight loss of the six subjects during the study was 7.56 kg.[10] Kayser and his colleagues studied dietary energy assimilation in six subjects for three weeks at 18,000 feet (5,000 m). During this period body fat decreased by 8 percent and body weight by 3 percent. Dietary gross energy intake was 3,235 ± 631 K cal/day. It was concluded that during the period of altitude exposure dietary energy assimilation was normal.[43]

The studies cited above fairly consistently show that during expeditionary climbing at altitudes between 17,000 feet (5,185 m) and 20,000 feet (6,100 m) the average daily caloric intake is about 3,000 K cal. At higher altitudes this is usually reduced to about 1,000 K cal per day.

Several theories concerning diets at high altitude have been proposed and deserve critical analysis: (1) a daily caloric intake of 5,000-6,000 calories is desirable; (2) a high caloric intake that prevents weight loss improves climbing performance and prevents burnout; (3) the stress and energy demands of high altitude climbing require multivitamins to help improve performance or as a safety factor.[41,42]

The assumption that a daily caloric intake of 5,000-6,000 calories is essential for high altitude climbing is probably erroneous; this recommendation is based on caloric requirements for sea-level endurance runners, whereas at altitudes around 18,000 feet (5,500 m) daily energy requirements are probably considerably less.[37,38] (1) Maximum oxygen consumption is decreased in proportion to the altitude. (2) During heavy exercise at high altitude climbers use a climb rate well below their maximum O_2 consumption and rest stops are frequent. Ward has estimated that at about 22,000 feet (6,710 m) the energy expended in climbing is equivalent to a walking on level ground at sea level of about 6.5 kilometers per hour.[44] (3) Total hours per day spent climbing may be few. (4) Many hours must be spent in descending, which requires much less energy, and many hours are spent resting, especially during bad weather. (5) Despite earlier contradictory reports, basal metabolic rate is probably only slightly increased at high altitude after acclimatization.[45,46] In a recent Pikes Peak study the basal metabolic rate was increased by 16 percent over sea-level values after three weeks (Fig. 8.5).[11]

Basal Metabolic Rate

Grover measured the basal metabolic rate in six normal subjects at 5,200 feet (1,586 m) and on Mount Evans, 14,150 feet (4,316 m), over a three-day period. Basal metabolic rate increased slightly (+6.7 percent) and it was speculated that this small rise could be explained by the increase in ventilation.[45] These results may be questioned, however, because the sea-level studies were not done under basal conditions whereas the altitude studies were. Gill and Pugh measured basal oxygen consumption in eight normal subjects who had been living for several months at 19,000 feet (5,800 m). The mean basal metabolic rate was increased by about 10 percent over predicted normal values. The subjects were not studied at sea level. The increase could only partly be attributed to an increase in the oxygen cost of ventilation, weight loss, a change in body composition, or cold exposure.[37,46]

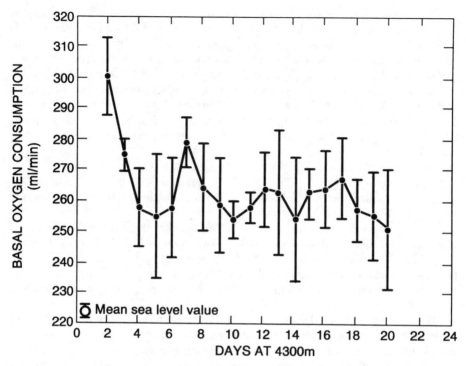

Figure 8.5. Basal oxygen consumption at sea-level and 14,104 feet (4,300 m). Values are means + SEM for seven subjects. From Butterfield, ref. 12.

Neither of the two studies considered an increase in cardiac work as an additional factor that might slightly increase oxygen consumption. For example, in the study of Gill and Pugh the mean heart rate at high altitude was 73 beats/ minute compared with 56 beats/minute at sea level. This degree of increase in heart rate alone could increase oxygen consumption by about 3-4 percent. One should also consider the increase in right ventricular work due to the presence of pulmonary hypertension.

A transient increase in basal metabolism does occur during the first few days of high altitude exposure (Fig. 8.5).[11] The increase is associated with an increase in ventilation. The effect may be largely due to beta-sympathetic activity. In a short-term study Huang and his associates showed that ascent to Pikes Peak resulted in an increase in metabolic rate of 20 percent and an increase in pulmonary ventilation of 28 percent. These two changes were almost completely blocked by beta-blockade using propranolol.[47,48]

Although shivering will increase the metabolic rate by as much as 50 percent, there is no evidence that people living and working in a cold environment have an increased caloric requirement, provided that they wear adequate clothing and are protected from wind and cold while they sleep. For example, daily caloric intake per man, per day varied from 3,400 calories to 3,800 calories at Fort Churchill, Hudson Bay, where temperatures varied from -12°F to -25°F. In the United States in temperate conditions caloric intake averaged 3,800 calories.[49]

Expedition caloric requirements are usually estimated from food consumed, which is subject to error. Few measurements have been made of daily oxygen consumption. Rogers measured the caloric cost of twelve men who spent five days in a sea-level survival situation in the subarctic winter. Daily oxygen consumption was measured by period collections of expired air in a gas bag carried on the subject's back. Light to heavy work was performed daily. Each subject was wearing 3.5 clo units* of winter clothing. The mean air temperature was -30°C. (Everest climbers usually wear about 3.0 clo units.) The energy expenditure per man on the first day averaged about 4,000 calories and then decreased to about 3,600 calories for the subsequent days. Weight loss over five days was about 5 percent of body weight.[50] At altitudes above 18,000 feet (5,490 m) the caloric requirements will probably be considerably less, hence a daily intake of 2,500-3,000 calories may be desirable.

It is clear that the effect of cold should be considered in estimating daily caloric needs, but an exact estimation is difficult owing to the lack of systematic studies. There is no convincing evidence that forced consumption of food to prevent weight loss improves climbing performance or prevents burnout. Many anecdotes relate instances of climbers who attained the summit of Everest and lost little or no weight in the process; they may, of course, have been able to eat more simply because they were more fit and acclimatized. One must consider that there is a much larger number of climbers who made successful ascents despite weight loss.

Vitamins and Food Supplements

In 1936 Dr. Walter Alvarez of the Mayo Clinic expressed concern over the excessive use of vitamins in adults and children. The situation is worse today largely as a result of drug company advertising, which suggests that vitamins are important to relieve "stress," as an insurance against deficiency or to enhance athletic ability. Sales of vitamins in the United States in 1985 were close to $3 billion, or twice the amount expended for coronary bypass surgery.[51]

Most climbing expeditions include multiple vitamins in the daily diet. The American expedition to Mount Everest, for example, used two vitamin preparations— "vitamin C and a high level water soluble therapeutic vitamin high in ascorbic acid and other water soluble ingredients." The justification for the vitamins was to prevent depletion of vitamin reserves during strenuous activity.[40] There is no evidence that, if a proper diet is consumed, vitamin supplements are necessary to improve performance, relieve stress, or prevent deficiencies. Large amounts of vitamin C have not been shown to prevent or modify upper respiratory infections or the common cold. The excessive use of vitamins A or D can cause distinct toxic manifestations. Chronic vitamin A toxicity is characterized by dryness of the skin, itching, desquamation, hair loss, weakness, fatigue, loss of appetite, headaches, and blurred vision. Symptoms of hypervitaminosis A occur most often in persons taking multiple vitamins. Excessive use of vitamin D (in excess of 50,000 IU per day) causes an elevation of serum calcium, nausea, vomiting, dehydration, and itching. Excessive amounts of nicotinic acid can cause flushing, itching, and gastric disease.

Supplemental substances such as biotin, minerals, vitamin E, vitamin K, and other substances are of no value except to the profits of pharmaceutical companies.[51,52,53] The cost of such preparations is not trivial. A typical single multivitamin preparation with several added substances will cost 15 cents a day per tablet, and if three tablets are taken daily with added vitamin C the cost could be as high as 75

---

*One clo unit is equivalent to a business suit or one-quarter-inch thickness of clothing.

cents a day; thus for a 30-man expedition of 100 days' duration the cost of vitamin supplements could range from $450 to as much as $2,250. Nevertheless, most expedition climbers use a simple multivitamin preparation above base camp to provide optimal vitamin intake when dietary deficiencies may be present.

Iron

Iron supplements are probably not necessary except in women, where iron losses may be significant. In rats and mice a response to hypoxia is a rapid increase in intestinal iron absorption before plasma iron turnover is changed.[54,55,56] This suggests that iron stores of the body can be increased before depletion occurs. Hannon[56] has shown that women who take supplemental iron will exhibit a greater increase in hematocrit than women who do not take iron during a 60 day exposure to 14,100 feet (4,300 m).

In summary, several general conclusions can be drawn from the above data regarding nutrition at high altitude: Weight loss is common during exposure to high altitude and consists of a loss of body fat and lean body mass. Insufficient caloric intake to balance daily energy consumption is probably responsible for most of the weight loss. It is unlikely that any degree of malabsorption occurs at extreme altitudes. Daily caloric needs at very high and extreme altitudes are substantially less than those of long distance runners at sea level and are in the range of 2,500-3,600 calories. The decreases in VO_2 max and lower levels of daily physical activity are probably responsible factors. A high carbohydrate diet appears to diminish symptoms of acute mountain sickness and may improve physical performance. A wide variety of foods that appeal to individual tastes is important in reducing the magnitude of high altitude weight loss. There is no evidence that supplemental vitamins, minerals, or other substances are necessary during expedition climbs.

References

1. CONSOLAZIO C, MATOUSH L, JOHNSON H, and DAWS T. Protein and water balances of young adults during prolonged exposure to high altitude (4300 meters). *Am. J. Clin. Nutrit.* 1968; 21:154-61.
2. CONSOLAZIO C, MATOUSH L, JOHNSON H, et al. Effects of high carbohydrate diet on performance and clinical symptomatology after rapid ascent to high altitude. *Fed. Proc.* 1969; 28:937-43.
3. CONSOLAZIO C, JOHNSON H, and KRZYWICKI H. Body fluids, body composition, and metabolic aspects of high altitude adapation. In M Yousef, S Horvath, and R Bullard, eds., *Physiologic adaptations*. New York: Academic Press, 1972.
4. JOHNSON H, CONSOLAZIO C, MATOUSH L, and KRZYWICKI H. Nitrogen and mineral metabolism at altitude. *Fed. Proc.* 1969; 28:1195-98.
5. SURKS M. Metabolism of human serum albumen in man during acute exposure to high altitude (14,000 ft). *J. Clin. Invest.* 1966; 45:1442-51.
6. BOYER S, and BLUME D. Weight loss and changes in body composition at high altitude. *J. Appl. Physiol.* 1984; 57:1580-85.
7. HARVEY T, JAMES H, and CHETTLE D. Birmingham Medical Research Expeditionary Society 1977 Expedition: Effect of a Himalayan trek on whole body composition, nitrogen, and potassium. *Postgrad. Med. J.* 1979; 55:475-77.
8. LICKTEIG J. Nutrition for high altitudes and mountain sports. In M. Casey, C. Foster, and E. Hixson, eds., *Winter sports medicine*. Philadelphia: F.A. Davis, 1990: 383-92.
9. PUGH L. The Silver Hut: Physiologic and medical aspects of the Himalayan Scientific and Mountaineering Expedition, 1960-61. *Sem. Respir. Med.* 1983; 5:113-21.
10. ROSE M, HOUSTON C, FULCO C, et al. Operation Everest II: Nutrition and body composition, *J. Appl. Physiol.* 1988;: 65:2545-51.

11. MACDOUGALL J, GREEN H, SUTTON J, et al. Operation Everest iI. Structural adaptations in skeletal muscle in response to extreme simulated altitude. *Acta. Physiologica Scand.* 1991; 142:421-27.

12. BUTTERFIELD G, GATES J, FLEMING S, et al. Increased energy intake minimizes weight loss in men at high altitude. *J. Appl. Physiol.* 1992; 72:1741-48.

13. CERRETELLI P, and de PRAMPERO O. Aerobic and anaerobic metabolism during exercise at altitude. In J Rivolier, P Cerretelli, J Foray, and P Segantine, eds., *High altitude deterioration.* Basel: S. Karger, 1985.

14. GLOSTER J, HEATH D, and HARRIS P. The influence of diet on the effects of a reduced atmospheric pressure in the rat. *Environ. Physiol. Biochem.* 1972; 2:117-24.

15. CHINN K, and HANNON J. Efficiency of food utilization at high altitude. *Fed. Proc.* 1969; 28:944-48.

16. BLUME F. Metabolic and endocrine changes at altitude. In J. Westt and S. Lahiri, eds., *High altitude and man.* Bethesda, Md.: American Physiological Society, 1984: 37-45.

17. GRAY G. Maldigestion and malabsorption: Clinical manifestations and specific diagnosis. In M. Sleisenger and J. Fordtran, eds., *Gastrointestinal disease.* Philadelphia: W.B. Saunders, 1983: 228- 56.

18. MILLEDGE J. Arterial oxygen desaturation and intestinal absorption of glucose. *Brit. Med. J.,* 1972; 3:557-58.

19. RAI R, MALHOTRA T, DIMRI G, and SAMPATHKUMAR I. Utilization of different quantities of fat at high altitude. *Am. J. Clin. Nutrit.,* 1975; 28:242-45.

20. CHESLER J, SMALL N, and DYKES P. Intestinal absorption at high altitude. *Postgrad. Med. J.* 1987; 63: 173-75.

21. SRIDHARAN K, MALHOTRA T, VPADHAYAY T, et al. Changes in gastrointestinal function in humans at an altitude of 3500 m (11,500 ft). *J. Appl. Physiol.* 1982; 50:145-54.

22. IMRAY C, CHESNER I, WRIGHT A, et al. Fat absorption at altitude: A reappraisal: *Proceedings,* Seventh International Hypoxia Symposium, 1991; 103. Abstract.

23. KAYSER B, DÉCOMBAZ J, FERN E, et al. Protein digestibility at 5,000 m. *Proceedings,* Seventh International Hypoxia Sympoisum, 1991: 103. Abstract.

24. WILLIAMS E. Mountaineering and the endocrine system. In C Clark, M Ward, and E. Williams, eds., *Mountain medicine and physiology.* London: Alpine Club, 1975: 38-44.

25. AMTRUBA J, RICHESON F, WHITE S, et al. The safety and efficacy of a controlled low-energy (very low- calorie) diet in the treatment of non-insulin dependent diabetes and obesity. *Arch. Int. Med.* 1988; 148:873-77.

26. SUTTON J. The hormonal responses to exercise at sea level. In J Sutton, C Houston, and N Jones, eds., *Hypoxia, exercise, and altitude.* New York: A. R. Liss, 1983: 325-41.

27. WHITTEN B, and JANOSKI A. Effects of high altitude and diet on lipid components of human serum. *Fed. Proc.* 1969; 28:983-86.

28. BERENDSOHN S. Hepatic function in chronic hypoxia of high altitude. *Arch. Intern. Med.* 1962; 109: 256-64.

29. HULTGREN H. Personal observation.

30. CAMPBELL J. Increase of resistance to oxygen want in animals on certain diets. *Quart. J. Exptl. Physiol.* 1938; 28:231-41.

31. CAMPBELL J. Diet and resistance to oxygen want. *Quart. J. Exptl. Physiol.* 1939; 29:259-75.

32. ANHOLM J, ESTES-BRUFF, ANDERSON C, and PETERS J. A controlled study of carbohydrate intake on acute mountain sickness at 3780 m altitude. In J Sutton, C Houston, and N Jones, eds., *Hypoxia, exercise, and altitude.* New York: A. R. Liss, 1987: 449.

33. KING C, BICKERMAN H, BOUVET W, et al. Aviation nutrition studies: Effect of pre-flight and in-flight meals of varying composition with respect to carbohydrate, protein, and fat. *J. Aviat. Med.* 1945; 16:69-84.

34. ECKMAN M, BARACH B, FOX C, et al. Effect of diet on altitude tolerance. *J. Aviat. Med.* 1945; 16: 328-40.

35. MITCHELL H, and EDMAN M. *Nutrition and resistance to climatic stress with particular reference to man.* Chicago: Research and Development Branch OQMG QM Food and Container Institute for the Armed Forces, 1949.

36. ASTRAND P, and BERGSTROM A. Diet and athletic performance. *Fed. Proc.* 1967; 26:1772.

37. POTERA C. Update on nutrition for mountaineers. *Summit,* 1985; 31:1-5.

38. POTERA C. Mountain nutrition: Common sense may prevent cachexia. *Physicians and Sports Med.* 1986; 14:233-37.

39. PUGH L, and WARD M. Some effects of high altitude on man. *Lancet* 1956; 271:1115.

40. PUGH L. Mount Cho Oyu, 1952; Mount Everest, 1953. *Sem. Resp. Med.* 1983; 5:109-12.

156

41. WEST J. *Everest the testing place.* New York: McGraw-Hill, 1985.
42. ULLMAN J. *Americans on Everest.* Philadelphia: Lippincott. 1964: 323-29.
43. KAYSER B, ACHESON K. BEMINI A, et al. Dietary energy assimilaiton at 5,000 m. *Proceedings,* Seventh International Hypoxia Symposium, 1991: 103. Abstract.
44. WARD M. *Mountain medicine.* London: Crosby, Lockwood, Staples, 1975.
45. GROVER R. Basal oxygen uptake of man at high altitude. J. Appl. Physiol. 1963; 18:909-12.
46. GILL M, and PUGH L. Basal metabolism and respiration in men living at 5,800 m (19,000 ft). *J. Appl. Physiol.* 1964; 19:949-54.
47. HUANG S, ALEXANDER J, GROVER R, et al. Increased metabolism contributes to increased resting ventilation at high altitude. *Resp. Physiol.* 1981; 57: 377-85.
48. MOORE L, CYMERMAN A, HUANG S, et al. Propranolol blocks metabolic rate increase, but not ventilatory acclimatization. *Respir. Physiol.* 1987; 70:195-204.
49. LeBLANC J. *Man in the cold.* Springfield, Ill: Charles C. Thomas, 1975: 38-40.
50. ROGERS T, SETLIFF J, and KLOPPING J. Energy cost, fluid, and electrolyte balance in subarctic survival situations. *J. Appl. Physiol.* 1964; 19:1-8.
51. The vitamin pushers. *Consumer Reports* 1986; 51:170-75.
52. HERBERT B, and BARRET S. *Vitamins and "health" foods: The great American hustle.* Philadelphia: Stickley, 1981.
53. JUKES T. Megavitamin therapy. *JAMA* 1975; 233:550- 51.
54. HATHORN M. The influence of hypoxia on iron absorption in the rat. *Gastroenterology,* 1971; 60:76-81.
55. RAJA K, PIPPARD M, SIMPSON R, and PETERS T. Relationship between erythropoiesis and enhanced intestinal uptake of ferric iron in hypoxia in the mouse. *Brit. J. Haematol.* 1986; 64:587-93.
56. HANNON J. Comparative altitude adaptability in young men and women. In L Follingsbee, and J. Wagner, eds., *Environmental stress.* New York: Academic Press, 1978.

CHAPTER 9

Water and Electrolytes

SUMMARY

Ascent to high altitude is accompanied by a prompt decrease in body weight during the first few days, as a result primarily of a decreased water intake and, to a lesser extent, an increased fluid loss from the respiratory tract. In some subjects a diuresis may occur that further adds to the negative water balance. Water loss via the respiratory tract becomes severe during heavy exercise at extreme altitudes and when combined with diminished thirst and the difficulty of melting snow and ice may seriously impair physical performance. Continued dehydration when associated with a decreased food intake results in orthostatic hypotension, weakness, apathy, and acidosis. Optimal water intake at extreme altitudes may require four to six liters of fluid per day to maintain a urine output of at least one liter per day. There is little evidence that salt tablets are necessary at high altitude, since sodium loss by the respiratory tract and sweating is minimal. There is disagreement about serum potassium levels at high altitude. An initial increase has been reported by most workers, which is probably related in part to the fall in aldosterone. Some workers have reported a decrease in serum potassium associated with symptoms of acute mountain sickness, but an increased potassium intake had little beneficial effect.

• • •

Acute effects

Ascent to high altitude is associated with a prompt decrease in body weight, related to a decrease in water intake as well as to an increased urine output. Janoski and his associates studied ten normal subjects living for nine days at 14,110 feet (4,300 m). Dietary intake including carbohydrates, protein, fat, and electrolytes was controlled by a liquid diet of constant composition administered at sea level prior to ascent and throughout the altitude stay.[1] Fluid intake decreased during the first days at altitude, accompanied by a significant reduction in urine volume. In a similar study, Johnson and his associates reported a 2.4 kg (mean) weight loss during the first four days at an altitude of 14,111 feet (4,300 m) in fifteen normal subjects. The weight loss was attributed to water loss and not to a decreased caloric intake (Fig. 9.1). Physical activity was maintained at a high level. A negative nitrogen balance also occurred, owing to a diminished food intake.[2] Studies of body composition by a determination of body density revealed a mean loss of 2.3 kg of body water after twelve days at altitude.[3] Upon return to sea level, water retention occurred and a positive nitrogen balance appeared. Krzywicki and his associates in a similar study also observed a mean weight loss of 3.75 kg in fifteen subjects at 14,110 feet (4,300 m) over a twelve-day period. Body water loss accounted for 1.81 kg (48 percent) of the weight loss. Blood and plasma volumes decreased.[4] Malhotra and his associates airlifted ten subjects to 11,400 feet (3,500 m), where studies were made for two to four days. All ten subjects were on a controlled diet

158

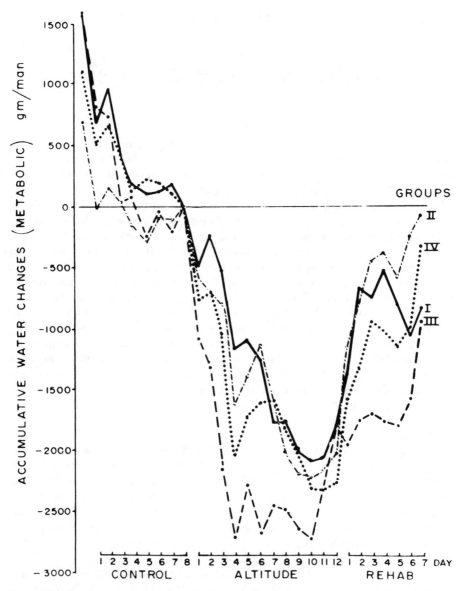

Figure 9.1. Cumulative water balances calculated from metabolic balances in fifteen normal subjects exposed to 14,110 feet (4,300 m). Water changes are assumed to be the differences between observed and calculated weight changes. Group I consisted of five men receiving a normal diet of 48 percent of calories as carbohydrate and 40 percent as fat; Groups II, III, and IV each consisted of ten men on a high carbohydrate (68 percent) and a low fat (20 percent) diet. The decrease in weight during the control period was due to a change from a standard Army ad libitum diet to an all-liquid diet. From Johnson et al., ref. 2.

that was started at sea level seven days before ascent. Fluid intake decreased by 100-300 ml per day at altitude.[5] Recently, Hoyt and his associates studied nine subjects in a hypobaric chamber for ten days at a simulated altitude of 14,100 feet (4,300 m). Significant decreases were observed in body mass (4.4 kg), total body water (1.7 liters), intracellular fluid (3 liters), and plasma volume (20 percent decrease). Extracellular fluid volume did not change significantly.[6]

The negative water balance at high altitude is not entirely due to a decreased water intake. Some persons may experience a spontaneous diuresis (hohendiuresis), but in controlled studies this appears to be a rare phenomenon. With a decrease in caloric intake or fasting, a negative water balance has been observed, with an isotonic contraction of extracellular fluid volume.[7] Exposure to cold may result in a diuresis.[8] In some persons an antidiuresis occurs at high altitude, and clinical evidence of systemic edema has been observed.[9]

Honig, using controlled animal experiments, has evaluated the effect of acute hypoxia on salt and water metabolism.[10] He points out that hypoxic stimulation of the peripheral arterial chemoreceptors results in an increased excretion of sodium by inhibiting renal tubular reabsorption. Excitation of the carotid and aortic body chemoreceptors informs the medulla oblongata, and therefore the brain, that arterial oxygen tension has decreased. Because renal nerve section does not prevent the increased loss of sodium by the kidney, hormonal mechanisms are probably involved, either adrenocortical hormones, vasopressin, or atrial natriuretic factor. In addition to the diuresis and increased sodium loss induced by hypoxia, there is also a transient inhibition of food and water intake. In animals this is greatly attenuated by carotid body nerve section, indicating that the effect is also mediated by the peripheral chemoreceptors. The mechanisms are probably also applicable to man: studies in human subjects have shown similar effects of high altitude exposure, that is, diuresis, negative water balance, and decreased intake of food and water.

Water Loss

At very high and extreme altitudes the increased loss of water from the respiratory tract will contribute to dehydration. Pugh reported that during non-climbing activity at the Silver Hut in the Himalayas, at an altitude of 17,660 feet (5,790 m), the mean water turnover was 3.9 liters per day, compared with 2.9 liters at sea level. During five to seven hours of climbing per day at higher altitudes, the water turnover was estimated at 5 liters per day.[11] The higher value was largely due to increased water loss via the lungs, which was estimated to be 2.9 ml per 100 liters of respiration at 16,300 feet (5,480 m). Calculated water losses via the respiratory tract at 20,000 feet (6,100 m) varied from 760 ml to 1,530 ml per 24 hours, depending upon the level of daily physical activity. Above 22,000 feet (6,710 m), climbers became progressively dehydrated, especially when not using oxygen. The sensation of thirst was blunted and urine output was decreased to as little as 500 ml per day. On Mount Everest, Hillary and Lowe, climbing between 18,300 feet (6,000 m) and 21,350 feet (7,000 m), drank three to five liters of fluid per day with urine outputs of 1.2 to 1.5 liters of fluid per day.[12] Many investigators have noted that at high altitude and during survival situations, thirst is not increased, despite considerable negative water balances.[13] Because of the intense solar radiation water, loss may also occur by perspiration. At very high and extreme altitudes, especially when using alpine-style summit techniques, the combined effects of cold and low food and water intake may result in uncompensated water loss, comparable to the contraction of extracellular fluids that occurs in a survival situation.

Metabolic effects

The hemodynamic and metabolic consequences of dehydration and an inadequate food intake can be serious. It has been shown that a water deficit of as little as 2 percent can decrease physical performance.[14] In another experiment, Rogers and Setliff exposed volunteer subjects to a 48-hour fast in a simulated survival situation on a frozen river.[15] Half the subjects could drink as much water as they wanted and half the subjects were given 1,920 ml of water per day. Weight loss was the same in both groups, indicating that the increased water intake did not prevent the dehydration attributed to fasting and an isotonic contraction of extracellular fluid volume. The administration of 115 mEq of sodium chloride per day resulted in less weight loss and maintained sodium balance. Further studies by Rogers and Setliff of twelve men exposed to five days of starvation under similar conditions revealed a loss of 8 percent of body weight, of which one-third was estimated to be due to an isotonic contraction of extracellular fluid.[7] Changes in heart rate, pulse pressure, and hematocrit were consistent with this degree of contraction. A moderately severe degree of acidosis was observed. The authors concluded that this amount of dehydration predisposed the subjects to syncope, induced lethargy and apathy, and could increase the susceptibility to peripheral cold injury and phlebothrombosis. The subjects did not experience thirst. If one applies these observations to alpine-style ascents, one must conclude that an adequate intake of calories and electrolytes is equally as important as an adequate fluid intake.

Blume and his associates reported a persistent increase in serum osmolality in thirteen mountaineers after a mean stay of 16.5 days above 17,700 feet (5,400 m). Serum osmolality rose from 290 ± 1 mOsm/kg at sea level to 295 ± 2 mOsm/kg T at 16,470 feet (5,040 m) and finally to 302 ± 4 mOsm/kg at 20,500 feet (6,300 m). Normal sea level values are 285-295 mOsm/kg. Serum concentrations of potassium, phosphate, and creatinine were elevated above sea level values. Mean twelve-hour urinary outputs were similar at both altitudes and higher than at sea level. Creatinine clearance was unchanged from sea-level values. Thirst was not experienced. Since urinary vasopressin excretion was also similar at all three altitudes, it was concluded that prolonged exposure to high altitude may result in persistent impairment in osmoregulation caused in part by an inappropriate arginine-vasopressin response to hyperosmolality.[16] The decreased sense of thirst at high altitude can lead to dehydration. This may also occur in elderly patients at sea level if adequate fluids are not taken, and may result in serious life-threatening dehydration.[17]

West has speculated that renal compensation for respiratory alkalosis is decreased in the presence of dehydration. This may result in a greater degree of alkalosis with a further leftward shift of the oxygen dissociation curve and a higher oxygen saturation for a given decrease in arterial PO_2. This may provide some advantage in climbing at extreme altitudes.[18]

Electrolytes

Acute exposure to high altitude will result in an increase in serum chlorides secondary to the decrease in blood bicarbonate. This is an expected compensation to maintain total anion concentration near normal levels. Endogenous creatinine clearance is decreased, owing to a decrease in renal blood flow.[1] There is disagreement about altitude-associated changes in serum electrolytes. Janoski and Slater observed

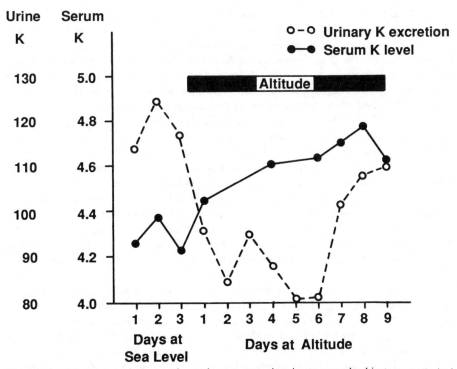

Figure 9.2. Urinary potassium excretion and serum potassium in ten normal subjects on a constant electrolyte intake and a controlled diet at sea level and during nine days on Pikes Peak, 14,110 feet (4,300 m). Urinary potassium excretion decreases as serum potassium rises. Potassium excretion expressed as milliequivalents per day and serum potassium as milliequivalents per liter. From Janoski et al., ref. 1.

a decreased urinary excretion of potassium and a rise in serum potassium during a nine-day stay at 14,110 feet (4,300 m) (Fig. 9.2). Serum chloride levels were increased, and no change occurred in serum sodium.[1,19] Malhotra,[5] Axelrod,[20] and Burrill[21] all observed an increased renal excretion of potassium and a fall in serum potassium with exposure to high altitude or during acute hypoxia. Waterlow postulated that some of the symptoms of acute mountain sickness might be due to a fall in serum potassium and gave members of his climbing group potassium supplements with some beneficial effect.[22]

The reasons for the differences in the results of these studies are not clear. Respiratory alkalosis will result in a fall in serum potassium, owing to potassium moving into the cells. Opposing this effect is the well-known fall in aldosterone secretion with acute exposure to high altitude, which would decrease potassium loss and increase serum potassium. Evidence supporting the latter concept is found in studies of high altitude residents by Ayres, who observed a rise in body potassium along with increased Na/K ratio in the saliva and a decrease in urine aldosterone excretion by the kidneys.[23] Sodium chloride supplements in the form of salt tablets are not necessary during most climbs at high altitude, because sweating is minimal in the cold, dry atmosphere and most of the excess water loss via the respiratory tract represents a pure water loss. Expedition and climbing diets usually contain adequate amounts of sodium and especially potassium in the form of soups and concentrated foods. Salt tablets may be helpful, however, during approach marches at lower elevations, where temperatures and humidity may be high and marked sweating occurs. The concentration of sodium chloride in sweat is about three grams per liter, or approximately six salt tablets per quart of water. An indication for salt tablets is copious sweating while exercising in a hot, humid climate. The use of other supplementary electrolytes such as potassium is not necessary, notwithstanding the advertising claims of many purveyors of beverages designed to replace electrolytes. An exception is when a climber is taking a diuretic for medical reasons or to prevent mountain sickness; in this case, the possibility of a marked loss of potassium, with resulting muscular weakness, can be prevented by potassium replacements either in the diet or in the form of potassium salts.

Salt tablets may even be dangerous at high altitude, where thirst is blunted, pure water loss occurs, renal function is diminished, and hemoconcentration is already present. Hypernatremia can cause profound mental changes, including coma.[17] Fatal hypernatremia has been reported due to exogenous salt intake.[24] Caution should also be observed in the use of certain antacids such as Rolaids, which are high in sodium.

It is apparent that increased water loss occurs at high altitude and that the loss is greater if there is increased physical effort. Thirst is a poor indicator of water deficit, and for that reason climbers are often unaware that their fluid intake is inadequate. Complicating this problem is a disturbance of osmoregulation. The altitude-induced hyperosmotic state is associated with a decrease in aldosterone. Vasopressin is not increased. Therefore, climbers should drink at least one quart of water or liquids per day, and as much as four quarts during days of heavy physical activity, so that they maintain a urine output of at least one quart a day. Studies have shown that during a strenuous march water replacement is inadequate if it is left up to the desires of the climbers, and that sufficient replacement can only be achieved by drinking a predetermined volume hourly.[25] Water intake volume must be judicious, however, and suited to the conditions of altitude, exertion, and temperature. Water intoxication has been described where the individual (at sea level and not exercising) drank three liters of water over a three-hour period. Seven other similar cases have been reported.[26] Hyponatremia due to exertion and excessive water intake has been described in recreational hikers in the Grand Canyon and in an ultramarathon runner.[27,28] Usually there is an associated inappropriate secretion of vasopressin, due to medications (acetaminophen), stress, nausea, or vomiting.

Acid-Base Changes
Ascent to high altitude is accompanied by an increase in ventilation with a resulting respiratory alkalosis, a decrease in arterial PCO_2, and an increase in pH. Renal compensation then occurs over several days with excretion of bicarbonate and a more alkaline urine. The time course of renal compensation is about four to eight days. In one study, ascent to 14,850 feet (4,500 m) resulted in a pH rise from 7.40 at sea level to 7.47 within 24 hours. The pH then slowly declined to 7.45 at the end of four days. Arterial PCO_2 and bicarbonate continued to fall, however.[29] Upon return to sea level, normal values were attained after about 48 hours.

Many workers have reported normal pH values in high altitude natives, suggesting complete renal compensation. Winslow, however, has shown that a mild respiratory alkalosis was present in 46 high altitude natives living at 14,980 feet (4,540 m). The mean plasma pH was 7.439±0.065.[30] The plasma pH values from two other investigators varied from 7.426 to 7.431.[30,31,32] These results indicate the presence of a respiratory alkalosis in high altitude natives and inadequate renal compensation for pH change. Arterial PCO_2 values from seven studies at a similar altitude varied from 31.6 mm to 34.0 mm.[31] Cruz and Recavarren reported a mean PCO_2 of 32.5 mm ± 2.5 mm in 159 high altitude residents.[32] In one observation at the Chulec General Hospital in La Oroya, Peru, 12,323 feet (3,730 m), the normal arterial PCO_2 in 90 male subjects aged 20-60 years was 32 mm.[33] These values are important in the diagnosis of chronic mountain sickness, where arterial PCO_2 may be abnormally high and respiratory acidosis may occur.

In lowlanders who acclimatize to high altitude, the arterial pH slowly returns to the normal value of 7.4. This is true of altitudes up to 9,900 feet (3,000 m), but at higher altitudes a respiratory alkalosis may persist and become more severe. At 20,000 feet (6,300 m) the mean arterial pH of acclimatized lowlanders was 7.47, and the mean arterial pH of two climbers at 26,600 feet (8,050 m) was 7.55.[31] In the latter cases, an uncompensated respiratory alkalosis was present; climbers like these two are probably not completely acclimatized, and the alkalosis may become less with a longer period of acclimatization. One cannot spend much time at this altitude, however, without experiencing altitude deterioration.

It has been speculated that metabolic compensation for respiratory alkalosis is slow and incomplete at very high and extreme altitudes. The possible mechanisms are yet to be determined, but volume depletion and hypoxia of the kidneys have been suggested.[31]

References

1. JANOSKI W, WITTEN B, SHIELDS J, and HANNON J. Electrolyte patterns and regulation in man during acute exposure to high altitude. *Fed. Proc.* 1969; 28:1185-89.
2. JOHNSON H, CONSOLAZIO C, MATOUSH L, and KRZYWICKI H. Nitrogen and mineral metabolism at high altitude. *Fed. Proc.* 1969; 28:1195-98.
3. KRZYWICKI H, CONSOLAZIO C, MATOUSH L, and JOHNSON H. Metabolic aspects of acute starvation-body composition changes. *Am. J. Clin. Nutrit.* 1968; 21:87-97.
4. KRZYWICKI H, CONSOLAZIO C, MATOUSH L, JOHNSON H, and BARNHART R. Body composition changes during exposure to altitude. *Fed. Proc.* 1969; 28:1190-94.
5. MALHOTRA M, BRAHMACHARI K, SRIDHARAN T, et al. Electrolyte changes at 3,500 m in males with and without high altitude pulmonary edema. *Aviat. Space Environ. Med.* 1975; 46:409-12.
6. HOYT R, DURKOT M, KAMIMORI G, et al. Chronic altitude exposure (4,300 m) decreases intra-cellular and total body water in humans. In *Hypoxia and Mountain Medicine*, ed. J Sutton, G Coates and C Houston, Burlington VT, Queen City Printers Inc. 1992; 306.
7. ROGERS T, SETLIFF J, and KLOPPING J. Energy cost, fluid, an electrolyte balance in subarctic survival situations. *J. Appl. Physiol.* 1964; 19:1-8.
8. BADER R, ELIOT J and BASS D. Hormonal and renal mechanisms of cold diuresis. *J. Appl. Physiol.* 1952; 4:649-58.
9. WARD M. *Mountain medicine.* London: Crosby, Lockwood, Staples, 1975:65.
10. HONIG A. Salt and water metabolism in acute high altitude hypoxia: Role of peripheral arterial chemoreceptors. *The Physiologist* 1989; 4:109-11.
11. PUGH L. The Silver Hut: Physiological and medical aspects of the Himalayan Scientific and Mountaineering Expedition, 1960. *Seminars in Respir. Med.* 1983; 5:113-21.
12. PUGH L. Physiological and medical aspects of the Himalayan Scientific and Mountaineering Expedition, 1960. *Brit. Med. J.* 1962; 2:621-27.
13. KRZYWICKI H, CONSOLAZIO C, JOHNSON H, et al. Water metabolism in humans during acute high altitude exposure. *J. Appl. Physiol.* 1971; 30:806-9.

164

14. WRIGHT E. Fluid and electrolyte requirements during exercise. *Nutrition* 1988; 7:33-37.
15. ROGERS T, and SETLIFF J. Value of fluid and electrolyte supplements in subarctic survival situations. *J. Appl. Physiol.* 1964; 19:580-82.
16. BLUME F, BOYER S, et al. Impaired osmoregulation at high altitude: studies on Mt. Everest. *JAMA* 1984; 252:524-26.
17. PHILLIPS R, ROLLS B, LEDINGHAM J, et al. Reduced thirst after water deprivation in healthy elderly men. *N. Engl. J. Med.* 1984; 311:753-59.
18. WEST J. Does dehydration at extreme altitude enhance tissue oxygenation. *Fed. Proc.* 1984; 43:419.
19. SLATER J, WILLIAMS E, EDWARDS R, et al. Potassium retention during the respiratory alkalosis of mild hypoxia in man. *Clin. Sci.* 1969; 37:311-26.
20. AXELROD D, and PITTS R. Effects of hypoxia on renal tubular function. *J. Appl. Physiol.* 1952; 4:493-601.
21. BURRILL M, FREEMAN S, and IVY A. Sodium, potassium, and chloride excretion of human subjects exposed to a simulated altitude of 18,000 feet. *J. Biol. Chem.* 1945; 157:297-302.
22. WATERLOW J, and BUNJE H. Observations on mountain sickness in the Colombian Andes. *Lancet* 1966; Sept. 24:655-61.
23. AYRES P, HUNTER R, WILLIAMS E, and RUNDO J. Aldosterone excretion and potassium retention in subjects living at high altitude. *Nature* 1961; 191:78.
24. MODER K and HURLEY D. Fatal hypernatremia from exogenous salt intake. Report of a case and review of the literature. *Mayo Clin. Proc.* 1990; 65:1587-94.
25. SYROTUCK J, R.N. Nutrition: Fluid and salt needs. *Off Belay* 1976; 24:24-31.
26. KLONOFF D, and JUROW A. Acute water intoxication as a complication of urine testing in the workplace. *JAMA* 1991; 265:84-85.
27. BACKER H, SHOPES E and COLLINS S. Hyponatremia in recreational hikers in Grand Canyon National Park. *J. Wilderness Med.* 1993; 4:391-406.
28. CLARK J, and GENNARI F. Encephalopathy due to severe Hyponatremia in an ultramarathon runner. *West. J. Med.* 1993; 159:188-89.
29. LENFANT C, and SULLIVAN K. Adaptation to high altitude. *N. Engl. J. Med.* 1971; 284:1298-1309.
30. WINSLOW R, MONGE C, STATHAM N, et al. Variability of oxygen affinity of blood: Human subjects native to altitude. *J. Appl. Physiol.* 1981; 51:1411-16.
31. WARD M, MILLEDGE J, and WEST J. *High altitude physiology and medicine.* Philadelphia: University of Pennsylvania Press, 1989:180-200.
32. CRUZ A, and RECAVARREN S. Chronic mountain sickness: A pulmonary vascular disease. In W Brendel and R Zink, eds., *High altitude physiology and medicine.* New York: Springer Verlag, 1982:271-77.
33. MARTICORENA E. Personal communication, 1982.

CHAPTER 10

Acclimatization

SUMMARY

Acclimatization is the process that takes place when sea-level dwellers ascend to high altitude and gradually improve their ability to tolerate the new environment. Natural acclimatization refers to the altitude tolerance of high altitude natives, which has been acquired by generations of exposure. Acquired acclimatization acts by reducing the oxygen gradient from inspired air to the interior of the cell by several processes. An important factor is the immediate and continued increase in ventilation, which is a highly sensitive, rapidly responding system. Other factors that reduce the gradient are a slight decrease in the A-a gradient, a left shift of the oxygen dissociation curve, increased tissue capillary density and enzyme changes within the cell. The increase in red cell mass acts to permit optimum oxygen transport without an undue increase in cardiac work. Acclimatization before ascent to altitudes exceeding 10,000 feet (3,050 m), either by a gradual ascent or by intermediate staging, is important not only for physical well-being but, also for the prevention of mountain illness. A gradual ascent over several days is commonly dictated by the terrain, such as the long approach marches necessary in the Himalayas. This is not simply an efficient method of acclimatization; it also improves physical working capacity. Above 14,000 feet (4,270 m), an ascent of 1,000-2,000 feet (305-610 m) per day should be alternated with rest days. Intermediate staging consists of spending several days at an altitude of 7,000-8,000 feet (2,135-2,440 m) before sojourns at higher altitudes.

Acetazolamide taken for a few days during ascent may prevent acute mountain sickness, facilitate sleep, and improve well-being. Physical working capacity at high altitude improves rapidly during the first few weeks of exposure, but little further improvement occurs after six weeks. Loss of acclimatization will occur during descent to lower altitudes or sea level of two to four weeks' duration. Training for competetive athletic events is best done at the altitude where competition will be held. Training at high altitude does not improve athletic performance at sea level. Training at an intermediate altitude may improve sea-level performance in long-distance races probably by the resulting increase in hematocrit.

· · ·

Definitions

Acclimatization to high altitude is achieved by three general processes: accomodation, acquired acclimatization, and natural acclimatization. *Accommodation*: a term proposed by Von Muralt, describes the immediate response of the body to rapid, passive transfer to high altitude.[1] *Acquired acclimatization*: a term suggested by Hurtado is the acclimatization that occurs when sea-level dwellers spend weeks or months at high altitude; this is the most common variety of acclimatization.[2]

Natural acclimatization: a term also suggested by Hurtado, describes the acclimatization or adaptation achieved by high altitude natives as a result of generations of exposure.[2,3] Some workers refer to this process as adaptation rather than acclimatization, but both terms mean the process, possibly by natural selection, by which those who survive are those who are most able to tolerate the stresses of high altitude life. A genetic change may be a factor.

Physiology

The primary effects of high altitude on the body are due to the decrease in inspired oxygen tension with a consequent decrease in arterial oxygen tension. There is considerable variation in the minimum cellular PO_2 at which normal oxidative enzyme function occurs; the critical PO_2 below which oxidative enzyme function is impaired may be as low as 3.5 mm Hg.[4] This value can be estimated by the PO_2 of venous blood leaving the tissue which may be 15-18 mm for the brain, 28 mm for resting muscle, and as low as 10 mm for myocardium. The rapidity with which cellular function deteriorates because of hypoxia is variable and may be only a few seconds for the retina or up to several minutes for the myocardium.

The processes of accommodation and acclimatization serve to maintain intracellular oxygen tension at a functional level, despite the decrease in the PO_2 of inspired air.[3] To analyze these processes it is important to understand the transport system of oxygen from the atmosphere to the interior of the cell. This system can be considered as a series of gradients (see Fig. 10.1), which are modified by exposure to high altitude.[4,5]

1. *Inspired air to alveolus.* Inspired air becomes warmed and fully saturated with water vapor as it passes through the nose, mouth, and trachea to the smaller airways and alveoli. The partial pressure of oxygen in the atmosphere of 150 mm Hg is thus reduced by the addition of water vapor and carbon dioxide. As a result, the sea-level inspired oxygen tension of 150 mm Hg is reduced to about 100-103 mm in the alveoli. This will vary with the amount of ventilation: hyperventilation will reduce this gradient primarily by decreasing the CO_2 and increasing the O_2 tension thus achieving higher partial pressure of oxygen in the alveoli. The increase in ventilation is one of the first adjustments to be made upon exposure to high altitude. The increase is due to response of the peripheral chemoreceptors to hypoxia. As a result of the increase in ventilation, the carbon dioxide pressure in the blood falls and the pH rises. This has an inhibitory effect on the respiratory centers but the stimulatory effect of hypoxia prevails. Hypocapnea and alkalosis persist for several days. During this time renal conservation of hydrogen ions and excretion of fixed base restores the blood pH to normal. There also occurs a gradual shift in the sensitivity of the respiratory centers so that once again the primary respiratory control is exerted by carbon dioxide. The increase in respiratory response to carbon dioxide is retained by long-term residents and is a sign of acclimatization. During muscular exercise the hypoxic stimulus is clearly dominant as evidenced by the very high ventilatory rates during exercise at extreme altitudes in the presence of respiratory alkalosis.

2. *Alveolus to capillary blood.* Oxygen in the alveoli moves across the alveolar and capillary membranes by a process of passive diffusion. The barrier between alveolar air and pulmonary capillary blood consists of the alveolar membrane, interstitial space, and capillary endothelium. Within the capillary, oxygen must diffuse through plasma and then through the red cell membrane. The total diffusion

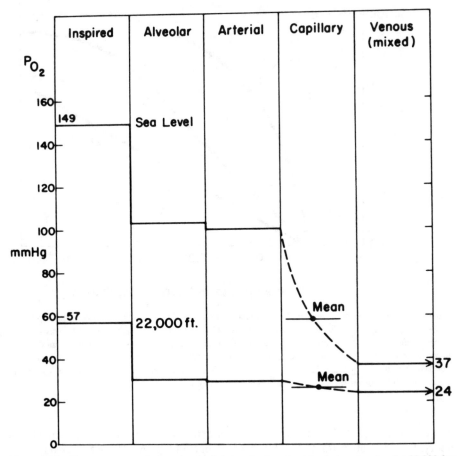

Figure 10.1. The oxygen cascade from inspired air to mixed venous blood at sea level and at 22,000 feet (6,710 m). The largest gradient from inspired air to alveolar air is partly under voluntary control. From Luft, ref. 5.

distance is very small-0.5 mu. The alveolar capillary membranes are extremely thin, measuring about 0.2 mu in thickness. Equilibration of alveolar oxygen with capillary blood is rapid, and about 80 percent complete in about 0.002 seconds (Fig. 10.2).[6] At high altitude oxygenation of capillary blood may be impaired by several factors: (1) Since alveolar PO_2 is low, the pressure gradient for diffusion is reduced and equilibration will occur more slowly. (2) If the rate of blood flow through the capillaries is increased there may be insufficient time of equilibration to occur.[6,7] Together, these factors probably account for the decrease in arterial oxygen saturation that occurs during exercise at high altitude.[7,8]

The mechanism of movement of oxygen from the alveolus to capillary blood was the basis for a historical controversy. In 1870 Ludwig suggested that the lung might secrete oxygen into the blood against a pressure gradient much as fish secrete air into a swim bladder. Haldane became convinced of the possibility of oxygen secretion when he conducted experiments on Pikes Peak with his Oxford colleague, Douglas. In fifteen experiments on five subjects he found arterial PO_2 to be higher

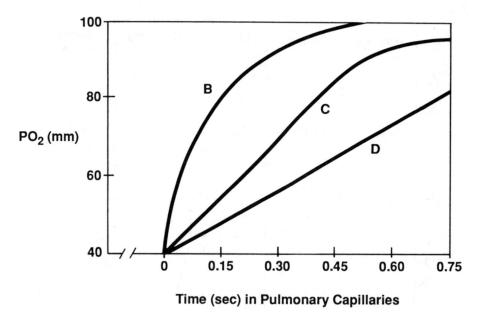

Figure 10.2. Exchange of oxygen in the pulmonary capillaries. The time the blood is in the capillaries for absorbing oxygen is indicated in seconds below. The vertical axis indicate the partial pressure of oxygen in the alveoli, breathing air at sea level. If diffusion from alveolus to capillary is moderately impaired, as shown in C, the uptake of oxygen is slower. When impairment is severe, as shown in D, arterial unsaturation is present. High altitude will have a similar effect, since the pressure of oxygen in the alveoli will be lower. B represents the normal sea level curve. From Comroe, ref. 6.

than alveolar PO_2 by 36 mm Hg. Barcroft's experiment on himself disproved this theory. He sat in an airtight glass box with a controlled atmosphere for six days and via a cannula arterial blood samples were obtained. His arterial PO_2 was always lower than his alveolar PO_2. Barcroft later confirmed these observations in the Peruvian Andes where his arterial blood was dark. If oxygen secretion had occurred the blood would have been bright red.[9]

3. *Alveolus to arterial blood.* A small A-a gradient between alveolar and peripheral arterial blood at sea level in normal upright man amounts to about 10 mm Hg. This gradient is due to a very small membrane component of about 1-2 mm Hg along with a larger venous admixture component of about 1-8 mm. The venous admixture component results from two actions: (1) some venous blood enters the pulmonary veins and left ventricle without passing through the pulmonary capillaries for oxygenation, the major sources being bronchial veins entering the pulmonary veins and Thebesian veins draining venous blood from the left ventricular myocardium; and (2) ventilation and perfusion inequalities result in some pulmonary capillary blood traversing areas of the lung that either are not ventilated or are poorly ventilated.

At high altitude the effect of a venous admixture upon arterial PO_2 is reduced. Inspection of the O_2 dissociation curve (Fig. 10.3) will show that at sea level a small decrease in arterial oxygen saturation due to a venous admixture will lower arterial PO_2 more than at high altitudes; where one is on the steep limb of the curve.[10]

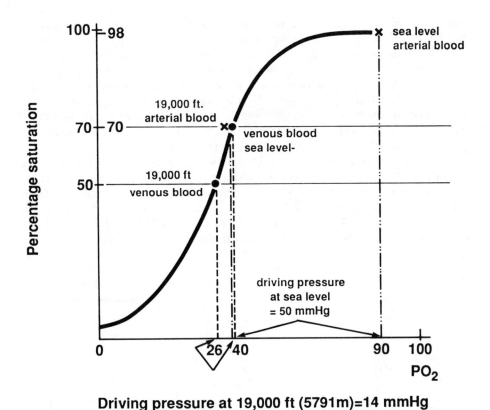

Driving pressure at 19,000 ft (5791m)=14 mmHg

Figure 10.3. The effect of a veno-arterial shunt at sea level, showing a considerable fall in arterial PO_2 with little change in arterial saturation. The decrease in PO_2 from arterial to venous blood is 50 mm with a drop in saturation of 28 percent. At high altitude a drop in arterial saturation of 20 percent results in a fall in PO_2 of only 14 mm Hg, due to the shape of the O_2 dissociation curve. From Ward, ref. 10.

4. *The oxygen dissociation curve*. The total amount of oxygen carried by each ml of blood is determined in part by the oxygen dissociation curve. This is a standard method of relating the partial pressure of oxygen in the blood to the oxygen content, or oxygen saturation, of the blood. The amount of oxygen in the blood is also determined by the amount of hemoglobin in the blood. One gram of hemoglobin when fully saturated contains 1.4 ml of oxygen.

Several factors alter the affinity of blood for oxygen. The effect of changes in pH upon the O_2 dissociation curve is shown in Figure 10.4. With a pH of 7.6 (alkalosis), arterial saturation at a PO_2 of 30 mm is about 56 percent, at a pH of 7.2 (acidosis), saturation at the same PO_2 is only about 30 percent. Thus in active metabolizing tissues, carbon dioxide release and acidosis will facilitate oxygen unloading, whereas in the more alkaline lung capillaries where carbon dioxide tension is low, oxygen loading is facilitated.

The O_2 dissociation curve has several important effects on oxygen transport at high altitude in addition to its effect on minimizing the fall in arterial oxygen tension due to venous shunts that have just been discussed. As one ascends from sea level to about 12,000 feet (3,600 m), arterial oxygen tension falls proportionally more than arterial oxygen saturation. Arterial PO_2 drops from 100 mm to about 72 mm while saturation decreases from 96 percent to 89 percent. The oxygen content of the blood is therefore only slightly reduced in comparison with the pressure of oxygen in the blood. At about 12,000 feet (3,660 m) on the steep part of the curve, small decreases in oxygen tension will now cause great decreases in oxygen saturation. This effect is partly diminished by a leftward shift of the dissociation curve owing to the respiratory alkalosis of high altitude (Fig. 10.4). At an arterial PO_2 of 30 mm and a normal pH of 7.4 the arterial saturation is about 45 percent, but at a pH of 7.6 the saturation now becomes 58 percent. During heavy exercise at extreme altitudes marked alkalosis permits O_2 saturation to be well maintained despite very low arterial PO_2 values. For example, on Mount Everest it was estimated that arterial O_2 saturation was about 70 percent which was nearly the same value that was present at the lower altitude of 20,600 feet (6,300 m).[7] In Operation Everest II, heavy exercise at 25,000 feet (7,625 m) caused the arterial PO_2 to fall from 52 mm (at rest) to 42 mm; arterial oxygen saturation also fell, from 85 percent to 72 per-

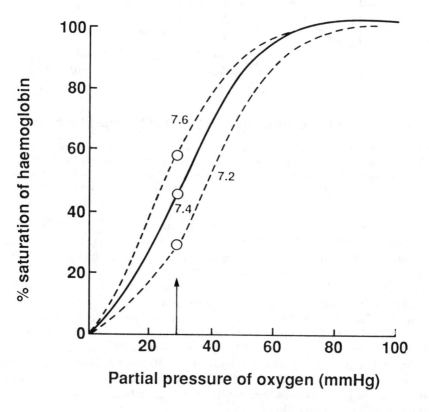

Figure 10.4. The effect of respiratory alkalosis at high altitude, showing an increase in arterial oxygen saturation. At an arterial PO_2 of 30 mm, raising the pH from 7.2 to 7.6 will increase arterial oxygen saturation from 28 percent to 57 percent. The indicated changes in pH are large to illustrate the phenomenon. It was estimated that on the summit on Mount Everest the arterial pH was 7.76. From Ward, ref. 10.

cent. The resting pH was 7.46.[8] Under such conditions oxygen saturation is more important than oxygen tension because the level of saturation is a measure of the oxygen available for the tissues, whereas the O_2 tension is the driving force that moves oxygen from blood to cells. For example, if the blood contained no red cells but the PO_2 of dissolved oxygen was normal, 100 ml of this blood would deliver only 0.3 ml of oxygen (in solution).[6]

5. *Arterial to mixed venous blood.* As blood passes from the arterial to the venous side of the perfused tissues of the body, the fall in oxygen partial pressure will be determined by the metabolic rate of the tissues, the rate of blood flow and the part of the oxygen dissociation curve over which these changes occur. Low flow rates as in heart failure and high tissue metabolism will result in marked venous unsaturation, while high flow rates and low tissue metabolism will result in less venous unsaturation.[11]

6. *Capillary blood to cell.* The oxygen tension of any single cell will depend upon its relative distance from a nutrient capillary. The mean oxygen tension of tissue cells will depend upon the cell/capillary ratio for that tissue. For example, during acclimatization more capillaries in muscle tissue may open up for blood flow. Capillary density may be a function of muscle atrophy rather than a growth of new capillaries.[12,13,14] More recent studies suggest that diffusion may also occur from arterioles and venules where the vessel walls are thin and the tissue oxygen tension is low.[6] The passage of oxygen from capillaries to cells may also be aided by myoglobin, a protein that can combine with oxygen even when tissue PO_2 is very low.[14] Ward has pointed out that at a PO_2 of 10 mm Hg, hemoglobin is only 10 percent saturated while myoglobin is 70 percent saturated. Some 10-12 percent of the total body iron is in the form of myoglobin, located primarily in the muscles and myocardium.[10] Increased amounts of myoglobin have been demonstrated in muscle tissues of man and animals at high altitude.[15,16] Myoglobin can act as a store of oxygen, but this function is limited by the fact that it gives up oxygen slowly.[14]

A more important function of myoglobin may be to speed the diffusion of oxygen by a physico-chemical process at the molecular level. This phenomenon was discovered by Wittenberg and Scholander.[17,18] These investigators suggested that myoglobin facilitated oxygen flux by about six times the rate of ordinary diffusion, and that it may account for most of the oxygen reaching the mitochondria, which are the energy-producing factories of the body.

7. *Intracellular gradients.* Robin has pointed out that 80 percent of cellular oxygen consumption occurs in the mitochondria with the remaining 20 percent occurring in other intracellular elements.[19] In high altitude cattle, Ou and Tenney have described an increase in the number of mitochondria per myocardial cell but no increase in mitochondrial size.[20] An increase in number rather than in size would facilitate oxygen transfer, just as an increase in the number of capillaries does. Kearny obtained different results from a study of myocardial mitochondria from high altitude rabbits and guinea pigs.[21] In his study, mitochondrial volume, numbers of mitochondria, and the estimated surface area of mitochondria were the same as in sea-level animals. The difference between these two studies may, however, be due to differences in methods or animal species.

An increase in myocardial succinic dehydrogenase in high altitude rabbits has been described by Harris.[22] High altitude animal tissues also contain higher concentrations of high-energy phosphates, exhibit more ATPase activity, and have an

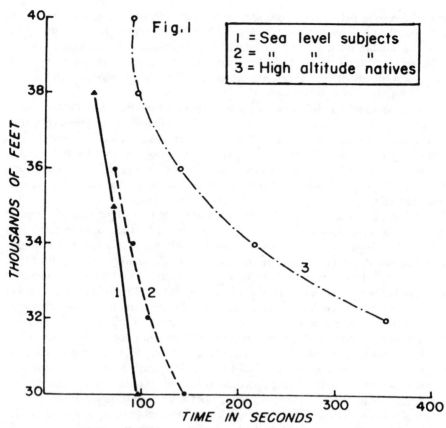

Figure 10.5. Time to unconsciousness in three groups of human beings subjected to rapid exposure to altitudes of 30,000 feet (9,150 m) and higher in a hypobaric chamber. Groups 1 and 2 were unacclimatized sea-level dwellers. Group 3 consisted of acclimatized high altitude Andean natives. Note that Group 3 subjects did not lose consciousness at an altitude of 32,000 feet (9,760 m). From Velasquez, ref. 23.

increased rate of glycolysis.[4] The importance of cellular acclimatization may be illustrated by the experiments of Velasquez, who subjected Peruvian highlanders, dwelling at an altitude of 14,900 feet (4,545 m), to simulated ascents in a hypobaric chamber to altitudes of 30,000-40,000 feet (9,150-12,200 m) in order to determine the duration of consciousness.[23] The pressure in the chamber was lowered at a simulated ascent of 3,000 feet/min (915 m/min) while the subjects were breathing oxygen via a face mask; when the selected altitude was attained the mask was removed. In sixteen subjects exposed to a simulated altitude of 30,000 feet (9,150 m) eight (50 percent) had an indefinite consciousness time. One of these subjects remained conscious for 120 seconds at 40,000 feet (12,200 m). The other eight (50 percent) remained conscious for 240-885 seconds (mean, 554 seconds). Two control groups of subjects living at sea level remained conscious for only 90-100 seconds at 30,000 feet (9,150 m) (Fig. 10.5). Syncope was preceded by only moderate hyperventilation. The factors that could preserve consciousness in the acclimatized subjects for only a few seconds include an increased diffusing capacity, increased hematocrit, increased pulmonary blood volume, and oxygen stores in the lungs and tissues. The major factor preserving consciousness was probably acclimatization at the cellular level.

8. *Pulmonary changes.* The pulmonary diffusing capacity may be increased in high altitude acclimatized individuals. This may be especially important during exercise.

9. *Polycythemia.* Historically the polycythemia of prolonged residence at high altitude was the first adaptive adjustment to be described. The increased red cell mass with a minimal change in plasma volume provides several advantages. Oxygen delivery to the tissues can be maintained with a lower cardiac output and less cardiac work. The lower pulmonary capillary blood flow will facilitate oxygen delivery to the blood in the lung. Increased pulmonary red cell volume may facilitate oxygen delivery. Marked increases in red cell mass, however, may have unfavorable effects by the increase in viscosity leading to thromboses and decreases in circulation in several organ systems.

Practical Aspects

A major problem in the assessment of acclimatization is the lack of any simple, precise measurement that will determine when a person is fully acclimatized. Maximum exercise capacity under controlled conditions gradually increases during a long stay at altitude, but this type of exercise does not measure many other important aspects of acclimatization. Arterial blood gas studies and respiratory and circulatory tests cannot identify the acclimatized person from the unacclimatized. Of even greater practical importance is the inability to detect at sea level those who will acclimatize quickly and completely as well as the individual who will do poorly at high altitude. Finally, there is great individual variation in altitude tolerance. Some persons may ascend rapidly to considerable elevations and still be able to perform heavy exercise soon after arrival with a minimum of discomfort. Others, though equally fit at sea level, may be miserable for many days, even at moderate altitudes, and may not attain effective physical performance levels until days or even weeks after ascent.

Simple practical indices of acclimatization include: (1) severity and duration of symptoms of acute mountain sickness: this can be evaluated by a simple symptom questionnaire or assessment of a climber's performance by other party members[24]; (2) the ability to function normally, sleep well, and maintain an optimum calorie and fluid intake; (3) minimum impairment of physical performance with gradual improvement during the altitude stay; (4) competent mental functioning and a stable emotional state. There are several methods of achieving acclimatization that will attenuate high altitude discomfort and illness.

Intermediate staging. For the average trekker or climber who plans to climb and sleep at altitudes between 10,000 feet (3,050 m) and 14,000 feet (4,270 m) two to four days spent walking and climbing at an intermediate altitude, between 6,000 feet (1,830 m) and 8,000 feet (2,440 m), will be beneficial.[24,25] Persons who have a history of acute mountain sickness may be helped by taking acetazolamide 125-250 mg every twelve hours before going up to higher altitudes. The medication should be started the day of ascent and continued for three to five days after arrival. Acetazolamide may also have a generally beneficial effect on physical performance.[26] A high carbohydrate diet started a few days before ascent and continued during the altitude stay may also be helpful.[27,28] Setting up camps to sleep as low as possible if peaks are to be climbed is always a useful strategy.

Anyone who plans to go to very high altitudes, of 14,000-18,000 feet (4,270-5,490 m), will benefit by a second stage of two to four days at 12,000-13,000 feet (3,660-3,965 m). For example, before climbing the Mexican volcanoes, 17,600-18,700 feet (5,368-5,704 m), two or three days spent in Mexico City (7,300 feet/2,227 m) and two to three days days at the Tlamacus Lodge on Popocatepetl (13,000 feet/3,965 m) will enable one to climb these summits with a minimum of altitude problems. Most climbers who fail to reach these summits have made the mistake of going directly from sea level to the start of their climb.

One stage ascent. Going to 9,000 feet (2,750 m) or even 14,000 feet (4,270 m) from sea level in one day is a common experience for South American tourists visiting Ecuador, Peru, and Bolivia. The risk of mountain sickness under these conditions is high. If it is not possible to spend a few days at an intermediate altitude, one should be prepared to experience some discomfort for the first few days after arrival. Only light activity should be carried out during this time, and the use of acetazolamide may be helpful. In larger cities, hotels will provide oxygen if symptoms become too uncomfortable. With a light plastic face mask, a flow rate of 2-4 liters per minute while one is quietly resting or sleeping is adequate. Oxygen should be used for at least fifteen minutes; it is of no benefit to take an occasional few breaths of oxygen.

Graded ascent. In areas such as the Himalayas long approach marches are usually required to reach high elevations, and acclimatization takes place gradually during the approach to base camp. Commercial airline flights to landing strips about 8,000 feet (2,440 m) may save time, but they greatly increase the risk of high altitude illness. At altitudes above 14,000 feet (4,270 m), Houston recommends that ascents should be limited to 500-1,000 feet (150-300 m) per day, and every third day should be a rest day.[29] Ascending to altitudes greater than 14,000 feet (4,270 m) and starting to climb immediately is both foolhardy and hazardous. Acetazalomide, as mentioned earlier, is helpful in cases of headache, mountain sickness, or insomnia during the first few days at high altitude. Continued acclimatization will occur up to 18,000 feet (5,490 m), but a prolonged stay above this altitude does not appear to enhance acclimatization and may, on the contrary, result in deterioration.

Acclimatization for extreme altitudes. No systematic studies have been made of what constitutes ideal acclimatization programs for climbs above 18,000 feet (5,490 m), but field experience provides some information. Most climbers in the Himalayas are well acclimatized after the long approach march from 5,000 feet (1,525 m), Katmandu, to 17,500 feet (5,338 m), the Everest base camp. Additional acclimatization occurs during the two-to-three week period of establishing higher camps up to 24,000 feet (7,320 m). To avoid altitude deterioration above 18,000 feet (5,490 m), only short stays at these altitudes are usually allowed followed by several rest days at lower altitudes. West has proposed that summit climbers who spend several days at a lower altitude and then make a rapid climb to the summit may achieve some physiological benefit from the greater degree of respiratory alkalosis that may be attained, as compared with summit climbers who spend several days at very high camps[30], but one must balance this theoretical advantage with the potential disadvantage of developing pulmonary edema.

High altitude deterioration. It is well known that a prolonged stay above 18,000 feet (6,000 m) does not result in improved acclimatization but instead brings progressive weight loss and a decrease in physical working capacity. In 1960-61 during the Himalayan Scientific and Mountaineering Expedition eight physiologists lived for up to 100 days at 19,024 feet (5,800 m). Weight loss at the rate of 0.5 to 1.5 kg per week occurred. At the end of the sojourn the physiologists were less fit than recently acclimatized climbers.[31] Ward has described features of the high altitude deterioration that is usually seen with a prolonged stay at altitudes over 18,000 feet (5,490 m). These include progressive increase in lassitude, decreased capacity for intellectual work, dulled senses, weight loss, poor appetite, insomnia, and a decrease in physical working capacity.[32]

Time required for acclimatization. The time required for acclimatization is variable and depends upon the altitude at which acclimatization is occurring as well as

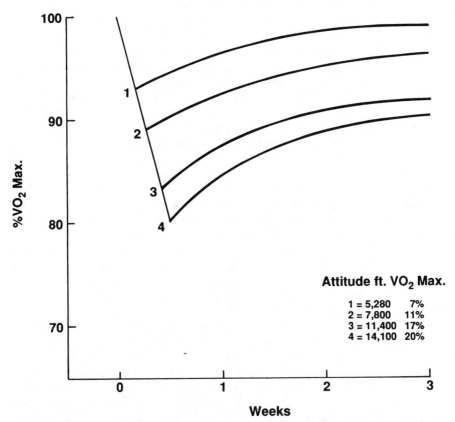

Figure 10.6. Theoretical time course of acclimatization of man to altitude during and at the peak of training. Upon arrival at altitude VO₂ max is decreased proportional to the altitude, being about 20 percent lower at 14,100 feet (4,272 m). By the second week most of the acclimatization has occurred, as indicated by increased performance. Little further gain is achieved by the third week. Note that even when maximum acclimatization has occurred, maximum performance still remains below sea-level values. The diagonal line indicates the number of days required to attain each altitude level. Data from Weihe, ref. 34; Consolazio, ref. 35; and Sime et al., ref. 36.

the physical activity carried out. The higher the altitude, the greater the decrement in performance from sea-level values and the longer the time required for acclimatization. At higher altitudes, sea-level performance levels are rarely attained even after complete acclimatization (Fig. 10.6).[33-36] West has estimated that acclimatization to extreme altitude is not complete at 30-36 days of exposure but may be nearly complete at 77 days.[37,38] This estimate is based on the relation between ventilation, arterial PCO_2, and PO_2. As ventilation reaches a plateau, arterial PCO_2 and arterial PO_2 will also reach a steady level. This process may occur as rapidly as four to eight days at the lower elevation of Pikes Peak, 14,100 feet (4,300 m).[39] Symptoms of acute mountain sickness rarely last more than seven days. Workers at the telescope on Mauna Kea at 13,800 feet (4,200 m) who arrive from sea level require five to seven days for symptoms of acute mountain sickness to subside and to attain improvement in psychometric tests.[14,40] It usually takes about four to six weeks at very high altitudes before one can climb and function effectively. Studies of exercise performance in athletes at sea level who were transported to 7,540 feet (2,300 m) revealed a gradual improvement in performance over a four-to-five-week period after an initial decrement during the first week. Even after five weeks of training at altitude, the maximum aerobic capacity is 10-14 percent less than at sea level.[33] Weihe reported that endurance runners exposed to 6,560-12,140 feet (2,000-3,700 m) experienced an increase in running time at altitudes of as much as 20 percent during the first week.[34] Training at this altitude improved performance over a two-to-three-week period, after which little additional improvement was noted (Fig. 10.6). Faulkner noted that even after eight months of training at 14,000 feet (4,270 m), sea-level performance was not regained.[41]

Loss of acclimatization. Although most of the physiologic changes that occur at high altitude will regress within two to six weeks at sea level, brief sojourns of a few days at sea level will not result in loss of acclimatization sufficient to develop altitude illness upon return to high altitude. Importantly, however, studies in Peru have indicated that a sea-level stay of greater than ten to fourteen days can apparently result in a susceptibility to high altitude pulmonary edema during re-ascent. Studies at Leadville, Colorado (10,300 feet/3,142 m), corroborate these observations. Children and young adolescents spending a stay as short as five days at a lower altitude often experienced pulmonary edema upon re-ascent.[42]

Intermittent altitude exposure. Occasional but regular short sojourns at high altitude may provide some degree of acclimatization, but no systematic studies have been made of this phenomenon. Airline pilots and crew members spend 20-30 hours a week at cabin altitudes of 5,000-8,000 feet (1,525-2,440 m) without developing a significant rise in hematocrit or red cell count. It is possible, however, that some degree of acclimatization has occurred.[43] Burse and Forte found that repeated eight-hour exposures to a low oxygen mixture-12.8 percent oxygen equivalent to 13,000 feet (3,960 m) for ten successive days in normal subjects was not sufficient to prevent symptoms of acute mountain sickness. Symptoms were similar to those of a control group breathing air in a similar manner.[44] Residents of sea-level South American cities such as Lima, Peru, frequently spend short sojourns at altitudes of 10,000 to 15,000 feet (3,050-4,575 m) on business or pleasure, and most of them report little effect of high altitude upon performance provided the altitude stay is only one to three days in duration. A physician who lives in Mérida, Venezuela, at 5,500 feet (1,680 m), nearly every weekend rides the cable car teleférico up to the top station at 15,600 feet (4,758 m), where he spends one to two days hiking and camping. Unacclimatized friends who have joined him on these excursions attest to the fact that he is well acclimatized, since he climbs rapidly with little evidence of impairment due to the altitude.

Repeated altitude exposure. The ability to acclimatize appears to improve with successive exposures to very high altitudes over several years. Climbers who have visited the Himalayas annually have noted that with each visit symptoms were less severe and physical performance improved more rapidly. Many climbers had no symptoms at all and only a slight decrease in physical performance up to 20,000 feet.

Hypobaric Chambers

The classic study by Houston and Riley in 1946 exposed four men in a low-pressure chamber to a gradually increasing simulated altitude of 22,000 feet (6,710 m) over 25 days. The subjects were reasonably comfortable and were capable of participating in research studies and cycle exercise. During the fourth week the subjects were exposed to an altitude of 29,150 feet (8,890 m). Two of the subjects remained at this altitude for 30 minutes and were able to perform cycle exercise.[45] In October-November 1985 Houston and his associates completed a second hypobaric pressure chamber study of eight subjects who were exposed to progressively higher simulated altitudes over a 40-day period. Two subjects dropped out at 18,000 feet (5,490 m) and 25,000 feet (7,620 m) but six were able to tolerate 25,000 feet (7,620 m) for 10 days and on several days were able to tolerate 29,000 feet (8,845 m) for three to four hours, during which they exercised on a treadmill and cycle ergometer and underwent a series of tests.[46]

At Nagoya University in Japan, climbers have used exposures in a hypobaric chamber for one to two hours per day over fourteen days combined with cycle ergometer exercise to acclimatize. After such a program one climber, Kamuro, was able to climb Mount McKinley from 13,045 feet (4,100 m) to the summit, 21,320 feet (6,500 m), in seven hours, which is a climb rate of about 1,125 feet (340 m) per hour. Kamuro spent two weeks at sea level after his chamber runs before he climbed McKinley, so he may have been only partially acclimatized.[47] Galen Rowell and Ned Gillette, two experienced mountaineers, took seven hours to climb the final 2,000 feet (610 m) of McKinley. Both were relatively unacclimatized and Rowell developed HAPE during descent. Their time from 2,500 feet (763 m), lower than Kamuro's starting point, to the summit was nineteen hours, or a climb rate of about 550 feet per hour.[48] Richalet and his colleagues reported on the effect of pre-acclimatization in five elite alpinists before a climb on Mount Everest. The group spent one week on Mont. Blanc, 15,766 feet (4,807 m), and 38 hours over three and a half consecutive days in a hypobaric chamber. In six days they were at the Everest base camp. They climbed to 25,584 feet (7,800 m) in five days—a rate significantly faster than that of previous climbers.[49]

In sum, the value of hypobaric chambers in acclimatization has yet to be demonstrated. It would seem that a prolonged period at base camp is more efficient, although more time consuming. After such periods of acclimatization remarkably fast alpine style ascents have been made such as Mount Everest, in 44 hours and K-2 in 27 hours to the summit and back to camp.

Age and Gender

Young individuals appear to be more susceptible to acute altitude illness than older, experienced climbers. Ward has stated that the early thirties appear to be the best age for climbing at extreme altitudes.[10] However, older climbers have attained several 8,000-meter summits including Mount Everest notably by Kurt Diemberger and William Read, both at age 50 years. Julius Boehm climbed Mount Rainier in July 1978 when he was 80 years old.[50,51]

Young women acclimatize to altitude more readily than men in several aspects. After the initial weight loss and decreased food intake during the first few days at altitude women exhibit a higher energy intake and less weight loss than men, and these differences persist for at least two weeks. Arterial PCO_2 is lower in women than in men throughout the altitude stay and this is accompanied by a higher arterial PO_2. These data indicate that women have a higher pulmonary ventilation than men. Young women exhibit a greater increase in hemoglobin during ascent than men and thus have a greater increase in arterial oxygen content, despite the fact that women have a lower hemoglobin level before ascent (13.7 gms/100 ml compared with 14.9 gms/100 ml).[52] Several women have climbed Mount Everest without oxygen.

Smoking

Smoking apparently impairs acclimatization. In a Swedish study of 109 men working on an irrigation project in Peru at an altitude of 10,500 feet (3,200 m), fourteen men had to terminate their contract and return to sea level. Ten of the fourteen were smokers and smoking appeared to be the only reason for their inability to tolerate the altitude. The smokers compared to non-smokers had a higher Hgb (18 gm vs 17 gms) and a higher hematocrit (57 percent vs 54 percent); and their oxygen dissociation curve was shifted to the left, which suggested a decreased capacity for oxygen delivery.[53]

Physical Conditioning at Sea Level

Physical training at sea level does not protect one against altitude illness nor does it appear to improve one's ability to acclimatize. Once acclimatized, however, the physically trained climber will be able to perform better than the untrained.

The effects of training at high altitude for competition at high altitude became the subject of interest and research following the Pan American games in Mexico City (altitude 7,200 feet/2,200 m) in 1955 and also before the Olympic Games in Mexico City in 1968. Most studies have shown that two to six weeks of training at the altitude at which competition will occur was beneficial, but training at altitudes higher than the altitude of competition was not helpful, nor does training at high altitude for competition at sea level improve sea-level performance.[35,54-59] Adams and his workers studied twelve middle-distance runners at sea level and high altitude, 7,540 feet (2,300 m). Maximum oxygen consumption during treadmill exercise and running time for two miles was determined in six subjects, who trained for three weeks at sea level and were then brought to altitude, where they continued training for another three weeks. A second group of six subjects carried out a reverse training process: three weeks at altitude followed by three weeks at sea level. The experiment showed that when runners who trained at sea level went to altitude they experienced an initial decrease in VO_2 max and an increase in running time for two miles; although these performances improved during the altitude stay, they did not

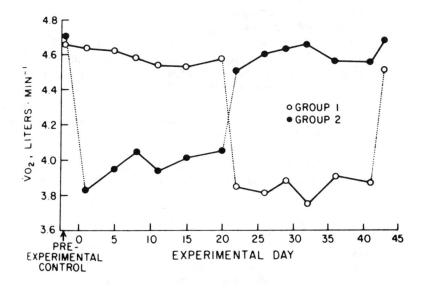

Figure 10.7. Maximum oxygen consumption using a treadmill in six middle-distance runners (Group 1), who trained for three weeks at sea level and then continued training for three weeks at 7,540 feet (2,300 m). Group 2 consisted of six runners who trained for three weeks at the same altitude and then continued training at sea level. Broken lines indicate the change in training site. From Adams et al., ref. 59.

attain sea-level values. Training at altitude, on the other hand, did not improve times at sea level.[59] (Fig. 10.7)

Adams' well-planned study convincingly showed that training at high altitude did not improve sea-level running times. Training at intermediate altitude above 5,000 feet may, however, be effective for distance runners and marathon runners, for whom endurance is critical. Top runners from many parts of the world live and train at Boulder, Colorado 6,000 feet (1,830 m).[60] Runners born and living at intermediate altitudes such as Kenya and Mexico City have done very well in marathons and long races at sea level. The commanding performance of the East German swimmers in the 1988 Olympic Games may have been due, in part, to their training in a hypobaric gymnasium and swimming facility.

Levine and his workers investigated the effect of living at altitude 8,200 feet (2,500 m) and training at 4,200 feet (1,280 m) in two groups of trained runners (n=10). Training intensity was carefully controlled and evaluated by recording heart rate, lactate, and VO_2 in the field during training. The athletes living at the higher altitude improved their VO_2 max by approximately 5 percent and could run a 5,000-meter race 30 seconds faster. They also had a 500 ml increase in blood volume, which may have accounted for their increase in performance; living at altitude probably represents a natural form of blood doping. No changes were seen in the athletes who lived and trained at the lower altitude.[61] Another method of increasing red cell mass is the use of erythropoietin to increase endurance capacity and maximum oxygen consumption[62], but it is suspected that the use of erythropoietin may have contributed to the deaths of world-class cyclists.[63] To my knowledge, the use of erythropoietin in preparation for high altitude climbing has not been reported.

This chapter has emphasized the oxygen transport system from inspired air to the interior of the cell. Other aspects of acclimatization involving specific organ systems are presented elsewhere in this volume. The most important adjustment to high altitude is the increase in ventilation, which minimizes the decrease in alveolar PO_2 due to the decrease in atmospheric PO_2. Other adjustments also contribute to the maintenance of intracellular oxygen tension at a viable level. It is a curious fact that oxygen delivery is not increased by an increase in cardiac output in the acclimatized person. The disadvantages of such an adjustment appear to outweigh any possible advantages. An increase in circulating hemoglobin allows oxygen transport to occur without requiring an undue increase in cardiac output. Important processes of acclimatization occur at the cellular level, but our understanding of these mechanisms is limited.

References

1. VON MURALT A. Acquired acclimation to high altitudes. In *Life at high altitudes.* Washington, D.C.: Pan American Health Association, 1966; 140: 53-57.
2. HURTADO A. Animals in high altitude: Resident man. In *Handbook of physiology: Adaptation to the environment,* ed. D Dill. Washington, D.C.: American Physiological Society, 1964: 843-60.
3. HURTADO A, et al. *Mechanisms of natural acclimatization: Studies on the native residents of Morococha, Peru, at an altitude of 14,000 feet, 4500 m.* School of Aviation Medicine, 1956; USAF Project No. 56-1.
4. TENNEY S. Physiological adaptations to life at high altitude. *Modern Concepts CV Dis.* 1962; 31: 713-18.
5. LUFT U. Aviation physiology: The effects of altitude. In *Handbook of physiology: Respiration II.* Washington, D.C.: American Physiological Society, 1965: 1099-1147.
6. COMROE J. *Physiology of respiration,* 2d ed. Chicago: Yearbook Medical Publishers, 1975.
7. WEST J. Man on the summit of Mount Everest. In J. West and S Lahiri, eds., *High altitude and man.* Bethesda, Md.: American Physiological Society, 1984: 5-17.
8. SUTTON J, REEVES J, WAGNER P, et al. Operation Everest II: Oxygen transport during exercise at extreme simulated altitude. *J. Appl. Physiol.* 1988; 64:1309-21.
9. MILLEDGE J. The great oxygen secretion controversy. *Lancet* 1985: Dec. 21-28: 1408-11.
10. WARD M. *Mountain medicine.* London: Crosby Lockwood Staples, 1975: 236-44.
11. WHITE M, ROULEAU J, RUDDY T, et al. Decreased coronary sinus oxygen content: A predictor of adverse prognosis in patients with severe congestive heart failure. *J. Am. Coll. Cardiol.* 1991; 18:1631-37.
12. MacDOUGALL D, GREEN H, SUTTON J, et al. Operation Everest II: Structural adaptations in skeletal muscle in response to extreme simulated altitude. *Acta Physiol. Scand.* 1991; 142:421-27.
13. BANCHERO N. Long term adaptation of skeletal muscle capillarity. *Physiologist* 1982; 25:385-89.
14. HEATH D, and WILLIAMS D. *High altitude medicine and pathology.* London: Butterworth's, 1989: 67-69.
15. REYNAFARJE B. Myoglobin content and enzymatic activity of muscle and altitude adaptation. *J. Appl. Physiol.* 1962; 17:301-05.
16. TAPPAN D, and REYNAFARJE B. Tissue pigment manifestations of adaptation to high altitude. *Am. J. Physiol.* 1957; 190:99-103.
17. WITTENBERG J. Myoglobin facilitated diffusion of oxygen. *J. Gen. Physiol.* 1965; 49:57-75.
18. SCHOLANDER P. Oxygen transport through hemoglobin solutions. *Science* 1960; 131:585-90.
19. ROBIN E. Of man and mitochondria: Coping with hypoxic dysoxia. *Am. Rev. Resp. Dis.,* 1980; 122: 517-31.
20. OU L, and TENNEY S. Properties of mitochondria from hearts of cattle acclimatized to high altitude. *Respir. Physiol.* 1970; 8:151-59.
21. KEARNY M. Ultrastructional changes in the heart at high altitude. *Pathologia et Microbiologia* 1973; 39:258.

22. HARRIS P, CASTELLO Y, GIBSON D, HEATH D, and ARIAS-STELLA J. Succinic and lactic dehydrogenase activity in myocardial hemogenates from animals at high and low altitudes. *J. Mol. & Cellular Cardiol.* 1970; 1:189.

23. VELASQUEZ T. Tolerance to acute anoxia in high altitude natives. *J. Appl. Physiol.* 1959; 14:357-62.

24. SAMPSON G. Procedures for the measurement of acute mountain sickness. *Aviat. Space Environ. Med.* 1983; 54:1063-73.

25. HANSEN J, HARRIS C, and EVANS W. Influence of elevation of origin, rate of ascent, and a physical conditioning program on symptoms of acute mountain sickness. *Military Med.* 1967; 132:585-92.

26. BRADWELL A, DYKES P, COOTE J, et al. Effect of acetazolamide on extreme performance at high altitude. *Lancet* 1986; May 3:1001-5.

27. CONSOLAZIO C, MATOUSH L, JOHNSON H, et al. Effects of high carbohydrate diets on performance and clinical symptomatology after rapid ascent to high altitude. *Fed. Proc.* 1969; 28:937-43.

28. HANSEN J, HARTLEY H, and HOGAN R. Arterial oxygen increase by high carbohydrate diet. *J. Appl. Physiol.* 1972; 33:441-45.

29. HOUSTON C. Acclimatization. In *Hypoxia: Man at altitude*, J Sutton, N Jones, and C Houston. New York: Thieme-Stratton, 1982: 158-60.

30. WEST J. Oxygenless climbs and barometric pressure. *Am. Alpine C.* 1984; 26:126-33.

31. PUGH L. Physiological and medical aspects of the Himalayan Scientific and Mountaineering Expedition, 1960-61. *Brit. Med. J.* 1962; 2:621-27.

32. WARD M, MILLEDGE J, and WEST J. *High altitude medicine and physiology.* Philadelphia: University of Pennsylvania Press, 1989.

33. BALKE B, DANIELS J, and FAULKNER J. Training for maximum performance at altitude. In R Margaria, ed., *Exercise at altitude.* New York: Excerpta Medica Foundation, 1967: 179-86.

34. WEIHE W. Time course of acclimatization to high altitude. In R Goddard, ed., *The effects of altitude on physical performance.* Chicago: Chicago Athletic Institute, 1967: 33-36.

35. CONSOLAZIO C. Submaximal and maximal performance at high altitude. In R Goddard, ed., *The effects of altitude on physical performance.* Chicago: Chicago Athletic Institute, 1967: 91-96.

36. SIME F, PENALOZA D, RUIZ L, et al. Hypoxemia, pulmonary hypertension, and low cardiac output in newcomers at low altitude. *J. Appl. Physiol.* 1974; 36:561-65.

37. WEST J. Tolerable limits to hypoxia on high mountains. In *Hypoxia: The tolerable limits*, ed. J Sutton, C Houston, and G Coates. Indianapolis: Benchmark Press, 1988: 353.

38. WEST J. Rate of ventilatory acclimatization to extreme altitude. *Respir. Physiol.* 1988; 74:323-53.

39. REEVES J. Personal communication.

40. FORSTER P. Telescopes in high places. In D Heath, ed., *Aspects of hypoxia.* Liverpool: Liverpool University Press, 1986: 217-22.

41. FAULKNER J, KOLLIAS J, FAVOUR C, et al. Maximum aerobic capacity and running performance at altitude. *J. Appl. Physiol.* 1968: 24:685-91.

42. SCOGGIN C, HYERS T, REEVES J, and GROVER R. High altitude pulmonary edema in the children and young adults of Leadville, Colorado. *N. Engl. J. Med.* 1977; 297:1269-72.

43. HURTADO A, ASTE-SALAZAR H, MERINO C, et al. Physiological characteristics of flight personnel. *J. Aviat. Med.* 1947; 18:406-16.

44. BURSE R, and FORTE V. Acute mountain sickness at 4500 m is not altered by repeated eight-hour exposures to 3200-3550 m normobaric hypoxic equivalent. *Aviat. Space Environ. Med.* 1988; 59:942-49.

45. HOUSTON C, and RILEY R. Respiratory and circulatory changes during acclimatization to high altitude. *Am. J. Physiol.* 1947; 149:565-88.

46. HOUSTON C, SUTTON J, and CYMERMAN A. Operation Everest II: Man at extreme altitude. *J. Appl. Physiol.* 1987; 63:877-82.

47. NAKASHIMA N. High altitude medical research in Japan. In *Hypoxia: Exercise and altitude*, ed., J Sutton, C Houston, and N Jones. New York: A.R. Liss, 1983: 170-73.

48. ROWELL G. High altitude pulmonary edema during rapid ascent. In *Hypoxia: Man at altitude*, ed., J Sutton, N Jones, and C Houston. New York: Thieme- Stratton, 1982: 168-70.

49. RICHALET J-P, BITTEL J, HERR J-P, et al. Pre-acclimatization to high altitude in a hypobaric chamber: Everest Turbo. In *Hypoxia and mountain medicine*, ed J Sutton, G Coates, and C Houston. Burlington, Vt: Queen City Printers, 1992: 202-12.

50. Off Belay, 1979; 44:29. *Notation.

51. Am. Alpine News 1979; 149:15.

52. HANNON J. Comparative altitude adaptability of young men and women. In *Environmental stress*, ed., L Folinsbee, J Wagner, J Borgia, B Drinkwater, J Gliner, and J Bedi. New York: Academic Press, 1978: 335-50.

53. LINDGARD F, and LILLJEKVIST R. Failure of long-term acclimatization in smokers moving to altitude. *Acta. Med. Scand.* 1984; 216:317-22.

54. BALKE B. Summary of Magglingen Symposium on sports at medium altitude. In R Goddard, ed., *The effects of altitude on physical performance*. Albuquerque, N. Mex.: Athletic Institute, 1967: 165-69.

55. GROVER R, and REEVES J. Exercise performance of athletes at sea level and 3,100 m, 10,200 feet altitude. In R Goddard, ed., *The effects of altitude on physical performance*. Albuquerque, N. Mex.: Athletic Institute, 1967: 80-87.

56. GROVER R, REEVES J, GROVER E, and LEATHERS J. Muscular exercise in young men native to 3,100 m, 10,200 feet altitude. *J. Appl. Physiol.* 1967; 22:555-64.

57. BUSKIRK E, KOLIAS J, PICON-REATIQUE J, et al. Physiology and performance of track athletes at various altitudes in the United States and Peru. In R Goddard, ed., *The effects of altitude on physical performance*. Albuquerque, N. Mex.: Athletic Institute, 1967: 65-71.

58. HANSEN J, VOGEL J, STELTER G, et al. Oxygen uptake in men during exhaustive work at sea level and high altitude. *J. Appl. Physiol.* 1967; 23:511-22.

59. ADAMS W, BERNGUER M, DILL D, et al. Effects of equivalent sea-level and altitude training in VO_2 max and running performance. *J. Appl. Physiol.* 1975; 39:262-66.

60. NODEN M. Bolder: Ideal terrain for training. *Sports Illustrated*, March 1990.

61. LEVINE B, STRAY-GUNDERSON J, DUHAIME G, et al. Living high-training low: the effect of altitude acclimatization/normoxic training in trained runners. *Med. Sci. Sports Exer.* 1991: 23, in press.

62. EKBLOM B, and BERGLUND B. Effect of recombinant erythropoietin on physical performance and maximal aerobic power in man. *Med. Sci. Sports Exer.* In Press.

63. ADAMSON J, and VAPNEK D. Recombinant erythropoietin to improve athletic performance. *N. Engl. J. Med.* 1991; 324: 698-99.

CHAPTER 11

Exercise

SUMMARY

A familiar aspect of altitude exposure is the progressive decrease in physical performance with increasing elevation. Normal climb rates of 2,000-3,000 feet (610-915 m) per hour can be maintained up to 15,000 feet (4,575 m), but thereafter the rate decreases markedly, to only about 500 feet per hour at 24,000 feet (7,320 m). Among the many conditions responsible for limiting the work rate at high altitude, perhaps the most important is hypoxemia, the severity of which increases in proportion to the altitude and level of exercise. Hypoxemia is related to the ventilatory response to hypoxia as well as to the capacity of the lung to transport oxygen to the capillaries. This capacity may be diminished by ventilation-perfusion abnormalities and possibly also by subclinical pulmonary edema.

Cardiac function remains normal even during maximum exercise. Cardiac output is decreased in proportion to the decrease in physical working capacity. Cardiac output during exercise may be limited by pulmonary hypertension, right ventricular dysfunction, and possibly tricuspid regurgitation. A decrease in plasma volume and, occasionally, severe dehydration may also limit cardiac output. Acclimatization, climbing skill, and physical fitness at high altitude are important adaptive mechanisms, and climbing effectiveness is also aided by adequate fluid and food intake, the use of oxygen, and acetazolamide. At extreme altitudes such as near the summit of Mount Everest, hypoxic cerebral dysfunction may be the limiting factor to physical performance.

• • •

Reduction in Performance

A familiar aspect of exercise at high altitude is the progressive limitation of physical performance with increasing altitude. Climbing rates and the elevation gained per day by expedition climbers begin to decrease sharply above 15,000 feet (4,575 m) (Figs. 11.1 and 11.2). Although acclimatized climbers may be able to maintain a climbing pace with an altitude gain of 2,000 to 3,000 feet (610-915 m) per hour up to 15,000 feet (4,575 m), at higher elevations the maximum rate of climb decreases sharply. Climbing rates at 24,000 feet (7,320 m) may be only 500 feet (150 m) per hour. At higher elevations the rates can be even slower: at 27,000 feet on Mount Everest (8,235 m), Somervell, climbing without oxygen, could manage only 80 feet (24 m) in one hour over relatively easy terrain; every twenty yards he had to rest for a minute or more, and he took seven to ten breaths per step.[1] Similar slow climb rates were observed by other oxygenless Everest summit climbers. Messner, whose climb rate at 3,000 feet (915 m) was nearly 6,600 feet (2,013 m) per hour, required more than one hour to climb the final 330 vertical feet (100 m) to the summit.[2] The maximum physical effort that can be expended above 25,000 feet

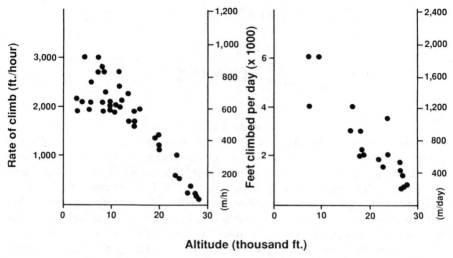

Figure 11.1. Climbing rates—feet per hour and feet climbed per day—reported from various expeditions. Redrawn from Pugh, ref. 37.

(7,625 m) is only about 40 percent of sea level values and is equivalent to walking about two miles per hour on level terrain. Descent requires about 50 percent less oxygen uptake. The decrease in climbing rates is a reflection of the decrease in maximum oxygen uptake at high altitude (Figs. 11.3 and 11.4).[3,4]

Running performances in distance races are also impaired even at modest altitudes.[5,6,7] At Mexico City (altitude 7,300 feet/2,226 m) during the Pan American games in 1955, running times for distances exceeding 1,500 meters were about 10 percent longer than at sea level (Fig. 11.5).

Decrements in physical performance at extreme altitudes are related in various ways to a number of conditions, as described below.

Cardiac output

Upon ascent to high altitude cardiac output is transiently increased both at rest and during exercise, sometimes by as much as 23 percent over sea level values. The increase is due to sympathetic stimulation initiated by hypoxia.[5] Over the first week at altitude cardiac output decreases so that at the end of ten days stroke volume and cardiac output during submaximum exercise are about 14 percent lower than at sea level.[8,9] The initial studies on this subject by Alexander and his colleagues utilizing the Fick principle were subsequently confirmed by echocardiography.[10] Wolfel and his associates found a 25 percent decrease in cardiac output during exercise in seven normal men after 21 days at 14,110 feet (4,300 m); resting cardiac output decreased by 17 percent.[11] The decrease in cardiac output was not due to a decrease in plasma volume, since by 21 days, red cell volume had increased so that total blood volume was the same as it was at sea level. Leg blood flow was decreased during exercise by 18 percent which is proportional to the decrease in cardiac output.[11]

Conflicting results have been reported on whether or not the decrease in cardiac output persists over longer periods of time at high altitude. During Operation Ever-

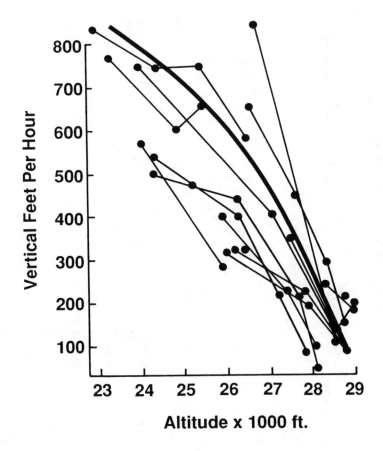

Fiure. 11.2. Climbing rates from 23,000 feet (7,015 m) to 29,000 feet (8,850 m) compiled from various expeditions. Although some of the climbers used oxygen, there was no significant difference in their climb rate and those data points are not identified. Heavy line = mean. Redrawn from T. Holzel, "Oxygen Use on Mt. Everest: An Atlantic Alpine Club report," Summit 1984; March-April:20-25.

est II (OE II) cardiac output was determined by the Fick method and two dimensional echocardiography at rest and during exercise at extreme altitudes in a hypobaric chamber.[10,12] Although stroke volume was reduced, an increase in heart rate maintained cardiac output within normal limits both at rest and during a given work load of exercise even as high as a simulated altitude of 25,000 feet (7,625 m). The subjects in OE II were well acclimatized, which may explain the discrepancy between Wolfel's studies[11] and the studies of Alexander and Grover.[8,9] Pugh and his associates also reported that cardiac output at 19,000 feet (5,800 m) in acclimatized subjects was the same as at sea level for a given work intensity.[13] These data indicate that, even though cardiac output at rest and during exercise may be reduced

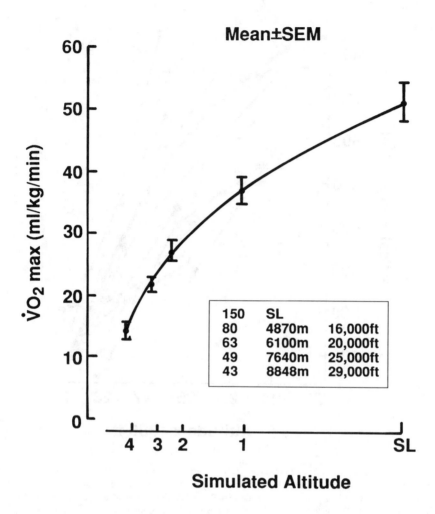

Figure 11.3. Maximum oxygen consumption (VO_{2max}) at sea level and four simulated altitudes in eight normal subjects. SL = sea level. Redrawn from Sutton et al., ref. 4.

after several days at high altitude, there is no evidence that a low cardiac output is responsible for a limitation of exercise performance. There is also no evidence that left ventricular function is impaired. In OE II, for example, during maximum exercise at a simulated altitude of 25,000 feet (7,625 m), left ventricular function remained normal.[10,12]

Pulmonary Hypertension

The above observations, as explained, apply to physically fit subjects who can tolerate extreme altitudes without difficulty. It is possible that persons who tolerate

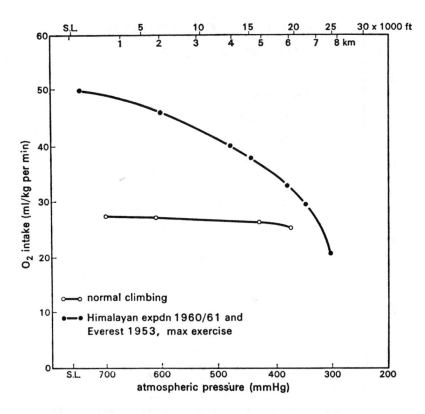

Figure 11.4. Maximum oxygen uptake at various altitudes and oxygen uptake of men walking uphill at their usual pace. This pace can be maintained in acclimatized men up to about 20,000 feet (6,100 m). Redrawn from Pugh, ref. 3.

altitude poorly may have physiological abnormalities that limit their cardiac output response to exercise. One of these is marked pulmonary hypertension. At extreme altitude pulmonary hypertension may be severe, especially during exercise. In OE II mean pulmonary artery pressures of 54 mm Hg were observed during exercise at a simulated altitude of 25,000 feet (7,625 m). Pulmonary vascular resistance at rest was 4.3 units compared with 1.3 units at sea level.[12] Even at the modest altitude of 13,400 feet (4,090 m) a mean exercise pulmonary artery pressure of 29 mm Hg was recorded by Vogel.[14] The obstruction to blood flow by the pulmonary vascular bed under these conditions could limit cardiac output and thus exercise performance. A sea-level analogy of this phenomenon is primary pulmonary hypertension or thromboembolic pulmonary hypertension, where both resting and exercise cardiac outputs are reduced.[15] The effect of pulmonary vascular obstruction in limiting cardiac output is illustrated by the observation that in thromboembolic pulmonary hypertension, cardiac output increases when pulmonary artery pressure is lowered by thrombectomy. In 34 patients with thromboembolic pulmonary hypertension, thrombectomy lowered the mean pulmonary artery pressure from 49 mm Hg to 27 mm with a fall in pulmonary vascular resistance from 997 dynes/sec/cm^{-5}. Cardiac

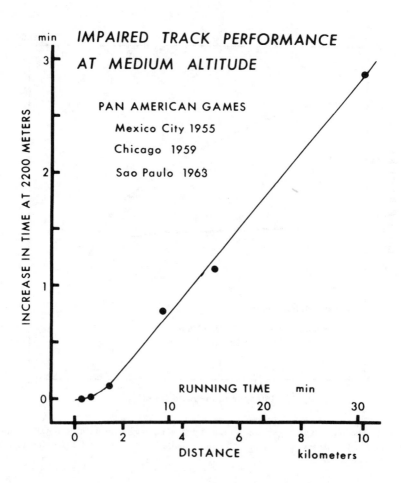

Figure 11.5. Average time in minutes (abscissa) for running distances from 100 to 1,000 meters as established at sea level during the Pan American Games in Chicago, 1959, and Saó Paulo, 1963. Times were significantly increased (ordinate) at the medium altitude in Mexico City, 7,216 feet (2,200 m). Reprinted with permission from Grover and Reeves, ref. 7.

output increased from 3.8 to 5.92 L/min (p = 0.001).[16] In primary pulmonary hypertension diltiazem inhibits hypoxic pulmonary vasoconstriction and this is accompanied by an increase in cardiac output.[17] In pulmonary hypertension due to chronic obstructive pulmonary disease, pulmonary artery pressure is lowered by hydralazine. This is accompanied by an increase in cardiac output at rest and during exercise.[18]

Adenosine has recently been shown to be a potent vasodilator of the pulmonary circulation in primary pulmonary hypertension. Adenosine has no effect on the systemic circulation. The administration of adenosine results in a rapid decrease in pulmonary artery pressure and resistance with an increase in cardiac output.[19] The increase in cardiac output could be related to an acute reduction in right ventricular afterload, as suggested by the authors. McKenzie and his colleagues observed an increase in right ventricular ejection fraction from 38 percent to 48 percent in Peruvian natives brought from 13,780 feet (4,200 m) to sea level.[20] They suggested that the improvement in right ventricular function was due to a decrease in afterload, that is, a fall in pulmonary artery pressure.

Right ventricular dysfunction. One result of pulmonary hypertension at high altitude is an increase in the work of the right ventricle. Enlargement of the right ventricle and paradoxial septal motion have been demonstrated by echocardiography.[10] Is it possible that the high pressure work load of the right ventricle during exercise at high altitude may result in right ventricular failure or dysfunction and thus limit cardiac output? Khaja and Parker's studies at sea level in patients with pulmonary hypertension and pulmonary disease suggest such a connection.[21] They found that right ventricular diastolic pressure was normal at rest but became elevated during exercise. Left ventricular diastolic pressure remained normal. The cardiac output increased by 27 percent in normal subjects but by only 4 percent in the patients with pulmonary disease; in the latter group, the mean pulmonary artery pressure was 30 mm Hg at rest and 52 mm Hg during exercise. Berger found a decrease in right ventricular ejection fraction during exercise in a similar study.[22] The effect of severe exercise at 9,318 feet (2,842 m) upon right ventricular function was studied in 23 runners participating in a 100-mile race. In five runners evidence of right ventricular dysfunction was found as evident by right ventricular dilatation, depressed function of the right ventricular free wall and paradoxical septal motion compatible with right ventricular pressure and volume overload. Pulmonary artery systolic pressure increased from 28 to 55 mm Hg. One runner with severe right ventricular dysfunction had a pulmonary artery systolic pressure of 65 mm Hg. The ventricular dysfunction resolved in 24 hours.[23]

Few studies have been made of right ventricular function at high altitude. In OE II right ventricular diastolic pressure was normal at rest and during exercise.[12] Hemodynamic studies in patients with high altitude pulmonary edema have revealed normal resting right atrial and right ventricular diastolic pressure.[24] I have seen one patient with high altitude pulmonary edema who had transient atrial flutter. This arrhythmia is commonly associated with an increased right atrial pressure.[25] In view of the limited amount of data, the concept that transient right ventricular dysfunction may limit cardiac output and exercise performance at high altitude must, for the time being, remain speculative.

Tricuspid insufficiency. Recent Doppler echocardiographic studies have shown that in patients with pulmonary hypertension tricuspid insufficiency of a variable degree is almost always present.[26] Exercise may increase the degree of regurgitation if pulmonary hypertension is present. The effect of tricuspid regurgitation during exercise would be to limit the normal increase in cardiac output. Tricuspid insufficiency was not observed in the OE II subjects at rest but no determinations were made during exercise.[10] Doppler studies during exercise at high altitude are clearly indicated to determine whether or not significant tricuspid regurgitation is present.

Reflex effects. Pressure sensitive receptors are present in the walls of the main pulmonary artery and right ventricle, and could reflexly decrease cardiac contractility and systemic vascular resistance when the intravascular pressure during exercise reaches a threshold value. Coleridge and his associates demonstrated pressure sensitive receptors in the pulmonary arteries of rabbits that reflexly lowered peripheral resistance when stimulated.[27] In patients with primary pulmonary hypertension, exercise often results in a fall in systemic blood pressure resulting in dizziness or syncope due to the effect of increased pressure on the right sided baroceptors. It should be noted that the importance of the baroceptors in the human heart and central vessels in circulatory control is still controversial.

Pulmonary Edema

It is possible that during maximum physical exertion at extreme altitudes varying degrees of pulmonary edema occur and may limit climbing ability. Subjects with a history of high altitude pulmonary edema who are brought to high altitude (10,200 feet/3,110 m) have exhibited an abnormal rise in pulmonary artery pressure and an abnormal fall in arterial oxygen saturation during exercise, despite the absence of symptoms or signs of high altitude pulmonary edema.[28] Even at medium altitudes distance runners will exhibit an increase in lung water after completion of a race, suggesting the presence of pulmonary edema.[29] Normal subjects brought to 14,000 feet (4,270 m) and exercising daily exhibit a decrease in vital capacity and transthoracic electrical impedance compatible with an increase in intrathoracic vascular fluid volume followed by a more gradual increase in extravascular fluid volume.[29,30]

Pulmonary edema limiting climbing performance has been noted by several experienced climbers. One climber who never before had high altitude pulmonary edema developed mild high altitude pulmonary edema on a rapid climb of Mount McKinley (20,300 feet/6,190 m) from Kalhitna Pass, 10,000 feet (3,050 m). The final 2,000 feet (610 m) of easy climbing required seven hours. During the descent and later that night typical gurgling pulmonary sounds of high altitude pulmonary edema were noted.[31] Recurrent pulmonary edema limiting climbing performance has been described by Irvin.[32] On the American Medical Research Expedition to Everest one experienced, acclimatized climber developed high altitude pulmonary edema during a rapid ascent to about 20,000 feet (6,100 m) and recovered when he was assisted to a lower altitude.[33] Two of the most important symptoms of high altitude pulmonary edema are marked weakness and fatigue associated with severe dyspnea. Some Everest climbers have noted that such symptoms and signs of high altitude pulmonary edema may be present in many climbers in the evening after returning from a strenuous day of climbing. These manifestations are absent in the morning after sleeping with low flow oxygen. Vachiery and associates studied hypoxic vasoconstriction in seven subjects with a prior history of HAPE. Only two had an abnormal hypoxic rise in pulmonary artery pressure. Of greater interest was the response of nine climbers who had successfully climbed to 19,680 feet (6,000 m) and 29,000 feet (8,842 m). Their response to hypoxia was less than normal subjects suggesting that successful climbers to extreme altitudes have a lower pulmonary artery pressure than others.[34] It is possible that these climbers do not develop subclinical pulmonary edema which would limit their exercise capacity.

Pugh and his associates observed large individual variations in calculated alveolar-arterial PO_2 gradients in acclimatized subjects who exercised at 19,000 feet (5,795 m) at Mingbo in the Himalayas.[13] These large gradients could be due to subclinical high altitude pulmonary edema, and this possibility is supported by the observations of one of the authors, who had a low diffusing capacity and raced a companion uphill for fifteen minutes starting at 15,300 feet (4,667 m); toward the end of the race he felt as though he could not expand his lungs fully, and on resting he developed a cough with sputum. Studies of OE II have also provided a valuable insight into the possibility that subclinical pulmonary edema is common in normal subjects at extreme altitudes and can limit physical performance. All subjects in OE II had a wide alveolar-arterial oxygen difference that was compatible with a right-to-left intrapulmonary shunt equivalent to approximately 25 percent of the cardiac output. The gradient also increased after rapid ascent from one altitude level to a higher level. The gradient increased during exercise. Oxygen breathing did not reverse the abnormality. Considerable individual differences were noted.[35,4] These observations suggest that even acclimatized high altitude climbers may be close to high altitude pulmonary edema that could reduce climbing speed and could become severe if a period of unusually heavy exertion were carried out.

Pulmonary Ventilation

The importance of pulmonary ventilation at extreme altitudes is illustrated by the observation that intense dyspnea and very high respiratory rates accompany physical exercise and these are major factors limiting one's climbing rate. At high altitude, ventilation during maximum exercise increases in proportion to the altitude

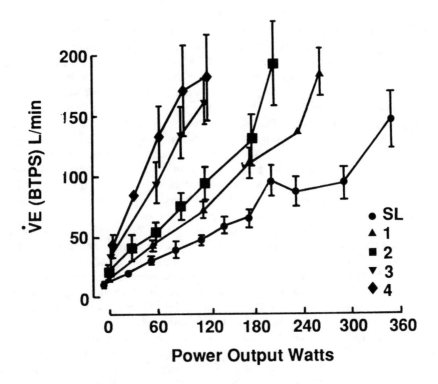

Figure 11.6. Ventilation during exercise in normal subjects at various simulated altitudes. SL - sea level; 1 - 16,000 feet; 2 - 20,000 feet; 3 - 25,000 feet; 4 - 29,000 feet. Redrawn from Wagner et al., ref. 35.

(Fig. 11.6). Very high ventilatory volumes occur during exercise at extreme altitudes. At 21,000 feet (6,400 m) on Mount Everest during maximum exertion on a cycle ergometer, a ventilation volume of 207 L/min was recorded at a work load of 1,200 kg/m/minute. Performing the same work at sea level ventilation was only 160 L/min. At 27,000 feet (8,235 m) during climbing one climber had a ventilatory volume of 107 L/min per minute BTP's and a respiratory rate of 86 per minute. This level of ventilation is lower than the 159 L/min that was achieved during maximum work on a cycle ergometer at a simulated similar altitude.[36] Pugh has pointed out that climbers usually select an oxygen uptake of 50-75 percent of their maximum for normal climbing at altitudes up to 19,680 feet (6,000 m).[37] Pulmonary ventilation may limit exercise performance at extreme altitude by several mechanisms, including respiratory muscle fatigue, the work of breathing, and hypoxic ventilatory response.

Respiratory muscle fatigue. A traditional concept proposes that, since maximum voluntary ventilation at rest is about twice the ventilatory rate during exercise at high altitude, a considerable respiratory reserve is available to the climber and therefore ventilation is not a factor that limits physical performance under these conditions. In addition, during heavy exercise, the pressure changes in the thorax are less than 30 percent of those attained during maximum voluntary ventilation. This concept has an inherent fallacy in that it assumes that high levels of maximum voluntary ventilation can be sustained. In fact, such levels cannot be sustained for more than a few seconds. Even levels of 55-80 percent of maximum voluntary ventilation can be maintained for only four or five minutes. At such levels of ventilation both inspiratory and expiratory muscles become fatigued. Thus, under conditions of hypoxia at high altitude, it is quite possible that respiratory muscle fatigue limits the amount of ventilation that can be performed for extended periods of time.

Work of breathing. Muscles of ventilation constitute about 6.7 percent of total body weight and require about 2.5 ml oxygen per minute at rest or about 1-2 percent of total body oxygen consumption. During voluntary hyperventilation at rest at a level of approximately 130 L/min per minute the oxygen consumption of the ventilatory pump increases to about 570 ml/min, or about 14 percent of the total body oxygen consumption, assuming a cardiac output of 6 L/min. During running or other heavy exercise at sea level, ventilation rarely approaches 130 L/min for long periods of time. Under such conditions total body oxygen consumption may be increased by as much as ten times, but the oxygen required for ventilation is still only a relatively small percentage of total body oxygen consumption.[38] Johnson and his workers examined the oxygen cost of breathing in trained endurance athletes and concluded that during maximum exercise such individuals often reach mechanical limits for lung and respiratory muscles in producing adequate alveolar ventilation. They suggested that respiratory muscle fatigue could occur at high ventilatory rates with a significant steal of oxygen from muscles of locomotion amounting to as much as 13 percent of VO_2 max. (range 11-16 percent.[39]

At high altitude, ventilation increases over sea level values for each work level and may be as high as 200 L/min for short, maximum exercise periods. For example, at sea level a work rate requiring 1.5 liters of oxygen per minute requires a ventilation of approximately 36 L/min. At 24,000 feet (7,320 m) a ventilation of approximately 122 L/min is associated with the same level of exercise. This high level of ventilation is partly due to hypoxic stimulation. The lower air density at high altitude decreases the work of breathing compared with sea level values at similar levels of ventilation; but, at high altitude the maximum oxygen capacity or working capacity of the body decreases, so that the oxygen cost of ventilation occupies a greater percentage of total oxygen consumption. It has been estimated that on the summit of Mount Everest, the oxygen cost of breathing at rest may require more than half the total oxygen consumed, so that very little oxygen is left over for sustained physical activity. The work of breathing may be further increased by the lower compliance of the lungs, owing to subclinical pulmonary edema.

Hypoxic ventilatory response. The level of ventilation attained during acute hypoxia at rest and during exercise with arterial PCO_2 kept constant is a measure of the "hypoxic ventilatory response." There was considerable individual variation in this response in members of the American Medical Research Expedition to Mount Everest and its relation to exercise performance.[40] Subjects were grouped according to high or low responders to hypoxia during sea level studies. After acclimatization at 21,000 feet (6,405 m), exercise ventilation was higher in the high-responder group and the decrease in blood oxygen saturation during exercise was less: 8.3 percent versus a 20.0 percent decrease. The climbers with the highest hypoxic ventilatory response reached and slept at higher altitudes. The response to hypoxia was not changed at altitude. Schoene and Masuyama also reported that a high hypoxic ventilatory response was associated with better function at extreme altitudes.[40,41]

These results must be interpreted with caution. Milledge and coworkers found that the ventilatory response of experienced high altitude climbers to hypoxic exercise at sea level was lower that that of nonclimbing scientists, and they concluded that there is little relationship between the hypoxic ventilatory response and the ability to perform well at extreme altitude.[42] Also, several studies have shown that men native to high altitude have a reduced hypoxic ventilatory response, and Hackett and his workers showed that Sherpas, too, have a reduced hypoxic ventilatory response.[43] A low hypoxic ventilatory response has been associated with an increased susceptibility to acute mountain sickness and high altitude pulmonary edema.[44,45]

A low hypoxic ventilatory response will be accompanied by a decreased work of breathing and will result in a lower arterial oxygen saturation during exercise. These studies indicate that maintaining a higher arterial oxygen saturation during climbing is probably more important than the additional work of breathing incurred with a high response.

Central Nervous System

There are, however, two important factors that may limit exercise performance: hypoxemia and the work of breathing, and both may affect the central nervous system and efferent impulses to exercising muscles.

Arterial PO_2 during exercise at a hypobaric chamber altitude equivalent to that of Mount Everest was 28 mm Hg.[12] This degree of hypoxemia combined with the associated severe alkalosis (pH 7.52) could adversely affect central nervous system control over muscle performance and result in weakness, fatigue, and lack of coordinations.[46] Saltin and his coworkers also suggested that exercise at high altitude may be limited by a centrally controlled reduction in leg blood flow owing to regional vasoconstriction. This would conserve cardiac output and direct blood flow to the muscles of respiration and vital organs. The reduction in leg blood flow induced by this mechanism could result in leg weakness and fatigue.[46] Support for this concept is derived from experiments by Secher and his workers, who determined cardiac output and leg blood flow during cycle exercise for ten minutes after which arm exercise was added. The final oxygen uptake was approximately 80 percent of maximum O_2 uptake. After arm exercise began, leg blood flow was reduced by almost 2 L/min despite an elevated leg muscle tissue concentration of lactate.[47] The results of the experiment are shown in Figure 11.7. Bigland-Ritchie and Vollestad have proposed a similar mechanism.[48]

Patients with congestive heart failure and left ventricular dysfunction exhibit a reduction in blood flow to the legs during exercise compared with subjects without

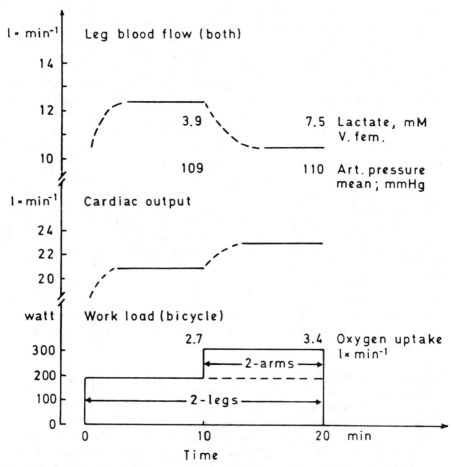

Figure 11.7. A possible explanation of leg weakness limiting exercise at high altitudes. Secher and his workers measured cardiac output and leg blood flow during exercise on a cycle ergometer. Exercise was performed with both legs for ten minutes after which arm exercise was added. The final oxygen uptake during the end of exercise was about 3.4 L/min, representing about 80 percent of the subject's maximum oxygen uptake. Cardiac output increased by about 2 L/min. when arm exercise was added. At that time leg blood flow was reduced by almost 2 L/min to supply the upper body with blood. Leg muscle tissue lactate increased but still leg flow decreased. Redrawn from Secher et al., ref. 47.

% Cardiac Output to Legs

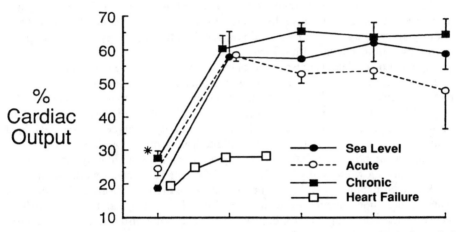

Figure 11.8. Leg blood flow as a percentage of cardiac output during exercise at sea level, after arrival at 14,110 feet (4,300 m) (open circles, acute), and after 21 days at altitude (solid squares, chronic). No change in the percentage of the cardiac output going to the exercising legs occurred at high altitude.[11] The open squares (heart failure) represent the reduction in leg blood flow during exercise in patients with congestive failure. Redrawn from Roubin et al., ref. 49.

failure. The reduction in leg blood flow is greater than the reduction in total cardiac output (Fig. 11.8). This mechanism also serves to divert blood flow to other vascular beds.[49]

In another experiment, Wolfel and his associates measured cardiac output at rest and during exercise in seven men at sea level, upon arrival at 14,110 feet (4,300 m), and after 21 days at that altitude.[11] Leg blood flow was also measured. Cardiac output at rest and during exercise (to the same level as at sea level) was decreased at 21 days by about 18 percent and exercise cardiac output was decreased by about 21 percent. The percentage of the cardiac output measured as leg blood flow was, however, the same as at sea level, upon arrival at high altitude, and at 21 days. The results of Wolfel's studies are shown in Figure 11.8. Unlike Secher's experiment, arm exercise was not added during leg exercise so the conditions of the study were different. Secher's concept is interesting and further studies are needed to support his theory.

Maximum Oxygen Consumption

Maximum oxygen consumption (VO_2 max) is a commonly used measure of physical working capacity, measured usually during treadmill or cycle ergometric exercise. The O_2 consumption can be roughly estimated by nomograms from the speed, grade and duration of exercise or the work load. In the Bruce continuous exercise treadmill protocol, a VO_2 max of 50 ml/kg/min is achieved by three minutes of jogging or running on a 16 percent grade at 4.2 miles per hour. This can be attained only by active, physically fit persons. Sedentary persons usually reach a VO_2 max of about 35-38 ml/kg/min.[50] For comparison, easy walking on the level requires a VO$_2$ of 7-10 ml/kg/min. Some workers report VO$_2$ max in terms of L/min. Thus an active person weighing 80 kg will have a VO$_2$ max of 50 ml/kg/min or about 4 liters of O$_2$ per minute. Some long distance runners can attain a VO$_2$max of over 80 ml/kg/min. Because this exercise involves both arm and leg work, cross country skiers may attain slightly higher levels. Maximum oxygen consumption decreases with increasing altitude (Fig. 11.3).

Application of data from treadmill or cycle tests to climbing performance should be made with caution, since climbing with a pack and using arm muscles involves more isometric work of legs, trunk, and arms than running does (Fig. 11-9). If, for example, one pedals an upright cycle ergometer using only arm and shoulder muscles, the peak work load that can be attained is only 41 percent of the peak load while pedaling the cycle with the legs. Fatigue from arm work will occur at a lower oxygen consumption than fatigue from leg work; and the circulatory effect of arm work versus leg work is also considerably different. For a given work output, arm work is accompanied by a higher heart rate and a higher systolic blood pressure than those attained during leg work, meaning, of course, greater cardiac work.[51] These observations apply particularly to rock and ice climbing, which require strenuous arm work.

A high VO$_2$ max can usually identify persons with greater endurance during a climb, but an important additional factor is the actual amount of energy used in

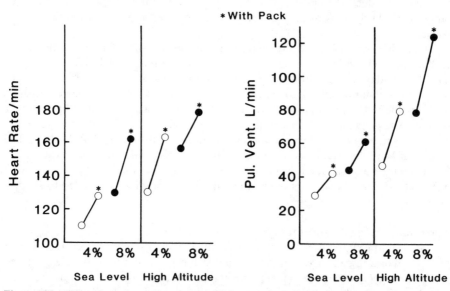

Effect of Carrying a 20Kg Pack on a Treadmill at 4% to 8% Grade 3.4 mph at Sea Level and 14,000 ft

Figure 11.9. Effect of carrying a 40 pound (20 kg) load on the back while walking on a treadmill at a steady pace at sea level and at 14,110 feet (4,300 m). A 4 percent grade is compared with an 8 percent grade. Treadmill speed is constant at 3.4 miles per hour. Note the marked increases in heart rate and ventilation. The first point in each panel represents walking without a pack. These conditions simulate climbing activity more accurately then walking without a pack. Redrawn from Consolazio et al., ref. 81.

climbing or the energy efficiency of the climber. For example, during a marathon run the fraction of VO_2 max that is utilized for most of the distance is about 75 percent. Fast running times in marathons are related not only to VO_2 max but also to running economy, that is, using substantially less oxygen during the race.[52] It is believed that climbers at extreme altitudes must have a VO_2 max at sea level of at least 50 ml/kg/min to be able to attain major summits with safety during daylight hours. Climbers usually choose an oxygen uptake of one-half to three-fourths of their maximum for normal climbing at extreme altitudes.[13]

The VO_2 max measured at or near sea level in six climbers who have made 27 summits higher than 26,240 feet (8,000 m) had a mean value of 56.5 ml/kg/min. The lowest value was 46 ml/kg/min.[42] During training before the climb, one of the climbers who reached the top of Everest without oxygen was able to run a distance of 4.38 km while ascending 3,000 feet (822 m) in 35 minutes with a calculated oxygen uptake of 64 ml/kg/min. If one assumes that no more than 70-80 percent of VO_2 can be sustained for more than a few minutes, this would result in a VO_2 of about 80 ml/min—this is about 25-30 percent higher than that of top Himalayan mountaineers of the 1980's.[42] Studies from the American Research Expedition to Everest indicate that at an equivalent altitude of 29,028 feet (8,848 m) the mean maximum oxygen uptake of two subjects was 1.07 L/min or 15.3 ml/kg^{-1}/min^{-1}. At sea level the mean value in five subjects was 4.63 L/min or 61.3 ml/kg^{-1}/ min^{-1}.[36] Climbers with a VO_2 max of >50 ml/kg/ min at sea level might be able to sustain as much as 10-12 ml/kg/min on the summit of Everest, which would permit the summit to be attained without oxygen.[53]

Attractive though it may be to consider that persons with a high VO_2 max at sea level will perform better at extreme altitudes, this has not been consistently demonstrated. Several top Himalayan climbers have sea level VO_2 values that are in the average range. Messner, for example, had a VO_2 max of 46 ml/ kg/min. In OE II, two of the subjects with the highest VO_2 max values at sea level (64 ml and 61 ml) developed the greatest VA/Q mismatches at 25,000 feet (7,625 m) and had to be withdrawn from the study.[35]

Pulmonary Gas Exchange

At high altitude arterial oxygen tension is decreased at rest and is further decreased during exercise. The decrease observed during exercise at extreme altitudes is so marked that this may an important factor limiting physical performance. (Fig. 11.10). Four general features of pulmonary gas exchange are involved in this phenomenon:

1. The low PO_2 of inspired air, which is proportional to the altitude and only partly compensated for by an increase in ventilation.

2. The diffusing capacity of the lung. There is a wide range of diffusing capacities in normal subjects with a mean value of about 40/ml/min/mm Hg (range 37- 59). The Sherpa Dawa Tensing had a diffusing capacity of 100 ml/min/mm Hg. Compared with normal values this would almost double the effective oxygen transfer on the summit of Everest from approximately 450 ml/min/ mm Hg to 750 ml.[54] It is likely that successful Himalayan climbers have higher than normal diffusing capacities.

3. The A-a gradient, that is, the pressure gradient of oxygen from the alveolus to the arterialized end of the pulmonary capillary is small at rest (6-8 mm) and becomes

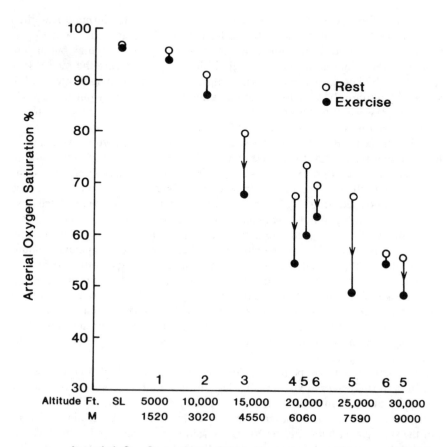

Arterial O$_2$ Saturation Rest–Exercise at Various Altitudes

Figure 11.10. Decrease in arterial oxygen saturation at rest (open circles), and during exercise (closed circles) at various altitudes. The other values were obtained during submaximum exercise. From J Wilkerson, ed., *Medicine for Mountaineering*, 3rd ed., Seattle: Mountaineers; and other references.

even smaller with exercise (2-3 mm). At extreme altitude this gradient becomes greater during exercise, probably because the velocity of the red cells traversing the capillaries is so great that complete oxygenation of the red cells cannot occur. It has been estimated that on the summit of Everest a 7 mm gradient is present between alveolar gas and capillary blood. This is particularly important because at that altitude arterial PO$_2$ is only 28 mm Hg. The marked decrease in arterial PO$_2$ is partly compensated for by the severe respiratory alkalosis and the resulting left shift of the oxygen dissociation curve, which maintains the arterial oxygen saturation; a saturation of 72 percent was estimated to be present on the summit of Mount Everest, a value similar to that determined at 24,000 feet (7,320 m).[53,54,55]

4. Ventilation/Perfusion mismatch (VA/Q). In the normally functioning lung all ventilated areas are perfused, so that ventilation and perfusion are "matched." A

mismatch occurs when ventilated areas are not perfused or when perfused areas are not ventilated. The latter problem occurs at high altitude especially in patients with high altitude pulmonary edema (HAPE), in which fluid in the interstitial tissues or alveoli of the lung blocks oxygen transfer. In OE II a VA/Q mismatch was present in all eight subjects and amounted to the equivalent of approximately 25 percent of the cardiac output transversing the lungs without oxygenation. The abnormality was greater with higher altitudes and was more pronounced after a rapid ascent, and it was increased during exercise.[35,4] As discussed earlier, the most likely explanation for the abnormality was interstitial pulmonary edema.

Blood Viscosity

There is little evidence that modest changes in blood viscosity observed in climbers at extreme altitudes significantly affect physical performance. Hematocrits above 60 percent are rarely present under these conditions. Peruvian natives with chronic mountain polycythemia may have hematocrits as high as 70 percent without any evidence of impaired physical performance. *In vitro* studies have shown no impairment in oxygen delivery to perfused canine hind limbs with hematocrits up to 70 percent.[56] On the basis of these observations, it was suggested that the ideal hematocrit for oxygen delivery during exercise might be 50-60 percent instead of the generally accepted value of 40-45 percent.

Hemodilution

Hemodilution at high altitude may affect exercise performance.[58] Horstman and colleagues reduced the hematocrit of five subjects by removal of 450 ml of blood and replacement with Ringer's lactate solution after two weeks at 4,300 mm. They observed a decrease in VO_2 max and an 8 percent increase in cardiac output during maximal exercise.[58] The oxygen carrying capacity of the blood had been reduced by 13 percent. The changes in hematocrit achieved in these studies were small, however: a decrease from 52.7 percent to 47.7 percent compared with a sea level value of 46.4 percent.

Sarnquist and his associates performed isovolumetric hemodilution in four acclimatized climbers at 17,700 feet (5,400 m) at the Mount Everest base camp. Approximately 15 percent of blood volume was removed and replaced with an equal volume of 5 percent human albumen solution with a reduction in hematocrit from 58 percent to 51 percent. Cycle ergometry was performed before and after the procedure. There were no changes in maximum work level, oxygen uptake, minute ventilation, or blood oxygen saturation (earpiece oximetry), and heart rate increased insignificantly, from 140 to 144 beats per minute. A significant but small improvement was observed in psychological tests. One subject developed a transient allergic reaction to the albumen infusion.[59] These studies indicate that hemodilution confers little significant advantage in physical performance to high altitude climbers and may be dangerous. In addition it appears that at hematocrit levels of 50-60 percent blood viscosity does not limit physical performance. Cardiac output increases after hemodilution in persons with a high hematocrit.[57] This does not indicate that viscosity has impaired cardiac output. Lindenfeld and her colleagues have shown that systemic oxygen transport is well preserved in dogs at rest and during exercise with increasing hematocrits up to 65 percent.[60] The increase in cardiac output following hemodilution is a normal response to maintain optimum oxygen delivery. For high altitude residents with chronic mountain sickness, hemodilution may have more beneficial effects upon exercise performance.[61]

Plasma Volume

A decrease in plasma volume occurs during ascent to high altitude, but over the course of the high altitude stay, red cell mass increases so that total blood volume is restored to normal. This was the finding of Wolfel and his associates, who tested subjects for 21 days at 14,110 feet (4,300 m); after that time, red cell volume had increased and total blood volume had been restored to the sea level, pre-ascent value.[11] After one to two months plasma volume may also be restored to pre-ascent values. The effect of the initial decrease in plasma volume upon physical performance appears to be partly responsible for the decrease in cardiac output during the first two weeks at high altitude.[5] Dehydration during strenuous climbs at extreme altitude, often a consequence of increased water loss and inadequate fluid replacement, may result in a decrease in plasma volume, which could in turn result in a reduced cardiac output during exercise. The magnitude of the decrease in plasma volume under these conditions is not known, but it can be inferred from changes in the hematocrit. Zink has reported an increase in hematocrit from 55 to 61 percent in one subject during a six-day climb from 18,200 feet (5,550 m) to 27,683 feet (8,440 m) with an associated weight loss of 6 kg. Plasma volume was estimated to have decreased by 25 percent and total body water decreased by 16 percent.[57] Hackett has recorded hematocrits exceeding 70 percent in four New Zealand climbers on Mount Everest.[62] Zink has recommended hemodilution to avoid this problem. It has been shown that a decrease in blood volume in normal subjects by bed rest or venesection or in cardiac patients by diuretics will lower cardiac output during exercise and will result in a decrease in physical working capacity.[5,63,64] Further studies of blood volume changes during climbing are necessary to determine the prevalence and magnitude of decreases in plasma volume, to examine the effect of dehydration upon such changes, and to determine the effect of changes in plasma volume on the cardiac output response to exercise.

Lactic Acid-Blood Lactate

The most abundant product of anaerobic metabolism in the exercising muscles is lactic acid, which diffuses into and accumulates in the blood during exercise. The level of blood lactate is proportional to the severity of exercise.[65] A rise in blood lactate and lactic acid indicates that the circulation to the exercising muscles is insufficient to meet the metabolic demands of the energy-producing pathways. In severe shock with a reduced blood flow to resting muscle, lactate and a lactic acidosis may also occur. Lactate is cleared from the blood largely by metabolism in the liver and also by other tissues, including inactive muscle. With exhausting exercise, blood lactate may rise rapidly and is cleared from the blood more slowly. For example, a champion athlete after a one-mile race had a rise in blood lactate to 175 mg/ml/100 ml. Forty minutes after the race the blood lactate had fallen to the pre-race level of 10 mg/100 ml. Following exhausting exercise arterial pH may fall to as low as 7.0.[65] One might have expected that exhausting exercise at extreme altitudes and under conditions of severe hypoxia would result in abnormal elevations of lactic acid that might limit performance, but this does not occur.

In 1936 Edwards first noted that exhaustive exercise at very high altitude was accompanied by only a very small rise in blood lactate.[66] This observation has since been confirmed by many workers and the phenomenon is known as "the lactate paradox." During exhausting exercise blood and muscle lactate are progressively reduced as altitude increases. For example, at sea level blood lactate at maximum exercise increases to about 13 mmol/L, whereas at 25,000 feet (7,600 m) in a hypobaric chamber blood lactate was only 5 mmol/L.[67] In high altitude natives even within the first few weeks after descent to sea level blood lactate does not rise during exercise. Intracellular pH in these natives did not decrease as much as in sea level natives during exercise.[68]

The mechanism of the lactate paradox remains unknown, but several factors may be involved: (1) maximum exercise at very high altitude is substantially less than at sea level[67]; (2) the rate of efflux from muscle to blood and the rate of clearance by the liver and other tissues may be different; (3) the markedly reduced bicarbonate may inhibit efflux of lactate to the blood; (4) there may be a reduced level of glycogenolysis in muscle.[69]

Acclimatization

Major aspects of man's adaptation to exercise at extreme altitudes have been studied by Sutton and his colleagues in OE II, with the help of eight normal young men who were placed in a hypobaric chamber in a 40-day simulated ascent to an altitude equivalent to the summit of Mount Everest and who performed maximum exercise at several simulated altitudes using a cycle ergometer.[12,35,4] It was found that as the oxygen pressure in inspired air (PIO_2) decreased, maximum oxygen uptake also decreased, from 3.98 L/min to 1.17 L/min. At 60 Watts of exercise (oxygen consumption 927 ml/min) at a PIO_2 of 43 mm, arterial PO_2 was 28 mm, PCO_2 was 11 mm, and mixed venous PO_2 was 14.8 mm. Arterial oxygen saturation was 51 percent and pH 7.55. The most important adaptations to such extreme conditions were: (1) a fourfold increase in alveolar ventilation, (2) increased diffusion of oxygen from capillaries to tissue mitochondria, (3) no change in cardiac output compared with sea level except for a moderate increase at the highest altitude, and (4) no change in diffusion from alveolar air to capillary blood. Significant tissue adaptations coupled with the above responses permitted acclimatized man to exercise efficiently at 29,000 feet (8,845 m).

Most successful climbers of the 26,240 feet (8,000 m) peaks in the Himalayas achieve adequate acclimatization during the four-to-eight week period of gradual ascent to elevations of 17,000-21,000 feet (5,185-6,400 m), including load carrying and the establishment of higher camps. Since it is well known that deterioration occurs at elevations above 18,000 feet (5,490 m), current climbing strategies involve short stays at high camps and periodic visits to lower elevations. The most effective acclimatization altitude for efficient climbing at extreme altitudes has not been determined, but it is probably between 14,000 and 16,000 feet (4,270-4,880 m). Pre-ascent exposure in hypobaric chambers such as those used by the Japanese and the French may provide rapid acclimatization with resulting more rapid ascent.[70,71] It has been shown that persons born and living at altitudes of 4,000-6,000 feet (1,220-1,830 m) in the United States are less susceptible than sea level residents to acute mountain sickness during acute exposure to 14,000 feet (4,270 m) in a chamber,[72] but there are no data to indicate that such persons are any more or less successful than sea-level residents in climbing at extreme altitudes.

Physical Conditioning

Clearly, physical conditioning is an important aspect of climbing ability, but opinions vary as to the degree of physical fitness and type of training that are needed. Some successful climbers have very vigorous training schedules before an expedition; others gain most of their physical fitness during the several weeks of the approach march and the setting up of routes and camps. Running may not be the most effective training exercise, since it involves primarily isotonic aerobic exercise. Muscle biopsies have shown that climbers and athletes engaged in heavy resistance or isometric exercise have more slow-twitch muscle fibers compared with runners or jumpers, who have a preponderance of fast-twitch fibers.[73] In general, training should consist of the type of exercise that will be performed during actual climbing: carrying a moderate load in a backpack up and down hills would seem preferable to running. It is not known whether such a training regimen is equally effective at sea level or at high altitude, but logistics usually dictate that most of the training will be done at the altitude of the climber's home residence.

The Heart at High Altitude

Many climbers, though certainly not all, train for a climb by running at sea level either on a level surface or in the hills. Theoretically, running at sea level should not necessarily result in improved performance at high altitude for the reason that at sea level the usual limiting factor in running is the cardiac output. When cardiac output reaches its limit during exercise, muscle oxygen delivery is compromised and lactic acidosis occurs. Arterial oxygen saturation is maintained except during maximum exertion, when it may fall. Competitive distance runners and athletes have an increased cardiac size, including the left ventricle. At high altitude, however, maximum effort is limited not by the cardiac output but by other conditions, including the capacity of the respiratory system to maintain arterial oxygen tension. At maximum effort the cardiac output and cardiac work are less than at sea level and lactic acidosis does not occur, although arterial PO_2 is markedly decreased. Left ventricular dimensions are decreased correspondingly throughout the altitude stay. In normal subjects living for six weeks at 17,500 feet (5,340 m) on Mount Logan left ventricular dimensions were less than those at sea level.[74] This phenomenon of decreased left ventricular work at high altitude deconditions left ventricular performance and may account in part for the adverse effect of training at high altitude for sea level distance running. A crude analogy can be made by comparing swimming on the surface and swimming under water: swimming on the surface is limited by the cardiac output; swimming under water is limited by progressive hypoxia long before the cardiac output is stressed.

Carrying Weight

For sustained climbing it is evident that the rate of work must be minimized. The work rate depends upon the grade of ascent, rate of climb, type of terrain, climbing efficiency, and weight carried. Too few studies have examined these factors in the field to permit general recommendations. One study performed on seven male Sherpa highlanders climbing with variable loads to 12,000 feet (3,660 m) suggested that for day-to-day operations work should be undertaken at no more than 30-40 percent of maximum work capacity. A rate of work equivalent to carrying a 25-30 kg load at 3.0-3.5 km/hr was considered optimal.[75] Oxygen consumption, energy expenditure, and efficiency of climbing with loads at low altitudes have been evaluated by Durin, who studied five men carrying loads of zero, 8 percent, and 16 percent of body weight at 1.12 m/sec for ten minutes.[76] Cymerman and his colleagues also evaluated energy expenditure during load carrying at high altitude.[77] Heart rate and pulmonary ventilation are greatly increased over sea level values during load carrying at high altitude (Fig. 11.9).

Climbing Skill

Climbing ability will influence the success of a climb by two mechanisms. A skillful climber will be able to climb fast and thus achieve a summit with ample time to descend before darkness makes the descent dangerous or requires a bivouac. An experienced climber is more efficient and uses less oxygen to climb a given distance, and therefore can climb faster with fewer rest stops.

Cold Tolerance

Exercise under cold conditions probably requires a greater amount of oxygen than exercise under normal temperatures, and severe cold will limit climbing performance. During ascent, heavy exertion will probably maintain an adequate body temperature, but during descent, which requires 50 percent less effort, body temperature may fall and hypothermia may occur. Some climbers have attempted to adapt to cold temperatures by performing training climbs carrying snowballs in their bare hands. It is true that fishermen in Arctic waters can, over one year, attain an unusual degree of cold adaptation by exposure of their hands to freezing water, and experimental studies of fishermen demonstrate a greater skin temperature of the hand immersed in cold water due to increased blood flow. In addition to the physiological adaptation, repeated exposure to cold will increase cold tolerance without objective physiological changes.[78]

Dehydration

Dehydration at high altitude is due to a combination of increased water loss and decreased fluid intake. Several things contribute to fluid loss: increased ventilation, dry cold air, breathing through the mouth, and, to some extent, sweating in the high ambient temperatures and under intense solar radiation. Water loss rather than sodium loss is predominant. Diminished thirst, which appears to be common at high altitude, is a contributing cause. Parenthetically, diminished thirst has been reported to be a cause of unexpected dehydration in the elderly.[79] The result is a decrease in plasma volume, an increase in plasma osmolality; and a rise in serum sodium, all of which impair physical performance and lower mental acuity. Dehydration must be avoided if climbing performance is to be maintained. Some degree of overhydration does not affect physical performance, but dehydration will. Normally hydrated man has a reservoir of body water that constitutes a valuable emergency source, and one can lose as much as 2.5 liters of body water before physical performance is affected. "Tanking up" on fluids before a climb would ensure that body water stores are sufficient. During a climb, an average intake of two to three liters per 24 hours is recommended, although Pugh has shown that an intake of three to four liters per day was necessary to obtain normal urinary volumes even in climbers at 18,000 feet (5,500 m).[13]

A urinary output of at least 500 ml per day should be achieved. At extreme altitudes fluid intake by climbers has often been deficient simply because of the time and fuel required to melt snow and ice; the weight of fluid that must be carried and protected from freezing and, as mentioned, decreased thirst, are additional causative factors. Some members of early assault parties on Mount Everest reported passing no urine for 24 hours. Attempting to become adjusted to dehydration by purposely not drinking fluids during training climbs, as some climbers have done, is useless: there is no evidence whatsoever that adaptation to dehydration can be achieved in this fashion.

Nutrition

The weight loss that is common at very high and extreme altitudes as a result of high energy expenditure and a diminished caloric intake because of a decrease in appetite may also possibly be due to the effect of hypoxemia on the gastrointestinal tract.[80] Members of early Mount Everest expeditions returned considerably emaciated, partly, from an inadequate diet. An analysis of dietary records from the 1935 British Everest expedition showed intakes of less than 1,500 kilo-cal/day for all the time spent above 18,000 feet (5,490 m). Subsequent expeditions encouraged a high fluid intake and an adequate diet, and that may have greatly improved climbing performances, but still a modest weight loss during climbs continues to be observed. This weight loss is partly due to loss of body fat, but muscle atrophy has also been documented. During acute exposure to high altitude a high carbohydrate diet has been shown to result in a lower incidence of mountain sickness and an increased work capacity.[81] During long ascents and descents as well as in bivouac situations that may last for several days an adequate fluid intake with frequent carbohydrate feedings will prevent acidosis and susceptibility to orthostatic hypotension, collapse, or shock.[82]

Psychological Factors

An intense desire to attain a summit is clearly necessary for a successful climb, but there must be a critical balance between desire and obsession, and between desire and caution. Too many fatalities have occurred when the compulsion to succeed has overcome sensible judgment. Judgment and decision making may be impaired by hypoxia, as we know from many anecdotes from climbers and subjects in hypobaric chambers.

Pharmacologic Aids

Acetazolamide is useful in the prevention of acute mountain sickness and in the amelioration of sleep hypoxia, including periodic breathing; it may also, I believe, prevent and minimize high altitude pulmonary edema. Experimental studies have shown that acetazolamide can increase cerebral blood flow and brain oxygen tension.[83] The magnitude of this increase in oxygen tension is equivalent to a descent from 1,600 to 2,300 feet (488-700 m). In a few studies that have been made of the effect of acetazolamide upon physical performance of acclimatized subjects at high altitude using a cycle ergometer, no improvement in maximum exercise capacity has been demonstrated.[84] Moreover, the duration of the beneficial effect of acetazolamide is limited to four to six days because continued administration often results in unpleasant side effects. Most physicians agree that acetazolamide should be only used for persons who are susceptible to acute mountain sickness or disturbed sleep, and even then for not more than five or six days.

There are some anecdotal claims that climbing performance at extreme altitudes may be improved by the temporary use of acetazolamide. To examine this possibility, Bradwell and his associates studied the effect of 500 mg of acetazolamide daily for up to 23 days upon exercise performance at 15,750 feet (4,846 m) in eleven climbers during an expedition to Rupino La in Nepal.[85] Ten other climbers were given placebos. Exercise performance at 85 percent maximum heart rate fell 37 percent in the acetazolamide group and 45 percent in the placebo group (p <.05). Weight loss, too, was less in the acetazolamide group and was correlated with greater daily exercise capacity (p <0.001). Muscle thickness decreased 8.5 percent in the acetazolamide group and 13 percent in the placebo group (p <0.001). The increase in muscle thickness was also attributed to greater physical activity. Physical well-being was better in the acetazolamide group. This is an important study and needs to be confirmed by others.

It is generally agreed that acetazolamide has a brief but beneficial effect by its increase in ventilation and arterial PO_2. Bradwell's study suggests that acetazolamide may have a long-term beneficial effect that is perhaps independent of its effect upon ventilation and the decrease in nocturnal periodic breathing. It should be remembered, however, that acetazolamide is a diuretic that will increase the loss of water, salt, and potassium and could contribute to serious dehydration and electrolyte disturbances unless adequate replacements are taken. Respiratory stimulants such as Provera have been shown to increase ventilation during sleep and exercise, but no beneficial effect has been demonstrated during exercise due to the increased ventilation.[86] In patients with high altitude polycythemia the administration of Provera for several weeks has resulted in a decrease in hematocrit, suggesting a continued stimulation of ventilation. Side effects are few.[87] No data are available regarding the use of such preparations in climbing.

Some climbers use barbiturates and tranquilizers to promote sound sleep. This is a highly individual choice, and usually climbers avoid such preparations. Barbiturates and Valium (diazepam) depress ventilation and may intensify sleep hypoxia and bring on more severe symptoms of mountain sickness. Valium has been reported to result in disorientation, agitation, and hallucinations 21-22 hours after a 10 mg dose at altitudes of 14,000-18,000 feet (4,270-5,490 m).[88] Dubowitz reported on the effect of low doses of temazepam (a benzodiazepine) upon sleep at 17,700 feet (5,400 m) in members of the British Mount Everest Medical Expedition 1994. All subjects showed an improvement in quality of sleep compared to placebo, and oscillations of arterial oxygen saturation were reduced, but the mean saturation was not reduced. A 10 mg dose was employed but the effect of larger doses was not examined.[89] Caffeine has been shown to increase the duration of running at 80 percent of VO_{2max} on a treadmill by 19.5 percent compared with a placebo.[90] Caffeine improves physical performance in cross country skiers.[91] The effect of caffeine upon exercise performance was evaluated by Fulco and his colleagues in 15 soldiers exercising at sea level and again on Pikes Peak 14,110 feet (4,300 m).[92] Little change in performance at sea level was noted but a 54 percent increase in performance was noted at altitude both with acute and more prolonged exposure. It was postulated that the effect was either due to an increase in exercise tidal volume or a reversal of altitude induced decrease in muscular force. Caffeine also has been shown to increase contractility of the diaphragm in normal subjects.[93] Total carbohydrate consumption was unchanged but fat metabolism was increased. It was postulated that by raising free fatty acid level caffeine can spare the early use of glycogen, which then can be utilized later.[90] Caffeine is a diuretic and fluid balance must be maintained.

Oxygen

Oxygen is now used by most climbers at extreme altitudes both during climbing and in sleep. Although oxygen was used for climbing as early as 1922 by a British Everest expedition, it took 31 years to develop the sufficiently light and reliable oxygen-breathing apparatus that was used in the first American ascents of Everest in 1963. The most successful system employs an open-circuit method whereby the climber breathes largely ambient air enriched by a small percentage of oxygen. Flow rates of oxygen are usually adjusted to an oxygen-air mixture roughly simulating an altitude of 17,000-19,000 feet (5,185-5,795 m). At 28,000 feet (8,540 m) during exercise a climber may breathe as much as 100 liters per minute. At an oxygen flow of 4 L/min (STP) only 12 percent of his ventilation would be pure

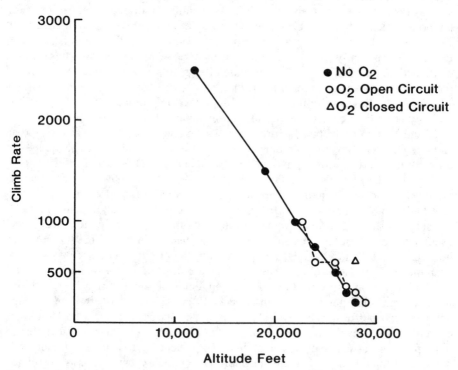

Figure 11.11. Approximate climbing rates for high altitude visitors from 12,000 feet (3,660 m) to 28,500 feet (8,693 m). Open circles and triangle represent climbers using oxygen; solid dark circles are climbers without oxygen. Although oxygen appears to offer no advantage in terms of increasing climbing rates, one might argue that it is possible, because of individual differences, that climbers using oxygen might not have been able to climb at all if they had not used oxygen. Redrawn from Ward, ref. 1.

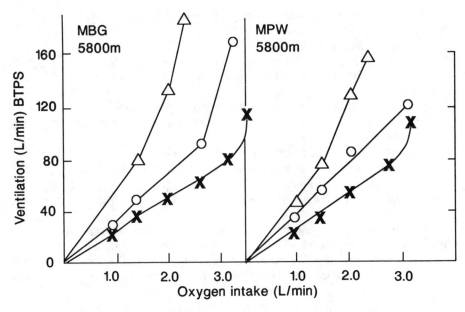

Figure 11.12. The effect of oxygen breathing upon minute ventilation during exercise in two acclimatized subjects at high altitude (open circles) compared with exercise while breathing air at high altitude (open triangles) and breathing air at sea level (X). Oxygen thus reduces the work of breathing at high altitude but sea level values are not achieved. Altitude 19,000 feet (5,800 m). Redrawn from Milledge, ref. 98.

oxygen, and without a reservoir it would be even less than this value. Flow rates commonly employed were 2 L/min from 23,000 to 26,000 feet (7,015 to 7,390 m) and 3 or 4 L/min above that altitude. There is observational evidence that climbing rates above 20,000 feet (6,100 m) are improved by oxygen, but this is difficult to assess (Fig. 11.11).

It is well established that nocturnal oxygen promotes sound sleep, reduces periods of awakening, reduces sleep hypoxia, and helps periodic breathing, and because of the sound sleep, climbing efficiency during the day is improved. High altitude deterioration is probably minimized.[94,95,96] Bourdillon in an experiment in the early 1950's tested sleeping oxygen masks made of light plastic that utilized the rebreathing method to store and conserve oxygen.[94] The flow rate used was 0.5 to 1 liter per minute.

Sea level values of VO_{2max} are not achieved even while breathing an oxygen mixture of 40 percent higher than sea level concentrations. Cardiac output is decreased by 12 percent.[97] Oxygen breathing at altitude reduces exercise ventilation but sea level values are not achieved (Fig.11.12).[98] These results indicate that factors other than hypoxemia limit physical performance at extreme altitudes.

Conclusions

This chapter has examined some of the conditions that limit exercise performance from high to extreme altitude. A systematic examination of the possible limiting factors involves several mechanisms.

Despite the presence of substantial pulmonary hypertension right ventricular failure has not been demonstrated.

Pulmonary vasoconstriction and pulmonary hypertension may restrict blood flow through the lungs and thus limit cardiac output especially during exercise. However, cardiac output appears to be appropriate for tissue oxygen delivery at levels of exercise.

Left ventricular function is normal at rest and during exercise.

Ventilation is adequate for oxygen transfer from lungs to capillaries since arterial PCO_2 remains low.

Diffusion from alveolus to end-capillary blood remains low.

Diffusion of oxygen from the capillary to the tissue mitochondria reflected by mixed venous PO_2 is not impaired.

Blood lactate is progressively reduced during exercise after acclimatization at high altitude.

Hypoxemia of the central nervous system could result in decreased efferent impulses to exercising muscles with consequent weakness and fatigue.

Fatigue of the muscles of respiration and diaphragms could by means of afferent impulses to the central nervous system initiate efferent impulses to decrease muscle contraction.

Shunting of blood flow from legs to control organs and muscles of respiration may result in leg weakness and fatigue.

Most exercise studies involving interventions have examined maximum exercise performance. There is a clear need to study also the effect of interventions upon submaximum performance, which is more clearly related to actual exercise activity.

References

1. WARD M. *Mountain medicine*. London: Crosby Lockwood Staples, 1975: 181.
2. MESSNER R. The mountain. In. J West, ed., *High altitude physiology*. Stroudsburg, Pa: Hutchinson Ross, 1981: 43-49.
3. PUGH L. High altitudes. In O Edholm and A Bacharach, eds, *Physiology of human survival*. New York: Academic Press, 1965: 121-145.
4. SUTTON J, REEVES J and WAGNER P. Tolerable limits of hypoxia for the lungs: Oxygen transport. In J Sutton, C Houston, and G Coates, eds., *Hypoxia: The tolerable limits*. Indianapolis: Benchmark Press, 1988: 123-32.
5. GROVER R, WEIL J, and REEVES J. Cardiovascular adaptaiton to exercise at high altitude. K Pandolf, ed., *Exercise and sport science review*, Vol. 14, New York: Macmillan, 1986.
6. GROVER R. Exercise performance of athletes at sea level and 3,100 meters altitude. *International Symposium on the Effects of Altitude on Physical Performance*. Albuquerque, N. Mex.: Athletic Institute, 1967: 80-87.
7. GROVER R, and REEVES J. Exercise performance at sea level and 3,100 meters altitude. *Med. Thorac.* 1966; 23:129-43.
8. ALEXANDER J, HARTLEY H, MODELSKI M, and GROVER R. Reduction of stroke volume during exercise in man following ascent to 3,100 m altitude. *J. Appl. Physiol.* 1967; 23:849-54.
9. ALEXANDER J, and GROVER R. Mechanism of reduced cardiac stroke volume at high altitude. *Circulation*, 1982; 66; Suppl. II:176. Abstract.
10. SUAREZ J, ALEXANDER J, and HOUSTON C. Operation Everest II: Enhanced left ventricular systolic performance in man at high altitude during operation Everest II. *Am. J. Cardiol.*, 1987; 60:137-42.
11. WOLFEL E, GROVES B, BROOKS G, et al. Oxygen transport during steady state submaximal exercise in chronic hypoxia. *J. Appl. Physiol.* 1991; 70:1129- 36.
12. GROVES B, REEVES J, SUTTON J, et al. Elevated high altitude pulmonary resistance unresponsive to oxygen. *J. Appl. Physiol.* 1987; 63:521-30.
13. PUGH L, GILL M, LAHIRI S, et al. Muscular exercise at great altitudes. *J. Appl. Physiol.* 1964; 19:431-40.

14. VOGEL J, GOSS J, MORI M, and BRAMMELL H. Pulmonary circulation in normal man with acute exposure to high altitude, 14,260 ft. (4,350 m). *Circulation* 1966; 34; Suppl III:223. Abstract.
15. KUIDA H, GAMMIN G, HAYNES F, et al. Primary pulmonary hypertension. *Am. J. Med.* 1957; 23:166-82.
16. MOSER K, AUGER W, and FEDULLO F. Chronic major vessel thromboembolic pulmonary hypertension. *Circulation* 1990; 81:1735-43.
17. GROVES B, DANNELLAN K, ROBERTSON A, and REEVES J. Diltiazem inhibits hypoxic pulmonary vasoconstriction in primary pulmonary hypertension. In J Sutton, G Coates, and J Remmers, eds., *Hypoxia: The adaptations.* Toronto: B.C. Decker, 1990: 163-68.
18. NAGARE A, and RUBIN L. The effects of hydralazine on exercise capacity in pulmonary hypertension secondary to chronic obstructive pulmonary disease. *Am. Rev. Resp. Dis.* 1986; 133:385-86.
19. MORGAN J, MCCORMACK D, GRIFFITHS M, et al. Adenosine as a vasodilator in primary pulmonary hypertension. *Circulation* 1991; 84:1145-49.
20. MCKENZIE D, GOODMAN L, NOTH C, et al. Cardiovascular adaptations in Andean natives after 6 weeks of exposure to sea level. *J. Appl. Physiol.* 1991; 70: 2650-55.
21. KHAJA F, and PARKER J. Right and left ventricular performance in chronic obstructive pulmonary disease. *Am. Heart J.* 1971; 82:319-27.
22. BERGER H. MATTHAY R, LOKE J, et al. Assessment of cardiac performance with quantitative radionuclide angiocardiography: Right ventricular ejection fraction with reference to findings in chronic obstructive pulmonary disease. *Am. J. Cardiol.* 1978; 41: 897-905.
23. DAVILA-ROMÀN V, GUEST T, ROWE W, et al. Ultra exercise induces right ventricular dysfunction. *J. Am. Coll. Card.* 1995; 25:Supplement 260A. Abstract.
24. HULTGREN H, LOPEZ C, LUNDBERG E, and MILLER H. Physiologic studies of pulmonary edema at high altitude. *Circulation* 1964; 29:393-408.
25. HULTGREN H. Personal observations.
26. KITABATAKE M, INOYE M, ASAS M, et al. Noninvasive evaluation of pulmonary hypertension by a pulsed Doppler technique. *Circulation* 1983; 68:302-09.
27. COLERIDGE J, and KIDD C. Reflex effects of stimulating baroceptors in the pulmonary artery. *J. Physiol.* 1963; 166:197-210.
28. HULTGREN H, GROVER R, and HARTLEY L. Abnormal circulatory responses to high altitude in subjects with a previous history of high altitude pulmonary edema. *Circulation* 1971; 44:759-70.
29. COATES G, GRAY G, MANSELL A, et al. Changes in lung volume and lung ventilation during hypobaric decompression. *J. Appl. Physiol.* 1979; 46:752-55.
30. JAEGER J, SYLVESTER J, CYMERMAN A, et al. Evidence for increased intrathoracic fluid volume in man at high altitude. *J. Appl. Physiol.* 1979; 47:670-76.
31. ROWELL G. High altitude pulmonary edema during rapid ascent. In J Sutton, N Jones, and C Houston, eds., *Hypoxia: Man at altitude.* New York: Thieme-Stratton, 1982: 168-70.
32. IRVIN R. Frequently recurring high altitude pulmonary edema. In J Sutton, N Jones, and C Houston, eds., *Hypoxia: Man at altitude.* New York: Thieme-Stratton, 1982: 171-72.
33. SARNQUIST F. Physicians on Mt. Everest. *West. J. Med.* 1983; 139:480-85.
34. VACHIERY J, MCDONAGH T, MORAINE J, et al. Doppler assessment of hypoxic pulmonary vasoconstriction and susceptibility to high altitude pulmonary vasoconstriction and susceptibility to high altitude pulmonary edema. *Thorax* 1995; 50:22-7.
35. WAGNER P, SUTTON J, REEVES J, et al. Pulmonary gas exchange during a simulated ascent of Mt. Everest. *J. Appl. Physiol.* 1987; 63:2348-59.
36. WEST J, BOYER S, GRABER D, et al. Maximal exercise at extreme altitude on Mt. Everest. *J. Appl. Physiol.* 1983; 55:688-98.
37. PUGH L. Muscular exercise on Mt. Everest. *J. Physiol.* (London) 1958; 141:233-61.
38. PARDY R, HUSSAIN S, and MACKLEM P. The ventilatory pump in exercise. *Clinics in Chest Med.* 1984; 5: 35-48.
39. JOHNSON B, SAUPE K and DEMPSEY J. Mechanical constraints on exercise hyperpnea in endurance athletes. *J. Appl. Physiol.* 1992; 73:874-78.
40. SCHOENE R, LAHIRI S, HACKETT P, et al. The relationship of hypoxic ventilatory response to exercise performance on Mt. Everest. *J. Appl. Physiol.* 1984; 56:1379-85.
41. MASUYAMA S, KIMURA H, SUGITA T, et al. Control of ventilation in extreme altitude climbers. *J. Appl. Physiol.* 1986; 61:500-06.
42. MILLEDGE J, WARD M, WILLIAMS E, and CLARKE C. Cardio-respiratory response to exercise in men repeatedly exposed to extreme altitude. *J. Appl. Physiol.* 1983; 55:1379-85.
43. HACKETT P, REEVES J, REEVES C, et al. Control of breathing in Sherpas at low and high altitude. *J. Appl. Physiol.* 1980; 49:374-79.

44. MOORE L, HARRISON R, MCCULLOUGH R, et al. Low hypoxic ventilatory response and hypoxic depression in acute altitude sickness. *J. Appl. Physiol.* 1986; 60:1407-12.

45. HACKETT P, ROACH R, SCHOENE R, et al. Abnormal control of ventilation in high altitude pulmonary edema. *J. Appl. Physiol.* 1988; 64:1268-72.

46. SALTIN B. Limitations to performance at altitude. In J Sutton, C Houston, and G Coates, eds., *Hypoxia: The tolerable limits.* Indianapolis: Benchmark Press, 1988: 9-34.

47. SECHER N, CLAUSEN J, and KLAUSEN K. Central and regional circulatory effects of adding arm exercise to leg exercise. *Acta. Physiol. Scand.* 1977; 100: 288-97.

48. BIGLAND-RITCHIE B, and VOLLESTAD N. Hypoxia and fatigue: How are they related? In J Sutton, C Houston, and G Coates, eds., *Hypoxia: The tolerable limits.* Indianapolis: Benchmark Press, 1988: 315-28.

49. ROUBIN G, ANDERSON S, SHEN W, et al. Hemodynamic and metabolic basis of impaired exericse tolerance in patients with severe left ventricular dysfunction. *J. Am. Coll. Cardiol.* 1990; 15:986-94.

50. BRUCE R, KUSUMI F, and HOSMER O. Maximal oxygen intake and nomographic assessment of functional aerobic impairment in cardiovascular disease. *Am. Heart J.* 1973; 85:546-62.

51. SCHWADE J, BLOMQUIST G, and SHAPIRO W. A comparison of the response to arm and leg work in patients with ischemic heart disease. *Am. Heart J.* 1977; 94:203-08.

52. SNELL P, and MITCHELL J. The role of maximal oxygen uptake in exercise performance. *Clinics in Chest Med.* 1984; 5:51-62.

53. WEST J, and WAGNER P. Predicted gas exchange on the summit of Mt. Everest. *Respir. Physiol.* 1980; 42:1-16.

54. SUTTON J, JONES N, and PUGH L. Exercise at altitude. *Ann. Rev. Physiol.* 1983; 45:427-37.

55. WEST J, HACKETT P, MARET K, et al. Pulmonary gas exchange on the summit of Mt. Everest. *J. Appl. Physiol.* 1983; 55:678-87.

56. GACHTGENS P, KREVTZ F, and ALBRECHT K. Optimal hematocrit for canine skeletal muscle during rhythmic isotonic exercise. *Eur. J. Appl. Physiol.* 1979; 41:27-39.

57. ZINK R. Haemodilution bei Hochgebirgsexpeditionen als Erfrierungsprophylake. *Artzliche Praxis* 1977; 29:2-6.

58. HORSTMAN D, WEISKOPF R, and JACKSON R. Work capacity during a 3 week sojourn at 4,300 m: Effects of relative polycythemia. *J. Appl. Physiol.* 1980; 49:311-18.

59. SARNQUIST F, SCHOENE R, HACKETT P, and TOWNES B. Hemodilution of polycythemic mountaineers: Effects on exercise and mental function. *Aviat. Space and Eviron. Med.* 1986; 57:313-17.

60. LINDENFELD J, WEIL J, TRAVIS V, and HORWITZ L. Hemodynamic response to normovolemic polycythemia at rest and during exercise in dogs. *Circ. Res.* 1985; 56:793-800.

61. WINSLOW R, MONGE C, BROWN H, et al. The effect of hemodilution on oxygen transport in high altitude polycythemia. *J. Appl. Physiol.* 1985; 59:1495-1502.

62. HACKETT P. Personal communication.

63. STAMPFER M, EPSTEIN S, BEISER G, and BRAUNWALD E. Hemodynamic effects of diuresis at rest and during intense upright exercise in patients with impaired cardiac function. *Circulation* 1968; 37:900-11.

64. SALTIN B, BLOMQUIST G, MITCHELL J, et al. Response to submaximal and maximal exercise after bed rest and training. *Circulation* 1968; 38; Suppl VII:1-78.

65. ROBINSON S. Physiology of muscular exercise. In V Mountcastle, ed., *Medical physiology*, 12th ed., St. Louis: C.V. Mosby, 1968: 520-52.

66. EDWARDS H. Lactic acid in rest and work at high altitude. *Am. J. Physiol.* 1936; 116:367-75.

67. SUTTON J, and HEIGENHAUSE G. Lactate at altitude. In J Sutton, G Coates, and J Remmers, eds., *Hypoxia: The adaptations.* Toronto: B.C. Decker, 1990: 94-97.

68. HOCHACHKA P, STANLEY C, MATHESON D. et al. Metabolic work efficiencies during exercise in Andean natives. *J. Appl. Physiol.* 1991; 70:1720-30.

69. YOUNG A. EVANS W, CYMERMAN A, et al. Sparing effort of chronic high-altitude exposure on muscle glycogen utilization. *J. Appl. Physiol.* 1982; 52:857-62.

70. ASANO K, MATSUZAKA A, KIKUCHI K, et al. Effects of simulated high altitude training on aerobic work capacity in Himalayan climbers (abstract). In J Sutton, G Coates, and J Remmers, eds., *Hypoxia: The adaptations.* Toronto: B.C. Decker, 1990: 287.

71. RICHALET J, BITTEL J, HERRY J, et al. Pre-acclimatization to high altitude in a hypobaric chamber: Everest turbo. In *Hypoxia and Mountain Medicine* eds Sutton J, Coates G, and Houston C. Burlington Vt./Queen City Printers. 1992: 202-12.

72. MARESH C, NOBLE C, ROBERTSON K, and SIME W. Maximal exercise during hypobaric hypoxia (447 torr) in moderate altitude natives. *Med. Sci. Sports Exer.* 1983; 5:360-65.

73. ARMSTRONG R. Skeletal muscle physiology. In R Strauss, ed., *Sports medicine and physiology.* Philadelphia: W.B. Saunders, 1979.

74. HULTGREN H, and FOWLES R. Left ventricular function at high altitude examined by systolic time intervals and M-mode echo-cardiography. *Am. J. Cardiol.* 1982; 52:862-66.

75. NAG P, SEN R, and RAY U. Optimal rate of work of mountaineers. *J. Appl. Physiol.* 1978; 44:952-55.

76. DURIN J. The oxygen consumption, energy expenditure, and efficiency of climbing with loads at low altitudes. *J. Physiol.* 1955; 128:294-309.

77. CYMERMAN A, PANDOLF K, YOUNG A, and MAHER J. Energy expenditure during load carriage at high altitude. *J. Appl. Physiol.* 1981; 51:14-18.

78. BLANC J. *Man in the cold.* Springfield, ILL: Charles C. Thomas, 1975: 1133-39.

79. PHILLIPS P, ROLLS B, LEDINGHAM J, et al. Reduced thirst after water deprivation in healthy elderly men. *N. Engl. J. Med.* 1984; 311:752-59.

80. BOYER S, and BLUME D. Weight loss and changes in body composition at high altitude. *J. Appl. Physiol.* 1984; 57:1580-85.

81. CONSOLAZIO C, MATOUSH L, et al. Effects of high carbohydrate diets on performance and clinical symptomatology after rapid ascent to high altitude. *Fed. Proc.* 1969; 28:937-43.

82. ROGERS T, SETLIFF J, and KLOPPING J. Energy cost, fluid, and electrolyte balance in subarctic survival situations. *J. Appl. Physiol.* 1964; 19:1-8.

83. LASSEN N, FRIBERG L, KASTRUP J, et al. Effects of acetazolamide on cerebral blood flow and brain tissue oxygenation. *Postgrad. Med. J.* 1987; 63:185- 87.

84. HACKETT P, SCHOENE R, PETERS R, and WINSLOW R. Acetazolamide and exercise in subjects acclimatized to 6,300 meters-a preliminary study. *Med. Sci. Sports Exerc.* 1985; 17:593-97.

85. BRADWELL A, DYKES P, COOTE J, et al. Effect of acetazolamide on exercise performance at high altitude. *Lancet,* 1986; May 3:1001-05.

86. ROBERTSON H, SCHOENE R, and PIERSON D. Augmentation of exercise ventilation by medroxyprogesterone acetate. *Clin. Physiol.* 1982; 2:269-76.

87. KRYGER M, GLAS R, JACKSON D, et al. Impaired oxygenation during sleep in excessive polycythemia of high altitude: Improvement with respiratory stimulation. *Sleep* 1978; 1:1-13.

88. ABERNATHY C, and MEEHAN R. Valium at high altitude: The Genet effect. In J Sutton, N Jones, and C Houston, eds., *Hypoxia: Man at altitude.* New York: Thieme-Stratton, 1982: 204. Abstract.

89. DUBOWITZ L. Oxygen saturation during sleep at high altitude and the effect of the benzodiazepine hypnotic temazepam. *Proceedings Second World Congress on Wilderness Medicine,* 1995, p. 18. Abstract.

90. COSTILL D, DALSKY G, and FINK W. Effects of caffeine ingestion on metabolism and exercise performance. *Med. Sci. Sports* 1978; 10:155-58.

91. BERGLUND B, and HEMMINGSON P. Effects of caffeine ingestion on exercise performance at low and high altitudes in cross country skiers. *Int. J. Sports Med.* 1982; 3:234-36.

92. FULCO C, ROCK P, TRAD L, et al. Effect of caffeine on submaximal exercise performance at altitude. *Aviat. Space Environ. Med.* 1994; 65:539-45.

93. SUPINSKI G, and HELSEN S. Comparison of the effects of aminophylline and caffeine on diaphragm contractility in man. *Am. Rev. Resp. Dis. Suppl.* 1983; 127:231. Abstract.

94. BOURDILLON B. Supplementary oxygen slows the rate of high altitude deterioration. *Proc. Royal Soc.* 1954; 143:24-32.

95. PUGH L. Mount Cho Oyu, 1952; Mount Everest, 1953. *Seminars in Resp. Med.* 1982; 5:109-12.

96. PUGH L. The Silver Hut. *Seminars in Resp. Med.* 1982; 5:113-21.

97. CERETELLI P. Limiting factors to oxygen transport on Mount Everest. *J. Appl. Physiol.* 1976; 40:658- 66.

98. MILLEDGE J. The control of breathing at high altitude. M.D. thesis. University of Birmingham, 1968.

CHAPTER 12

Acute and Subacute Mountain Sickness

Part 1: Acute Mountain Sickness

SUMMARY

Acute mountain sickness is the most common discomfort experienced by newcomers to high altitude. The incidence can vary widely according to the speed of ascent, the altitude attained, and individual susceptibility. Following rapid ascent to 8,000-9,000 feet (2,440-2,745 m), about 25 percent of visitors will have three or more symptoms and about 5 percent will require bed rest and a cessation of normal activity. Ascent to 10,000-12,000 feet (3,050-3,660 m) will result in symptoms in nearly everybody and about 10 percent will be incapacitated. In some symptoms may occur as low as 7,000 feet (2,135 m). Headache, insomnia, lassitude, and anorexia, which may be associated with nausea and vomiting, are major discomforts. Symptoms are most intense on the second and third days after arrival and disappear in five to eight days. Symptoms are worse in the morning hours and are probably related to increased hypoxemia during sleep. The young and physically fit may be more susceptible than older, experienced altitude travelers. Cerebral hypoxia, and increased cerebral flow are present, but the exact cause of specific symptoms such as headache is unknown. Prevention by acclimatization is too often neglected by the foolhardy, who rush to high altitude too fast only to be stricken by the dreaded soroche agudo. Acclimatization at an intermediate altitude or a slow ascent with a few days of rest upon arrival may be all that is necessary to prevent unpleasant symptoms. The use of acetazolamide 125-250 mg twice daily, started the day before ascent and continued for four to five days after arrival, is the only well-established preventative and therapeutic agent. Low-flow oxygen at night is helpful, and it is available in many high altitude hotels and resorts. Steroids, such as dexamethasone, when given with acetazolamide may be more effective, but the potential side effect of depression following cessation of the drug makes their use unwise. Furosemide and other diuretics are of no value and can result in unpleasant side effects, including hypotension and weakness. In severe cases, high flow oxygen or the use of a hyperbaric bag and descent will be necessary. Acute mountain sickness, although unpleasant and alarming, is not a serious illness, but severe cases may occasionally progress to high altitude pulmonary edema or cerebral edema, and therefore continued observation and appropriate management should not be neglected.

• • •

Acute mountain sickness consists of a group of unpleasant symptoms beginning 6 to 48 hours after rapid ascent to high altitude. The most common symptoms are headache, anorexia, nausea, fatigue, dizziness, and insomnia-discomforts not unlike those of motion sickness or of an alcoholic hangover. Depending upon the altitude, severe symptoms rarely last more than three to five days. The incidence and severity are dependent upon the speed of ascent, the altitude attained, and individual susceptibility. Severe episodes of acute mountain sickness (AMS) may be totally incapacitating and may be associated with high altitude pulmonary edema (HAPE) or cerebral edema (HACE). Some workers have suggested that AMS should be a generic term to include both high altitude pulmonary edema and cerebral edema. However, for purposes of descriptive accuracy, the use of separate terms is more convenient since some patients with AMS may also have HAPE, HACE or both. It is quite evident that each of these three conditions may occur as separate, distinct entities. "High altitude illness" is suggested as a single descriptive term for the several conditions related to high altitude exposure that may result in unpleasant symptoms or impair normal function.

Historical Aspects

The earliest description of AMS, and probably HAPE as well, is found in Chinese writing from 37 and 32 B.C., which refer to the mountain passes on the eastern border to China as Great Headache Mountain and Little Headache Mountain, where "Man's bodies become feverish, [and] they lose color and are attacked with headache and vomiting."[1] One of these passes was probably the Kilik Pass on the Afghanistan border, 15,837 feet (4,827 m). There is also a record of one person in a caravan who coughed up bright red blood, perhaps indicative of high altitude pulmonary edema.

In the sixteenth century a more complete description of AMS was made by José de Acosta, a Jesuit priest who lived in Peru from 1572 to 1587.[2] In the book of his experiences in the New World (1590), he described symptoms that he observed while crossing high Andean passes on his journey to Cuzco from the Pacific Coast:

"There is in Peru a very high mountain range that they call Pariacaca. I had heard tell of this malady that it caused in one, and so I went prepared as best I could in accordance with the instructions that those who they call guides or pathfinders provide thereabout; and with all my preparations, when I climbed the Escaleras de Pariacaca, as they are called, which is the highest part of that mountain range, almost suddenly I felt such a deadly pain that I was ready to hurl myself from the horse onto the ground; and, although there were many of us, each one hastened his pace without waiting for his companion in order to leave quickly from that evil spot; I found myself alone with an Indian, whom I begged to help me stay on the beast. And immediately there followed as much retching and vomiting that I thought I would lose my soul, because after what I ate and the phlegm, there followed bile and more bile both yellow and green, so that I brought up blood from the violence that I felt in my stomach. Finally, I must say that if that had continued, I would have understood death to be certain, but it did not last more than about three or four hours, until we went a long way downward and arrived at a more agreeable atmosphere; where I found all my companions, about fourteen or fifteen, all extremely tired, some going about pleading for confession thinking that they were really going to die. Others dismounted, vomiting and experiencing diarrhea, going completely astray; and I was told that some had lost their lives from that accident. I saw another who threw himself on the ground screaming from the ravaging pain that the passage of Pariacaca had caused him. Yet, ordinarily it does no injury of importance, besides that temporary fatigue and distressing grief." [Acosta, 1590; English translation by Jarcho.[3]

Acosta seems to have been aware of the effect of acclimatization upon AMS, for he observed that symptoms were less severe crossing the Andes from the east than when crossing from the west. The ascent from the east is more gradual, moving from the Altiplano, 8,000-13,000 feet (2,440-3,965 m), and then to the high passes. The route Acosta describes here probably crossed the Pariacaca Pass, approximately 15,570 feet (4,750 m), located about 40 miles south of Morococha in the La Oroya area.[2] It is of interest that this description has been referred to as an early description of AMS, yet upon close analysis the illness was probably acute gastroenteritis as pointed out by several Peruvian investigators.[4] Nevertheless, Acosta should be credited with several observations regarding high altitude such as the relative immunity of high altitude dwellers to AMS and the effect of a slow ascent in lessening symptoms of AMS.

DeSaussure had climbed extensively in the Alps from 1760 to 1787 when he climbed Mount Blanc, the third recorded climb of this highest mountain in Europe. He made many observations of the pulse and respiration on mountain summits and published a description of his travels and experiments in four volumes entitled *Voyages dans les Alpes*. He was one of the first to suggest that the symptoms of AMS were probably due to a decrease in oxygen in the blood.[5] DeSaussure's hypothesis was subsequently borne out by Paul Bert, the father of altitude physiology, who in 1878 proved that the symptoms of AMS, especially headache, could be relieved by breathing oxygen. At about the same time, Angelo Mosso (1897) carried out extensive studies of the effects of high altitude in man in his laboratory on Monte Rosa in the Pennine Alps (the Regina Margherita Hut), at 14,960 feet (4,560 m). He described most of the clinical features of AMS and concluded on the basis of his experiments that many of the symptoms of AMS were related to the decrease in arterial PCO_2. Mosso coined the term "acapnia."[6]

In 1913 T. M. Ravenhill, a physician to a mining company in the Andes, published the following accurate clinical description of the symptoms of AMS (Puna) as experienced by visitors to his village at an elevation of 15,400 feet (5,050 m). The trip from sea level by train required 42 hours, or two and a half days, depending upon whether the traveler took an overnight train or made a one-night stopover in a town at a lower altitude:

"It is a curious fact that the symptoms of puna do not usually evidence themselves at once. The majority of newcomers have expressed themselves as being quite well on first arrival. As a rule, towards evening the patients begins to feel rather slack and disinclined for exertion. He goes to bed, but has a restless and troubled night, and wakes up next morning with a severe frontal headache. There may be vomiting. Frequently there is a sense of oppression in the chest, but there is rarely any respiratory distress or alteration in the normal rate of breathing so long as the patient is at rest. The patient may feel slightly giddy on arising from bed and any attempt at exertion increases the headache which is nearly always confined to the frontal region. The patient feels cold and shivery. The headache increases toward evening, so also does the pulse rate. All appetite is lost and the patient wishes to be left alone—to sleep if possible. Generally during the second night he is able to do so and as a rule wakes next morning feeling better; the pulse-rate has probably dropped to about 90; the headache is only slight. As the day draws on he probably feels worse again, the symptoms all tending to reappear on any exertion; if, however he keeps to his bed, by the fourth day after arrival he is probably very much better, and at the end of a week he is fit again."[7]

Six years later, in 1919, Barcroft carried out his famous experiment in which he spent ten days in a glass house so constructed as to allow the chamber to be reduced in oxygen content gradually over the duration of the experiment. The interior atmosphere consisted of approximately 10 percent oxygen. On the sixth day, after a slow simulated ascent to 18,000 feet (5,490 m), he experienced symptoms of AMS which he described as follows:

"On the morning of the sixth day I awoke with typical symptoms of mountain sickness: vomiting, intense headache and difficulty of vision. I have recollections of very acute headache accompanied by vomiting as a child, but never in adult life or even in my boyhood can I think of any such attack as occurred in the chamber. In the chamber I lived an easy though normal life, reading, writing, making observations, doing the gas analyses, seeing to the air scrubbers, taking exercise on the bicycle ergometer and so forth. There was no cause other than oxygen want to which my sickness could be attributed. The partial pressure of oxygen corresponded to about 18,000 feet (5,490 m), much higher than the Peak of Teneriffe, but, on the other hand, I had not precipitated matters by performance of any such exacting feat as the ascent of a sandhill 1,500 feet (460 m) in height."[8]

This experiment added further proof to the concept that lack of oxygen was the major cause of AMS. Haldane then, also in 1919, performed a similar experiment using a hypobaric chamber. He made a rapid simulated ascent with a companion (A.M. Kellas) to the equivalent of 23,500 feet (7,168 m). Both men experienced severe symptoms of acute hypoxia and might well have died or suffered severe cerebral damage had it not been for the caution observed by the assistants outside the chamber.[9]

Between 1920 and the start of World War II several important field studies were made by Haldane, Dill, Barcroft and others, on Pikes Peak in Colorado, at Cerro de Pasco in Peru, and in Chile. Their reports were valuable for describing clinical symptoms of AMS, and they also explored—with equivocal results—the arterial PCO_2 as an important etiologic factor, including the administration of ammonium chloride and breathing 3 percent CO_2.[10,11,12]

In 1965 and 1969 Menon and Singh in two landmark papers described the occurrence of HAPE and AMS in Indian troops that were moved rapidly to high altitude during the border dispute with China.[13,14] In 1976 Hackett and Rennie carried out careful studies of AMS occurring in 278 trekkers at Pheriche in Nepal, 14,245 feet (4,343 m), and added many clinical details to previous observations.[15] Recently, several studies of AMS made in various parts of the world and in hypobaric chambers have examined etiologic mechanisms as well as methods of prevention and treatment. Historical aspects of AMS have been reported by Sutton.[16]

Clinical Features

Symptoms of AMS are rarely observed at altitudes of less than 7,000 feet (2,135 m) and when present at lower elevations are usually mild. I have observed occasional episodes of anorexia, postprandial vomiting, and headache in teenagers following heavy exertion at elevations as low as 7,000 feet (2,135 m). Although it has been suggested that patients with pulmonary or cardiovascular disease with a low arterial oxygen saturation experience AMS at lower elevations, there are no data to support this contention. Indeed, such persons may be less susceptible to AMS, because they are in one respect already acclimatized at sea level. Rapid ascent to elevations above 10,000 feet (3,050 m) will usually result in some symptoms in nearly all unacclimatized persons.

Symptoms usually do not appear until 6 to 48 hours after arrival. Earlier symptoms occur in persons who carry out heavy physical effort immediately upon arrival or when the altitude attained is very high, that is, greater than 14,000 feet (4,270 m). Symptoms usually increase in severity and reach a peak of intensity at 48 to 72 hours, after which they subside over the next five to six days (Fig. 12.1).

Barcroft's following account of AMS during ascent by train from Lima to La Oroya, 12,230 feet (3,730 m), and Cerro de Pasco, 14,200 feet (4,330 m), in Peru in 1924 well describes the symptoms than can be experienced even today on the same railroad:

"Making the ascent by train, one is lightly touched by soroche and experiences his first symptoms at an altitude of 10,000 feet (3,050 m) or more. Subjectively lassitude, then headache, usually frontal, growing in severity and perhaps nausea are felt. One feels cold, particularly in the extremities, the pulse quickens, respiration becomes deeper and more frequent, the face is pallid, lips and nails are cyanotic. On descending from the summit to La Oroya at 12,230 feet (3,730 m), though a marked improvement is felt, one finds himself reduced to a helpless condition of weakness which renders the least muscular effort irksome and productive of shortness of

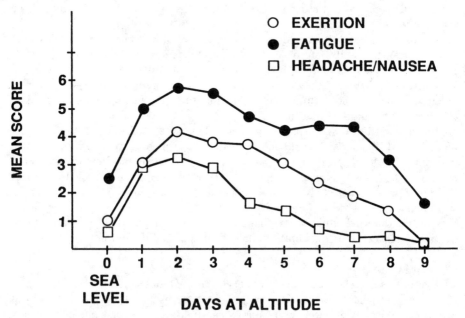

Figure 12.1. Duration, severity, and nature of symptoms of AMS during exposure of eight soldiers to an altitude of 14,100 feet (4,300 m) on Pikes Peak. From Sampson and Kobrick, ref. 31.

breath, dizziness, and palpitation. The night's sleep is restless and on waking one feels much as one does on venturing on to his feet after recovering from an acute infection. In two or three days, strength returns, the color improves somewhat and all but the more severe forms of exertion may be undertaken without distress. The minority are less fortunate than this. During the ascent the symptoms are qualitatively the same, but frequently more severe and the nausea gives way to vomiting. The night's sleep fails to bring relief; severe headache, gastrointestinal instability, and weakness continue for several days; the body temperature may be supranormal (102° F. by rectum), and at times one is aware of palpitation. Cyanosis is marked. After three or four days in bed, relief comes and in a week normal activity may be resumed."[17]

Symptoms

An analysis of nine reports of AMS reveals that the most common symptoms are headache, insomnia, nausea-anorexia, lassitude, fatigue or weakness, malaise, and dizziness or light-headedness (Table 12.1). Headaches, in particular, may be so severe that normal activities become impossible. Among the 200 trekkers studied by Hackett and Rennie at Pheriche, 65 percent experienced headache.[15] Hackett reported on the relative frequency of symptoms in climbers.[18] Exertional dyspnea was noted by 38 percent of the subjects and was second only to headache (46 percent), probably because these climbers were physically very active.

Honigman and his associates in a survey of 3,158 visitors to Colorado ski resorts 6,300-9,700 feet (1,922-2,959 m) elevation found the following prevalence of symptoms in patients with AMS: mild headache 54 percent, (severe 8 percent), sleep disturbances 31 percent, fatigue 26 percent, dyspnea 21 percent, dizziness 21 percent, anorexia 11 percent and vomiting 3 percent.[19]

Headache. Headache associated with AMS is usually diffuse and steady, less often of the throbbing sort. Frontal headaches are most common but occasionally occipital or parietal headaches are experienced. The headache may be intense and has been described as the sensation to a tight band compressing the skull. Others have felt as if their head would burst. The pain is worse upon arising in the morning and may abate during the day. Heavy activity may be followed by a more severe headache. Usually the discomfort is worse lying flat and is lessened in the erect position. Headache is exacerbated temporarily by straining, lifting, or coughing. Recumbency and sleep may intensify the headache; light activity in the open air may provide relief. Conditions that decrease arterial oxygen saturation tend to make headaches worse: sleep, recumbency, and heavy exercise; and conditions that increase arterial oxygen saturation will diminish the intensity of the headache: hyperventilation, light activity in the open air, erect position, etc.

Anorexia, nausea, vomiting. Appetite is commonly impaired and food intake is reduced during the first week at altitude. Strong foods such as salt herring, for example, are usually much more distasteful than fruit juices or foods of a bland but light consistency. In severe cases nausea and vomiting are common, and vomiting may sometimes occur quite suddenly after eating without any preceding nausea. Vomiting is common in children who ascend rapidly. Nausea and vomiting are central in origin, arising in the chemoreceptor trigger zone or the emetic center. Medications that stimulate the zone to cause emesis are apomorphine, digitalis, and morphine. Vomiting may also be caused by afferent impulses from the pharynx and

Table 12.1
Rank Order of Frequency of Symptoms of AMS by Various Investigators

Billings[46] - 12,470 feet (3,800 m)
   Headache
   Light-headedness
   Nausea
   Dyspnea
   Fatigue
   Insomnia

Favour[45] - 14,150 feet (4,316 m)
   Headache
   Insomnia
   Lassitude
   Anorexia, nausea
   Mental impairment
   Malaise

Hansen[40] - 10,000-13,000 feet
(3,050-3,965 m)
   Dyspnea
   Headache
   Dizziness
   Palpitations
   Insomnia
   Nausea

Hultgren[c] - 12,470 feet (3,800 m)

   Insomnia
   Fatigue
   Malaise
   Dyspnea
   Anorexia, nausea
   Headache

Hackett[15] - 13,917 feet (4,243 m)
   Headache
   Insomnia
   Anorexia, nausea
   Dizziness
   Dyspnea
   Lassitude

Evans[39] - 15,000 feet (4,575 m)
   Headache
   Insomnia
   Malaise
   Lassitude
   Sleepiness
   Dizziness

Hall[22] - 17,500 feet (5,338 m)
   Headache
   Insomnia
   Dyspnea
   Nausea
   Vomiting
   Decreased physical activity

Singh[14] - 11,000-18,000 feet (3,355-5,490 m)
   Headache
   Nausea, anorexia
   Dyspnea
   Insomnia
   Muscular weakness
   Dizziness

Hackett[24][a] - 14,000 feet (4,270 m)[b]

Headache	46%
Exertional dyspnea	38%
Periodic breathing	25%
Anorexia	22%
Nausea	18%
Dry cough	14%
Lethargy	14%
Edema, hands and feet	7%

Hultgren[c] - 10,000 feet (3,050 m)[c]

Insomnia	83%
Weakness	50%
Dyspnea	42%
Headache	33%
Memory loss	33%
Anorexia	25%

NOTES: [a]Data from trekkers; 42 percent spent 13 days walking into Pheriche, 58 percent flew to 9,184 feet (2,800 m) and walked to Pheriche in 3-4 days.

[b]Data from climbers on Mount Denali; 70 percent experienced lack of coordination or visual difficulties.
[c]Personal observations at Crooked Creek Altitude Station, California and Barcroft White Mt. Research Station.

hypopharynx, stomach, peritoneum, cerebral vessels, and labyrinth. Rhythmic labyrinthine stimulation result in the nausea and vomiting of motion sickness.

Lassitude, fatigue, malaise, laziness. Symptoms of a prevailing inertia or lassitude are difficult to describe accurately. Some have compared them to having a hangover or experiencing a bout of the flu. Some of these symptoms may be due to inadequate nighttime sleep.

Dizziness, light-headedness, syncope. Feeling faint, dizzy, or unsteady especially upon arising in the morning or standing after recumbency is common in AMS. Some persons may actually faint or collapse and require support. Such symptoms are usually a consequence of either of two conditions: (a) a postural fall in blood pressure owing to the decrease in plasma volume that occurs during ascent; or (b) hyperventilation and alkalosis, which by decreasing cerebral blood flow can result in a centrally mediated faint. Patients at sea level who have the hyperventilation syndrome may experience syncope via a similar mechanism.

Insomnia. An inability to sleep soundly is experienced by nearly all newcomers who sleep above 8,000 feet (2,440 m). Disturbed sleep may not be associated with severe daytime symptoms, however, and it therefore should not be regarded as a diagnostic symptom of AMS if it is the only significant discomfort. Sleep disturbances at altitude consist of frequent arousals, periodic breathing, episodes of dyspnea, which may be related to periodic breathing, strange dreams, and a sensation that the night is 24 hours long. Severe sleep disturbances or "white nights" may be followed by fatigue and sleepiness during daytime hours.

Central nervous system. Impairment of memory and difficulty in performing tasks requiring mental concentration may occur, and there may also be irritability, depression, abnormal behavior, and hysterical outbursts. One so afflicted usually prefers to be alone and secluded. Ataxia and incoordination are rare, but when present should suggest the presence of cerebral edema. All these symptoms are probably related to the effect of hypoxia upon the central nervous system, which may result in changes in cerebral blood flow and cerebral edema.

Dyspnea, breathlessness, increase in respiratory rate. Dyspnea at rest is rare in AMS, but marked dyspnea on slight exertion is common. Episodes of dyspnea at night may be due to periodic breathing. Dyspnea at rest with an associated increase in respiratory rate and heart rate should suggest the possibility of pulmonary edema. Several reports have described in detail the symptoms of AMS, including severity and duration.[18-24]

The following diagnostic criteria for AMS were proposed by a consensus committee that met at the 1991 International Hypoxia symposium: . . . "in the setting of a recent gain in altitude, the presence of headache, and at least one of the following symptoms: gastrointestinal (anorexia, nausea, or vomiting), fatigue or weakness, dizziness or light-headedness, difficulty sleeping".[25]

Definition

Severity grades. Classifying the severity of AMS by the effect of symptoms upon normal daily functions is useful for medical and scientific purposes as well as for accurate communication. Most clinical classifications of functional impairment make use of four grades of severity, from mild symptoms that do not interfere with normal activity (Grade 1) to severe symptoms that require bed rest or hospitalization (Grade 4). The following classification, graded 1-4, was proposed by a consensus committee at the 1990 Hypoxia Conference at Lake Louise, Canada[25]:

Grade 1. Symptoms are present, but do not interfere with normal daily activity. The patient can continue the trek.

Grade 2. Symptoms impair normal function. The patient is able to continue, but only with some difficulty.

Grade 3. Severe symptoms that make the patient reduce activity. Cannot continue. Rest is required. Symptoms are stable and nonprogressive.

Grade 4. The patient is unable to ambulate, cannot care for personal needs, bed rest is required, symptoms are progressive, and disturbances of consciousness or gait may be present. AMS of this severity is a medical emergency and requires prompt therapy with oxygen and descent. Such patients frequently have associated problems included HAPE and HACE.

A similar simple classification of severity of AMS has been used by Hackett and is quite applicable to trekkers and climbers.[15,18] Hackett's system has three grades of incapacity: (1) symptomatic, but able to continue, (2) unable to continue, and (3) must be carried down. In 200 trekkers evaluated at Pheriche, 14,245 feet (4,343 m), the following groups of severity were reported: 22 percent, feeling normal; 59 percent, symptomatic but able to continue; 16 percent, unable to continue. Three percent had to be carried or transported down. This group of trekkers was acclimatized: 42 percent had spent thirteen days walking from Katmandu, and 58 percent had flown to Lukla, 9,275 feet (2,827 m), and spent four to five days walking to Pheriche. Symptoms were more common and severe in those who had flown to Lukla.

Incidence

The incidence of AMS and severity classifications from five published papers are shown in Table 12.2.[15,21,22,26,46] At 11,500 feet (3,506 m) and 10,000 feet (3,050 m), the lowest altitudes studied, 21-25 percent of the subjects had no symptoms. Above this altitude nearly all subjects had some symptoms, but most symptoms were not incapacitating. In 10-25 percent symptoms were severe but did not require descent or hospitalization; descent or hospitalization was required in about 3 to 8 percent of patients. The highest incidence of Class 3 patients was observed by Hall: of 18-20 subjects, 90 percent of those who were transported to 17,000 feet (5,185 m) had Class 3 symptoms and were described as "grossly impaired," but none required hospitalization.[22]

Kayser evaluated the incidence of AMS in 530 trekkers climbing a 17,700 foot (5,400 m) pass in Nepal over eight days; 371 questionnaires were returned and 353 were evaluated. The overall prevalence of AMS was 63 percent. Symptoms were positively correlated with rate of ascent. More symptoms were present in women and obese men and fewer symptoms were present in persons with pre-trek acclimatization.[23]

AMS at Moderate Altitudes

Some particularly interesting observations have been made on reactions to moderate altitudes around or below 10,000 feet (3,050 m), to which most skiers and amateur trekkers ascend. Houston interviewed 3,906 visitors to six Colorado ski resorts at altitudes of 8,000-9,500 feet (2,440-2,900 m). He found that three or more

Table 12.2
Severity Classification of AMS

| Carson[21] n=23 | | Billings[46] n=25 | |
14,130 feet (4,310 m)		12,470 feet (3,800 m)	
Class	0 none	Class	0 none
	1 17%		1 8%
	2 65%		2 76%
	3 17%		3 12%
	4 0%		4 4%
Kamat[26] n=24		Hall[22] n=20	
11.500 feet (3,508 m)		17,500 feet (5,338 m)	
Class	0 21%	Class	0 none
	1 25%		1 0
	2 21%		2 2
	3 25%		3 90%
	4 8% (HAPE)		4 0
Hackett[a] n=200		Hultgren[b] n=12	
13,917 feet (4,243 m)		10,000 feet (3,050 m)	
Class	0 33%	Class	0 25%
	1-2 62%		1 75%
	3 30%		2 0
	4 8%		3 0
			4 0

NOTES: Severity is graded as: 0=none; 1=mild, able to carry out normal activity; 2=moderate, limits normal activity; 3=severe, cannot carry out normal activity, cannot continue to trek; 4=serious, cannot ambulate, may have disturbed consciousness, must descend.

[a] Data from trekkers, 42 percent of whom spent 13 days walking in and 58 percent of whom flew to 9,184 feet (2,800 m) and walked into Pheriche in three to four days; symptoms of 148 of 278 (53 percent) who had AMS.[18]

[b] Hultgren. Personal observations at Crooked Creek Altitude Station, California.

symptoms of AMS were experienced by 12 percent, and 27 percent had a history of previous episodes of AMS.[27]

Montgomery and his associates examined the incidence of AMS in 454 men and women who attended a week-long meeting at a ski resort in the Rocky Mountains at an elevation of 6,560 feet (2,000 m). The presence of three or more of the five possible symptoms of AMS with a severity of at least Grade 2 occurred in 25 percent of the subjects.[28] The minimum estimate of symptomatic individuals was 12 percent. Symptoms had subsided in nearly all subjects by the third day.

Honigman and his associates interviewed 3,158 adult tourists (mean age 45±12 years) at altitudes of 6,900-9,700 feet (2,104-2,958 m) in the Colorado Rockies to determine the incidence of symptoms of acute mountain sickness.[19] Sixty-nine percent were males and 90 percent had traveled from sea level. Seventy-one percent of the subjects experienced at least one of various adverse symptoms: headache, 69 percent; sleep disturbance, 31 percent; unusual fatigue, 27 percent; dyspnea, 21 percent; dizziness, 20 percent; loss of appetite, 11 percent; and vomiting, 3 percent. In 63 percent of the subjects there was no reduction in recreational activity; in 35 percent there was a moderate reduction; 2 percent were confined to bed rest. Severe headache and fatigue were the most likely symptoms to predict a reduction in activity (odds ratio = 15.7 and 6.1, respectively). Three or more symptoms were present in 23 percent of subjects. Fewer symptoms were reported from a lower altitude, 6,900 feet (2,105 m), than from the highest area, 9,712 feet (2,960 m). Also, fewer symptoms were reported by persons who were in excellent physical condition and had spent one to two days in Denver before going on to the mountains. Obese persons had a higher incidence of symptoms than did others. The authors concluded that some symptoms of acute mountain sickness will be experienced by a majority of visitors to Rocky Mountain resorts, and that in about 30 percent these symptoms will cause a moderate reduction in recreational activity for one or two days. Similar results were obtained in a survey of visitors to the Swiss Alps.[30]

In summary, any study of the incidence of AMS must include the number of important symptoms as well as their severity. The threshold altitude for mild AMS appears to be a sleeping altitude of about 8,000 feet (2,440 m). At this elevation about 12-25 percent of subjects will experience three or more symptoms of AMS of mild to moderate severity, which will then disappear after the third day. Above this threshold elevation, the incidence and severity of AMS increase rapidly: at 12,470 feet (3,800 m) all subjects experience symptoms, severe (Grade 3-4) in about 15-30 percent, and longer lasting than at lower altitudes. The comparative incidence of AMS and high altitude pulmonary edema from field surveys is summarized in Table 12.3

The following symptoms in patients with AMS should be regarded as serious, and possible indications of the presence of HAPE or HACE: ataxia, incoordination, severe headache not relieved by medication, marked dyspnea, sounds of fluid in the chest and an altered mental state. Such patients should be treated promptly by rest and oxygen and transported to a lower altitude. Physical findings in serious cases include tachypnea and tachycardia at rest, cyanosis, rales, and abnormal neurological signs. A common, serious neurological sign is truncal ataxia.

AMS Questionnaires

Questionnaires that evaluate symptoms of AMS, their variety, severity, and time course, have proved particularly useful in assessing the effect of interventions such as medications that may prevent or ameliorate symptoms. The questionnaire is usually administered at sea level before ascent and then daily after ascent at the same time of day. A numerical score of severity can be derived from all or selected symptoms, each of which is graded by the subject in terms of intensity. A commonly employed questionnaire was developed and later modified by Sampson.[31] Fifty-five symptoms are evaluated and severity is scored using a five-point scale. The major symptoms can be classified into five groups: discomfort associated with exertion, fatigue, symptoms related to ear, nose, and throat, headache-nausea, and general malaise. A modified questionnaire that has been employed in our laboratory for several years is shown in Table 12.4. Each of the nine symptoms is scored from zero through ten relating to the degree of discomfort. By adding all the numbers one arrives at the total score. For example, a score of zero indicates that none of the symptoms was present, while a score of 90 indicates severe symptoms in all

Table 12.3
Recent Surveys of the Incidence of AMS
in Various Groups at Different Altitudes

Data base	Location	Altitude		Numbers of Subjects	Incidence (percent)
		Feet	Meters		
Climbers[a]	Swiss Alps	9,350	2,850	47	9
	Swiss Alps	10,000	3,050	128	13
	Swiss Alps	11,970	3,650	82	34
	Swiss Alps	14,953	4,559	209*	53
Meeting attendees[b]	Colorado Rockies	6,560	2,000	454	12
Visitors[c]	Colorado ski areas	8,000-9,500	2,440-2,745	3,906	12
Visitors[d]	Colorado ski areas	6,300-9,700	1,922-2,959	1,909	15
Climbers[e]	Nepal	15,800	4,815	63	37
Trekkers[f]	Nepal	17,712	5,400	353	63

SOURCES: [a]Maggiorini et al., ref. 30; [b]Montgomery et al., ref. 28; [c]Houston, ref. 27; [d]Honigman et al., ref 19; [e]Hirata et al., ref. 48; [f]Kayser, ref. 23.
*Eleven climbers at 14,953 feet (4,559 m) had HAPE (~5.3 percent.)

categories. The most common symptoms experienced by 45 subjects exposed for four days to an altitude of 12,470 feet (3,800 m) after a rapid ascent by auto were: poor sleep, tiredness, sleepiness during the day, uncomfortable feeling, shortness of breath, anorexia or nausea, and headache.

Despite their seeming objectivity and accuracy, questionnaire methods do have several limitations. Too many items may be evaluated and the severity score may be complicated by symptoms not related to AMS. Most questionnaires only evaluated symptoms at rest and do not contain any evaluation of mental of physical performance ability. In studies on small numbers of subjects a peer rating of severity of symptoms by the subjects themselves can be of additional value in assessing severity. Another method, but only applicable to small groups, is a careful assessment by a physician based on interviews and daily observation.

At the 1990 International Hypoxia Conference at Lake Louise, Canada, a consensus committee proposed two special questionnaires: a systematic self-assessment questionnaire (Table 12.5) and a physician's form (Table 12.6). These forms, if adopted and widely used, will permit a more accurate and complete assessment of symptoms, clinical data, and degree of disability than the widely differing forms previously and currently in use.[25] The self-assessment questionnaire is useful for surveys and for patients to fill out before being seen by a physician. The physician's form, including symptoms, physical findings, and laboratory test results, is designed to be completed by a physician, a physician's assistant, or a nurse. Physical signs, laboratory data, and symptoms that may indicate the presence of pulmonary and/or cerebral edema are included.

Table 12.4
General High Altitude Questionnaire

INSTRUCTIONS: You are to put a circle around the number that best describes how you feel *right at this moment*. Put down what first comes into your mind. Don't try to analyze too closely.

	0	2	4	6	10
1.	not nauseated at all	a little nausea	some nausea	quite nauseated	severely nauseated
2.	not short of breath at all	a little short of breath	some shortness of breath	quite short of breath	severely short of breath
3.	not tired at all	slightly tired	about average tiredness	a little tired	very tired
4.	no headache at all	a little headache	some headache	bad headache	severe headache
5.	weak on walking	some weakness on walking	quite weak on walking	severe weakness on walking	very severe weakness, could hardly walk
6.	very good appetite for all food	did not feel like eating as much as usual	appetite definitely poor	very poor appetite but ate some food	no appetite at all, could rarely eat
7.	mind and memory very sharp	some loss of memory	moderate loss of memory and made errors	poor memory, forgot many things	very poor memory, could hardly remember simple things

Last night I slept:

8.	very well	quite well	about average	not very well	hardly at all

Last night I

9.	did not awaken	woke up once or twice	woke up several times	was awake more than I slept	was awake all night

Last night I had:

10.	no trouble breathing	a little trouble breathing	some trouble breathing	a lot of trouble breathing	severe trouble breathing

Table 12.5
Self-Assessment Questionnaire for AMS

All responses should describe the most severe symptoms
experienced over the past 48 hours

Circle the appropriate descriptor.

1. **HEADACHE**
   0-none at all
   1-mild, no problem
   2-very definite, somewhat
     unpleasant, bothersome
   3-severe, very unpleasant,
     can't do anything

2. **APPETITE - NAUSEA**
   0-good appetite, no nausea
   1-fair appetite, some nausea
   2-can hardly eat, moderate nausea
   3-cannot eat, severe nausea and
     vomiting, incapacitated

3. **FATIGUE, WEAKNESS**
   0-none at all
   1-a bit tired and weak
   2-definitely tired and weak,
     can't do several things
   3-severe weakness and tiredness
     can't do any activities

4. **DIZZY OR LIGHT-HEADED**
   0-not at all
   1-occasionally feel dizzy or
     light-headed
   2-very definitely dizzy or
     light-headed, a bit bothersome
   3-severely dizzy, light-headed,
     feel faint, can't do anything

5. **DIFFICULTY SLEEPING**
   0-slept soundly
   1-awake a few times which is
     unusual for me
   2-definitely poor sleep, awake
     many times
   3-very poor sleep, awake nearly
     all night

6. **CHANGE IN MENTAL STATUS**
   0-no problems
   1-a little slow thinking
     a little forgetful
   2-definitely confused listless,
     can't concentrate
   3-very confused, can't remember much
     had to be aroused several times

7. **ATAXIA PROBLEMS WITH BALANCE**
   0-no problem with balance
   1-some problems but not bad
   2-definite problems, unsteady walking
   3-severe balance problems, can
     hardly walk without help

8. **EDEMA (SWELLING UP)**
   0-no swelling
   1-face puffy in morning
   2-face and hands definitely swollen
   3-face, hands, ankles, and legs
     swollen, can't put on shoes-boots

9. **FEELING SICK, MALAISE, FEEL LOUSY**
   0-I feel OK
   1-a little ill but I can do anything
   2-I definitely feel bad, ill,
     it is unpleasant
   3-I am very sick as if I have the flu
     or something serious. I can hardly
     function

Table 12.6
Clinical Evaluation of AMS

Responses to be obtained by interview

Severity Score for Each Symptom

0-no symptoms
1-mild but no problem
2-moderately unpleasant
3-severely unpleasant
4-terrible worst I have had

Final Functional Score
Effect of symptoms upon activity level

0-no effect on any level of activity
1-minor-no change or some decrease
or no change in activity
2-moderate-can only do light activity
3-severe-cannot do anything, must
rest
4-very severe, totally incapacitated

SYMPTOMS SCORED BY NUMBERS ABOVE

1. HEADACHE   0 1 2 3 4

2. NAUSEA, NO APPETITE   0 1 2 3 4

     VOMITING (circle one)   Yes No

3. FATIGUE, WEAKNESS   0 1 2 3 4

4. DIZZY, LIGHT-HEADED   0 1 2 3 4

5. DIFFICULTY SLEEPING   0 1 2 3 4

6. CHANGE IN MENTAL STATUS
     0-none
     1-lethargy lassitude slow
     2-disoriented confused
     3-stupor semiconscious

7. ATAXIA
     0-none
     1-some trouble walking
     2-can't walk straight at all
     3-needs help to walk or stand

8. PERIPHERAL EDEMA
     0-none
     1-face in morning
     2-face, hands
     3-face, hands, feet, legs
     can't put on shoes

9. FEEL SICK, MALAISE   0 1 2 3 4

Physical and Objective Findings

1. RALES
     0-none
     1-one quadrant only
     2-two quadrants
     3-three quadrants
     4-all lung fields

     Audible fluid in airways
     (circle one)   Yes No

2. CHEST X-RAY FINDINGS
     0-clear
     1-infiltrate present
     2-increased vascularity only
     3-doubtful for HAPE

3. VITAL SIGNS

     Temp H. Rate   Resp. Rate

     BP. Vital Cap. $\%FEV_1$ $\%O_2$ Sat.
     Predicted   Predicted

SYMPTOMS (NOT FOR AMS SCORE)
     (circle one)

1. SHORT OF BREATH   Yes No

2. COUGH
     Bloody or pink sputum   Yes No

3. CHEST TIGHT OR CONGESTED
     Sounds of fluid in lungs   Yes No

One useful finding that can be evaluated by scores obtained from questionnaires is the time course of AMS. Most symptoms are at their most severe within 24 to 36 hours after arrival and then quickly subside, so that most travelers or climbers are symptom-free by the end of one week. An example of the severity of symptoms and time course after an ascent to 12,470 feet (3,800 m) in 46 subjects studied by the author is shown in Figure 12.2. Symptoms at 10,000 feet (3,050 m) on day 1 were substantially less than on day 1 at the higher altitude.

Robinson reported that a questionnaire give similar results in evaluating severity and duration of symptoms in nine of eleven subjects who were studied during two separate exposures to 14,000 feet (4,270 m).[32] Forster obtained similar results in the evaluation of symptoms in workers who ascended to the Mauna Kea Observatory,

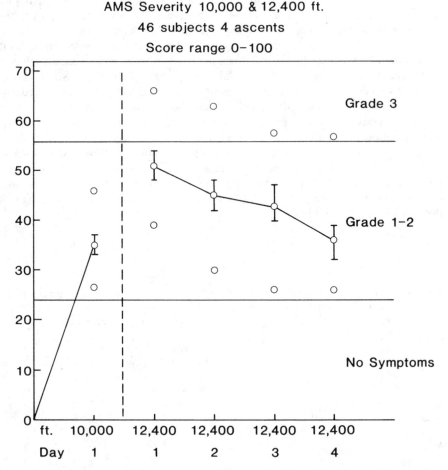

Figure 12.2. The right panel shows the severity of AMS in 46 subjects during four rapid ascents from sea level to 12,400 feet (3,780 m); mean scores and one standard deviation are shown, as well as the range (open circles). The range of scores from no symptoms to multiple severe symptoms 0-90. Assessment was made in the morning after breakfast. Twelve subjects spent one night at 10,000 feet (3,050 m). The same symptoms were experienced by all subjects. Symptoms subsided over four days. Graded system and the questionnaire used are defined in the text. Hultgren, unpublished data.

13,800 feet (4,200 m), every five days. Symptoms were similar but less severe after repeated ascents.[33] The severity of symptoms during repeat ascents to 12,747 feet (3,800 m) one year apart in eleven subjects was evaluated by comparing the severity scores of individual symptoms. Two subjects made five ascents, four made three ascents and five made two ascents. In 74 of 110 scores the mean variation was three or less out of a total score of ten indicating recurrences of the same symptoms with the same severity on repeat ascents (Table 12.7).

Physical Examination

There are no specific diagnostic physical signs of acute mountain sickness, and the value of a careful physical examination is primarily to detect other coexisting conditions. The following physical signs may be observed in patients with AMS: cyanosis of mucous membranes and extremities associated with pallor, tachypnea and tachycardia at rest; often, a decreased urine output and evidence of dehydration may be present if nausea or vomiting has occurred. The presence of rales, cyanosis, tachypnea, and tachycardia should suggest the diagnosis of pulmonary edema. Hackett and Rennie noted rales in 23 percent of 200 trekkers who were examined at Pheriche, and of all the patients with rales, 60 percent had AMS.[15] Singh and his associates noted rales in about 33 percent of soldiers with AMS.[14] Severe headache, ataxia, and neurological signs should suggest the presence of cerebral edema, but this complication is less common than pulmonary edema. Systemic edema and weight gain may be present in trekkers and was observed in 18 percent of 200 subjects at Pheriche.[15] Twice as many women had edema as men. AMS was more common in those with edema (61 percent) than in those without edema (43 percent). Bärtsch and his associates reported that weight gain and facial edema were more common in patients with AMS than in those without symptoms. Studies were done at 14,950 feet (4,559 m).[34,35]

Table 12.7

Recurrent symptom severity scores in two ascents by three subjects one year apart to 12,470 feet (3,800 m). Symptoms severity was scored from 0 to 10 (Table 4). Symptom severity was similar in the nine symptoms shown above during the second ascent.

	L.		W.		K.	
	Scores	Difference	Scores	Difference	Scores	Difference
Dizzy	2 - 2	0	3 - 6	3	2 - 2	0
Headache	2 - 3	1	3 - 5	2	3 - 5	2
Awake	3 - 4	1	4 - 4	0	6 - 6	0
DOE	3 - 3	0	3 - 4	1	3 - 4	1
Weak	2 - 2	0	3 - 4	1	5 - 3	2
Nausea	2 - 2	0	2 - 5	3	3 - 3	0
Palpitations	3 - 2	1	5 - 6	1	6 - 4	2
Depressed	2 - 2	0	2 - 4	2	2 - 2	0
Fatigue	5 - 4	1	4 - 9	5	5 - 5	0
Mean difference		0.4		1.8		.7

Laboratory Studies

Simple clinical laboratory tests provide little diagnostic information of AMS. Common findings in any newcomer to high altitude include a modest rise in hematocrit, a reduction in arterial oxygen saturation, a decreased arterial PCO_2, and a decrease in bicarbonate. A small decrease in vital capacity is usually present. Body temperature may be slightly elevated.[36] Some studies have shown that a higher arterial PCO_2 is associated more consistently with severe symptoms than the degree of fall in arterial oxygen saturation.

Persons with AMS appear to have a lower arterial oxygen saturation than those who are free of symptoms.[18,37] Bärtsch and his workers studied 13 patients with severe AMS at 14,810 feet (4,557 m). The mean arterial PO_2 was 34 mm Hg with an A-a gradient of 7.9 mm Hg, compared with an arterial PO_2 of 40 mm Hg and an A-a gradient of 7.9 mm Hg in 25 healthy subjects.[20] A low arterial PO_2 upon ascent may therefore be predictive of the subsequent occurrence of AMS.

Hackett and his associates reported that in 45 arrivals at high altitude (Mount McKinley, 14,430 feet/4,400 m) who subsequently developed AMS, the mean arterial oxygen saturation was 74.2 percent, compared with 81.5 percent in 115 other arrivals who did not develop AMS; A-a gradients were higher (12.5 mm Hg) in 13 patients who became sick, compared with 8 mm in 25 subjects who kept well.[37] These results illustrate that hypoxemia is an important factor in the etiology of symptoms of AMS, but because of wide individual variations blood gas studies will probably be of limited diagnostic or predictive value.

Incidence and Severity

All studies have shown that the incidence and severity of AMS are dependent upon the speed of ascent, the altitude attained, previous acclimatization, age and sex, physical fitness (including obesity), physical activity upon arrival, and history of AMS.

Speed of ascent. In Merida, Venezuela, 5,500 feet (1,680 m), a teleférico carries people from the center of town to the top station at 15,600 feet (4,760 m) in about 45 minutes. The top station has a restaurant, curio shop; and tourist walkway. Most of the tourists and local inhabitants who take this ride to the top are ill upon arrival, and symptoms become worse the longer they stay. Yawning and somnolence are the earliest signs. Exertional dyspnea, headache, nausea and vomiting, malaise, and light-headedness are common. Cyanosis is marked. All these symptoms subside upon descent except for headache, which may persist for many hours. I know of no other place in the world where one can ascend so rapidly to such a high altitude. Mount Rainier at 14,410 feet (4,395 m) is usually climbed from near sea level by spending the first night in a hut or camp at about 10,000 feet (3,050 m) and completing the climb and descent on the next day. The incidence of AMS (severity not defined) is about 50-75 percent.[38] During one ascent of 45 climbers, 10 climbers (22 percent) had to go down because of AMS.

Ascent to a similar or higher altitude over many days of gradual climbing results in sufficient acclimatization so that AMS is less common and less severe. Thus, trekkers who walked to Pheriche at 14,245 feet (4,343 m) had fewer symptoms than those who flew to Lukla at 9,275 feet (2,827 m) and walked from there to Pheriche.[15]

Altitude attained. Symptoms are rare below 7,000 feet (2,135 m) and if present are usually mild and of short duration. Montgomery and his workers reported AMS occurring as low as 6,560 feet (2,000 m), but only 12 percent had significant symptoms.[28] At 11,500 feet (3,660 m), 79 percent of subjects had symptoms (Table 12.2). Studies from our laboratory have shown that at 10,000 feet (3,050 m), only 25 percent of subjects were free of symptoms. At 12,000 feet (3,660 m) and 14,000 feet (4,270 m) nearly all unacclimatized subjects will have some symptoms, and at these altitudes severe illness requires descent in 4-8 percent.

Previous acclimatization. It has long been understood, even since the late 1600's, when Acosta wrote, that gradual acclimatization over a period of several days is preferable to rapid ascent. Hackett's studies in Nepal showed this, as did earlier studies of troops brought to Pikes Peak, which indicated that a preliminary stay of several days at 7,500 feet (2,290 m) greatly reduced the incidence and severity of AMS.[39,40] Residents of Rocky Mountain areas at 6,000-7,000 feet (1,830-2,135 m) who are rapidly exposed to an altitude of 14,000 feet (4,270 m) experience less severe symptoms of AMS than do sea level residents.[41] Honigman has reported that Colorado residents who visit ski areas in the Rocky Mountains have less severe symptoms of AMS than do those who come from sea level.[19] Permanent residents at 5,400 feet (1,650 m), however, are not immune to severe AMS or HAPE when they ascend to a substantially higher elevation. After a stay at sea level or a lower elevation for several days or weeks, such medium-high altitude residents will have lost enough acclimatization to have acquired a susceptibility to AMS and HAPE upon return to high altitude.

Age and gender. Little information is available regarding age and sex differences in susceptibility to AMS, largely because most observations have been made in a relatively homogenous population group, that is, young males. Hackett found a negative correlation with age in trekkers in Nepal. The mean age of 200 patients with AMS was 35.2 years ± 13.3 years, and 31.4 years ± 9.7 years in those without symptoms (p=0.029). One cannot accurately interpret age differences however, without knowing the age and sex distribution of the study population. Elderly persons who visited Vail, Colorado, 8,200 feet (2,500 m) had an incidence of AMS of 16 percent which is slightly lower than that reported for younger persons.[42,19] Men are slightly more affected by AMS than women (58 percent versus 42 percent p <0.01).[19] The difference is more striking in HAPE where only 16 percent of women are affected.[47] Harris reported that women on Pikes Peak tolerated high altitude better than men.[43]

Physical fitness and physical activity. Despite a prevailing notion that physical fitness achieved through regular aerobic exercise such as running before going to high altitude will present AMS, there are no data to support this theory. Ravenhill in 1913 stated, "There is in my experience no type of man of whom one can say he will or will not suffer from puna. Most of the cases I have instanced were young men to all appearances perfectly sound. Young, strong and healthy men may be completely overcome. Stout, plethoric individuals of the chronic bronchitic type may not even have a headache."[7] Cymerman and his associates reported that symptoms of AMS were actually more severe in young men with the highest VO_{2max} measured before ascent to 14,100 feet (4,300 m) than in subjects with lower VO_{2max}.[44] Favour studied two groups of soldiers brought to 14,150 feet (4,316 m). One group consisted of middle-distance runners at a high level of physical fitness induced by a regular training program; the other group consisted of normal sedentary subjects. Both groups had similar symptoms of AMS with a similar degree of severity.[45] Billings and his workers made similar observations at 12,470 feet

(3,800 m).[46] Honigman reported that among visitors to Rocky Mountain ski resorts those who considered themselves to be in excellent physical condition had fewer symptoms of AMS than those who considered themselves to be in only average or good physical condition.[19] Bias on the part of the persons interviewed could not be excluded. Milledge and his associates made similar observations in 17 climbers at 14,760 feet (4,500 m).[29]

Heavy physical activity upon arrival at high altitude probably accentuates the symptoms of AMS, but few systematic studies have been made of this phenomenon. Traditionally, upon arrival from Lima at Chulec General Hospital in the Peruvian Andes, 12,230 feet (3,730 m), the visitor is guided to a comfortable bed, given tea and toast, and told to avoid heavy physical activity during the next 24 hours. A group of physiologists had previously driven by car up to the Barcroft Laboratory, 12,470 feet (3,800 m), in previous years without any significant altitude illness. One year their truck developed a flat tire about 10,000 feet (3,050 m) and the group had to work hard to jack up the vehicle and change the tire. The next day all members of the group had severe AMS and could not conduct their planned experiments. On previous and subsequent ascents without vehicle problems symptoms were only mild.

Obesity. Three separate studies have indicated that obese individuals may experience symptoms of acute mountain sickness that are more frequent and more severe than those of average-weight persons. Kayser reviewed 353 questionnaires to trekkers climbing a 17,710 foot (5,400 m) pass in the Nepalese Himalaya.[23] The overall prevalence of acute mountain sickness was 63 percent. Body mass index (weight/length^2) was significantly correlated with mountain sickness in men (p= <0.05) but not in women. Hirata found a similar correlation in 63 Japanese climbers, 23 of whom experienced mountain sickness at 15,800 feet (4,815 m). In the obese climbers symptoms were more frequent and severe than in those with a normal or thin habitus.[48] Honigman and his associates reported that in visitors to Rocky Mountain ski resorts obese persons had a higher number of symptoms and more severe symptoms of AMS than non-obese persons.[19]

Prediction of AMS. At sea level there is no simple method of predicting the occurrence of AMS. In general, previous episodes of AMS will usually be repeated during subsequent altitude exposures, and persons who tolerate high altitude without symptoms will usually not develop AMS during return visits. It has been shown that persons who are likely to develop AMS will have a higher prevalence of certain physiological features than those who do not develop symptoms. These include a lower vital capacity,[37,49,50] and a lower hypoxic ventilatory drive[51-54] at sea level. Milledge and his associates, however, found no correlation between the hypoxic ventilatory drive measured before going to altitude and symptom scores for AMS after arrival.[55] Upon exposure to altitude AMS-susceptible subjects will exhibit a lower minute ventilation, a higher arterial CO_2 tension, and a lower arterial PO_2.[37,49,51,56] Susceptible subjects also appear to have a greater degree of relative hypoventilation upon continued exposure to altitude.[21] Individuals who have experienced symptoms of AMS will be very likely to experience similar symptoms upon repeat exposures (Table 12.7).

Etiology

It is evident that the important cause of AMS is hypoxia, but it should also be recognized that hypoxia may result in symptoms via several pathways.

Hypocapnia. Mosso in 1897 proposed that the hypocapnia of acute high altitude exposure may be the cause of some of the symptoms of AMS.[6] Childs and McFarland reported that inhalation of 3 percent carbon dioxide may be beneficial in the relief of symptoms.[10,11] The hypocapnia concept is difficult to support, because maximum hypocapnia is not achieved until several days after arrival at high altitude, at a time when symptoms of AMS have largely subsided. An important refutation of Mosso's concept was provided by Maher, who maintained normocapnia in five subjects exposed to a simulated high altitude with 3.8 percent CO_2 added to the atmosphere.[57] Four other subjects were exposed to the same altitude without added CO_2 and became hypocapneic. The severity of symptoms was greater in the normocapneic subjects (Fig. 12.3). These data do not exclude the possibility that some of the symptoms of AMS may be related to alkalosis, including dizziness, light-headedness, weakness, fatigue, and tremor. Such symptoms are commonly observed at sea level in anxiety states and the hyperventilation syndrome. The breathing of lower concentrations of CO_2 up to 3 percent for short periods of time may be beneficial in AMS by virtue of the resulting increase in ventilation.[58]

Hypercapnia. Forwand reported a positive correlation between the arterial PCO_2 and the occurrence and severity of headache, insomnia, and gastrointestinal symptoms in 22 subjects at 12,790 feet (3,900 m).[59] King and Robinson found an inverse relationship between the ventilatory response to hypoxia and symptoms of AMS.[51] A consequence of a low ventilatory response to hypoxia would be a higher PCO_2; this may not be a causative factor, however, but simply a marker of a decreased ventilatory response to hypoxia.

Fluid retention. Singh and his colleagues were aware of the association of HAPE and HACE with AMS in military personnel brought to altitudes between 11,000 and 18,000 feet (3,355-5,490 m). They were also aware of the lag period of several hours or days before symptoms of these illnesses appeared, which seemed to refute the possibility that acute hypoxia alone was an important causative factor. They proposed that a major cause of AMS as well as of HAPE and HACE was fluid retention due to a "sudden discharge" of antidiuretic hormone triggered by central nervous system hypoxia.[14] Retention of water and sodium would facilitate systemic edema formation as well as edema of the lung and brain. As a result of this concept the liberal use of diuretics, morphine, and steroids was advocated to prevent and treat AMS. Subsequent studies by Aoki and Robinson showed that the degree of hydration could not be correlated with the presence and severity of AMS.[60] Hackett's study at Pheriche provided indirect evidence of an antidiuretic effect upon symptoms. He observed that less weight loss occurred in trekkers with AMS than in those without symptoms (p=0.07). He also noted that more symptoms were present in those who had lost little weight. Of the subjects who had AMS, 19 percent reported a reduced urine output, but in those without AMS only 3 percent reported a reduced urine output.[18]

Bärtsch and his associates have shown that persons susceptible to acute mountain sickness who ascended to 14,950 feet (4,559 m) exhibited a rise in aldosterone, ADH, and ANF that was greater than the increase in nonsusceptible persons.[20,34,35] Sodium excretion was decreased and facial edema was more common in the AMS-susceptible subjects. Thirty minutes of exercise on a cycle ergometer resulted in greater increases in these hormones than at rest in the susceptible subjects. The changes occurred before the onset of acute mountain sickness. Although a rise in

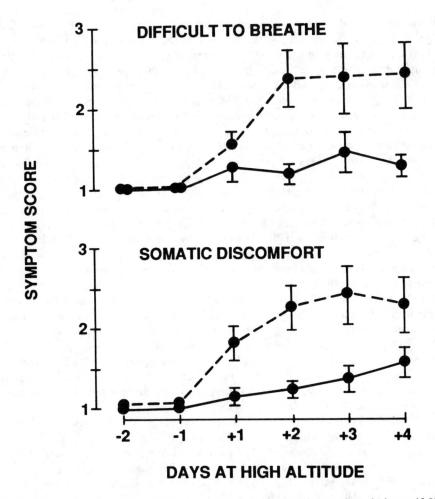

Figure 12.3. Score of symptoms of AMS during four days of hypobaric hypoxia equivalent to 13,000 feet (4,000 m) in ten normal subjects. The dashed lines indicate the effect of adding 3.8 percent CO_2 to the chamber atmosphere and repeating the study. Note that symptoms are more severe when CO_2 is added. Somatic discomfort scores represent the average of scores for headache, nausea, dizziness, and difficulty in breathing. Values are mean + S.E. 1 = not present; 2 = slight; 3 = moderate. From Maher et al, ref. 57.

ANF would tend to increase sodium and water excretion, the authors suggested that this effect of ANF was overcome by the combined effect of aldosterone and ADH.[35] If fluid retention is an important factor in producing the symptoms of AMS, one must inquire why it is not present in all patients with AMS, and why furosemide does not prevent AMS or result in symptomatic relief.

The vasogenic theory. The hypoxic-vasogenic theory proposes that the primary conditions responsible for the varied symptoms of AMS involve the central nervous system by means of a hypoxia-mediated increase in cerebral blood flow that results in vasogenic cerebral edema. The vasodilatation and high cerebral blood flow may overcome regional areas of vasoconstriction and make it possible for abnormally high flows and pressure to be transmitted to the capillary bed, with resulting interstitial edema and capillary injury. This process is a pressure breakthrough analogous to the high-pressure breakthrough that is probably responsible for the clinical manifestations of hypertensive encephalopathy.[61,62] Visual evidence of increased flow and capillary injury is seen in engorgement of retinal vessels by high flow and retinal hemorrhages. The same changes are probably occurring in the brain.[16]

This concept of the pathogenesis of AMS proposed by Sutton and Lassen[61] is supported by several observations. (a) High altitude exposure is accompanied by a prompt increase in cerebral blood flow of 25-50 percent, which gradually subsides over five to seven days. This is the average time course of the symptoms of AMS.[63-66] (b) Interventions that decrease cerebral blood flow relieve symptoms of AMS, including oxygen, descent, hyperventilation, and ergotamine. (c) Symptoms of AMS are worsened by factors that increase cerebral blood flow, such as 3.8-7 percent carbon dioxide inhalation.[57] (d) Nausea, vomiting, and periodic breathing have a central nervous system origin. (e) The headache of AMS may be due to dilatation and stretching of cerebral vessels.[67] (f) Autopsy studies and brain biopsies have demonstrated the common occurrence of cerebral edema and capillary injury in AMS, HAPE, and HACE. CT scans and MRI studies of the brain in AMS have demonstrated cerebral edema. MRI studies have revealed slightly increased intensity of the white matter compatible with vasogenic cerebral edema.[68,69] Some studies have raised doubts about the vasogenic theory of cerebral edema in AMS. For example, Reeves and his associates showed that headache at high altitude was not related to internal carotid arterial blood velocity.[70] However, Hackett and his workers showed that oxygenation improves high altitude headache with a decrease in middle cerebral artery blood flow velocity.[71]

Cellular edema. The major central nervous system abnormalities in AMS are known to be an increased cerebral blood flow, vascular dilatation, a low-pressure breakthrough with capillary injury, and interstitial edema, but the exact role of intracellular cerebral edema remains to be clarified. Hypoxia may interfere with the intracellular sodium pump, allowing sodium to enter the cells with an osmotic influx of water and resulting tissue edema.[72,73,74]

Severinghaus has suggested that cellular ion pump failure is an unlikely result of hypoxia-induced ATP depletion since this occurs only under very severe degrees of hypoxia.[75]

In summary, there are many unanswered questions about the etiology of symptoms in AMS, including the role of increased cerebral blood flow and the role of interstitial edema and intracellular edema. If an increase in cerebral blood flow or "vasogenic edema" results in symptoms, why is there a delay in the onset of symptoms of 12-24 hours after arrival when CBF increases promptly upon arrival? What role does interstitial edema play in producing symptoms? Cerebral edema from other causes does not predictably cause headache. The rapid relief of symptoms by oxygen or descent occurs too rapidly to be due to a decrease in cellular cerebral edema. Cerebral edema may persist after relief of symptoms. And what is the mechanism of capillary injury in AMS? Another unanswered question has to do with vascular constriction, which, in cerebral vessels can result in migraine-like headaches. What role does alkalosis play in the symptoms of AMS by producing cerebral vasoconstriction? Finally, although it is clear that oxygen, descent, and increased ventilation provide rapid relief of AMS symptoms, what are the mechanisms that are involved?

Prevention and Treatment of AMS

Many interventions have been tried to prevent or ameliorate symptoms of AMS, and some of these merit discussion.

Ammonium chloride. In 1932 during the successful ascent of Mount Kamet, 25,447 feet (7,760 m), Greene noted that he obtained some benefit from ammonium chloride, using a small dose of 0.45 grams, three times daily.[76] Following this observation Douglas and Greene evaluated the effect of ammonium chloride in one subject rapidly exposed to 20,000-22,000 feet (6,100- 6,710 m) in a hypobaric chamber.[77] Ammonium chloride was given in a large dose—10 grams the day before ascent and 5 grams the following day. The results suggested some benefit from the resulting acidosis by a slower heart rate and an increased working capacity. The arterial PCO_2 decreased by 2.5 mm and arterial PO_2 increased by 3.3 mm. The authors suggested that a dose of three grams per day might be adequate to obtain a beneficial effect.

Barron studied the effect of 15 grams of ammonium chloride given to six of twelve subjects before an ascent by auto to 15,500 feet (4,728 m) in Peru. Despite a decrease in alveolar PCO_2, no symptomatic benefit was noted. Gastric distress occurred in several subjects.[12] Singh and his associates gave ammonium chloride (6 gms per day) for three days to 30 patients with AMS. Seven were not affected and 23 felt worse! Intravenous ammonium chloride (10-20 gms) was given to ten patients; one felt better and nine were not affected or felt worse.[14]

It is evident that ammonium chloride will result in a rapid but slight acidosis with a decrease in PCO_2, a decrease in pH, and a resulting increase in arterial PO_2. One gram given intravenously will decrease arterial PCO_2 by about one mm.[78] But there are several disadvantages to ammonium chloride, the most important being gastric irritation. Also, the intravenous administration is dangerous; severe systemic reactions have been reported.[78] The concomitant administration of acetazolamide and ammonium chloride has not been evaluated.

Carbon dioxide. In 1935 Childs and his associates administered carbon dioxide to tourists with mountain sickness on Pikes Peak to reduce the respiratory alkalosis, and some systemic benefit was noted.[10] Later, McFarland and Dill demonstrated that 3 percent CO_2 added to low oxygen mixtures or used in a hypobaric chamber resulted in an increase in ventilation and a decrease in symptoms.[11] In 1975 Maher and his associates showed that 3.8 percent CO_2 added to the atmosphere of a hypobaric chamber at a simulated altitude of 11,500 feet (3,500 m) resulted in an increase in severity of mountain sickness in five subjects compared with four hypocapneic controls.[57] They speculated that symptoms including headaches were worsened by CO_2, possibly because of cerebral vasodilatation and an increase in cerebral blood flow. Recently a beneficial effect of adding 3 percent CO_2 to ambient air in patients with AMS was reported by Harvey and his associates.[58] Six patients were studied during a medical expedition to 17,700 feet (5,400 m). Arterial PCO_2 increased by 9-28 percent and respiratory alkalosis was reduced. Symptoms of AMS were rapidly relieved. In three subjects cerebral blood flow (measured by the radioactive xenon method) was increased by 17-39 percent. Hackett and his associates also reported that breathing 3 percent CO_2 produced hyperventilation, an increase in arterial O_2

saturation, and relief of headache. Estimated cerebral blood flow was not increased.[71] Reeves and his associates found that the administration of 7 percent CO_2 resulted in a large increase in estimated cerebral blood flow, but no change in headache.[70]

Bärtsch and his associates compared the effect of breathing 3 percent CO_2 with 33 percent O_2 in patients with AMS at 14,958 feet (4,559 m). Carbon dioxide was ineffective in reducing symptoms, although ventilation was increased with a slight rise in arterial PO_2. Oxygen breathing effectively relieved symptoms and was accompanied by a decrease in estimated blood flow velocity in the middle cerebral artery. The authors concluded that inhalation of 3 percent CO_2 cannot be recommended as an emergency treatment of AMS because it is no more effective than a placebo.[79]

Field studies of cerebral blood flow have been performed by Jensen and his associates using xenon-133.[80] Cerebral blood flow at 10,500 feet (3,200 m) was increased 24 percent at four days and by 47 percent above sea level values at 15,750-16,400 feet (4,800-5,000 m) at nine days. No difference in blood flow was noted between subjects who did and did not have symptoms of AMS. Acetazolamide and CO_2 inhalation reduced symptoms of AMS despite an increase in cerebral blood flow. Although these data might suggest that symptoms of AMS are not related to an increase in cerebral blood flow, the increase in arterial PO_2 produced by acetazolamide or CO_2 breathing may have relieved symptoms despite the increase in cerebral blood flow.

Rolaids and antacids. The use of Rolaids was publicized as a method of preventing AMS in 1977.[81] The hypothesis proposed was that metabolic acidosis is more prevalent during exercise at high altitude than at sea level and that the acidosis may aggravate symptoms of AMS. It was recommended that two to twelve tablets of Rolaids daily would be beneficial during climbs of short duration, such as on Mount Rainier.

There are several problems with this hypothesis and the recommendations. At high altitude the blood is alkaline, and there is no evidence that a metabolic acidosis is present or can be related to symptoms. It is not possible to affect serum pH by even large doses of alkali. Falchuk gave 50 grams of $NaHCO_2$ to three subjects for three days and achieved only a slight increase in alkalinity of the blood (pH rose from 7.44 to 7.47). One of the three subjects developed nausea and vomiting and could not be studied further.[82] Rolaids consist of dihydroxyaluminum sodium bicarbonate; one tablet contains 53 mg of sodium, which is the highest sodium content of twelve available tablet antacids. A placebo-controlled trial of Rolaids was carried out on Mount Rainier without benefit except a slight amelioration of headache at 13,000 feet (3,962 m), but not on the summit, 14,410 feet (4,395 m). No physiological differences were noted between the two treatment groups.[38] Twelve grams of Rolaids were given before the 48 hour climb (36 tablets—one-half the maximum safe dose as defined by the manufacturer).

Potassium supplements. Waterlow and Bunje suggested that potassium depletion may be a factor in the symptoms of AMS.[83] They carried out studies during four expeditions to Columbia at altitudes of 12,000-14,000 feet (3,660-4,270 m). Potassium supplements of 70 mEq per day were compared with placebos. Serum potassium levels were slightly increased by the supplements (5.20 mEq/L, and 4.88 mEq/L in the placebo group). Although symptoms appeared to be more severe in the placebo group, the results are difficult to interpret, especially since other workers have shown a rise in serum potassium associated with a decrease in potassium excretion at high altitude.[84] Singh and his associates gave potassium chloride (1.8 gms daily) for three days to 30 patients with AMS and gave an additional ten patients IV potassium. The results were disappointing.[14] This was a risky experiment, since intravenous potassium salts can cause cardiac arrest.

Furosemide. Treating and preventing AMS by furosemide has been subject of much controversy. The treatment was first tested by Singh and his associates in 1969.[14] They studied 1,925 patients with AMS who had arrived at altitudes between 11,500 feet (3,500 m) and 18,000 feet (5,490 m). A total of 840 patients who were not treated experienced a duration of symptoms of two to five days. Furosemide was given in a dose of 160 mg per day for two days or longer to 446 patients, with a reported relief of symptoms and signs (largely pulmonary rales) in 6 to 48 hours. This study had several flaws that make the interpretation of the results difficult. No criteria for the diagnosis of AMS were presented. The diagnosis was made by medical officers who were probably aware of the treatment, and this bias cannot be excluded. The incidence of AMS was low and the symptoms were not severe. Of the 200 subjects, only 24 (12 percent) developed AMS, and of these patients 64 percent were classified as mild with an average of only 2.1 symptoms. Singh also made a trial of a similar dose of furosemide started on the day of ascent to 11,500 feet (3,500 m) and continued for one day more, to determine whether or not AMS could be prevented. Symptoms were relieved in former residents who were returning to high altitude ($p<0.01$), but there was no significant effect in newcomers to high altitude ($p=.07$). Dyspnea was reportedly relieved by furosemide.

Aoki and Robinson[60] examined the state of body hydration in relation to symptoms in AMS in twelve subjects on three occasions in a hypobaric chamber at 14,000 feet (4,270 m). A placebo-controlled crossover protocol was employed and each subject acted as his own control. The effect of furosemide 80 mg (given on the day of ascent) was compared with a placebo as well as with vasopressin, which was employed to maintain body hydration. Furosemide resulted in a diuresis and a loss of 3.5 percent of body weight. A multiple-item symptom questionnaire revealed no differences in the scores of the three groups. The authors concluded that moderate dehydration resulting from a diuretic does not affect the occurrence or severity of AMS.[60]

Gray and his associates compared the effect of furosemide and acetazolamide in fourteen subjects who were brought to 17,500 feet (5,340 m) on Mount Logan.[85] Five were given 40 mg of furosemide twice daily for two days and five were given acetazolamide 250 mg every eight hours for 36 hours before hours before ascent. Four subjects were given placebos. The results were dramatic. The furosemide and placebo group all were completely incapacitated (Functional Class III). Three of the furosemide group showed severe ataxia, a fourth was unable to stand, and a fifth became comatose and was evacuated. Clinical signs of dehydration and falling blood pressure necessitated stopping furosemide and forcing fluids. In contrast, the acetazolamide group remained reasonably well and only suffered mild AMS. None were incapacitated (Functional Class I and II).

The author and his associates have studied plasma volume, symptoms and AMS, and the effect of furosemide upon ascent to 12,470 feet (3,800 m) to the White Mountain Research Station in California.[86] Twenty-two subjects were studied on separate occasions. Placebo controls were employed. Furosemide was given on the day of ascent and for two days after arrival at high altitude in a dose of 40 mg twice daily. Venous blood samples revealed a greater rise in hemoglobin in the furosemide-treated subjects compared with the placebo group. (Fig. 12.4). Postural hypotension (a decrease in systolic blood pressure >10 mm) occurred in four of ten furosemide-treated subjects. Two subjects experienced syncope preceded by an unobtainable blood pressure (Fig. 12.5). These effects were not present in the control group.

In the same experiment, the effect upon symptoms was also examined by the use of an AMS scoring system. Symptoms were slightly worse in the furosemide treated subjects on day 1, but no difference was noted on days 2 and 3. A crossover study was carried out in four subjects who were given furosemide during one ascent and a placebo during a second ascent one year later. A slight increase in severity score was present in the furosemide-treated group. One subject receiving furosemide was so weak that he was unable to complete the climb to 14,200 feet (4,330 m). Furosemide resulted in a prompt diuresis, moderate weight loss, and a slight decrease in serum sodium and potassium, but there were considerable individual differences. (Table 12.8)

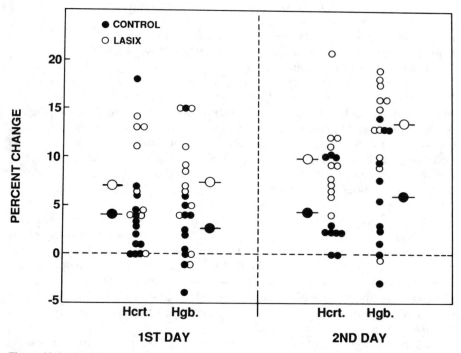

Figure 12.4. Changes in hematocrit and hemoglobin in 22 normal subjects brought to 12,400 feet (3,780 m). Studies were made in the mornings after the first and second night at altitude. Nine subjects received furosemide (Lasix), 40 mg on the day before ascent and on the arrival. Mean values are shown. Note that hematocrit and hemoglobin values are higher in the subjects who received furosemide, and these values are higher on the second day than on the first day. Thus furosemide results in a greater decrease in plasma volume than usually occurs with ascent to high altitude. From Hultgren et al, ref. 86.

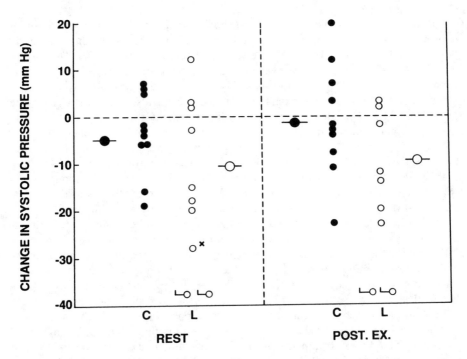

Figure 12.5. The effect of furosemide (Lasix) upon blood pressure during quiet standing and standing after two minutes of light exercise. The subjects were studied in the morning after spending the night at 12,400 feet (3,780 m). Open circles indicate subjects, who were given two doses of 40 mg of furosemide 24 hours before ascent; solid circles indicate placebo-treated control group. Note the lower systolic pressures in the furosemide-treated subjects. Two furosemide subjects during each study fainted (bottom of panels). Thus the diuretic results in postural hypotension in susceptible subjects. A decrease in systolic blood pressure of >20 mm Hg during 2 minutes of standing from supine position is usually defined as orthostatic hypotension. From Hultgren et al, ref. 86.

Table 12.8
Acute Mountain Sickness on Two Different Exposures to 12,400 feet (3,782 m) in Four Subjects Receiving a Placebo or Furosemide.

Subject	Placebo			Total	Furosemide			Total
	Day 1	Day 2	Day 3		Day 1	Day 2	Day 3	
HF	28	32	36	96	35	29	32	96
HH	39	41	52	132	28	51	61	140
NL	37	34	34	105	28	32	36	96
JP	45	55	39	139	47	42	45	134
Total score				472				466

SOURCE: Hultgren, unpublished data.

NOTES: The scoring system employed is described in the text. Scores for each of three days at altitude are shown as well as the total scores. No difference exists between the Furosemide and placebo treatments. The questionnaire employed is shown in Table 12.4. Scores on repeat exposures are similar.

In summary, furosemide has not been shown to be of value in the prevention or treatment of AMS, and even the original report advocating its use did not clearly demonstrate any benefit because of serious methodologic deficiencies. There is no question that furosemide is a dangerous drug to use at high altitude because of its capacity to reduce blood volume seriously, in a setting where plasma volume is already decreased by acute hypoxia. Spironolactone has also been employed in the prevention of AMS, but the reported studies were not controlled.[87,88] It can be concluded that diuretics are of no value in the prevention and treatment of AMS.

Morphine sulfate. Morphine sulfate was originally recommended by Singh and his associates for the treatment of HAPE.[89] Subsequently it was used in AMS (15 mg intravenously) as an adjunct to furosemide with the claim that the resulting diuresis was greater than that attained by furosemide alone.[14] No controlled trials of morphine in AMS have been reported, and its use in AMS does not seem justified.

Steroids. Betamethasone and dexamethasone are synthetic steroids of similar activity, and they are the most potent of the glucocorticoids. They are anti-inflammatory agents and are essentially devoid of mineral corticoid activity and sodium-retaining potency. Dexamethasone has been used in the treatment of vasogenic cerebral edema.[90,91] In the 1968 study by Singh and his associates betamethasone was given to 24 patients with AMS and neurological abnormalities with relief of headache and vomiting within three days. Furosemide was also given, and betamethasone appeared to have increased its diuretic effect.[14] In recent years, a number of studies of dexamethasone in the prevention and treatment of AMS have been reported.[92-94] Most of these were field trials, but hypobaric chamber studies were also performed.[68,92,93,96-100] The essential results of these studies to date are summarized below:

1. Dexamethasone 2 mg every six hours beginning on the day of ascent may reduce the symptoms of AMS, but it is less effective than acetazolamide.[103] Hackett and his workers found that AMS was not prevented when subjects ascended to 14,430 feet (4,400 m) in one hour by helicopter.[101]

2. Dexamethasone given with acetazolamide on a recreational climb from 4,400 feet (1,340 m) to 13,300 feet (4,050 m) did not prevent AMS, but when given with acetazolamide it appeared to result in more relief of symptoms than the latter drug alone.[95]

3. Ellsworth reported that dexamethasone was more effective than acetazolamide or a placebo in reducing symptoms of AMS in the ascent of Mount Rainier (14,405 feet, 4,392 m).[95]

4. Dexamethasone was employed in the treatment of severe AMS by Hackett and his associates.[101] When it was given in doses of 4 mg every 6 hours, all eleven patients were markedly improved at 12 hours, but symptoms rapidly increased 24 hours after the drug was discontinued. Dexamethasone in a dose of 4 mg every 6 hours started 34 hours before exposure to a chamber altitude of 14,000 feet (4,270 m) and continued for 52 hours after ascent had a positive effect upon cognitive performances and mood states compared with a placebo.[102]

5. Several clinical trials of dexamethasone in AMS contain problems in study design that make the interpretation of the results difficult. These include exposure to relatively low altitudes with a gradual ascent profile, the absence of severe mountain sickness, the possible bias of subjects, who may down-play symptoms because they are aware of being in a study, and the fact that blinding may not be complete, because acetazolamide usually causes a diuresis whereas dexamethasone does not.[103]

Studies in the Peruvian Andes twenty years ago indicated that prednisone, 40 mg twice daily started two days before ascent to high altitude, was of no value in preventing AMS. Acetazolamide was subsequently found to be effective and is now used extensively, with the result that the incidence of AMS and HAPE has been greatly reduced in the mining town of La Oroya. In a study of therapeutic modalities in patients in Peru with HAPE, dexamethasone 0.5 mg every eight hours after a loading dose of 1.5 mg was found to have no effect on heart rate, respiratory rate, or symptoms in six hospitalized patients. The administration of 150-200 mg of hydrocortisone intravenously to two patients had no effect on symptoms, heart rate, respiratory rate, or arterial blood gases.

Steroids are of no value in the treatment of high altitude pulmonary edema.[104] The use of steroids in AMS by Johnson and his associates was based on the hypothesis that symptoms are related to cerebral edema, and because steroids are useful in the treatment of cerebral edema a beneficial effect might be observed in AMS. There is no conclusive evidence that cerebral edema alone is the cause of symptoms of AMS. In patients with metastatic carcinoma of the brain, steroids are of established value in relieving symptoms, including headache, nausea, and vomiting.[90] The mechanism of action appears to involve a decrease in volume of the surrounding cerebral tissue by dehydration rather than by a effect on the neoplasm. Steroids have little effect upon cerebral blood flow or the cerebral circulation.[90,105] Intravenous methylprednisolone has been used in the emergency treatment of acute asthma with subjective improvement, but the mechanism of action is unknown.[106] The mechanism of action of steroids in AMS is likewise unknown since no changes in physiological variables have been observed.[96,104] It is possible, therefore, that euphoria and changes in mood may be an important explanation for their action in mild to moderate AMS. Rabold has recently reviewed the published studies of dexamethasone for prophylaxis and treatment of AMS.[107]

Phenytoin (Dilantin). Phenytoin has been advocated as a possible method of reducing symptoms of cerebral hypoxia.[108] The basis for this suggestion is the ability of phenytoin to reduce intracellular sodium concentrations in the brain during hypoxia and in that way to lessen cerebral edema. To test this suggestion, Burse and his associates studied six subjects in two separate experiments in a hypobaric chamber (15,000 feet/4,575 m) for a 56-hour period using placebo controls. Phenytoin 300 mg per day was started one day before ascent and continued for the duration of the altitude exposure. No beneficial effect upon symptoms was evident.[109]

Acetazolamide (Diamox). Experiments with acetazolamide have been conducted since the mid-1960's. In 1966, Cain and Dunn reported that the use of acetazolamide resulted in a decrease in bicarbonate, pH, and alveolar PCO_2 with an increase in ventilation, which was most significant on the second and third day of exposure; there was little effect on the fourth and fifth day.[110] The dose of acetazolamide was 750 mg, given in divided doses the night before and the morning of ascent. Placebo controls were employed. Symptoms were not evaluated.

In 1968, Forwand and his associates performed a study of the effect of acetazolamide upon symptoms and physiological variables in 43 subjects brought to Mount Evans, Colorado, at 12,800 feet (3,990 m). Acetazolamide 250 mg every eight hours was given for 32 hours before and continued for 40 hours after ascent. Placebo controls were employed and studies were carried out over five days on the mountain.[59] The results confirmed those made by Cain and Dunn and in addition showed

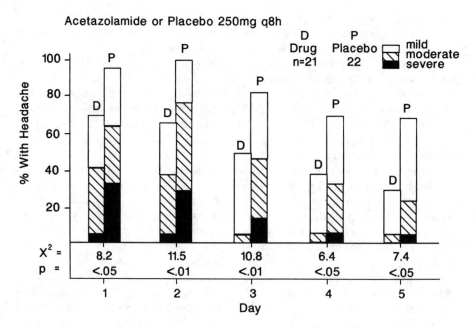

Figure 12.6. Patterns of headache during five days of exposure to 12,800 feet (3,900 m) in 21 subjects given acetazolamide and 22 subjects given a placebo. Acetazolamide was given in a dose of 250 mg every 8 hours for 72 hours starting 32 hours before ascent. Placebo tablets were given on the same schedule. The column heights refer to the percentage of subjects with headache. Severity of headache is indicated by shading. Values for chi square (X^2) and probability are shown below. Headache is less frequent and less severe in the treatment group. From Forwand et al, ref. 59.

a striking decrease in symptoms of AMS in the treatment group, with the greatest effect seen during the first three days at high altitude (Fig. 12.6). Minute ventilation and alveolar PO_2 were higher in the acetazolamide treated group (Fig. 12.7). Both pH and PCO_2 were decreased (Fig. 12.8). It was also noted that symptoms, especially headache, appeared more severe in subjects with the highest PCO_2 levels and had little relationship to alveolar PO_2.

At the same time, Kronenberg and Cain carried out similar studies on 23 subjects at a simulated altitude of 14,000 feet (4,270 m) for 72 hours with comparable results.[111] They also reported that benzolamide was less effective than acetazolamide and suggested that acetazolamide should be continued for 40 hours after arrival at high altitude.[112] More recently, Hackett and his associates compared benzolamide with acetazolamide in the control of periodic breathing during sleep. Both were effective in reducing periodic breathing and increasing oxygen saturation, but more side effects were noted with benzolamide.[37]

In 1971, Gray and his associates compared the effects of acetazolamide, furosemide, and a placebo at an altitude of 17,500 feet (5,340 m) on Mount Logan. Acetazolamide clearly suppressed most of the symptoms of AMS, while furosemide and a placebo were equally without effect.[85]

In 1976, Evans and his associates brought subjects from sea level to 5,400 feet (1,650 m) for four days, gave acetazolamide 500 mg twice daily for the final two

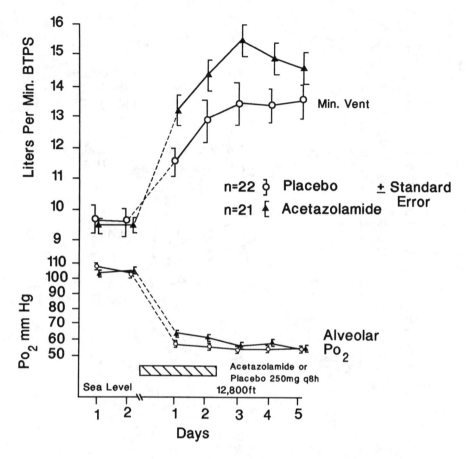

Figure 12.7. Time course of mean values for minute ventilation (top) and alveolar oxygen tension (bottom) in 22 subjects given a placebo and 21 subjects given acetazolamide in the same study illustrated in Figure 12.6. Minute ventilation and alveolar oxygen tension are significantly higher in the treatment group. From Forwand et al, ref. 59.

days before ascent to Pikes Peak, and continued acetazolamide for two more days. An 85 percent reduction in symptoms of AMS was observed in this group compared with a control group that ascended to Pikes Peak without staging or medication.[39]

In 1979, Sutton and his associates added additional important information regarding the effect of acetazolamide at high altitude in an experiment in which placebo-controlled studies of oxygen saturation during sleep were performed on nine subjects at 17,500 feet (5,340 m).[113] Despite the fact that the subjects had been at that altitude for 8 to 30 days and were partly acclimatized, acetazolamide (250 mg every 8 hours for 5 doses) greatly reduced the magnitude of sleep hypoxia with an increase in arterial oxygen saturation and pulmonary ventilation. The average arterial oxygen saturation during sleep at 72±2.1 percent was increased to 78.7 percent ±1.2. Numerous other papers have clearly established the value of acetazolamide in the prevention and treatment of AMS.[39,114,115]

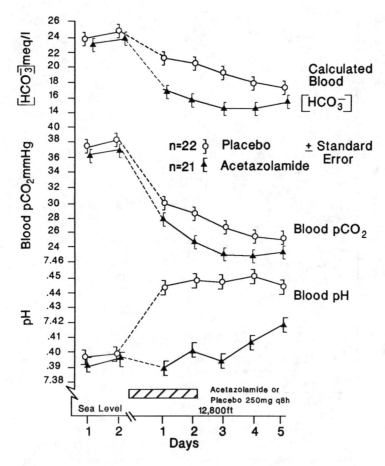

Figure 12.8. Time course of mean values of pH, CO_2 tension, and bicarbonate in arterialized blood of 22 subjects receiving placebo (circles) and 21 subjects receiving acetazolamide (triangles) during exposure to 12,800 feet (3,900 m). The same subjects are shown in Figures 12.6 and 12.7. From Forwand et al, ref. 59.

Acetazolamide has as its major pharmacological action the inhibition of the enzyme carbonic anhydrase. Its beneficial effect at high altitude is to diminish the degree of alkalosis with a resulting higher arterial PCO_2 and an increase in ventilation. Part of this effect is due to an increase in the urinary excretion of bicarbonate and fixed cations, mostly sodium. As a result, the concentration of bicarbonate in the extracellular fluid decreases and a metabolic acidosis results. Acetazolamide (0.5 gm intravenously) increases cerebral blood flow probably by producing a carbonic acidosis in brain tissue and extracellular fluid. These effects will stimulate respiration.[116] A modest diuresis also occurs, the magnitude of which exhibits considerable individual variation. Renal potassium loss is increased. The urine becomes alkaline, with a decrease in the excretion of titratable acid and ammonia. Acetazolamide has been used in the treatment of glaucoma by its capacity to reduce the rate of aqueous humor formation and thus the intraocular pressure.

Almitrine. Almitrine is a respiratory stimulant that has been used in the treatment of chronic pulmonary disease at sea level.[117,118] It is not approved for use in the United States. Hackett compared the effect of almitrine and acetazolamide during sleep on Mount McKinley at 14,500 feet (4,400 m). A double-blind randomized study was made on four normal subjects. Both drugs improved oxygenation during sleep. Acetazolamide diminished periodic breathing, but almitrine appeared to increase it, probably because of its effect in stimulating the peripheral chemoreceptors. Acetazolamide is therefore to be preferred to almitrine, not only because of its effect in stimulating respiration but also because it greatly decreases the periodic breathing that disturbs sleep.

Hyperbaric bag therapy. An important recent advance has been the development of a portable hyperbaric bag (Gamow bag) large enough to accommodate one patient and capable of maintaining a pressure of 2 psi (-104 mm Hg). The bag is a impermeable Cordura nylon cylinder with an internal polyurethane coating. An airtight zipper, vertically aligned, permits patient access. A pressure inlet valve is attached to a foot pump. A pressure-limited 2 psi gauge pop-off valve allows continuous venting of the bag with a steady bag pressure. A flow of 30 L/min can be maintained by 10-15 pumps per minute. The bag weighs seven kilograms and can be folded into a medium-size rucksack. A plastic face portal allows visual contact with the patient. The bag pressure results in a rapid drop in altitude: at 13,290 feet (4,027 m) inflation of the bag to 104 mm Hg is equivalent to an altitude drop to 8,400 feet (2,545 m). The bag seems to have a number of advantages. It is portable, lightweight, easily carried, and it can be used several times. It can be dropped from an aircraft. It avoids the expense, weight, and mechanical problems associated with oxygen. It is not harmful to the patient: unpleasant pain in the ears is the only complication that has been noted. Kasic and his associates compared the effect of two hours of simulated descent in the bag at 9,300 feet (2,834 m) with two hours of oxygen breathing at 4 L/min by mask in 24 patients with HAPE.[119] Bag treatment increased arterial oxygen saturation from 84 percent to 91 percent, whereas oxygen breathing increased saturation from 83 percent to 96 percent. The two methods of treatment were equally effective in reducing symptoms. Improvement persisted for at least one hour after treatment stopped. A placebo was not employed. Similar results have been reported by Forster[120], Bärtsch[121], Robertson[122], Taber[123], and King.[124]

Recommendations for Prevention

On the basis of the studies described above, including considerable practical field experience, the following recommendations for the prevention of AMS can be summarized:

1. Acclimatization at an intermediate altitude is the most physiological and harmless method of prevention. If one is going to spend several nights at an altitude of 9,000-12,000 feet (2,750-3,660 m), sleeping one or two nights at an altitude between 6,000 and 7,000 feet (1,830-2,135 m) will prevent symptoms in most persons. If one plans to spend several nights above 12,000 feet (3,660 m), two or three nights at an intermediate altitude should be observed.

For climbs or treks above 14,000 feet (4,270 m) where rapid ascent is necessary, one should spend four or five days at 9,000-12,000 feet (2,745-3,660 m) before ascent. At higher altitudes, it is advisable to limit ascents to no more than 1,500 feet per day (sleeping altitudes). Most treks or climbs, if wisely planned, will offer a period of acclimatization en route either by a gradual ascent or by a stay at an intermediate altitude. Unfortunately, some group leaders are unaware of the problems of rapid ascent, and even large groups are sometimes flown to high altitude areas without acclimatization, advice about altitude illness, any provision for treatment, and without the presence on the tour of any experienced medical personnel or physician. All too frequently, also, commercial trekking and tour companies do not provide sufficient time to overcome jet lag and to acclimatize. Legal action against such companies in the event of serious altitude illness is becoming more common. Physical conditioning at sea level before ascent will not reduce the chances of developing AMS nor will it ameliorate symptoms.[125]

2. The administration of acetazolamide is not advisable if the person has not experienced significant symptoms during previous high altitude exposures.

3. For trekkers who have not been to high altitude before, staying at an intermediate altitude should be observed and acetazolamide should be carried to be used if symptoms occur. The usual dose is 125 to 250 mg twice daily for five days. In my opinion, acetazolamide should not be given routinely to everyone going to high altitude. Many trekkers will have only mild symptoms and can avoid the inconvenience and potential side effects of this medication.

4. Acetazolamide is indicated for persons who have a history of significant symptoms of AMS, and for such persons the combination of staging and acetazolamide will be highly effective. A dose of 125 mg twice daily may be quite as effective and will have fewer side effects. Continuing acetazolamide for longer than five days after arrival is not advisable, because its effectiveness diminishes and there is an increasing chance of side effects. Some climbers prefer to continue taking 125 mg prior to sleep at high altitude because it prevents periodic breathing which may disturb sleep.

5. The most common side effect of acetazolamide is a diuresis, which will usually require nocturnal voiding, so a wide-mouth bottle in the tent is advisable. Paresthesias and a numb sensation of the fingers, toes, and circumoral area are usual and harmless. Beer and carbonated beverages may taste bad. Other side effects are less common, but include progressive myopia, gastric upsets, drowsiness, and malaise. At altitudes above 17,000 feet (5,185 m), acetazolamide should be used with caution, especially if it has not been started at lower elevations. Recently a climber in his sixties had ascended to the final camp on Aconcagua at 19,300 feet (5,890 m) without difficulty and without using acetazolamide. He was advised to start acetazolamide the evening before the summit attempt. After taking 500 mg, he developed a considerable diuresis and a gastric upset with resulting weakness and malaise, which became so severe that he could not start the summit climb. He recovered after a rest day and descended to the roadhead without difficulty.[125] Gastrointestinal symptoms at altitudes above 16,000 feet (4,880 m) have also been observed by Hackett.[126]

6. Considerable potassium is lost with the diuresis, and potassium intake should be increased during the use of acetazolamide. Natural high-potassium foods such as fruits, nuts, and soup are usually sufficient to replenish potassium losses.

7. A physician should be consulted before taking acetazolamide, since there are some contraindications, including sensitivity to sulfanilamides and liver or kidney disease. Serious side effects from acetazolamide are rare, but long-term use has

been associated with occasional instances of bone marrow depression and aplastic anemia.[110,127] Angle glaucoma is not a contraindication to acetazolamide.

8. At this time the use of steroids to prevent AMS seems unwise; acetazolamide is far more effective, and complications of the use of steroids may be serious in a mountain environment.

9. Other precautions that will ameliorate symptoms of AMS include the following: (a) light activity for two to three days after arrival. (b) Adequate fluid intake. (c) A high carbohydrate diet, preferably in frequent small feedings rather than in three heavy meals each day. (d) Avoidance of alcohol, codeine, sedatives, or medications that promote sleep, the use of which will depress respiration and increase hypoxia. Alcohol has been shown to inhibit the initial stages of adequate ventilatory adaptation to mild hypoxia at moderate altitude.[128] Hackett has reported that a majority of patients with HAPE seen on Mount Denali had used sleeping pills. Low dose (5 mg) benzodiazepine has been shown to inhibit ventilatory adaptation to moderate altitude with a decrease in oxygen saturation and an increase in PCO_2.[129] The use of Valium when taken to promote sleep has been shown to result in a state of confusion.[130] Respiratory depression may occur.[131] (Fig. 12.9). (e) Avoidance of

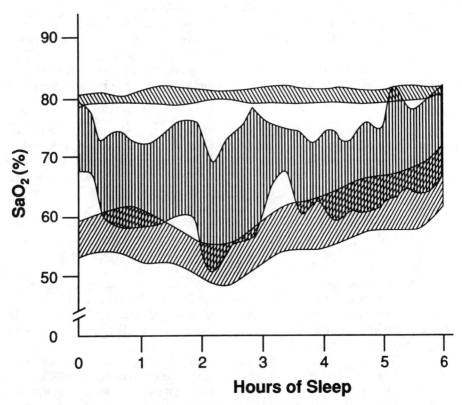

Figure 12.9. The effect of oxazepam, a benzodiazepine derivative (lowest panel) and acetazolamide (top panel) on arterial oxygen saturation during sleep at high altitude compared with no medication (center). From Sutton, ref. 131.

smoking. The carbon monoxide of cigarette smoke combines irreversibly with hemoglobin, thus making it impossible to transport oxygen. As much as 4 to 8 percent of available hemoglobin may be combined with carbon monoxide in heavy smokers. (f) Tea and coffee need not be avoided, since these are mild respiratory and central nervous system stimulants and will prevent daytime sleep. (g) Avoidance of sleeping or dozing during the day. Sleeping or dozing will decrease ventilation and increase hypoxia. Light physical activity is preferable.

Treatment

The following general recommendations can be made regarding the treatment of AMS.

1. Limited activity or bed rest should be advised. To continue normal activity or to continue a trek or a climb will usually make symptoms worse.

2. Sleep may not be beneficial since hypoventilation may occur during sleep. Medications that promote sleep should be avoided.

3. The following medications may be used to relieve headache and other symptoms: aspirin, acetaminophen with codeine if necessary; prochlorperazine (Compazine) or promethazine (Phenergan) may relieve nausea. The usual dose of Compazine is 10 mg every 6 hours. Phenergan can be given as 25-50 mg orally every 9 hours. Drowsiness usually occurs with Phenergan.

4. Acetazolamide (Diamox) should be administered, if it has not been used prophylactically. The usual dose is 125-250 mg every 8-12 hours. The dose for children is 5-10 mg/kg/day. A response is usually seen in 12-24 hours.

5. Low-flow oxygen (2-4 L/min) via nasal prongs or a plastic face mask will usually relieve symptoms and may be used during the night to promote sleep and rest. In most high altitude cities such as in Peru and Bolivia hotels will provide oxygen.

6. Dexamethasone 4 mg orally or parenterally every six hours may be used under certain conditions, including the failure to respond to accepted methods of treatment and when oxygen is not available or descent not possible. Once started, dexamethasone should be continued until symptoms are relieved, and occurs in six to twelve hours. This preparation should be used only when necessary because side effects are common.

7. If oxygen is not available and symptoms are severe, the hyperbaric Gamow bag may be employed. Preliminary studies indicate that the degree of improvement is comparable to the use of oxygen, and persistent relief of symptoms may occur after two to four hours in the bag.

8. Patients with severe symptoms that are not relieved promptly by the above methods should be examined carefully for the presence of HAPE or HACE. A rapid heart rate, increased respiratory rate, persistent cough, pulmonary rales, disturbance of consciousness, and ataxia are indications of these complications, and prompt descent should be instituted.

9. Assisted descent with continuous oxygen administration is mandatory in patients with persisting symptoms or clinical evidence of HAPE or HACE. This should be done as expeditiously as possible, since such patients may rapidly become helpless and require evacuation by litter, ambulance, or helicopter. A descent of even 3,000-4,000 feet (915-12,000 m) may result in rapid recovery. Most of the deaths from HAPE have been the result of undue delay in descending, when the patient has been able to walk or could have been transported with assistance.

Part 2: Subacute Mountain Sickness

Subacute mountain sickness is a syndrome originally described by Monge in Peru consisting of the persistence of the usual symptoms of acute mountain sickness for weeks or months after arrival at high altitude. Some individuals who move to altitudes exceeding 10,000 feet (3,050 m), may experience continuing symptoms which impair effective daily activities and necessitate a return to a lower altitude. The physiological characteristics of a high hematocrit, low arterial oxygen saturation, and hypoventilation that characterize chronic mountain sickness are absent. The term "subacute mountain sickness" was originally applied to this intermediate form of mountain sickness by Monge,[132,133,134] and in deference to his important original observations this designation should be continued. Hurtado and others subsequently recognized the occurrence of this form of mountain sickness and the validity of the diagnostic term employed by Monge.[135] These Peruvian investigators also referred to this condition essentially as a persistent failure to acclimatize.

Symptoms

Subacute mountain sickness is characterized by persisting unpleasant and often incapacitating symptoms, that are in some instances similar to those of acute mountain sickness, but are of much longer duration. One of the most common of these symptoms is the inability to obtain sound, restful sleep at night. This may vary in severity from mild insomnia to an almost total inability to sleep. Periodic breathing may be partly responsible for the insomnia. Nocturnal restlessness, sleeping for only short intervals through the night, and disturbing dreams are common.

Headache, depression, the inability to carry out sustained mental work, forgetfulness, and a decreased ability to do conceptual thinking are also frequently observed. Irritability and personality changes are occasionally noted. Fatigue, weakness, and exertional dyspnea may be a troublesome problem. Anorexia may be persistent and may contribute, along with insomnia, to the characteristic weight loss of from five to fifteen pounds. Indigestion, intolerance to fatty foods, and flatulence are commonly experienced. Fluid requirements are increased and dehydration is a common clinical problem. The low humidity at altitude creates problems for the person with dry skin. Cuts and abrasions heal slowly. Pruritus is common.

Most of the clinical information on subacute mountain sickness comes from mining companies in the Peruvian Andes, which employ a large population of workers, many of whom come from sea level. Work contracts may extend from three to five years. Common altitudes of residence for the Cerro Corporation were 12,230 feet (3,730 m) in the La Oroya area and 14,200 feet (4,330 m) in Cerro de Pasco. Some 5-10 percent of newcomers to these mines exhibited continuing symptoms of subacute mountain sickness as described above of sufficient severity to require their return to sea level. An equal percentage experienced mild continuing symptoms but were able to continue working at altitude, especially if they could return to a lower altitude on weekends and holidays. Hellriegel described the major symptoms as headache, forgetfulness, decreased intellectual function, dyspnea on slight exertion, anorexia, continued weight loss, increased thirst, and inability to sleep, with sleepiness and fatigue during the day.[136]

Hellriegel's observations are pertinent, since he was Medical Director of the Chulec General Hospital in La Oroya, Peru for 25 years. This was the central medical facility for the Cerro Corporation, which employed several thousand workers and thus provided a unique experience in many forms of high altitude medical problems.

Physical Findings

The physical findings and laboratory studies of subacute mountain sickness are essentially similar to those observed in acute mountain sickness—that is, cyanosis (usually), weight loss, moderate accentuation of the second sound at the pulmonic area, clear lungs, normal urinalysis although the urine may be of a high specific gravity, and elevation of the hematocrit to a variable degree depending upon the altitude, but not to the marked degree seen in chronic mountain sickness. The electrocardiogram may not show evidence of right ventricular hypertrophy. Cardiac enlargement by chest x-ray is absent and pulmonary edema is absent. Few clinical studies of subacute mountain sickness have been made, but the syndrome does not appear to be characterized by the marked cyanosis, clubbing of the digits, marked arterial unsaturation, episodic stupor, and heart failure that are seen in chronic mountain sickness. Subacute mountain sickness is rarely encountered in natives and most commonly occurs in sea-level dwellers who must live at high altitude. The problem may be seen among mountaineers at altitudes over 15,000 feet (4,575 m), and this is usually referred to as "high altitude deterioration".

Incidence

The incidence is low. Even in Peru, where non-native workers live at altitudes between 10,000 feet (3,050 m) and 14,200 feet (4,328 m), only a small number must leave the altitude because of intolerable symptoms. In Nepal Singh and his associates studied 840 untreated patients with AMS resulting from rapid exposure to elevations between 11,000 feet (3,355 m) and 18,000 feet (5,490 m). Twelve percent had symptoms that lasted for more than 29 days and only one percent still had symptoms after six months that were severe enough to require descent. Oxygen provided only temporary benefit.[14]

Etiology

I am not aware of any systematic epidemiological, clinical, or laboratory studies that have been made of subacute mountain sickness. Such studies are clearly needed to further understand the etiology of this syndrome.

Treatment and Management

Low-flow oxygen administered during the night may be useful in relieving the distress of severe insomnia. Pharmacological agents such as medroxyprogesterone acetate (Provera), methazolamide, and acetazolamide are of limited value because of side effects or a short duration of action.[117,137,138] One report, however, has described beneficial effects of acetazolamide over a 23-day period; exercise performance was enhanced and weight loss ameliorated.[139] Almitrine is a respiratory stimulant, but it does not diminish periodic breathing.[117] Sedatives should be avoided. Living at lower altitudes and commuting daily to higher altitudes is effective in many situations, and even descent to a lower altitude on weekends may relieve symptoms sufficiently to allow continued useful work at the high altitude. On Mauna Kea in Hawaii (13,800 feet/4,200 m) telescope workers avoid prolonged symptoms of mountain sickness by working five days on the mountain and spending five days at sea level for a work shift of 40 days. Then they spend 40 days at sea level. In these workers, over a two-year period, only one developed severe mountain sickness with every ascent and had to discontinue work on the mountain.[140] Smoking may increase symptoms. A study was made of workers recruited to work on an irrigation project at 10,500 feet (3,200 m) in Peru. Of 51 sea-level-dwelling employees there were 25 smokers and 26 nonsmokers. Fourteen had to terminate their contract because of persistent symptoms. Ten were smokers. Smokers had a higher hematocrit and hemoglobin level than nonsmokers.[141] Obesity may also be a risk factor as pointed out earlier in this chapter.

References

1. GILBERT D. The first documented report of mountain sickness: The China or Headache Mountain story. *Respir. Physiol.*, 1983; 52:315-16.
2. GILBERT D. The first documented description of mountain sickness: The Andean or Pariacaca story. *Respir. Physiol.*, 1983; 52:327-47.
3. JARCHO S. Mountain sickness as described by Fray Joseph de Acosta, 1589. *Am. J. Cardiol.* 1958; 2:246-47.
4. BONAVIA D, LEÓN VELARDE F, MONGE CC, SANCHEZ GRIÑAN MI, WHITTEMBURY J. Acute mountain sickness: critical appraisal of the Pariacaca story and on-site study. *Resp. Physiol.*, 1985; 62:125-34.
5. HOUSTON C. *Going higher: The story of man and altitude*. Little, Boston: Brown, 1987.
6. MOSSO A. *Life of man on the high Alps*, ed. A. Landon and T Fisher, London: Unwin, 1898.
7. RAVENHILL T. Some experiences of mountain sickness in the Andes. *J. Trop. Med. & Hyg.* 1913; 20:313-20.
8. BARCROFT J, COOKE A, HARTRIDGE H, et al. The flow of oxygen through the pulmonary epithelium. *J. Physiol.* 1920; 53:450-72.
9. HALDANE J, KELLAS A, and KENNAWAY E. Experiments on acclimatization to reduced atmospheric pressure. *J. Physiol.* 1920; 53:181-206.
10. CHILDS S, HAMLIN H, and HENDERSON Y. Possible value of inhalation of carbon dioxide in climbing great altitudes. *Nature* 1935; 135:457-458.
11. McFARLAND R, and DILL D. Comparative study of the effects of reduced oxygen pressure on man during acclimatization. *J. Aviat. Med.* 1938; 9:18-44.
12. BARRON E, DILL D, EDWARDS H, and HURTADO A. Acute mountain sickness: The effect of ammonium chloride. *J. Clin. Invest.* 1937; 16:541-46.
13. MENON N. High-altitude pulmonary edema. *N. Engl. Med.* 1965; 273:66-73.
14. SINGH I, KHANNA P, SRIVASTAVA M, et al. Acute mountain sickness. *N. Engl. J. Med.* 1969; 280: 175-84.
15. HACKETT P, and RENNIE D. The incidence, importance, and prophylaxis of acute mountain sickness. *Lancet* 1976; Nov. 27:1149-55.
16. SUTTON J. Acute mountain sickness: A historical review with some experiences from the Peruvian Andes. *Med. J. Australia* 1971; 2:243-48.
17. BARCROFT J. *Respiratory function of the blood. Part 1: Lessons from high altitude*. Cambridge University Press, 1925:14-15.
18. HACKETT P, and RENNIE D. Rales, peripheral edema, retinal hemorrhage, and acute mountain sickness. *Am. J. Med.* 1979; 67:214-18.
19. HONIGMAN B, THEIS M, KOZIOL-MCLAIN J, et al. Acute mountain sickness in a general tourist population at moderate altitude. *Ann. Int. Med.* 1993; 118:587-92.
20. BÄRTSCH P, VOCK P, MAGGIORINI M, et al. Respiratory symptoms, radiographic, and physiologic correlations at high altitude. In *Hypoxia: The adaptations*, ed. J Sutton, G. Coates, and J Remmers. Toronto: B.C. Decker, 1990:241-45.
21. CARSON R, EVANS O, SHEILDS J, and HANNON J. Symptomatology, pathophysiology, and treatment of acute mountain sickness. *Fed. Proc.* 1969; 28: 1085-91.
22. HALL W, BARILA T, MATZGER E, and GUPTA K. A clinical study of acute mountain sickness. *Arch. Environ. Health* 1965; 10:747-53.
23. KAYSER B. Acute mountain sickness in Western tourist around the Thorong pass (5,400 m) in Nepal. *J. Wilderness Med.* 1991; 2:110-17.

24. HACKETT P, and RENNIE D. Acute mountain sickness. In *Seminars in respiratory medicine*, New York: Thieme-Stratton, 1983; 5:132-40.

25. HACKETT P, and OELZ O. The Lake Louise consensus on the definition and quantification of altitude illness. In *Hypoxia and mountain medicine*, eds. J Sutton, G. Coates, and C Houston. Burlington, VT: Queen City Printers, 1992; 327-30.

26. KAMAT S, RAO T, SARMA S, et al. Study of cardiopulmonary function on exposure to high altitude. *Am. Rev. Resp. Dis.* 1972; 106:414- 31.

27. HOUSTON C. Incidence of acute mountain sickness: A study of winter visitors to six Colorado ski resorts. *Am. Alpine J.* 1985; 27: 162-65.

28. MONTGOMERY B, MILLS J, and LUCE J. Incidence of acute mountain sickness at intermediate altitude. *JAMA* 1989; 261:732-34.

29. MILLEDGE JS, BEELEY JM, BROOME J, et al. Acute mountain sickness and susceptibility, fitness and hypoxic ventilatory response. *Eur. Respir. J.* 1991; 4:1000-3.

30. MAGGIORINI M, BUHLER M, WAITER M, and OELZ O. Prevalence of acute mountain sickness in the Swiss Alps. *Brit. Med. J.* 1990; 301:853-55.

31. SAMPSON J, and KOBRICK J. The environmental symptoms questionnaire: Revision and new field data. *Aviat. Space Environ. Med.* 1980; 51:872-77.

32. ROBINSON S, KING A, and AOKI V. Acute mountain sickness: Reproducibility of its severity and duration in an individual. *Aero. Med.* 1971; 42:706-08.

33. FORSTER P. Reproducibility of individual response to exposure to high altitude. *Brit. Med. J.* 1984; 289:1269.

34. BÄRTSCH P, SHAW M, FRANCIOLLI M, et al. Atrial natriuretic peptide in acute mountain sickness. *J. Appl. Physiol.* 1988; 65:1929-37.

35. BÄRTSCH P, MAGGIORINI M, SCHOBERSBERGER W, et al. Enhanced exercise-induced rise of aldosterone and vasopressin preceding mountain sickness. *J. Appl. Physiol.* 1991; 71:136-43.

36. MAGGIORINI M, BÄRTSCH P, and OELZ O. Elevated body temperature in severe acute mountain sickness (AMS). In *Hypoxia and mountain medicine*, ed. J Sutton, G. Coates, and C Houston. Burlington, VT: Queen City Printers, 1992:311.

37. HACKETT P. The Denali research project, 1982- 1985. *Am. Alpine J.* 1986; 28:129-37.

38. ROACH R, LARSON E, HORNBEIN T, et al. Acute mountain sickness, antacids, and ventilation during rapid, active ascent of Mt. Rainier. *Aviat. Space Environ. Med.* 1983; 54:397-401.

39. EVANS W, ROBINSON S, HORSTMAN D, et al. Amelioration of the symptoms of acute mountain sickness by staging and acetazolamide. *Aviat. Space Environ. Med.* 1976; 47:512-16.

40. HANSEN J, HARRIS C, and EVANS W. Influence of elevation of origin, rate of ascent, and a physical conditioning program on symptoms of acute mountain sickness. *Mil. Med.* 1967; 132:585-92.

41. MARESH C. Influence of moderate altitude residents (2,200 meters) on acute mountain sickness and exercise response during early hypobaric hypoxia (4,270 meters). Ph.D. diss., University of Wyoming, 1981.

42. ROACH R, HOUSTON C, HONIGMAN B, et al. How well do older persons tolerate moderate altitude? *West. J. Med.* 1995; 162:32-36.

43. HARRIS C, SHIELD J, and HANNON J. Acute altitude sickness in females. *Aero. Med.* 1966; 37:1163-67.

44. CYMERMAN A, JAEGER J, KOBRICK J, and MAHER J. Physical fitness and acute mountain sickness (AMS). *Proceedings*, Hypoxia Symposium, Arctic Institute of North America, 1979:66.

45. FAVOUR C. Mountain sickness in fit and sedentary subjects exposed acutely to high altitude. Personal communication.

46. BILLINGS C, BRASHEAR R, BASON R, and MATHEWS D. Medical observations during prolonged residence at 3,800 m. Personal communication.

47. HULTGREN H, HONIGMAN B, THEIS K, and NICHOLAS D. High altitude pulmonary edema in a ski resort. *West. J. Med* (in press).

48. HIRATA K, MASUYAMA S, and SAITO A. Obesity as a risk factor for acute mountain sickness. *Lancet* 1989; Oct. 28:1040-41.

49. HACKETT P, RENNIE D, HOFMEISTER S, et al. Fluid retention and relative hypoventilation in acute mountain sickness. *Respiration* 1982; 43:321-29.

50. ANHOLM J, HOUSTON C, and HYERS T. The relationship between acute mountain sickness and pulmonary ventilation at 2835 meters (9,300 ft.). *Chest* 1979; 75:33-36.

51. KING A, and ROBINSON S. Ventilation response to hypoxia and acute mountain sickness. *Aero. Med.* 1972; 43:419-24.

52. SCHOENE R. Control of ventilation in climbers to extreme altitude. *J. Appl. Physiol.* 1982; 53:886- 90.

53. SUTTON J, BRYAN A, GRAY G, et al. Pulmonary gas exchange in acute mountain sickness. *Aviat. Space Environ. Med.* 1976; 47:1032-37.
54. MOORE L. HARRISON G, MCCULLOUGH R, et al. Low acute hypoxic ventilatory response and hypoxic depression in acute altitude sickness. *J. Appl. Physiol.* 1986; 60:1407-12.
55. MILLEDGE J, THOMAS P, BEELEY J, and ENGLISH J. Hypoxic ventilatory response and acute mountain sickness. *Eur. Respir J.* 1988; 1:948-51.
56. Birmingham Medical Research Expeditionary Society Mountain Sickness Study Group. Acetazolamide in control of acute mountain sickness. *Lancet* 1981; 24:180-83.
57. MAHER J, CYMERMAN A, REEVES J, et al. Acute mountain sickness: Increased severity in eucapneic hypoxia. *Aviat. Space Environ. Med.* 1975; 46:826-29.
58. HARVEY T, WINTERBORN M, LASSEN N, et al. Effect of carbon dioxide in acute mountain sickness: A rediscovery. *Lancet* 1988; Sept. 17:639-41.
59. FORWAND S, LANSDOWNE M, FOLANSBEE J, et al. Effect of acetazolamide on acute mountain sickness. *N. Engl. J. Med.* 1968; 279:839-45.
60. AOKI V, and ROBINSON S. Body hydration and the incidence and severity of acute mountain sickness. *J. Physiol.* 1971; 31:363-67.
61. SUTTON J, and LASSEN N. Pathophysiology of acute mountain sickness and high altitude pulmonary edema. *Bull. Europ. Physiol. Path. Resp.* (Nancy) 1979; 15:1045-52.
62. LASSEN N, and AGNOLI A. The upper limit of autoregulation of cerebral blood flow on the pathogenesis of encephalopathy. *Scand. J. Clin. Invest.* 1972; 30:113-15.
63. SHENKIN H, and BOUZARTH W. Clinical methods of reducing intracranial pressure: Role of the cerebral circulation. *N. Engl. J. Med.* 1970; 282: 1465-71.
64. SHAPIRO W, WASSERMAN A, BAKER J, and PATTERSON J, JR. Cerebrovascular response to acute hypocapnic an eucapnic hypoxia in normal man. *J. Clin. Invest.* 1970; 40:2362-68.
65. SEVERINGHAUS J, CHIODI H, EGER E, et al. Cerebral blood flow in man at high altitude: Role of cerebrospinal fluid pH in normalization of flow in chronic hypocapnia. *Clin. Res.* 1966; 19:274-84.
66. SEVERINGHAUS J, et al. Cerebral blood flow in man at high altitude. *Circ. Res.* 1900; 19:274-82.
67. *Wolff's Headache and other head pain*, 4th ed., ed. D. Dalessio, New York: Oxford University Press, 1980.
68. LEVINE B, YOSHIMURA K, KOBAYASHI T, et al. Dexamethasone in the treatment of acute mountain sickness. *N. Engl. J. Med.* 1989; 321:1707-13.
69. MATSUZAWA Y, KOBAYASHI T, FUJIMOTO K, et al. Cerebral edema in acute mountain sickness. In *High Altitude Medicine*, ed. G. Veda, J Reeves, and M Segiguchi. Matsumoto, Japan: Shinshu University, 1992:300-304.
70. REEVES J, MOORE L, MCCULLOUGH R, et al. Headache at high altitude is not related to internal carotid arterial blood velocity. *J. Appl. Physiol.* 1985; 59:909-15.
71. HACKETT P, ROACH R, and GREEN E. Oxygenation, but not increased cerebral blood flow improves high altitude headache. Abstract, *Proceedings*, Sixth International Hypoxia Symposium, 1989.
72. HANSON J, and EVANS W. A hypothesis regarding the pathophysiology of acute mountain sickness. *Arch. Environ. Health* 1970; 21:666-69.
73. JAMISON R, The role of cellular swelling in the pathogenesis of the organ ischemia. *West. J. Med.* 1974; 120:205-18.
74. HANNON J, CHINN K, and SHIELDS J. Effects of acute high altitude exposure on body fluids. *Fed. Proc.* 1969; 28:1178-84.
75. SEVERINGHAUS J. Hypothetical roles of angiogenesis, osmotic swelling, and ischemia in high-altitude cerebral edema. *J. Appl. Physiol.* 1995; 79: 375-79.
76. GREENE C. Camp Four. In *Kamet conquered*, ed. F Smythe. London: Gollanez, 1932:180-81.
77. DOUGLAS C, GREENE C, and KERGIN C. The influence of ammonium chloride on adaptation to low barometric pressures. *J. Physiol.* 1933; 78:404-14.
78. ZINTEL H, RHOADS J, and RAVDIN I. The use of intravenous ammonium chloride in the treatment of alkalosis. *Surgery* 1943; 41:728-31.
79. BÄRTSCH P, HAEBERLI A, FRANCIOLLI M, et al. Comparison of carbon dioxide-enriched, oxygen-enriched, and normal air in treatment of acute mountain sickness. *Lancet* 1990; 336:772-75.
80. JENSEN J, WRIGHT A, LASSEN N, et al. Cerebral blood flow at altitude. Abstract, *Proceedings*, Sixth International Hypoxia Symposium, 1989.
81. PENBERTHY L. *Acute mountain sickness-type R*. Seattle: Altitude Medical Publishing Co., 1977.
82. FALCHUK K, LAMB T, and TENNEY S. Ventilatory response to hypoxia and CO_2 following CO_2 exposure and $NaHCO_3$ ingestion. *J. Appl. Physiol.* 1966; 21:393-98.

254

83. WATERLOW J, and BUNJE H. Observations on mountain sickness in the Colombian Andes. *Lancet* 1966; 2:655-61.
84. JANOSKI A, WHITTEN B, SHIELDS J, and HANNON J. Electrolyte patterns and regulation in man during acute exposure to high altitude. *Fed. Proc.* 1969; 28:1185-89.
85. GRAY G, BRYAN A, FRAYSER R, et al. Control of acute mountain sickness. *Aero. Med.* 1971; 42:81-84.
86. HULTGREN H, BILISOLY J, FAILS H, et al. Plasma volume changes during acute exposure to high altitude. *Clin. Res.* 1973; 21:224; and unpublished observations.
87. JAIN S, SINGH M, SHARMA V, et al. Amelioration of acute mountain sickness: A comparative study of acetazolamide and spironolactone. *Int. J. Biometerol.* 1986; 30:293-300.
88. CURRIE T, CARTER P, CHAMPION W, et al. Spironolactone and acute mountain sickness. *Med. J. Australia* 1976; 2:168-70.
89. SINGH I, KAPILA C, KHANNA P, et al. High altitude pulmonary edema. *Lancet* 1965; 1:229-34.
90. FISHMAN R. Brain edema. *N. Engl. J. Med.* 1975; 293:706-11.
91. CASSILETH P, LUSH E, TORRI S, and GERSON S. Antiemetic efficacy of dexamethasone therapy in patients receiving cancer chemotherapy. *Arch. Int. Med.* 1983; 143:1347-49.
92. JOHNSON T, ROCK P, FULCA C, et al. Prevention of acute mountain sickness by dexamethasone. *N. Engl. J. Med.* 1984; 310:683-86.
93. FERRIERA P, and GRUNDY P. Dexamethasone in the treatment of acute mountain sickness. *N. Engl. J. Med.* 1985; 312:1390.
94. HACKETT P, and ROACH R. Medical therapy of altitude illness. *Annals Emerg. Med.* 1987; 16:980-86.
95. ZELL S, and GOODMAN P. Acetazolamide and dexamethasone in the prevention of acute mountain sickness. *West. J. Med.* 1988; 148:541-45.
96. ELLSWORTH A, MEYER E, and LARSON E. Acetazolamide or dexamethasone use versus placebo to prevent acute mountain sickness on Mount Rainier. *West. J. Med.* 1991; 154:289-93.
97. ROCK P, JOHNSON T, CYMERMAN A, et al. Effect of dexamethasone on symptoms of acute mountain sickness at Pikes Peak, Colorado. *Aviat. Space Environ. Med.* 1987; 58:668-72.
98. SHLIM D. Treatment of acute mountain sickness. (Letter) *N. Engl. J. Med.* 1985; 313:891-92.
99. ELLSWORTH A, LARSON E, and STRICKLAND D. A randomized trail of dexamethasone and acetazolamide for acute mountain sickness prophylaxis. *Am. J. Med.* 1987; 83:124-30.
100. FERRAZZINI G, MAGGIORINI M, KRIEMBER S, et al. Successful treatment of acute mountain sickness with dexamethasone. *Brit. Med. J.* 1987; 294:1380-82.
101. HACKETT P, ROACH R, WOOD R, et al. Dexamethasone for prevention and treatment of acute mountain sickness. *Aviat. Space Environ. Med.* 1988; 59:950-54.
102. JOBE J, SHUKITTHALE L, BANDERET L, and ROCK P. Effects of dexamethasone and high terrestrial altitude on cognitive performance and effect. *Aviat. Space Environ. Med.* 1991; 62: 727-32.
103. MONTGOMERY B, LUCE J, MICHAEL P, and MILLS J. Effects of dexamethasone on the incidence of acute mountain sickness at two intermediate altitudes. *JAMA* 1989; 261:734-36.
104. MARTICORENA E, and HULTGREN H. Evaluation of therapeutic methods in high altitude pulmonary edema. *Am. J. Cardiol.* 1979; 43:307-12.
105. GUDEMAN S. Failure of high-dose steroid therapy to influence intracranial pressure in patients with severe head injury. *Neurosurg.* 1979; 51:301-06.
106. LITTENBERG B, and GLUCK E. A controlled trail of methyl-prednisone in the emergency treatment of acute asthma. *N. Engl. J. Med.* 1986; 314:150-56.
107. RABOLD M. Dexamethasone for prophylaxis and treatment of acute mountain sickness. *J. Wilderness Med.* 1992; 3:54-60.
108. WOHNS R, and KERSTEIN M. The role of dilantin in the prevention of pulmonary edema associated with cerebral hypoxia. In *Hypoxia, exercise, and altitude*, ed. J Sutton, C Houston, and N Jones. New York: A.R. Liss, 1983. Abstract.
109. BURSE R, LANDOWNE M, CYMERMAN A, et al. Ineffectiveness of phenytoin in the control of acute mountain sickness (AMS). *Proceedings*, International Hypoxia Symposium, Banff, 1988. Abstract.
110. CAIN S, and DUNN J. Low doses of acetazolamide to aide accommodation of men to altitude. *J. Appl. Physiol.* 1966; 21:1195-2000.
111. KRONENBERG S, and CAIN M. Hastening respiratory acclimatization to altitude with benzolamide. *Aero. Med.* 1966; 39:296-302.
112. KRONENBERG R, and CAIN S. Letter to the Editor. *N. Engl. J. Med.* 1969; 280:49.
113. SUTTON J, HOUSTON C, MARSELL A, et al. Effect of acetazolamide on hypoxemia during sleep at high altitude. *N. Engl. J. Med.* 1979; 301:1329-31.

114. GREEN M, KEER A, MCINTOSH I, and PRESCOTT R. Acetazolamide in prevention of acute mountain sickness. *Brit. Med. J.* 1981; 283:811-13.

115. LARSON E, et al. Acute mountain sickness and acetazolamide: Clinical efficacy and effect on ventilation. *JAMA* 1982; 248:328-32.

116. LASSEN N, and SEVERINGHAUS J. Acute mountain sickness and acetazolamide. In *Hypoxia and cold*, ed. J. Sutton, C Houston, and G Coates. New York: Praeger, 1987:493-504.

117. HACKETT P, ROACH R, HARRISON G, et al. Respiratory stimulants and sleep periodic breathing at high altitude: Almitrine versus acetazolamide. *Am. Rev. Resp. Dis.* 1987; 135:896-98.

118. CONNAUGHTON J, DOUGLAS N, MORGAN A, et al. Almitrine improves oxygenation when both awake and asleep in patients with hypoxia and carbon dioxide retention caused by chronic bronchitis and emphysema. *Am. Rev. Resp. Dis.* 1985; 132:206-10.

119. KASIC J, YARON M, NICHOLAS R, et al. Treatment of acute mountain sickness: Hyperbaric versus oxygen therapy. *Ann. Emerg. Med.* 1991; 20:1109-12.

120. FORSTER P, BRADWELL A, WINTERBORN M, et al. Alleviation of hypoxia at high altitude: A comparison between oxygen and carbon dioxide inhalation, and hyperbaric compression (Gamow bag). In *Hypoxia and mountain medicine*. ed. J Sutton, G Coates, and C Houston. Burlington, VT: Queen City Printers, 1992: pp 303.

121. BÄRTSCH P, MERKI B, KAYSER B, et al. Controlled trial of the treatment of acute mountain sickness (AMS) with a portable hyperbaric chamber. In *Hypoxia and mountain medicine*, ed. J Sutton, G Coates, and C Houston. Burlington, VT: Queen City Printers, 1992: pp 299. Abstract.

122. ROBERTSON J, and SHLIM D. Treatment of moderate acute mountain sickness with pressurization in a portable (Gamow™) bag. *J. Wilderness Med.* 1991; 2:268-73.

123. TABER R. Protocols for the use of a portable hyperbaric chamber for the treatment of high altitude disorders. *J. Wilderness Med.* 1990; 1:181-92.

124. KING S, and GREENLEEE R. Successful use of the Gamow hyperbaric bag in the treatment of altitude illness at Mount Everest. *J. Wilderness Med.* 1990; 1:193-202.

125. HONIGMAN B, READ M, LEZOTTE D and ROACH R. Sea level physical activity and acute mountain sickness at moderate altitude. *West. J. Med.* 1995; 163:117-21.

126. HACKETT P. Personal communication.

127. FRAUNFELDER F, and BAGBY G, JR. Possible hematologic reactions associated with carbonic anhydrase inhibitors. *JAMA* 1989; 261:2257-58. Questions and Answers.

128. ROEGGLA G, ROEGGLA H, ROEGGLA M, et al. Effect of alcohol on acute ventilatory adaptation to mild hypoxia at moderate altitude. *Ann. Int. Med.* 1995; 122:925-27.

129. ROEGGLA G, ROEGGLA M, WAGNER A, et al. Effect of low lose sedation with diazepam on ventilatory sedation response at moderate altitude. *Wien Klin. Wochenschr* 1994; 106:649-51.

130. ABERNATHY and MEEHAN R. Valium at high altitude: The Genet effect. In *Hypoxia: Man at altitude*, ed. J Sutton, N Jones, and C Houston. New York: Thieme-Stratton, 1982. Abstract.

131. SUTTON J. Sleep disturbances at high altitude. *Phys. Sports Medicine* 1982; 10:79-84.

132. MONGE C. High altitude disease. *Arch. Int. Med.* 1937; 59:32-40.

133. MONGE M and MONGE C. *Historical confirmation, high altitude diseases: Mechanism and management*. Springfield, IL: Charles C. Thomas, 1966.

134. WINSLOW R, and MONGE C. *Hypoxia, polycythemia, and chronic mountain sickness*, Baltimore, MD: Johns Hopkins University Press, 1987.

135. HURTADO A. Some clinical aspects of life in high altitudes. *Ann. Int. Med.* 1960; 53:247-58.

136. HELLRIEGEL K. Die Wirkung grosser und Mittlerer Höhen auf den Menschen bei seiner Ankunft und wahrend der ersten Wochen seines Aufenthaltes. *Schweizerische Zeitschrift fur Sportmedizine*, 1900; 00:191-203.

137. KRYGER M, MCCULLOUGH R, et al. Treatment of excessive polycythemia of high altitude with respiratory stimulant drugs. *Am. Rev. Resp. Dis.* 1978; 117:455-64.

138. HEATH D, and WILLIAMS D. *High altitude medicine and pathology*. London: Butterworth's, 1989: 282-94.

139. BRADWELL A, DYKES P, COOTE J, et al. Effect of acetazolamide on exercise performance at high altitude. *Lancet* 1986; May 3: 1001-05.

140. HEATH D, and WILLIAMS D. *High altitude medicine and pathology*. London: Butterworth's, 1989: 288-94.

141. LINDEGARDE E, and LILLJEKUIST R. Failure of long-term acclimatization in smokers moving to high altitude. *Acta. Med. Scand.* 1984; 216:317-22.

CHAPTER 13

High Altitude
Pulmonary Edema

SUMMARY

High altitude pulmonary edema (HAPE) occurs in unacclimatized individuals who are rapidly exposed to altitudes in excess of 8,000 feet (2,440 m). It is commonly seen in climbers and skiers who ascend to high altitude without previous acclimatization and upon arrival engage in heavy physical exertion. Initial symptoms of dyspnea, cough, weakness, chest tightness, and occasionally hemoptysis appear, usually within one to three days after arrival. Common physical signs are tachypnea, tachycardia, rales and cyanosis. In severe episodes, disturbances of consciousness or coma may be observed. Descent to a lower altitude, nifedipine, oxygen administration and bed rest result in rapid clinical improvement. Fatal episodes continue to occur in many parts of the world as access to high altitudes by unacclimatized visitors is made easier my modern means of travel. Most deaths occur when a prompt diagnosis is not made, when the victim is not moved to a lower altitude, or when oxygen is not available. Subjects who develop HAPE do not have demonstrable preexisting cardiac or pulmonary disease. Physiological studies during the acute stage have revealed a normal pulmonary artery wedge pressure, marked elevation of pulmonary artery pressure, severe arterial unsaturation, and usually a low cardiac output. Pulmonary arteriolar (precapillary) resistance is elevated. A working hypothesis of the etiology of HAPE suggests that hypoxic pulmonary vasoconstriction and possibly thrombotic occlusion of portions of the pulmonary vascular bed are extensive but not uniform. The result is overperfusion of the remaining patent vessels with transmission of the high pulmonary artery pressure to capillaries. Dilatation of the capillaries and high flow with resulting shear forces results in capillary injury with leakage of protein and red cells into the alveoli and airways. A sea-level analogue of this type of "overperfusion edema" is pulmonary edema following thromboendarterectomy for thromboembolic pulmonary hypertension. An individual susceptibility to HAPE is evident in view of repeat episodes in some persons. Persons with congenital absence of one pulmonary artery, children, and climbers who ascend rapidly and exercise heavily upon arrival are also susceptible.

The earliest hemodynamic abnormality in HAPE is a hypoxic increase of pulmonary arteriolar resistance and pulmonary artery pressure during the first hours of exposure to high altitude. HAPE represents one of the few varieties of pulmonary edema where left ventricular filling pressure is normal.

High-altitude pulmonary edema (HAPE) continues to be a hazard to mountaineers, trekkers, and skiers, with about 20 deaths reported annually throughout the world despite educational efforts directed toward prevention, early recognition, and treatment. HAPE is not uncommon in recreational visitors to the

Colorado Rockies, where many a vacation has been ruined by this illness. With increasing numbers of people going to high altitudes, HAPE will continue to be a problem.

• • •

Historical Aspects

High altitude pulmonary edema has probably been observed for centuries in high elevations throughout the world. The Chinese in 37-32 B.C. described acute mountain sickness occurring in traders who crossed the mountain passes in western China at elevations of 15,800 feet (4,820 m). Among these records is a report of one person in a caravan who was ill and coughed up bright red blood.[1] This was probably an episode of HAPE. In 1500 Mirza Haidar described cases of an illness called *damgiri* or *Yas* in the mountains of Central Asia. His description includes all the essential features of HAPE: severe dyspnea, insomnia, delirium, death shortly after onset or after a duration of several days, occurrence in recent arrivals at high altitude but not among natives unless they ascend to a higher altitude, and cure by descent.[2]

In 1879 a Swiss guide, Josef Brantschen, died of probable HAPE during an attempted traverse of the Matterhorn in one day from Brevil to Zermatt. After a 6,000-foot (1,830 m) climb the party bivouacked at the Cravate Hut at 13,500 feet (4,120 m). Toward evening, Brantschen became ill, was delirious, and groaned rhythmically. His pulse was rapid. Throughout the night he moaned and became worse. An attack of pain seized him, he turned about ceaselessly, and a "frightening rattle tore at his throat." Finally he slept, and in the morning he felt somewhat better. He was too weak to continue the climb, however, and stayed in the hut while his companions traversed the Matterhorn and descended to Zermatt. A rescue party found Brantschen dead in the hut the next day.[3]

A detailed description of another fatal case was published by Mosso in 1898.[4] A physician climber on his descent from the summit of Mount Blanc stopped at the Vallot Hut, 14,100 feet (4,300 m). Here, he became severely ill, developed progressive mental confusion, and coma. Before he lapsed into coma and died, a companion noted a respiratory rate of 50-70 breaths per minute. An autopsy was performed and the cause of death was ascribed to "suffocative catarrh accompanied by acute edema of the lungs due to pneumonitis."

In 1913 Ravenhill published accurate descriptions of cases of acute mountain sickness, high altitude cerebral edema, and HAPE that he observed while a medical officer for a mining company in the Chilean Andes.[5] He reported the clinical features of HAPE in three patients, one of whom died, and in addition described his own symptoms while experiencing an episode of HAPE. His report is of historical significance. One of his patients was described as follows:

"An Englishman visited the district, 15,400 feet (4,700 m) in February. He arrived in the usual way by train, a forty-two hour journey from sea level. He seemed in good health on arrival and said he felt quite well. Nevertheless, he kept quiet, ate sparingly and went to bed early. He woke next morning feeling ill with symptoms of the normal type of puna (mountain sickness). As the day drew on he began to feel very ill indeed. In the afternoon his pulse rate was 144, respirations 40. Later in the evening, he became very cyanosed, had acute dyspnea and evident air hunger with all the extraordinary muscles of respiration being called into play. The heart sounds were very faint, the pulse irregular and of a small tension. He seemed to present a typical picture of a failing heart. This condition persisted through the night. He coughed up with difficulty. He vomited at intervals. He had several inhalations of oxygen. Strychnine and digitalis were given. Towards morning, he recovered slightly and as there luckily was a train going down in the early morning, he was sent straight down. I heard that when he got down to 12,000 feet (3,660 m) he was considerably better and at 7,000 feet (2,135 m) he was nearly well. It seemed to me that he would have died had he stayed in the altitude for another day."

Although Ravenhill believed that the illness of this traveler was due to "an acute heart condition," and used the term "puna of a cardiac type" to describe what was probably HAPE. Ravenhill's report was published in the *Journal of Tropical Medicine and Hygiene* and received little attention; none of the early papers on HAPE from Peru and elsewhere refer to it. Physicians in Peru were familiar with occasional cases of HAPE, which they considered to be episodes of heart failure, and in 1927 Dr. H. Crane, the chief surgeon of Chulec General Hospital in La Oroya, Peru, 12,230 feet (3,730 m), described several patients who were admitted to the hospital with "acute cardiac insufficiency and mountain sickness" and subsequently recovered rapidly upon descent.[6]

In 1937 Hurtado described a high altitude resident who developed pulmonary edema upon returning from a sea-level visit.[7] The patient was a 58-year-old man who had been living at high altitude for 29 years and during those years had been to Lima many times without experiencing symptoms upon return. On this occasion, he became severely ill at Casapalca, 13,600 feet (4,150 m), while returning to La Oroya after a three-day visit to Lima. He had a cough productive of a large quantity of "black" blood, headache, severe dyspnea, and mental "incoordination." On examination he was orthopneic, anxious, and severely cyanotic, and rales were present over both lungs. He was coughing up abundant, foamy, red-tinged sputum. The heart rate was 120/min and his arterial oxygen saturation 77 percent (normal at Casapalca, 83-84 percent). A chest x-ray revealed diffuse infiltrates more intense at the bases. The vital capacity was 1.5 liters. When the patient returned to Lima the symptoms gradually abated, but after two months he returned to La Oroya and again became ill, this time showing symptoms of dyspnea, pulmonary congestion, and edema of the extremities, but not of mountain sickness. His arterial oxygen saturation was now 84 percent and the vital capacity was 2.7 liters. Hurtado proposed that this patient's pulmonary edema was probably related to rapid ascent and referred to the illness as a type of "soroche." He also proposed that the illness was due to preexisting myocardial disease resulting in transient acute heart failure. A careful review of the original case report suggests that the patient's illness was probably not an uncomplicated episode of HAPE, but it may well have been related to underlying cardiac disease or possibly a pulmonary embolus with pulmonary edema for the following reasons: the patient was older than the usual patient with HAPE; the sea-level stay was short, only three days; symptoms appeared abruptly a few hours after leaving sea level; the arterial oxygen saturation was not markedly decreased, i.e., only 77 percent; the patient improved slowly after descent and upon returning to La Oroya two months later the patient exhibited dyspnea, pulmonary congestion, and peripheral edema, suggesting the presence of cardiac disease. Nevertheless, Hurtado's case report is accepted by many as one of the earliest descriptions of HAPE in Peru.

Chulec General Hospital in La Oroya, Peru, was, at that time, the location of the earliest observations and systematic studies of HAPE by physicians. The hospital was in a most favorable location for these observations, being the central medical care facility for the workers and miners of the Cerro de Pasco Corporation, and being located on a major railroad and highway.* Over the years, Chulec Hospital has treated many cases of acute altitude illness, including HAPE, representing all age groups and newcomers to high altitude as well as permanent residents who were returning to high altitude after a sojourn of variable duration at sea level. Following Crane's 1927 report, other cases have been observed by Dr. A. J. Kerwin (1937), Dr. Einar Lundberg, and others. Kerwin noted that he saw several cases of HAPE, who were sent down to Lima by train or auto with oxygen "hoping that they would survive the trip." In 1952 Lundberg presented studies (still unpublished) on a series of cases of HAPE at a conference of the Medical Association of Yauli.[8] Lizarraga, in 1954, wrote his medical thesis on HAPE, describing fourteen cases observed at Chulec General Hospital from 1950 to 1954. This very complete report includes a summary of clinical symptoms, physical findings, and laboratory studies.[9] Since then other Peruvian physicians have published similar case reports.[10-13] In February 1959 I had the opportunity to visit the Chulec General Hospital. Together with Drs. Einar Lundberg and Kurt Hellriegel I reviewed 41 cases of HAPE and I reported this study in May 1960.[14] In September 1960 Dr. Charles Houston published a report of an episode of HAPE occurring in a skier in Aspen, Colorado and suggested that deaths in mountaineers previously ascribed to pneumonia were probable instances of HAPE.[15] Subsequently a more comprehensive description of HAPE was published in 1961 combining my observations with those of Dr. Houston.[16]

Fatal episodes of HAPE have occurred in climbers for many years, but before 1957 pneumonia was thought to be the cause. An example of the lack of awareness of the nature of HAPE was the response to a letter published in the British journal Practitioner in 1955 in which a climber gave a description of a fatal case of HAPE in a companion at 16,000 feet (4,880 m) on Mount Kenya. The letter described all the essential features, including the onset of the symptoms at 14,000 feet (4,270 m) on the second day of the climb, dyspnea, coughing, cyanosis, and finally, at 3:00 a.m. of the fifth day, the appearance of "pink froth about the nostrils," semicoma, and death. A year earlier the climber had experienced a similar episode but had recovered upon descent. The writer asked whether acute pulmonary edema was a common symptom of high altitude sickness. A reply by L. Pugh, the well-known British physiologist, stated that "I have not come across any other case of sudden death at high altiutde in an otherwise healthy individual nor have I read of any in the literature".[17] Residents in the Andean areas of South America still speak of the danger of "pneumonia of the mountains." When autopsies were performed on climbers who had died of HAPE, the gross diagnosis was usually pneumonia. Owing to the length of time between death and the autopsy and/or the lack of facilities, histologic studies were rarely done. A typical example of fatal HAPE in a climber in Peru is illustrated by the following report:

W.B. age 38, a healthy and experienced mountaineer, was climbing in the Cordillera Blanca in June 1958. In three days he climbed from 9,000 feet (2,745 m)

*The Cerro de Pasco Corporation was subsequently taken over by the Peruvian government and re-named the Centro Min de Peru.

to 14,000 feet (4,270 m) over a series of ridges, one of which was 16,000 feet (4,880 m) high. On the evening of June 26 he was more tired than other members of the party, and exhibited periodic breathing. On June 27 he engaged in little activity but on June 28, steep climbing to a higher camp with heavy packs was done. W.B. was far more short of breath than other members of the party. On arrival at the 16,000 feet (4,880 m) camp, he was tired, listless, and could not eat. He began to cough and one of his companions stated that he "obviously had fluid in his lungs." He was comfortable only in a seated position. Because of the impression that he had pneumonia, he was given penicillin, which he had previously received without reaction. His breathing rapidly became more labored, his cough more severe and frequent and his companion, who was not a physician, wrote in his diary — "over the next few hours W.B.'s breathing became progressively more congested and labored. He sounded as though he were literally drowning in his own fluid with an almost continuous loud bubbling sound as if he were breathing through liquid."

An attempt was made to obtain an emergency air drop of oxygen, and more penicillin was given. During the night his breathing became far worse, he lost consciousness, and became limp, dying at dawn on the second day of illness. His companion stated in his diary "a couple of hours after his death, when we got up to carry on the day's activities, I noticed a white froth resembling cotton candy had appeared to well up out of his mouth. This was even though he was sitting up with his head tilted back." The body was temporarily covered with rocks, and two days later was brought to Caras where an autopsy was performed five days after death. The verbal report of the autopsy diagnosis was as follows: "Bilateral fulminating pneumonia." Postmortem autolysis precluded microscopic examination.[16]

The clinical course, the description of his symptoms, and the rapid death of this climber are more characteristic of pulmonary edema than of any infectious process, which, indeed, would very likely not have been fatal but rather would have responded to the penicillin that was used in adequate doses early in the disease.

In 1962-63 during the border conflict between India and China, Indian troops that were transported rapidly to high altitude in the Himalayas suffered a high incidence of acute mountain sickness (AMS) and HAPE, and reports of clinical studies on these problems were published by Indian physicians.[18-19] From 1962 to 1964 Dr. N. Menon was stationed at a field hospital in Leh, Ladakh in India at 11,000 feet (3,413 m) when he began to see troops being admitted to the hospital with pulmonary edema. Nearly all had recently arrived at high altitude by air. The incidence was 5.7 per 1,000. Initially it was believed that these patients had bronchopneumonia and it was well known that "bronchopneumonia" at high altitude was invariably fatal. Later it was realized that the patients had pulmonary edema, and the treatment consisted of the standard methods used in cardiac failure, including bed rest, oxygen, digoxin, diuretics, antibiotics, and morphine. It is of interest that 101 patients with pulmonary edema were seen from 1962 to 1964 and only four deaths occurred despite the fact that the majority of the patients acquired pulmonary edema at the same altitude as the hospital. Descent was not possible. Dr. Menon's description of these cases is one of the landmark papers of the field of high altitude illness.[20] Subsequently many studies of HAPE have been published by investigators in Peru, India, and the United States. Historical aspects are reviewed in Table 13.1.

Table 13.1
HAPE—Historical Aspects

	Observations	Author-Reference	Date	Country
1.	Early descriptions of probable HAPE	Gilbert[1]	37 B.C.	China
		Haidar [2]	1500	Asia
		Mosso[4]	1898	Alps
		Gos[3]	1908	Alps
2.	Description by physicians	Ravenhill[5]	1913	Chile
		Hurtado[7]	1937	Peru
3.	Collected cases and analysis of clinical features	Lizarraga[9]	1955	Peru
		Bardales[11]	1957	Peru
		Alzamora-Castro[12]	1961	Peru
4.	First U.S. report of collected cases of HAPE	Hultgren[14]	1960	U.S.
5.	First report of HAPE in U.S.	Houston[15]	1960	U.S.
6.	Analysis of cases from Peru and in mountaineers	Hultgren[16]	1961	U.S.
7.	Analysis of cases	Singh[18]	1965	India
		Menon[19]	1965	India
8.	Hemodynamic studies	Fred[48]	1962	U.S.
		Hultgren[49]	1964	Peru
		Penaloza[50]	1969	Peru
9.	Autopsy studies	Hultgren[61]	1962	U.S.
		Arias-Stella[62]	1963	Peru
		Nayak[63]	1964	India
10.	Pulmonary hypertension the initial abnormality in HAPE	Hultgren[70]	1971	U.S.
11.	Overperfusion concept of the mechanism of HAPE	Hultgren[66]	1966	U.S.
		Hultgren[44]	1978	U.S.
12.	HAPE associated with absent right pulmonary artery	Hackett[47]	1980	U.S.

Clinical Features

Symptoms. The first symptoms of HAPE begin 24-72 hours after arrival at high altitude. In adults, symptoms commonly follow heavy physical exertion such as climbing, skiing, or hiking. In about half the cases, HAPE is accompanied by common symptoms of AMS, including malaise, headache, anorexia, and insomnia. Important initial symptoms of HAPE are dyspnea, cough, chest tightness, and fatigue or weakness. The cough is nonproductive but persistent, often continuing into the night. Later the cough becomes "loose" and productive of clear, watery sputum. In about ten percent of cases hemoptysis may appear. The sputum is rusty-colored or streaked with red blood. The patient may be aware of gurgling sounds in his chest during increased respiratory effort. Dyspnea is manifested first during exertion and progressively limits one's walking or climbing ability. Dyspnea at night is most fearful: the sensation is similar to that of a tight constricting band about one's chest, limiting the ability to take a deep, satisfying breath. Respiratory rate is increased but tidal volume is not, and dyspnea may not be evident upon inspection unless the respiratory rate is counted. Orthopnea is rare and only occurs in 5-10 percent of patients. The sitting position is not obligatory as in cardiac pulmonary edema.

Orthopnea in HAPE should provide a deeper tidal volume and more efficient use of the accessory muscles of respiration; however, some patients with HAPE have reported that they felt worse sitting up and that lying flat initiated coughing that brought up more fluid and made respiration easier. The supine or prone position probably brought on fluid drainage into the larger airways that resulted in coughing. The first case of HAPE described in North America was "not orthopneic but was coughing severely and was desperately dyspneic on the slightest exertion."[15] When first seen the patient was lying prone and even in the hospital preferred to be in the prone position.[21] The absence of orthopnea should exclude the possibility of cardiac pulmonary edema. Fatigue or weakness during physical effort is an insidious symptom and may precede dyspnea and cough. Characteristically, a person with HAPE begins to walk more slowly and stops frequently to rest. In severe cases the victim cannot walk, stand, or even get into a sleeping bag. Other symptoms include headache, nausea and vomiting, inability to sleep, palpitations, and precordial chest pain or a sense of precordial pressure. The precordial discomfort may suggest angina, but radiation to the neck or arms does not occur. Pleuritic pain is rare and when present should suggest the presence of pulmonary embolism. Symptoms of central nervous system involvement such as confusion, hallucinations, obtundation, or coma represent severe pulmonary edema with hypoxemia and antedate death within six to twelve hours unless oxygen is given and/or prompt descent is initiated. Occasionally syncope may occur, especially during effort. Cerebral function is very sensitive to hypoxia, and when obtundation or coma occurs, very low arterial oxygen tensions are present. Syncope during effort may also be related to the exercise-induced drop in arterial oxygen saturation with resulting acute cerebral hypoxia. A similar mechanism may occur in swimmers who hyperventilate before swimming under water. The decrease in arterial PCO_2 inhibits the drive to breathe, and arterial PO_2 falls to a level where unconsciousness occurs.[22] This may be related to a diminished ventilatory response to hypoxia which is present in cases of HAPE.[23,24] Ataxia is rare but when present indicates the presence of high altitude cerebral edema (HACE). Common symptoms are shown in Tables 13.2 and 13.3.

It is important to emphasize that the symptoms of HAPE may be quite variable and are due in part to the altitude attained, the rapidity of ascent, and the age of the patient. Patients without dyspnea have been observed.[23,24,25] In a few cases coma has occurred without significant preceding warning symptoms. Persons who have recently arrived from sea level have been found dead a day or two later, having expired during the night.

Table 13.2
Frequency of Symptoms of HAPE in Adults and Children

	Adults > 20 yrs. (40 patients)		Children <20 yrs. (51 patients)	
	Number	Percent	Number	Percent
Dyspnea	20	50	33	65
Cough	21	52	35	70*
Hemoptysis	10	25	18	35
Nonproductive cough	7	18	12	24
Watery sputum	4	10	5	10
Headache	11	27	8	16
Weakness fatigue (malaise)	9	23	27	53*
Fluid in lungs	7	18	3	6
Insomnia	4	10	3	6
Nausea-vomiting	3	8	14	28*
Orthopnea	3	8	8	16
Palpitations	2	5	4	8
Confusion	2	5	1	2
Precordial pressure	1	2.5	0	0
Syncope	1	2.5	1	2
Coma	1	2.5	2	4
Ataxia	1	2.5	0	0

SOURCES: Lopez, ref. 32 and Marticorena, ref. 33.

NOTES: Asterisks indicate symptoms that are more common in children. No fatal cases were included.

Table 13.3
Common symptoms in 286 Collected Cases of HAPE

Symptom	Lobenhoffer Percent	Hultgren Percent	Symptom	Lobenhoffer Percent	Hultgren Percent
Dyspnea	71	77	Vomiting	17	16
Cough	68	69	Orthopnea	13	9
Malaise	58	25	Insomnia	12	-
Headache	35	53	Apathy	11	-
Nausea	23	35	Confusion	10	14
Coma	24	-	Edema	7	-
Chest pain	21	1	Ataxia	6	2

SOURCES: Lobenhoffer, ref. 31 and Hultgren, ref. 25.

NOTES: Most of these cases are adults. Hemoptysis was not reported. Many fatal cases were included, hence coma was commonly observed. Lobenhoffer reported on 134 cases and Hultgren reported on 150 cases.

At lower altitudes, that is, 8,000-10,000 feet (2,440-3,050 m), symptoms may sometimes be present for several days with only moderate disability, or severe symptoms may appear within a few hours after ascent to higher altitude.

In 150 patients with HAPE observed at a ski resort in Colorado, 9,300 feet (2,840 m) the following symptoms were observed: dyspnea, 77 percent; orthopnea, 7 percent; cough, 69 percent; hemoptysis, 6 percent; headache, 53 percent; chest congestion, 41 percent, nausea, 35 percent; fever, chills, sweats, 30 percent; weakness or fatigue,[25] percent. The mean time from arrival at the resort to the onset of symptoms was 3 ± 1.3 days.[25]

On the whole, children exhibit the same symptoms as adults except for a higher frequency of malaise, nausea and vomiting (as noted in the Keystone data), and chest discomfort. In a child, the gradual onset of somnolence, cyanosis, and coma may indicate severe HAPE. For both adults and children, symptoms tend to become worse during the night, and it is not unusual in severe cases for coma to occur during sleeping hours.

Physical signs. The most common early sign of HAPE is an obvious limitation in physical performance. The patient walks or climbs at a progressively slower pace with more frequent rest stops to recover strength and to overcome exertional dyspnea. The patient arrives at camp late, does not wish to eat or drink, and retires early. The following morning the patient prefers to rest in the tent and may from time to time walk out feebly to relieve bodily functions. Urine is scanty. Specific symptoms such as cough or dyspnea may be absent or denied. Persons who show such behavior must be examined carefully and systematically for the characteristic signs of HAPE. Cyanosis is nearly always present but may not be evident unless the examination is carried out in daylight. (A blue tent can make anyone cyanotic!) Lips, nose, tongue, ears, sclerae, fingernails and fingertips are common sites of cyanosis. Even though the patient may not appear dyspneic, the respiratory rate is always increased and usually exceeds 20/min in adults and 30/min in children. The resting heart rate is also increased and usually exceeds 90/min in adults and 110/min in children. Physically fit adults with a normally low resting heart rate may exhibit a heart rate of less than 90-100 min. A rough correlation exists between the increase in heart rate and respiratory rate in HAPE (Fig. 14.1). A slight temperature elevation is common and is usually higher in HAPE than in AMS.[25,26] The temperature in uncomplicated HAPE rarely exceeds 101° F.

Higher temperatures associated with chills, sweats, or mucopurulent sputum should suggest pneumonia. The blood pressure may be elevated due to sympathetic stimulation.[25] Heart sounds may be faint but the second sound in the pulmonic area is usually prominent, especially in children, where pulmonic valve closure may even be palpable. The neck veins are flat. Rales are usually present and may be detected even without a stethoscope in some patients by placing one's ear to the back of the uncovered chest. Rales have been observed to be present most often only posteriorly, and usually over the middle lung fields. In some patients rales may be present when radiographic signs of HAPE are absent; occasionally, too, rales may be absent when radiographic signs of HAPE are present.[25,27] Bubbling sounds of fluid in the airways can often also be detected by listening to the patient's open mouth during deep respirations. The extremities are usually cold and pale and the patient presents the general picture of circulatory collapse or shock. Dyspnea may be less intense for a few minutes after coughing up fluid. Irrational behavior, hallucinations, obtundation, and coma indicate severe hypoxia with resultant effects upon the central nervous system.

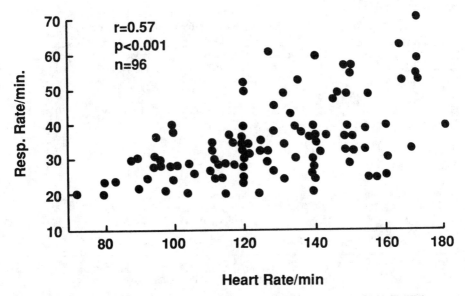

Figure 13.1. Relation between heart rate and respiratory rate in 96 patients with HAPE. Higher rates occur in children. Data collected from the literature. The increased heart rate is related to hypoxemia. The increased respiratory rate is a sensitive indicator of respiratory dysfunction as well as hypoxemia. From Hultgren, refs. 16, 25. From Gravelyn, ref. 45.

Physical signs in 150 patients with HAPE seen at a ski resort in Colorado were evaluated. The mean heart rate was 104 ± 18.5 beats per minute. Forty patients (26.7 percent) had a heart rate of ≥120 beats per minute. The mean respiratory rate was 22.9 ± 6.2 per minute. Thirty-nine (26 percent) had a rate of ≥24 per minute. The mean oral temperature was 99 ± 1.45 degrees Fahrenheit. In thirty patients (20 percent) the temperature exceeded 100°F. The blood pressure was frequently elevated. The mean systolic pressure was 132 ± 20 mm Hg. Twenty-six patients had a systolic blood pressure of ≥150 mm Hg. The mean diastolic pressure was 84 ± 13 mm Hg. Seventeen patients had blood pressures of ≥150/90 mm Hg.[25] Patients from higher altitudes have higher respiratory rates and heart rates but lower blood pressures. Tables 13.4 and 13.5.

It cannot be emphasized too strongly that trip leaders and trip physicians should be thoroughly familiar with the symptoms and signs of HAPE so that prompt descent with or without oxygen can be carried out before the patient is unable to walk down even with assistance. The common physical signs are reviewed in several papers,[18,19,25,27,28] and are summarized in Tables 13.4 and 13.5.

Diagnostic Criteria

A consensus committee that met at the 1991 International Hypoxia Symposium proposed the following diagnostic criteria for HAPE: In the setting of a recent gain in altitude the presence of the following: at least two of the following symptoms: dyspnea at rest, cough, weakness or decreased exercise performance, chest tightness or congestion; plus at least two of the following signs: rales or wheezing in at least one lung field, central cyanosis, tachypnea, and tachycardia.[29] In mountain resorts

Table 13.4
Vital Signs (Mean Values) in HAPE Observed in 239 Patients

Vital Sign	Lobenhoffer	Hultgren*	Kobayashi	Hultgren**
Temperature	99.8 ± 1.3	98.8 (97-105)	99.8 (98.4-102.4)	99 ± 1.5
Number of patients	49	26	18	150
Heart rate/min	119 ± 24	122 (70-160)	111 (76-160)	104 ± 19
Number of patients	71	34	20	150
Respiratory rate/min	36 ± 13	32 (20-54)	26 (12-55)	23 ± 6
Number of patients	32	12	16	150
Blood pressure mm Hg				
Systolic 119 ± 26	106 (78-142)	140 (98-170)	132 ± 20	
Diastolic	73 ± 20	69 (30-100)	89 (70-129)	84 ± 13
Number of patients	44	21	24	150

SOURCES: Lobenhoffer, ref. 31; Hultgren*, ref. 16, Kobayashi, ref. 35; and Hultgren**, ref. 25.

NOTES: Most of the patients are adults. Vital signs are taken from four separate reports.

± - one standard deviation, (___) range

Table 13.5
Heart and Respiratory Rates in HAPE in Children and Adults

	Children <20 years (mean age, 10 years)	Adults ≥ 20 years (mean age, 32 years)	Adults ≥ 20 years
Range	3 - 19 years	21 - 62 years	20 - 60 years
	≤ 10 years 27/46 58%	< 30 years 24/50 48%	<30 years 52/120 43%
n	n = 46	n = 50	n = 120
Heart rate m	130/min	120/min	104 ± 19/min
Range	70 - 170/min	80 - 180/min	64 - 148/min
≥ 120	38/46 83%	27/47 59%	37/120 31%
n	n = 46	n = 47	n = 120
Resp. rate m	35/min	31/min	23 ± 6/min
Range	20 - 54/min	20 - 60/min	12 - 44/min
≥ 30	19/25 76%	14/31 45%	25/120 21%
n	n = 25	n = 31	n = 120

SOURCES: Lopez, ref. 32, Marticorena, ref. 33 and Hultgren, ref. 25.

where medical facilities are available chest roentgenograms are usually recorded and provide some additional diagnostic values in evaluating severity and ruling out cardiac failure and other pulmonary conditions. Their cost effectiveness may be questioned, however, and many chest roentgenograms may be performed only for medicolegal reasons. A pulse oximeter is probably of greater value in the diagnosis and evaluation of severity and determining the effectiveness of therapy.

Severity Class and Clinical Course

In general, the severity of HAPE can be estimated by observation and a simple physical examination. Four grades of severity can be defined:

Grade 1. Mild. Minor symptoms with limitation of heavy effort only. Slight resting tachycardia and increased respiratory rate. No limitation on normal activities.

Grade 2. Moderate. Ordinary effort reproduces symptoms, and normal activities are reduced. Patient is ambulatory. Tachycardia and tachypnea present. Symptoms of dyspnea, weakness, cough are evident to others. Rales may be present.

Grade 3. Serious. Symptoms are present at rest. The patient can barely walk to take care of bodily functions and prefers to remain at bed rest. Sensorium may be dulled. Confusion and disorientation may be present. Tachycardia-tachypnea present. Rales are easily heard.

Grade 4. Severe. Patient is obtunded or comatose. Cannot respond logically to questions or commands. Unable to sit or stand. Noisy breathing with sounds of fluid in the airways. Marked tachycardia and tachypnea.

These clinical grades of severity can be roughly correlated with heart rate, respiratory rate, ECG changes, and chest x-rays (Table 13.6, Fig. 13.2). Heart rates and respiratory rates may be faster in children than in adults (Table 13.5) and are increased in a parallel fashion (Fig. 13.1).

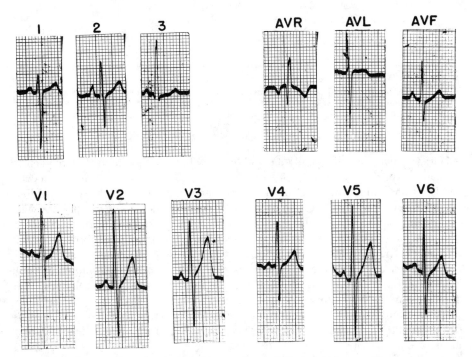

Figure 13.2. Electrocardiogram of a 8-year-old girl with HAPE. Note signs of right ventricular hypertrophy and right atrial strain, these signs regressed upon recovery. From Hultgren, ref. 16.

Table 13.6
Severity Classification of HAPE

Grade	Clinical	ECG	Chest film
1. Mild. Capable of normal activity	Minor symptoms with dyspnea only on heavy exertion	Tachycardia only. Heart rate at rest < 100	Minor infiltrates involving less than half of one lung field
2. Moderate. Patient is ambulatory	Symptoms of dyspnea, weakness, fatigue on ordinary effort. Headache, dry cough	Tachycardia with resting heart rate >100 - 110 P wave changes only	Infiltrates involving at least half of one lung field
3. Serious. Can barely attend to bodily functions, needs assistance	Symptoms of dyspnea, headache, weakness, nausea at rest. Loose recurrent productive cough	Tachycardia with heart rate 110-120 P wave and minor QRS-T wave changes	Bilateral infiltrates involving at least half of each lung field
4. Severe. Totally incapacitated in bed. Cannot get up	Stupor or coma. Unable to stand or walk. Severe cyanosis. Bubbling rales present with copious sputum, usually bloody	Tachycardia with heart rate > 120. Right axis deviation, QRS, T wave and P wave changes	Bilateral infiltrates involving more than half of each lung field

SOURCE: Hultgren, ref. 56.

NOTES: Table shows clinical severity classification and grading of heart rate, ECG changes, and the amount of infiltrate in the chest film. Higher heart rates will be present in children <20, add 10/min.

Grade 4 patients will usually die within a few hours unless high-flow oxygen is available or prompt descent to a lower altitude can be carried out. Death may occur suddenly and sometimes unexpectedly, probably as a result of hypoxic cardiac arrest. In severe hypoxia, failure of the central control centers for respiration and circulation may result in a decrease in both respiratory rate and heart rate with a terminal bradycardic-asystolic cardiac arrest. Terminal ventricular fibrillation may also occur. These events may be preceded by a slowing of the respiratory rate and heart rate and a fall in blood pressure. In such severe cases the administration of high flow oxygen may result in an increase in respiration, indicating that hypoxic depression of the respiratory center was present.

The clinical grading system is important in reporting cases of HAPE or in carrying out therapeutic interventions, since, in general, the prognosis depends upon the degree of severity.

Clinical assessment of HAPE. To develop standard methods of collecting data on patients with HAPE two forms have been developed for field trials. One form is a patient questionnaire listing symptoms and the severity of each. A second form is a clinical evaluation form to be completed by the physician. The purpose of this form is to verify presence and severity of symptoms, record objective findings, and estimate disability. The forms are illustrated in Tables 13.7 and 13.8.

Complications or associated conditions. Cerebral edema, cerebral thrombosis, bronchopneumonia, pulmonary embolism, and myocarditis have been found at autopsy in cases of HAPE.[30] Cerebral edema is the most common associated condition and is manifested clinically by the usual symptoms and signs of severe headache, vomiting, ataxia, confusion, hallucinations, and disturbances of

Table 13.7
Self-Assessment Questionnaire for HAPE

All responses should describe the most severe symptoms experienced over the past 48 hours.

Circle the appropriate descriptor

1. Dyspnea – Short of Breath
  0 - not short of breath at all
  1 - some trouble breathing, not bad
  2 - definite shortness of breath,
    had to slow down
  3 - very unpleasant shortness of
    breath, had to slow down, a
    lot of trouble breathing even
    at rest, can't walk.
  Did you have to sit up to breathe?
    Yes   No

2. Chest Congestion – Chest Tightness
  0 - not congested at all
  1 - a bit of congestion and chest
    tightness
  2 - definitely congested and
    feels tight a bit unpleasant
  3 - terrible, I can hardly
    breathe, I feel suffocated

3. Feeling Sick – Lousy – Malaise
  0 - I feel OK
  1 - a little bit ill but I can
    do anything
  2 - I definitely feel bad, ill
    it is unpleasant
  3 - a terrible cough - it won't
    stop even at night

  Did you have bloody or pink
  sputum (Circle one) Yes No

5. Weakness – Tiredness – Fatigue
  0 - none at all
  1 - a bit tired or weak
  2 - definitely tired and weak, I can't
    do many things
  3 - terrible, weak and tired, I can't
    do anything, totally incapacitated

6. Headache
  0 - none at all
  1 - mild headache, no problem
  2 - a definite headache, somewhat
    unpleasant
  3 - a severe headache, all day very
    unpleasant, I can't do much

7. Nausea – Loss of Appetite
  0 - none at all good appetite
  1 - not a good appetite, some nausea
  2 - definitely nauseated, could not
    eat much
  3 - bad nausea all day, ate hardly
    anything
  Did you vomit (Circle one)   Yes No

8. Change in Mental Status
  0 - no problems, thinking memory ok
  1 - a little slow in thinking and
    remembering
  2 - definitely confused at times,
    can't concentrate, listless
  3 - very confused, lethargic, had to
    be aroused a few times

Table 13.8
Clinical Evaluation of HAPE

Responses to be obtained by interview

Severity Score for Each Symptom

0 - no symptoms
1 - mild symptoms but no problem
2 - moderately unpleasant
3 - severely unpleasant
4 - terrible, the worst I have had

Final Functional Score
Effect of symptoms on activity level
0 - no effect on any level of activity
1 - minor effect, heavy activity decreased
2 - moderate effect, can do only light activity
3 - severe, unable to do planned activity
4 - very severe, totally incapacitated

Symptoms Scored by Numbers Above

1. Dyspnea   0 1 2 3 4
   Orthopnea   (circle one) Yes No

2. Cough   0 1 2 3 4
   Bloody sputum
            (circle one) Yes No

3. Congested - Tight Chest   0 1 2 3 4
   Sounds of fluid in lungs
            (circle one) Yes No

4. Weakness Fatigue   0 1 2 3 4
   (Can't walk far)

5. Feel Sick Malaise   0 1 2 3 4

6. Headache   0 1 2 3 4

7. Nausea   0 1 2 3 4
   Vomiting   (circle one) Yes No

8. Mental Status (circle one)
   0 - normal
   1 - lethargy, lassitude, slow
   2 - disoriented, confused
   3 - stupor, semiconscious

9. Ataxia (circle one)
   0 - none
   1 - balance maneuvers poor
   2 - steps off line
   3 - needs help to walk or stand

Physical and Objective Findings

1. Rales   0 1 2 3 4
   0 = none 1 = one quadrant
   4 = all over chest
   Sounds of fluid in air ways
      (circle one)   Yes No

2. Cyanosis   0 1 2 3 4

3. Chest X-ray
   0. clear
   1. infiltrate 1/4 lung fields
   2. infiltrate 1/2 lung fields
   3. infiltrate 3/4 lung fields
   4. infiltrate all lung fields

4. Other Chest X-ray findings
   (circle finding)
   1. increased vascularity only
   2. increased pul. arteries diameter
   3. Kerley lines
   4. pleural effusion
   5. increased heart size (CT >50%)

5. Respiratory Distress   0 1 2 3 4

6. Vital Signs
   Temp H. Rate   Resp. Rate
   BP   Vital Cap. FEV_1
         Predicted Predicted
   Oxygen Sat. PO_2

consciousness. In 150 cases of HAPE seen at a ski resort in Colorado 21 (14 percent) were confused, lethargic, drowsy or disoriented. Only three (2 percent) were ataxic.[25] Focal neurologic deficits such as hemiplegia suggest the presence of thrombotic lesions in the cerebral circulation. Bronchopneumonia may precede the onset of HAPE or may occur as an associated complication. Chills, fever, sweats, mucopurulent sputum and the presence of a febrile illness in other party members should indicate the possibility of bronchopneumonia. A temperature exceeding 102°F and a white count greater than 12,000/ml are common in bronchopneumonia but rare in uncomplicated HAPE.

Pulmonary embolism and infarction have been observed at autopsy in HAPE. Symptoms of cough, hemoptysis, pleuritic pain, and chest wall tenderness are useful clinical clues. Evidence of peripheral venous thrombosis or edema of the legs may be present. Occasional cases of viral myocarditis have accompanied HAPE. Such patients commonly have a history of an antecedent flu-like illness with chills and fever. On hospital entry shock has been present with marked tachycardia and unexpected cardiac arrest has occurred.[30] Details of clinical features of HAPE have been described in several recent publications.[27-36]

Table 13.9
Standard Laboratory Values in Reported Cases of HAPE

	Vail, Colorado[a] 8,200 ft. (2,500 m)	La Oroya, Peru[b] 12,400 ft (3,780 m)	La Oroya, Peru[c] 12,400 ft (3,780 m)	Japan[d] 9,627 ft (2,935 m)
Hematocrit				
n	28	17	not reported	26
mean	46%	48%		48%
range	37-53	40-64		±4.7%
Leucocytes				
n	31	26	36	26
mean	11,500	10,800		14,400
range	6,800-20,800	7,200-16,500	7,000-15,000	±4,400
Urine spec. gravity				
n	21	16	36	
mean	1.017	1.026	1.020	
range	1.005-1.035	1.006-1.035	1.005-1.030	
Sedimentation rate				
n	not reported	18	36	
mean		13 mm	14 mm	
range		4-31 mm	7-30 mm	

SOURCES: [a]Sophocles, ref. 34; [b]Hultgren, ref. 16; [c]Marticorena, ref. 33; [d]Kobayashi, ref. 35.

NOTES: Mild leucocytosis, a concentrated urine, and usually a normal sedimentation rate are present. Higher white cell counts and increased sedimentation rates could reflect varying degrees of associated pneumonia. Differential leucocyte counts done in 25 patients seen in Vail, Colorado, were: PMNs 74%, range 46-88%. Hematocrits were 48% ± 6. Leucocyte counts 13,000 ± 660 in 38 cases reported by Lobenhofer, et al., ref. 31.

Table 13.10
Arterial Blood Gas Values in HAPE

	Room air PO_2	Oxygen PO_2	Room air PCO_2	Oxygen PCO_2	Room air pH	HCO_3
Mean	40 mm	57 mm	28.5 mm	28 mm	7.45	19.7 mEq/L
	n = 41	n = 29	n = 41	n = 32	n = 32	n = 14
Range	18 - 56 mm	45 - 115 mm	21 - 38 mm	21 - 32 mm	7.31 - 58	15.5 - 23.0

Normal values, 12,400 feet (3,779 m)		Normal values, sea level	
PO_2	53 mm	PO_2	75 - 100 mm
PCO_2	32.5 + 2.5 mm	PCO_2	35 - 45 mm
pH	7.40	pH	7.35 - 7.45
		Bicarb	24 - 30 mEq/L

SOURCE: Hultgren, ref. 39.

NOTES: Arterial oxygen tension is markedly decreased with little rise during 100% O_2 administration. Arterial PCO_2 is low and is not changed during oxygen administration. Because many of these measurements were made in medical facilities at a lower altitude than that of the onset of HAPE, they tend to underestimate the values present before descent.

Table 13.11
Blood and Alveolar Gas Analysis (mean ± SD) at 14,953 feet (4,558 m) in Patients with AMS, with HAPE and Without Either

	Without AMS	Mild AMS	Severe AMS	HAPE
n	42	26	13	15
SaO_2 (%)	83.0±6.3[a]	78.4±8.2	75.6±9.4[b]	62.6±10.7
PaO_2 (torr)	45.8±6.9	41.1±5.4	40.7±6.2[b]	31.7±5.5
$PaCO_2$ (torr)	23.5±2.3	24.3±2.9	23.4±2.5	24.6±2.6
$(A-a)DO_2$ (torr)	6.2±3.5[c]	9.3±3.7	11.4±5.9[b]	18.6±6.9

SOURCE: Bartsch, ref. 40.

[a] p <0.05
[b] p <0.001 between adjacent values
[c] p <0.005 compared to values of severe AMS

Laboratory Studies

Routine laboratory studies in patients with HAPE admitted to hospitals are summarized in Table 13.9. The hematocrit and hemoglobin values are elevated in relation to the patient's duration of altitude exposure. The levels will usually fall slightly after recovery, since dehydration is common in HAPE.[37,38] A moderate leucocytosis is common, but values exceeding 14,000/ml should suggest the possibility of an associated infection such as pneumonia. Part of the rise in the white blood cell count could be due to hemoconcentration and sympathetic stimulation. The urine is concentrated and usually acid. The sedimentation rate is usually normal but may be moderately elevated in a few patients, either because of infection or because of tissue necrosis that may occur in the lungs.[16,34,35]

Arterial blood gas studies in HAPE have revealed a marked decrease in arterial PO_2 and a uniform decrease in arterial PCO_2. Data from several reports on patients with HAPE have shown a mean arterial PO_2 of 42 mm (range 23-65 mm Hg) and a mean arterial PCO_2 of 28 mm (range 21-32 mmg).[39] The results are shown in Table 13.10. Blood and alveolar gas analyses from fifteen patients with HAPE at 14,958 feet (4,559 m) have been reported by Bärtsch and his associates.[40] The results are shown in Table 13.11. The values for arterial PO_2 and PCO_2 are lower because all studies were done at high altitude whereas many of the studies in Table 13.10 were done at a lower altitude than where HAPE occurred. Other reports of blood gases in HAPE with essentially similar results have been published.[25,40,41,42,43] It is possible that in some cases right to left shunting is responsible, in part, for the occasional very low arterial PO_2 values.[43]

It is important to note that, despite the severe degree of hypoxemia and possible resulting respiratory depression, arterial PCO_2 is always decreased. In addition, the administration of 100 percent oxygen results in only a modest increase in PCO_2. These data are compatible with hyperventilation and a large right-to-left intrapulmonary shunt.

Computerized tomograms of the brain have been obtained in nine patients who had neurological signs and symptoms. The scans revealed small ventricles and cisterns, disappearance of sulci, and a diffuse low-density appearance of the entire cerebrum, indicating cerebral edema in eight of the nine patients. These abnormalities disappeared with clinical improvement. Cerebral edema is a recognized complication of HAPE and these data support this experience. Fukushima reported similar findings in one fatal case of HAPE. CPK was 4609 IU/liter with 6 percent MB and 90 percent MM. At autopsy cerebral edema with petechial hemorrhages was present.[41]

Studies of ventilatory function in HAPE have revealed an increase in respiratory rate, and a decrease in vital capacity and maximum breathing capacity with a decrease in maximum expiratory force.[33,45] The results are shown in Table 13.12. The abnormalities in pulmonary function promptly return to normal upon recovery. A significant decrease in vital capacity may be of diagnostic value in HAPE. For example, one adult subject with a previous history of HAPE was evaluated 24 hours after ascent to 10,200 feet (3,110 m) and 12,470 feet (3,800 m) on two different occasions. Vital capacity decreased by 19 percent and 11 percent respectively, and on the second occasion a mild pulmonary infiltrate was present in the chest x-ray despite absence of symptoms. Although vital capacity normally decreases slightly upon ascent to high altitude, the decrease is only about 3.0 percent ± 2 percent hence a decrease in vital capacity of >10 percent may indicate HAPE. The method is limited by the need to determine a control vital capacity at sea level.

The Electrocardiogram

The electrocardiogram in HAPE often shows changes compatible with acute pulmonary hypertension that resolve upon recovery.[16,44] These occur more commonly in children than in adults. The following changes have been observed: (1) increased right axis deviation, (2) peaked P waves in leads 2-3 and AVF and upward peaking of the initial portion of the P wave in leads V_1- V_2, and (3) increased depth of precordial S waves, which may extend to V_5-V_6. A representative ECG is shown in Figure 13.2. The heart rate is increased. I have personally observed one 41-year-

Table 13.12
Pulmonary Function in Five Cases of HAPE (Mean Values)

	HAPE	Recovery
Heart rate		
Children	110/min.	76/min.
Adults	114/min.	61/min.
Respiratory rate		
Children	30/min.	16/min.
Adults	29/min.	12/min.
Vital capacity		
Children	1200 ml	1970 ml
Adults	2100 ml	3350 ml
Maximum breathing capacity		
Children	41 ml/min.	70 ml/min.
Adults	77 ml/min.	110 ml/min.
Ventilation		
Children	6.66 L/min.	6.16 L/min.
Adults	9.10 L/min.	8.89 L/min.
Maximum expiratory Force		
Children	45 mm Hg	70 mm Hg
Adults	80 mm Hg	115 mm Hg

SOURCE: Marticorena, ref. 33.

NOTES: Three children (age 11-13 years) and two adults (age 32 and 40) with mild-moderate HAPE (grades 1 and 2) were studied at 12,400 feet (3,780 m) on entry to the hospital and one week after recovery. Note the faster heart rate and respiratory rate in children. Significant decreases in vital capacity and maximum breathing capacity are present during HAPE. Ventilation is only modestly increased. Maximum expiratory force was measured by having the patient blow into a mercury manometer.

old patient who developed transient atrial flutter with 2:1 AV block, which subsided spontaneously after hospital admission. A review of the heart rate in adults with HAPE revealed a few patients with heart rates of 140-150, suggesting that these patients may also have had atrial flutter. Atrial flutter is probably due to hypoxia and an acute rise in right atrial pressure. No ventricular arrhythmias have been reported in HAPE.

Radiologic Features

Roentgenograms of the chest are of diagnostic value in revealing pulmonary infiltrates and a normal heart size. Kerley lines and left atrial enlargement are absent. The most common location of small or moderate infiltrates is in the right mid-lung field. In severe cases both lungs may be nearly filled by infiltrates, but usually some clear areas can be seen between localized areas of opacification, including a small area above the diaphragms. Cardiac enlargement is usually not present and measurements of heart size during HAPE and after recovery have shown no systematic change in heart size.[16] Vock and his associates described the chest roentgenograms in 60 cases of HAPE. The diameters of the main and right pulmonary arteries were increased, but this was not a specific sign since a similar increase occurred during altitude exposure in persons without HAPE. Ninety-two percent had confluent infiltrate. In 40 cases (67 percent), the infiltrate was homogeneous and in 16 (26 percent) it was patchy. In five cases (8 percent) only increased vascularity was present. Most infiltrates were present in the right lung field and infiltrates present only in the left lung field were rare. Rales were present in some individuals with clear lung fields who later developed infiltrates, hence rales may be a particularly sensitive indicator of early HAPE.[27] Further studies by the same group indicated that early HAPE was not seen before 18 hours at altitude. It was interstitial in five or eight cases, mostly peripheral in four of eight, bilateral in six of eight and often patchy with upper lobe predominance more severe. HAPE was more often confluent, right sided and central. CT scans clearly demonstrated the patchy nature of early HAPE and was more sensitive than radiography in detecting small infiltrates.[28]

In 150 patients with HAPE seen at a Colorado ski resort, a pulmonary infiltrate was present in 132 patients (88 percent). Most of the infiltrates were bilateral involving the central portion of both lung fields. This was present in 80 patients (53 percent). The right mid-lung field only was involved in 51 patients (34 percent) and only one patient had a single infiltrate in the left lung. Infiltrate was absent in 18 patients (12 percent) but an abnormal degree of vascular congestion was present in each of their chest radiographs.[25]

A simple system of grading the severity of the pulmonary infiltrate is shown in Figure 13.3.

Kobayashi and his colleagues made careful measurements of cardiac size and volume in 27 patients with HAPE and found that a slight decrease in size and volume occurred with recovery, probably owing to a change in right ventricular volume.[35] Typical chest films are shown in Figures 13.4, 13.5, and 13.6. Prominence of the main pulmonary artery is occasionally present and may subside upon recovery. Pleural effusion is rare. Pulmonary edema confined to the left lung should raise the possibility of congenital absence of the right pulmonary artery.[47] The pulmonary infiltrates of HAPE are easily distinguished from the fine reticular infiltrates with a central "bat wing" distribution of cardiac pulmonary edema. An example of cardiac pulmonary edema is shown in Figure 13.7. In contrast, CT scans of the chest clearly show the patchy nature of the infiltrate in HAPE (Figs. 13.8 and 13.9).

Hemodynamics

Only a few hemodynamic studies of HAPE have been performed at high altitude during the acute stage before treatment,[35,41,42,46,49-51] but the results have been consistent in demonstrating the following abnormalities: (1) an elevated pulmonary artery mean pressure (mean = 46 mm Hg); (2) a normal or low pulmonary artery wedge pressure (mean 3.6 mm); (3) a moderately reduced cardiac index (mean 3.0 L/min/ m^2); (4) a decreased systemic blood pressure (mean = 79 mm); and (5) an increased pulmonary arteriolar resistance (mean = 13 units). The results of 21 cases

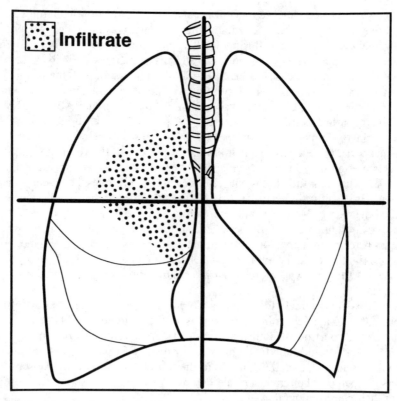

Figure 13.3. Method of scoring the amount of infiltrate in HAPE. The lung is divided into four quadrants in the AP chest roentgenogram. A Grade 1 infiltrate is indicated since the estimated area is equivalent to one quadrant.

are shown in Table 13.13. The pulmonary artery wedge pressure is probably an accurate reflection of the left atrial pressure, since in one patient the catheter fortuitously entered the left atrium via a foramen ovale and recorded a normal pressure.[48] The administration of 100 percent oxygen rapidly lowers pulmonary artery pressure but normal values are not always attained. Exercise and induced hypoxia will result in a marked rise in pulmonary artery pressure but without a change in pulmonary artery wedge pressure.[49] The hemodynamic data clearly indicate that HAPE is not due to left ventricular failure and that the abnormality resulting in edema must reside in the lung.

Epidemiology and Incidence

Altitude of occurrence. HAPE rarely occurs below 8,000 feet (2,440 m), and episodes, that occur between 8,000 (2,440 m) and 10,000 feet (3,050 m) are usually related to heavy physical effort such as skiing or climbing (Fig. 13.10). At higher altitudes HAPE may occur with only light or sedentary activity. The altitude of occurrence refers to the altitude at which one sleeps and not the altitude attained for a short period during daily activity. The threshold of approximately 8,000 feet (2,440 m) is well illustrated by the experience of skiers in California. Millions of visitors

Table 13.13
Hemodynamic and Blood Gas Data from 21 Cases of HAPE
Studied at High Altitude

Date	Hultgren	Autezana	Kobayashi	Normal*
Arterial O_2 sat.	71% (55-87)	74% (72-86)	(41)*	85%
PA mean mm Hg	46 mm (22-117)	62 mm (54-70)	26 mm (15-36)	22 mm
PA wedge mm Hg	4 mm (1-9)	5 mm (2-9)	6 mm (3-7)	8 mm
Cardiac index L/min/m²	3.0 (2.3-4.5)	2.1 (1.3-2.9)	3.8 (3.0-4.9)	3.4
PA resistance dynes. sec/cm⁻⁵	1035 (350-2900)	2680 (1520-4000)	514 (185-809)	220
BA mean mm Hg	79	87	ND	110
Arterial PC O_2	28 (24-35)	29 (24-36)	30.6	32
Number studied	13	5	5 (15-36)	21
Heart rate/min.	110* (75-140)	117 (110-130)	—	72
Altitude	12,400 ft (3,750 m)	12,045 ft (3,650 m)	9,626 ft (2,935 m)	12,400 ft (3,750 m)

SOURCES: Data from Hultgren, ref.13; Antezana, ref. 42; Kobayashi, ref. 35. Normal data from Hultgren, ref. 49.

NOTES: Values in Column 3 (Kobayashi) are more normal than the others because the altitude of occurrence was lower and studies were done within 4.5 hours after hospital entry and after descent to 2,000 feet (610 m).

ABBREVIATIONS: PA - pulmonary artery, BA - brachial artery, * Arterial PaO_2

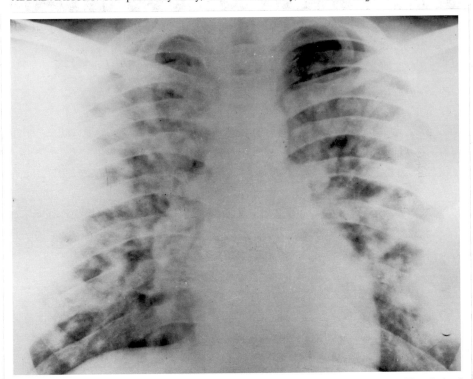

Figure 13.4. (A) Chest film of a 16-year-old boy with HAPE taken on hospital entry. Note lack of increase in heart size and irregular distribution of infiltrate with clear areas of lung above the diaphragm.

278

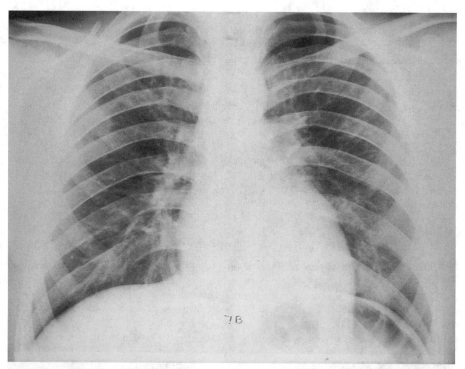

Figure 13.4. (B) Same patient four days later.

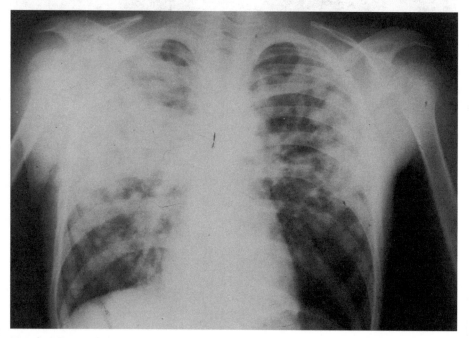

Figure 13.5. Chest film of a 14-year-old boy with HAPE. Note the presence of more infiltrate in the right mid-lung field. This is a common finding in HAPE.

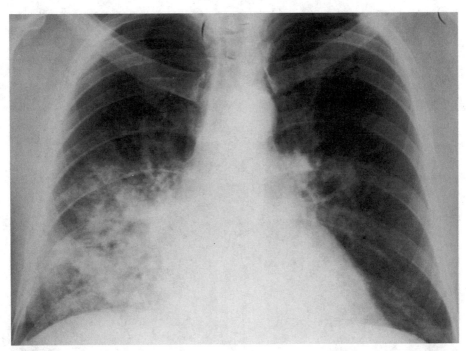

Figure 13.6. Chest film of a 30-year-old man with HAPE. This film was taken three days after the onset of HAPE and one day after descent. In some patients with HAPE, infiltrates may persist for several days after recovery.

ski in the Lake Tahoe area where most lodges and accommodations are below 6,500 feet (1,980 m). HAPE is almost unknown in this area. Farther south in the Mammoth Lakes area a similar large number of skiers stay at lodges and accommodations from 8,000 to 9,000 feet (2,440 m-2,750 m). A large new lodge at Mammoth is at 9,000 feet (2,750 m). A moderate number of cases of HAPE are seen in this area each year.

Fifty-six patients with HAPE and HACE (all males except one) were evacuated from the Swiss Alps between 1980 and 1984. Symptoms began on the second or third day after arrival and evacuation was necessary on the fourth to fifth day. The highest incidence of illness was at the Capanna Margherita refuge at 14,800 feet (4,559 m). No cases occurred below 8,125 feet (2,500 m). Only one in 588 climbers who stayed overnight at the refuge required evacuation. There were no fatalities.[52]

One can develop HAPE at lower altitudes under rare circumstances. A unique episode occurred in the Lake Tahoe area. A family had skied at Vail, Colorado, 8,200 feet (2,500 m), for several days until the thirteen-year-old daughter developed moderate HAPE. The family returned to California but stopped to ski at Soda Springs, 6,700 feet (2,044 m). After skiing hard all day the daughter noted a return of dyspnea, dizziness, nausea, cough, and insomnia. At 2:00 a.m. she was found semiconscious in the bathroom with gurgling respirations. In the emergency room the heart rate was 136/ min, respiratory rate 38/min. A chest x-ray revealed bilateral pulmonary infiltrates more marked in the right lung. The arterial PO_2 was 20 mm, PCO_2 39 mm, and pH 7.40. Treatment with 100 percent oxygen, bed rest,

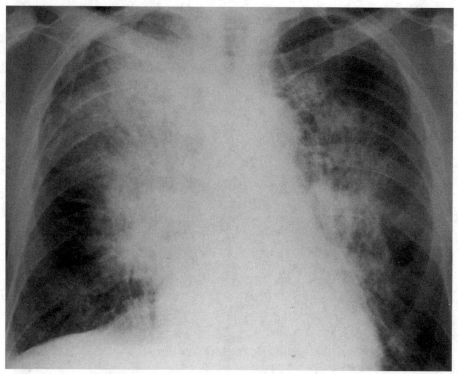

Figure 13.7. Chest film of a patient with acute cardiac pulmonary edema due to ruptured chordae of the mitral valve. The infiltrate has a fine, reticular pattern with a central "bat wing" distribution involving both lungs. This pattern is related to the central lymphatic drainage of the lung, which is more effective in draining fluid from the periphery of the lung as well as the greater central radiologic thickness of the central portion of the lung. From Levinson, ref. 91.

furosemide and morphine resulted in rapid recovery and clearing of the chest film in three days. This patient probably had mild, resolving HAPE that was made more severe by skiing at a lower altitude. Another case is that of a 22-year-old woman who had run several marathons. She flew to Salt Lake City 4,255 feet (1,298 m) where she stayed two nights and then flew to Colorado Springs, 6,500 feet (1,983 m). On the third day she ran seven miles with another marathon runner at a pace much faster than her usual pace. That evening she was weak, had difficulty even walking up or down a few flights of stairs, noted a headache, and had a persistent dry cough. During the night she had severe dyspnea with a viselike chest pressure making it difficult to take a breath. She sat up most of the night. Symptoms persisted for 24 hours and then subsided with rest. In this instance very heavy exertion soon after arrival was a precipitating factor despite spending three days in Salt Lake City where she did some running. Persons with a congenital absence of the right pulmonary artery may develop HAPE at altitudes as low as 5,200 feet (1,590 m).[53]

Acclimatization

Acclimatization at an intermediate altitude for several days will protect most persons from HAPE occurring at higher altitudes, but acclimatization may not pre-

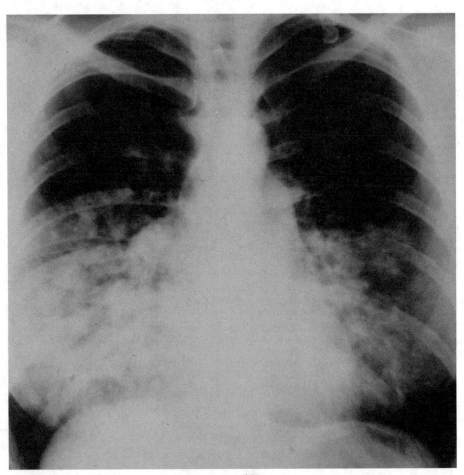

Figure 13.8. Chest film of a female patient with moderately severe HAPE - radiologic score 2. Note basal distribution of infiltrate. Apical areas are usually spared in HAPE. Reproduced by permission from Vock, refs. 27, 28.

vent HAPE if one ascends rapidly to a higher altitude. For example, a member of a trekking party in Peru spent eight days in Cuzco and Huaraz, 11,483 feet (3,500 m) and 9,935 feet (3,030 m), with the group before a climb of 4,000 feet (1,220 m) over a 15,400 foot (4,700 m) pass carrying a pack. During the next three days the party moved up to camp at 13,450 feet (4,100 m). Here the subject became ill with HAPE and expired suddenly, 36 hours after the onset of symptoms. HAPE has also occurred in well-acclimatized climbers on Mount Everest who climb high and fast from a base camp.[54] In this area in 1963 several acclimatized climbers noted signs and symptoms of HAPE after a day of strenuous climbing above 20,000 feet (6,100 m). These signs and symptoms disappeared during the night with the aid of low-flow, sleeping oxygen.[55] The altitude of occurrence of 100 reported cases of HAPE is shown in Figure 13.10.

Time of onset. The time from arrival at high altitude to the onset of symptoms depends upon many variables, but there is general agreement that a period of 24-72

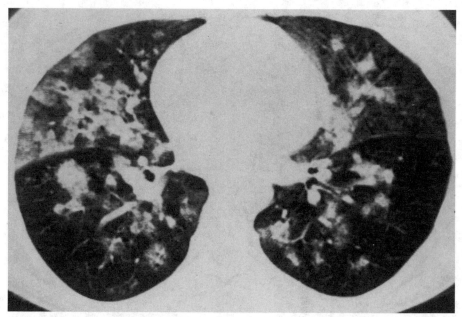

Figure 13.9. CT scan of the same patient with moderately severe HAPE - radiologic score 2 - showing a more anterior distribution of infiltrate. Reproduced by permission from Vock, refs. 27, 28.

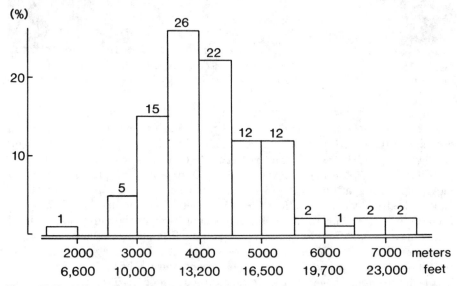

Figure 13.10. Altitude of occurrence in 100 cases of HAPE. Note that 68 percent occurred from 10,000 feet (3,050 m) to 14,800 feet (4,500 m). This is the altitude range visited most frequently. One case at 6,600 feet (2,000 m) may represent a person who lacked a right pulmonary artery. From Lobenhoffer, ref. 31.

hours of altitude exposure usually precedes the onset of symptoms. In Vail, Colorado, the mean time from arrival to the onset of cough and dyspnea in a predominately adult male population was 2.5 days ± 0.8 days, range 1 to 5 days.[34] At a ski resort in Colorado the mean time to onset of symptoms from arrival was 3 ± 1.3 days.[25] In children, the onset of symptoms may be more rapid: Lopez, for example, noted that in 50 percent of 117 children in Peru, symptoms began within 24 hours of ascending rapidly to 12,230 feet (3,730 m).[32] (See Table 13.14).

Incidence. The incidence of HAPE also depends upon many variables: altitude, time required for ascent, age, and activity engaged in upon arrival. In a survey that was carried out in La Oroya, Peru, 12,230 feet (3,730 m), to determine the incidence of HAPE during rapid ascent to this altitude by rail or auto, the overall incidence of HAPE was found to be 3.4 percent.[56] Only 2 of 50 adults making 458 ascents experienced HAPE (4 percent). Twenty-six episodes of HAPE occurred in 402 ascents by subjects under 21 years, therefore for a single ascent to 12,230 feet (3,730 m) the estimated incidence of HAPE was 60/1,000 for subjects under 21 and 4/1,000 for older patients. The incidence in Indian troops transported by air to an altitude of 11,500 feet (3,500 m) or higher was 5.7 percent. If travel was accomplished by truck the incidence was 0.3 percent.[18] In troops moved rapidly to altitudes between 11,000 and 18,000 feet (3,355- 5,500 m), the incidence of HAPE was 13-15 percent.[19] A survey of male visitors and skiers to Vail, Colorado, 8,200 feet (2,500 m), from 1979 through 1982 revealed an incidence of approximately 10 cases per 100,000.[34] In 200 trekkers evaluated by Hackett and Rennie at 14,000 feet (4,270 m) in Nepal, the incidence of HAPE was 4.5 percent.[57] The incidence of HAPE on Mount McKinley in Alaska is about 20-33 percent.[58] Maggiorini and his associates reported eleven case of HAPE in 209 climbers at 14,958 feet (4,559 m) in Switzerland, an incidence of 5.2 percent.[59] Snyder observed a similar incidence on Mount Kenya.[60]

Table 13.14
Time of Onset of Symptoms After Arrival at High Altitude

	Children & Adults (Lobenhoffer)		Adults (Hultgren)		Children (<19 years) (Lopez)	
	No.	Percent	No.	Percent	No.	Percent
0 (Day of Arrival)	20	20	12	9	64	51
1 (Day after Arrival)	21	21	30	22	37	30
2	11	11	43	32	18	14
3	12	12	23	17	4	3
4	9	9	11	8	0	0
5	5	5	11	8	1	1
6	4	4	1	1	0	0
7	1	1	2	2	1	1
> 7 days	17	2	2	1	1	
Total	100		135		125	

SOURCES: Data from Lobenhoffer et al, ref. 31; Lopez, ref. 32 and Hultgren, ref. 16.

NOTES: Lobenhoffer's cases were mostly adults. Note the higher number of children than adults exhibiting symptoms on the day of arrival. Many adults who exhibited the late onset of symptoms had moved from one altitude to a higher elevation, where HAPE developed.

Collected data on the incidence of HAPE are summarized in Table 13.15. In most of these surveys HAPE was serious enough to result in disability and to require treatment. In recent arrivees to high altitude systematic examination will reveal a larger number of subjects who have signs of subclinical or mildly symptomatic HAPE. Hackett and Rennie, for example, observed rales in 23 percent of 200

Table 13.15
Incidence of HAPE Reported from Various Studies

Risk group	Altitude	Incidence %	Authors
Mount Kenya; 7,500 trekkers	13,000 feet (3,965 m) to 14,500 feet (4,423 m)	0.44%	Houston[21]
Mount Kenya; 50,000 visitors	10,050 feet (3,063 m) to 14,500 feet (4,423 m)	0.10%	Snyder[60]
Mount Everest region; 522 trekkers	14,000 feet (4,270 m)	2.4 - 4.5%	Hackett[58]
India; thousands of soldiers	11,500 feet (3,508 m) to 18,000 feet (5,490 m)	2.3 - 15.5%	Singh[18]
India; thousands of soldiers	11,500 feet (3,508 m)	0.57%	Menon[20]
Peru; residents of La Oroya	12,400 feet (3,782 m)	0.6% adults 8.1% children	Hultgren[56]
Vail, Colorado; 268,872 male visitors	8,200 feet (2,500 m)	10/10,000	Sophocles[34]
Leadville, Colorado; residents	10,300 feet (3,142 m)	50/100,000 adults 140/100,000 children	Scoggin[46]
Swiss Alps; 209 climbers	14,953 feet	5.3%	Maggiorini[26]

NOTES: The highest incidence occurred in Indian soldiers brought rapidly to elevations above 14,000 feet (4,070 m). The lowest incidence was observed in males visitors to Vail, Colorado, at 8,200 feet (2,500 m). No cases were observed in women at this elevation.

Table 13.16
Age Distribution of 219 Patients with HAPE
Seen at Chulec General Hospital, La Oroya, Peru, 1950-1967

Age	Number	Percent
<3 years	23	9.0%
3 - 4 years	34	14.7%
5 - 9 years	107	46.7%
10 - 14 years	29	12.6%
15 - 19 years	13	5.6%
20 - 24 years	9	3.9%
>24 years	4	5.9%
Total	219	

SOURCE: Lopez, ref. 32.

NOTES: Six patients (2.6%) were less than one year of age and two patients (1.0%) were over 34 years.

trekkers of whom only 4.5 percent had clinical HAPE.[57] Houston examined climbers before and after an ascent of Mount Rainier 14,408 feet (4,400 m). In 140 subjects, 15 percent had pulmonary rales appearing after descent.[21] Singh noted that about one-third of patients with severe AMS had pulmonary rales.[18] These data suggest that subclinical pulmonary edema occurs at an incidence of about six to ten times that of symptomatic HAPE.

Age and gender. Studies in Peru have shown that HAPE is about six times as common in children as in adults, and it also appears to be more serious. In a study of 97 subjects exposed to a total of 1,157 rapid ascents to 12,230 feet (3,730 m), 81 percent of the episodes in children aged two to twelve years were severe, compared with only 22 percent in adults over twenty years.[33] The age distribution of 219 patients with HAPE seen at Chulec Hospital in La Oroya, 12,230 feet (3,730 m) from 1950 to 1967 is shown in Table 13.16 and Figure 13.11. The highest incidence, accounting for 46.7 percent of all cases, was in the five-to-nine-year age group. Only 10 percent of cases were over nineteen years. HAPE was rare in infants; however, only 5 percent of 219 cases were under two years of age.[32] The mean age of 46 patients with HAPE seen at Vail was 36 years, ± 10 years, with a range from 12 to 55 years.[34] The mean age of 150 patients with HAPE seen at a Colorado ski resort was 34 years ± 16.25

In young patients there is no sex predilection. Sixty percent of 200 cases seen at Chulec Hospital were males. The slight predominance of males is not significant and could be due to a greater level of physical activity engaged in after arrival in boys compared with girls.

In adults, HAPE appears to occur more frequently in men than in women. In visitors to Vail, Colorado, 8,200 feet (2,500 m), the incidence of HAPE in women was 0.74 per 100,000 women compared with 10.0 per 100,000 men.[34] In a Colorado ski resort 84 percent of 150 cases of HAPE were males.[25] The reason for the difference is not clear, but, again, it could be due to more physical exertion in men, or possibly to a greater degree of ventilation during sleep in women, most of whom were probably premenopausal.[34] HAPE has been reported in women climbers.[31]

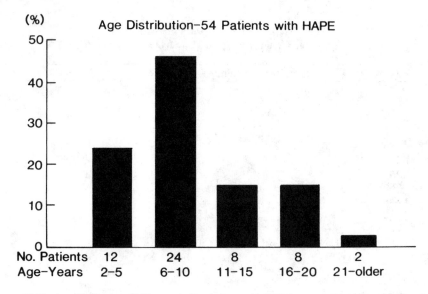

Figure 13.11. Age distribution of 54 consecutive patients with HAPE seen at Chulec General Hospital, La Oroya, Peru, altitude 12,230 feet (3,730 m). From Marticorena, ref. 33.

Severity

Because of the lack of a commonly used definition, there is little information available on the severity of cases of HAPE. In Peru, a grading system of clinical severity (described earlier in this chapter) was employed in classifying 52 cases of HAPE. The results are shown in Table 13.17. Half of the patients were grade 2 and only two patients were classified as having grade 4 HAPE.

HAPE During Reascent

It has long been observed in Peru that persons who live at high altitude may develop HAPE after a sojourn at sea level. The length of time spent at a lower altitude required to result in HAPE during reascent varies. Most studies have indicated that 10-14 days at a lower altitude are required, but for children the stay may be shorter.[16] In 200 cases of HAPE, twelve children (6 percent) developed HAPE after a sea level stay of less than seven days (Table 13.18).[32] Studies from Leadville, Colorado, 10,150 feet (3,100 m), have shown that children descending to Denver, 5,400 feet (1,635 m), or lower may develop HAPE after a stay at the lower altitude of only three to five days.[46] In Peru, employees of mining companies who live at altitudes of 11,000-14,900 feet (3,355-4,545 m) descend frequently to Lima at sea level for three to seven days without experiencing symptoms upon return.

Some authors have proposed that HAPE during reascent (Type II) differs from HAPE that occurs during a first ascent (Type I).[34] It has also been suggested that reascent HAPE occurs more commonly in children age nine to sixteen years with an approximately equal sex distribution, in contrast to the high predominance of males in the Vail, Colorado, cases; all of which occurred on first ascent.[34] This argument is weak, because the difference in the Vail cases may be due entirely to the age groups exposed and the frequency of travel from high to low altitudes.

Table 13.17
Severity Grade in 52 Consecutive Cases of HAPE
Admitted to Chulec General Hospital, La Oroya, Peru

Severity grade	Clinical		Radiologic		Electrocardiogram	
	No.	%	No.	%	No.	%
1. Mild	17	33	24	46	27	56
2. Moderae	26	50	12	23	16	33
3. Serious	3	15	14	27	3	6
4. Severe	1	2	2	4	2	4

SOURCE: Hultgren and Marticorena, ref. 125.

NOTES: There is an approximate correlation between each grading method. Grading method described in Table 13.6 and Figure 13.2.

Table 13.18
Duration of Sea-level Stay, Prior to Developing Reascent HAPE in 113 Patients

Sea-level stay, days	Number of patients	Percent
<7	12	10.5%
7 - 13	3	2.6%
14 - 20	63	55.0%
21 - 27	8	7.0%
28 - 56	13	11.4%
57 - 90	9	7.9%
>90	5	4.5%
Total	113	

SOURCE: Lopez, ref. 32.

Individual Susceptibility

Recurrent episodes in the same person have been observed in Peruvian hospitals for many years.[11,16,32] Some 10-20 percent of the patients seen at Chulec Hospital in La Oroya will have had one previous episode of HAPE, and an additional 10-20 percent will have had more than one previous episode. Four patients had had six or more episodes (Table 13.19).[32] Although systematic data are not available from climbers, there are many individual reports of recurrent episodes. In one study, 3 of 19 fatal cases of HAPE had experienced previous episodes.[31] Recurrent episodes may be less common in adults, however, than in children. In Vail, Colorado, only one of 46 patients had experienced a previous episode of HAPE.[34] A similar observation was made of another nearby ski resort.[25]

There is no evidence of racial susceptibility or immunity to HAPE either in children or in adults.

Table 13.19
Single and Repeat Episodes of HAPE in
111 Patients at Chulec General Hospital, La Oroya, Peru

Number of episodes	Number of patients	Percent
1	68	61.2%
2	22	19.8%
3	10	9.0%
4	6	5.4%
6	2	1.8%
7	2	1.8%
8	1	0.9%
Total	111	

SOURCE: Lopez, ref. 32.

NOTES: The marked decrease after two episodes is partly due to the family's taking precautions to prevent a third attack.

Pathology

Knowledge of the pathology of HAPE is limited by the paucity of well-conducted autopsy studies.[30,41,61-64] Table 13.20 summarizes 25 autopsy reports. The mean age was 31 years (range 9-62 years). All were males. The duration of symptoms before death was two days (range 1-3 days). The following gross findings were present:

1. All lungs showed diffuse pulmonary edema with bloody, foamy fluid being readily expressed from the cut surfaces and usually filling the airways. Mean total lung weight was 1,960 grams (range 1,200-3,000 grams). Normal combined weight of normal lungs is between 750 and 800 grams. Grossly evident pulmonary emboli or thrombosis was present in two cases, one of which had pulmonary infarcts. There were no areas of substantial purulent consolidation indicating extensive pneumonia.

2. There was no evidence of left ventricular failure including hypertrophy or dilatation of the left ventricle or left atrium. There was no myocardial infarction or coronary occlusion. The right ventricle, right atrium, and proximal pulmonary arteries were often distended.

3. Cerebral edema was present in three of eight cases in which the brain was examined, and petechial hemorrhages were present in three. No thrombotic cerebral lesions were seen. Two brains were weighed, with values of 1,750 and 1,610 grams (normal value, 1,350).

Histologic studies revealed the following:

1. Alveoli and airways were filled with pink staining edema fluid and moderate numbers of red cells.

2. Areas of hemorrhage with confluent masses of red cells in the alveoli were present in four cases.

3. Small foci of dense accumulations of PMN leucocytes indicating pneumonitis were present in four cases. Smaller focal areas of PMN leucocytes, monocytes, and lymphocytes were present in 3 additional cases.

4. In four cases small thrombi were seen in terminal pulmonary arterioles and capillaries.

5. In two cases hyaline membranes were found lining the walls of alveoli indicating a high protein exudate.

Table 13.20
Analysis of Autopsy Studies in 25 Cases of HAPE

Clinical data

Age	mean: 31 years	range: 21-42 years
Sex	mean: all males	
Duration symptoms	mean: 2.2 days	range: 1-12 days
Altitude		range: 8,400-17,200 feet (2,562-5,246 m)
Coma	5/12 (42%)	

Gross examination:

Lung weight: n=9		
right: n=7	mean: 1,080 gms.	range: 600-1,600
left: n=7	mean: 950 gms.	range: 460-1,400
combined: n=9	mean: 1,960 gms.	range: 1,200-3,000
Pulmonary edema	25/25	range: 100%
Pulmonary embolism-infarction	2/24 (8%)	
Cerebral edema	4/24 (17%)	
Brain wt. (n=3)	mean: 1,617 gms.	range: 1,490-1,750 gms.
Brain hemorrhages	4/21 (19%)	
Brain thrombi	none	

Histologic examination

Pulmonary thrombi	11/24 - (46%)
Pneumonitis	5/24 - (21%)
Leucocyte infiltrates	17/23 - (75%)
Hyaline membranes	9/24 - (37%)
Infarction	1/24 - (4%)
Hemorrhages (alveolar)	14/24 - (58%)

SOURCES: Data from Fukushina, ref. 41; Hultgren et al, ref. 61; Arias-Stella et al, ref. 62; Nayak et al, ref. 63.

NOTES: Epidemiological data regarding sex, age, duration of symptoms, altitude, and incidence of coma are similar to fatal cases described in Table 13.21. Histologic studies reveal a high incidence of pulmonary arteriolar and capillary thrombi, hyaline membranes, alveolar hemorrhages, and leucocyte infiltration compatible with vascular obstruction and injury. Normal brain weight 1,350 gms. Normal lung weight R-400 gms. L-350 gms. Presence or absence of coma was stated in only 12 reports.

Nayak and his workers reported the autopsy findings in thirteen patients with HAPE with similar results.[63] Seven cases had hyaline membranes and six had microscopic evidence of thrombi in small pulmonary arteries and capillaries. Focal pneumonitis were found in six cases. Acute severe hypoxia may result in acute pulmonary edema with similar findings.[64]

Arias-Stella and Kruger reported unusual vascular structures in two cases of HAPE.[63] These represented small muscular pulmonary arteries that continued into dilated preterminal arterioles connecting directly with septal capillaries. These vessels could transmit high pulmonary artery pressure directly to the pulmonary capillary bed and in that way result in high capillary pressure edema without postulating any changes in capillary permeability. Whether such arterio-capillary anastomoses are etiologic factors in HAPE or merely a consequence of pulmonary hypertension remains unanswered.

The above autopsy studies excluded patients who exhibited gross evidence of pneumonia or pulmonary embolism. Both these conditions can be fatal at high altitude and both can be accompanied by pulmonary edema.[65] Acute myocarditis and myocardial infarction may also result in fatal pulmonary edema in persons who were well and fit at the beginning of a trip.

Certain conclusions can be derived from these data:

1. There is no evidence of left ventricular failure or underlying cardiac disease.

2. The degree of pulmonary edema is severe, and widespread and can result in death by hypoxia.

3. Although small foci of pneumonitis may be demonstrated histologically, in about one-third to one-half of cases lung infection appears to be coincidental and not a causative factor.

4. The protein rich alveolar exudate with numerous areas of alveolar hemorrhage and the presence of alveolar hyaline membranes indicate that the edema fluid has a high protein content compatible with extensive capillary injury.

5. Thrombotic lesions in small pulmonary arteries and capillaries in half the cases suggest that in some patients thrombotic vascular obstruction may play a role in elevating the pulmonary artery pressure.

6. Cerebral edema is not universally present and therefore can be excluded as a causative factor.

Medicolegal Aspects

For medicolegal reasons a complete autopsy is essential in high altitude deaths even if several days have elapsed. In foreign countries the nearest U.S. Consulate should be notified at once. The autopsy should include a complete examination of the lungs, pulmonary arteries and branches, coronary arteries, and myocardium as well as the brain. All branches of major coronary arteries should be sectioned and dissected to detect disease or thrombi. Organs, including lungs, brain, and heart, should be weighed. Portions of lung, coronary arteries, myocardium, and brain should be fixed in formalin and Zenker's solution for histologic study. Gross photographs of dissected organs should be recorded and saved. These determinations are essential to establish the cause of death. Death due to HAPE or HACE may indicate negligence on the part of the trip leader or trip physician and can result in legal action. Death due to myocardial infarction or myocarditis or to preexisting disease does not usually result in legal action.

Mortality and Fatal Cases

The mortality of HAPE is difficult to determine, since there have been few surveys and there are many variables that would affect mortality, such as availability of medical care. In visitors to the Colorado Rockies, HAPE has resulted in very low mortality, probably because of mild episodes, prompt diagnosis, and easy access to medical care. Sophocles found that no deaths occurred in 75 cases of HAPE in Summit County and Vail, Colorado, 9,000-11,000 feet (2,743-3,554 m).[34,36] At Chulec General Hospital in Peru, the mortality was 6.2 percent in over 200 patients; most of the deaths were children whose parents did not seek medical attention promptly.[32] Menon reported a mortality of 3.9 percent in Indian troops.[20] The mortality is probably highest in mountaineers and trekkers who ascend too quickly to very high altitudes where the onset of HAPE may be rapid, descent difficult, and oxygen not available. A knowledge of epidemeological features of fatal cases is important for prompt recognition and treatment. A summary of 19 fatal cases is shown in Table 13.21. All were males, with a mean age of 35.4 years (range 17-62 years). The mean altitude of the occurrence of HAPE was 14,360 feet (4,380 m); and 13 of the 19 cases occurred above 14,000 feet (4,300 m). All but two patients ascended rapidly (one was actually flown to 13,000 feet (3,965 m) in a helicopter).

Table 13.21
Analysis of 19 Fatal Cases of HAPE

Age		
mean	35.4 yrs.	
range	17-62	
Sex	all males	
Altitude of onset		
mean	14,360 feet	
	(4,380 m)	
range	9,000 feet	
	(2,750 m)	
	to	
	24,000 feet	
	(7,320 m)	
Over 14,000 feet	13/19	68%
(4,300 m)		
Days at altitude		
mean	6.0	
range	1-19	
≤3 days	9/19	48%
Acclimatized	3/19	16%
Duration of symptoms		
mean	1.8	
≤2 days	16/19	84%
Prior HAPE	3/19	16%
Rapid ascent	17/19	90%
Symptoms ignored	8/19	42%
Treatment		
Rest only	10/19	53%
Oxygen	3/19	16%
Descent	5/19	26%
Oxygen + descent	1/19	5%
Coma	8/19	42%
Sudden death	5/19	26%

NOTES: Analysis of the epidemiological features of 19 fatal cases of HAPE collected from published reports by the author. Most reported fatalities are in adult males.

Only three had some degree of acclimatization, and two of these developed HAPE after ascending to a higher altitude. The mean number of days of symptoms before death was 1.8 days; 16 of the 19 cases had symptoms for only two days or less. Only four patients received oxygen, and in only six was descent initiated. Eight were in coma prior to death; and in five sudden death occurred. Circulatory collapse—faint heart sounds, unobtainable blood pressure, and shock—preceded death in three cases. It should be emphasized, however, that except for preterminal coma or collapse, the symptoms experienced by these patients were no different from those in the usual nonfatal cases: malaise, weakness, cough, hemoptysis, vomiting, gurgling noises in the chest, delirium, and somnolence. Lobenhoffer analyzed 19 deaths among 166 cases of HAPE. Of 61 patients who descended or were treated with oxygen or both only four died but there were 10 deaths among those who neither descended nor were given oxygen.[31] Several fatal cases of HAPE have occurred in persons who were traveling alone and retired to their hotel room when symptoms became severe. A companion might have been life saving, since the progression of symptoms to coma would have led to a call for medical assistance. This review illustrates some important clinical points relevant to mountaineers and trekkers. Fatal HAPE is more common above 12,000 feet (3,660 m). In over half the cases reviewed, symptoms appeared within four days of ascent. Once symptoms appear, death may occur within 24-48 hours; but the nature of the initial symptoms does not characterize potentially fatal cases. Mental changes, confusion, delirium, coma, and circulatory collapse commonly precede death, which, as the review shows, may occur suddenly and unexpectedly (20 percent of cases).

Etiology

The etiologic mechanisms of HAPE must be considered within the framework of certain well-established features of this unusual form of pulmonary edema: (1) presence of a rise in pulmonary artery pressure resulting from high altitude ascent, with a normal pulmonary artery wedge and left atrial pressure; (2) acute hypoxic pulmonary arteriolar vasoconstriction, which is reversed by breathing oxygen or descent; (3) absence of left ventricular failure or pneumonia; (4) marked pulmonary capillary congestion and presence of capillary and arterial thromboses in many fatal cases; (5) harmful effect of heavy exercise, but improvement on bed rest. (In 1966, the author suggested the following concept of the etiology of HAPE, which deserves comment.[66,67] It was proposed that the primary cause of HAPE was nonhomogeneous obstruction of the pulmonary vascular bed by hypoxic vasoconstriction and possibly intravascular thromboses. During periods of exercise with increased cardiac output, unobstructed areas of the pulmonary circulation would be subjected to high pressure and flow and the precapillary arterioles would be dilated, permitting the pressure to be transmitted directly to the capillary bed, with resulting interstitial and alveolar edema. With dilation of arterioles and capillaries, the pulmonary veins would then become the site of resistance to flow, which would also facilitate a high capillary pressure. Small pulmonary arteries and arterioles have relatively thin muscular walls and are easily dilated by small pressure elevations, thus an important mechanism of HAPE is a regional failure of hypoxic vasoconstriction and dilatation of nonconstricted vessels in local areas of the lung (Fig. 13.12).) A similar concept has been suggested for the mechanism of hypertensive encephalopathy in systemic hypertension. It has been proposed that in this condition cerebral edema

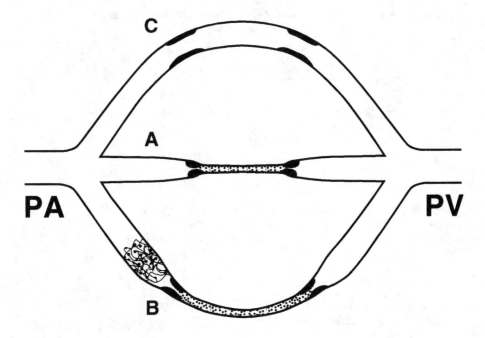

Figure 13.12. Diagram of the pulmonary circulation in HAPE according to the author's overperfusion concept.

A. Hypoxic arteriolar constriction closes off part of the pulmonary circulation.

B. Arteriolar constriction and obstruction of pre-capillary vessels by thrumbi obstruct the pulmonary circulation.

C. Remaining non-obstructed circulatory bed is subjected to high pressure and flow with a resulting increase in capillary pressure. Capillary wall injury increases capillary permeability. Pulmonary veins may now be the site of pressure drop due to high flow and/or venous constriction.

is due to failure of cerebral vasoconstriction, permitting high arterial pressure to be transmitted to the capillary bed with resultant edema. Failure of vasoconstriction is due to a very high arterial pressure. The degree of pressure elevation is thought to be the etiologic factor. Clinical and experimental evidence is available to support this concept.[68]

Overperfusion Concept. The overperfusion concept of HAPE can be supported by the following general lines of evidence.

1. A rise in pulmonary arterial pressure due to hypoxic pulmonary arteriolar constriction occurs in normal subjects acutely exposed to high altitude. During exercise a further rise in pressure occurs.[69]

2. Persons who have experienced previous episodes of HAPE respond to high altitude exposure by a greater rise in pulmonary pressure than normal subjects. Because this rise in pressure occurs in the absence of clinical evidence of pulmonary edema, it probably represents the initial abnormality in patients who develop HAPE[70] (See Fig. 13.11 and Table 13.22). Normal subjects acutely exposed to high

Table 13.22

Hemodynamics and Blood Gases During Acute Altitude Exposure of Subjects with a Previous History of HAPE

Number	Age in years	PCV %	O$_2$ Sat. %	PCO$_2$ mm	PAm mm Hg	PAw mm Hg	C.I.	PAR	BAM mm Hg	H. Rate
1	22	43	88	32	22	8	3.2	265	100	89
2	36	42	85	33	41	12	4.1	420	98	95
3	37	40	92	33	47	—	3.1	450	78	82
4	38	40	91	26	37	11	2.9	540	103	96
5	54	40	83	28	47	11	3.4	555	128	107
Mean	37.2	41	87.6	30.4	38.8	10.5	3.36	446	101	94

SOURCE: Hultgren et al., ref. 70.

NOTES: All five subjects were studied 24-48 hours after arrival at high altitude (10,150 feet, 3,095 m). None had clinical symptoms or signs of pulmonary edema. Pulmonary hypertension with a normal PA wedge pressure was present in all but one subject. These changes probably represent the initial stage of HAPE.

PCV = packed cell volume
PAm = pulmonary artery mean pressure
PAw = pulmonary artery wedge mean pressure
C.I. = cardiac index L/min/m^2
PAR = pulmonary arteriolar resistance dynes/sec/cm^2
BAM = brachial artery mean pressure

altitude have similar changes in pulmonary arterial pressure, A-a gradients, and ventilation-perfusion matching, but the responses are of a lesser magnitude.[71]

3. Additional obstruction of the pulmonary vascular bed may occur as the result of arterial and capillary thromboses, which have been observed in fatal cases at autopsy. Indirect evidence of intrapulmonary thrombosis includes a decrease in platelet count, shortening of the whole blood coagulation time, and possible accumulation of platelets in the lungs.[72,75] Kobayashi and his colleagues observed a slight decrease in platelets and a moderate prolongation of prothrombin time in 26 patients with HAPE.[35] Fukushima and his colleagues reported a fatal case of HAPE with a platelet count of 119.000/mm before death. Multiple microthrombi were present in pulmonary arterioles and alveolar capillaries.[41]

The overperfusion concept of HAPE is illustrated by the following experimental study in which increased flow through a portion of normal lung results in pulmonary edema with a normal left atrial pressure and a mean pulmonary artery pressure similar to that reported in cases of HAPE (Fig. 13.12). In the study, large mongrel dogs (mean weight 16 kg) were anesthetized with nembutal anesthesia and the chest was opened via a left thoractomy. Ventilation was controlled by a Bennett apparatus, which supplied room air. The pericardium was opened and the following measurements were made: (1) arterial and right atrial oxygen contents, blood gas tensions, and pH; (2) pressures from the femoral artery, right atrium, left atrium, and pulmonary artery, and pulmonary artery wedge pressure. Right and left atrial pressures were recorded via plastic cannulas tied into the atrial appendages. Pulmonary artery pressure and wedge pressures were recorded via a double-lumen catheter inserted into the left-upper-lobe pulmonary artery. After control measurements had been made, the right pulmonary artery was ligated, and following a ten-minute stabilization period, blood gas values and pressures were again determined. The right atrium was then cannulated via catheters from the femoral and jugular vein. A roller pump inflow cannula was inserted via a stab wound into the main pulmonary artery and secured by ligatures. A roller pump withdrew blood from the right atrium and delivered a constant flow to the main pulmonary artery, thus bypassing the right ventricle. Bypass of the right ventricle is necessary to prevent right ventricular failure and to maintain and vary the pulmonary flow. Initial bypass flow was started at 500 ml/ min. Blood samples and pressures were again recorded. Ligatures were then placed around the isolated branches of the pulmonary artery to the left lower lobe and the left middle lobe. The ligatures were then slowly tightened so that total pulmonary flow was diverted through the left upper lobe. After ten minutes, blood gas and pressure values were determined; this was repeated at ten-minute intervals. Similar measurements were made with bypass flows of 1.1 and 1.5 L/min. Cardiac output was determined by the Fick principle. Expired air was collected in a meteorological balloon and analyzed. All pressures were referred to the midchest.

At the termination of each experiment, the arteries, veins, and bronchi to each lobe were tied. The lobes were removed and weighed in air. The volume was determined by water displacement. Sections were taken for histologic study.

Results. Ligation of the right pulmonary artery resulted in a moderate increase in pulmonary arterial pressure from a control value of 16.2 to 30.5 mm Hg (mean). Femoral arterial pressure, left atrial pressure, and cardiac output did not change significantly.

Ligation of pulmonary arterial branches to left lower and left middle lobe was then performed. When perfusion of the left upper lobe along began, the lobe became engorged and a continuous palpable thrill and murmur appeared over the the upper lobe artery and surface of the lung. After ten to twenty minutes of perfusion the lobe became stiff and cyanotic, blood-tinged fluid filled the bronchi. Arterial oxygen saturation fell rapidly. Examination of the lobe after removal from the animal revealed diffuse pulmonary edema, and fluid oozed from the cut surface. The mean specific gravity of eight edematous lobes was 0.93, and the uninvolved, ligated lobes had a mean specific gravity of 0.56. The mean specific gravity of normal lobes of the lung removed immediately after ligation from three anesthetized dogs was 0.36. The protein content of the edema fluid removed from the bronchi was 4.3 to 5.3 grams/100 ml. Plasma proteins were not measured. Normal plasma protein concentration in mongrel dogs was reported by Vreim and her associates to be 5.9 ± .43 gms/100 ml.[76] Using this value the pulmonary edema fluid protein would be between 73 and 90 percent of the estimated plasma protein indicating increased capillary permeability. Histologic studies revealed marked capillary dilatation and engorgement with red cells and diffuse hemorrhagic pulmonary edema.

The hemodynamic data from eight dogs are summarized in Table 13.23. The left atrial and pulmonary arterial wedge pressures remained normal throughout each study and showed no significant changes from the control pressures. The mean pulmonary arterial pressure was 48 mm Hg (range 31-68 mean) just before gross pulmonary edema appeared. The cardiac output, i.e., total pulmonary flow, was not significantly different from control values. The calculated pulmonary vascular resistance rose from 9.6 units (following ligation of the right pulmonary artery) to

Table 13.23
Hemodynamics of Overperfusion Pulmonary Edema

	Dog	Sheep	Man
PA mean mm Hg	48	28	45
PA wedge mm Hg	6	11*	4
PA resistance dyne/sec/cm^5	800	320	1,500
Cardiac output L/min/50 kg.	4.2	4.4	2.2

SOURCES: Hultgren, ref. 44; Staub et al, ref. 77.

NOTES: The hemodynamics of overperfusion pulmonary edema in the dog model compared with pulmonary edema in the sheep produced by balloon catheter obstruction or glass bead embolization (Younes, ref. 79). The right-hand column represents mean data from eleven cases of HAPE in man. Pulmonary resistance has been corrected to cardiac output /50 kg.

ABBREVIATIONS: PA = Pulmonary artery.

* Left atrial pressure - unchanged from control.

20 units. From measurements of the weight of normal lung lobes, it was found that the left upper lobe consisted of approximately 25 percent of the weight of the total lung. Assuming that the capacity of the vascular bed is uniformly distributed in the dog lung, one can estimate that in these studies the blood flow through the left upper lobe was increased by 600 percent.

Conclusions. These data demonstrate that a sixfold increase in blood flow to a portion of the normal dog lung will result in severe pulmonary edema. Under the experimental conditions leading to pulmonary edema, the mean pulmonary artery pressure was 48 mm Hg and the pulmonary arterial and pulmonary artery wedge pressures were normal. Hemodynamic studies of HAPE have revealed similar values: pulmonary arterial mean pressures of 46 mm Hg with normal pulmonary artery wedge and left atrial pressures (Table 13.13). Staub and Landolt have obtained similar results by partially occluding the pulmonary circulation in sheep by ligation and embolism.[76,77] Similar studies have been done by Gibbon.[78]

Younes studied overperfusion pulmonary edema in dogs.[79] Pneumonectomy and removal of lung tissue left 33-55 percent of the lung intact; pulmonary blood flow through this portion of the lung was four to five times normal. Pulmonary artery mean pressure was 35 mm Hg and pulmonary capillary pressure was also increased. Younes speculated that the pulmonary venules and veins were relatively indistensible and thus acted as the locus of resistance to flow. High capillary pressure and pulmonary edema resulted. Left atrial pressure was not elevated. The protein content of the edema fluid was not determined.

The overperfusion concept depends upon nonhomogeneous obstruction in the pulmonary vascular bed. The most important initiating factor is hypoxic vasoconstriction. It is well known that unilateral hypoxia will result in vasoconstriction in the hypoxic lung with an increase in blood flow to the normoxic lung.[80] Even diffuse hypoxia may result in irregular areas of vasoconstriction. Lehr injected India ink into the veins of rabbits before and after acute hypoxia and examined the distribution of the ink particles in the lungs. With normoxia most particles had traversed the lung. With hypoxia irregular areas of the lung had trapped ink particles, suggesting local areas of vasoconstriction and blockage of blood flow, but other

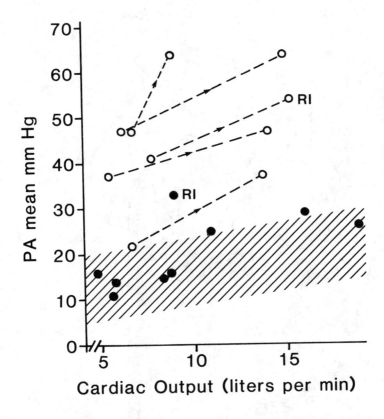

Figure 13.13. Pulmonary artery mean pressures in five subjects with a previous history of HAPE who were brought to 10,150 feet (3,096 m) and studied after a morning of hiking up to 12,500 feet (3,810 m). Studies were made at rest and during exercise at sea level (solid circles) and at altitude (open circles). Normal values for normal subjects at that altitude are indicated by the hatched area. Note that during exercise at sea level one subject (RI) had an abnormal pressure rise and two others were also probably abnormal. At high altitude, however, resting and exercise PA pressures were abnormal in all subjects. PA wedge pressures remained normal. The rise in PA pressure occurred despite a respiratory alkalosis in all subjects. Subject RI was not exercised at altitude. From Hultgren, ref. 70.

areas were free of particles, suggesting the absence of local vasoconstriction.[81] Fowler and Read obtained similar results using a different experimental model.[82] Dawson reported data suggesting that hypoxia results in heterogeneity of vascular perfusion in canine lungs.[83]

Viswanathan and his colleagues provided further evidence that hypoxia results in uneven pulmonary vascular constriction in HAPE. Twelve subjects with a prior history of HAPE and eight subjects who had been to high altitude without developing HAPE were studied by pulmonary regional perfusion and ventilation scanning

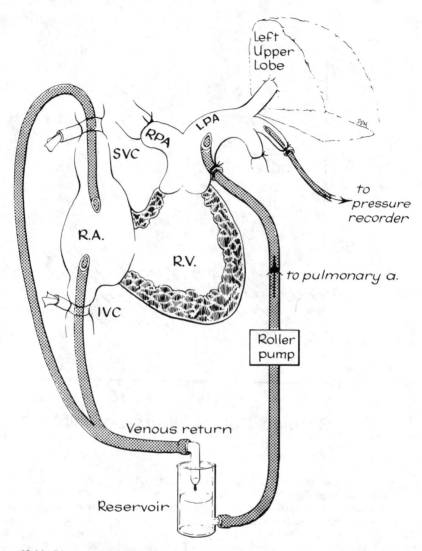

Figure 13.14. Diagram of experimental method producing pulmonary edema by increased blood flow through a single lobe of a canine lung. RA = right atrium, RV = right pulmonary artery, IVC = inferior vena cava, SVC = superior vena cava. The total cardiac output passes through the pulmonary vascular bed of the left upper lobe, resulting in pulmonary edema. Pressures are indicated in Table 13.23. From Hultgren, ref.44.

after 5 minutes of breathing 10 percent oxygen. The HAPE cases showed areas of increased perfusion more prominent in lower than upper areas with a marked increase in perfusion in localized areas. Control subjects showed a uniform decrease in perfusion in most areas with less reduction in lower than in upper areas.[84] The findings in the HAPE case are consistent with the radiologic distribution of infiltrate in HAPE which is more common in central and lower areas with less infiltrate in the upper areas of the lung.

Scherrer and his associates provided further evidence of the uneven blood flow in HAPE. They showed that inhaled nitric oxide in patients with HAPE lowered pulmonary artery pressure, improved oxygenation and shifted blood flow in the lung away from the edematous regions toward non-edematous areas, thereby improving the matching of ventilation and perfusion with a decrease in the alveolar-arterial oxygen difference. Nitric oxide is an endothelium derived relaxing factor synthesized locally in the pulmonary circulation.[85]

Other factors may be involved in uneven obstruction to pulmonary blood flow. Thrombotic obstruction by fibrin thrombi and clumps of platelets have been observed in autopsy specimens and in the previously described canine model.[44,63,64] Clumps of platelets entrapped in the small vessels of the pulmonary vascular bed may release vasoactive substances such as thromboxane metabolites which may cause vasoconstriction. Finally, pulmonary vasoconstriction by the sympathetic nervous system may play a role in view of the effect of nifedipine and the alpha blocker pentolamine in lowering pulmonary artery pressure (Fig. 13.15).

The patchy distribution of infiltrates in the chest x-rays of patients with HAPE also suggests that some areas of the lung are vasoconstricted (no edema) while other areas are overperfused and edematous owing to a failure of vasoconstriction (Figs. 13.4 and 13.5). This phenomenon is vividly illustrated by CT scans of the chest in HAPE where the areas of overperfusion edema are shown as white, circumscribed

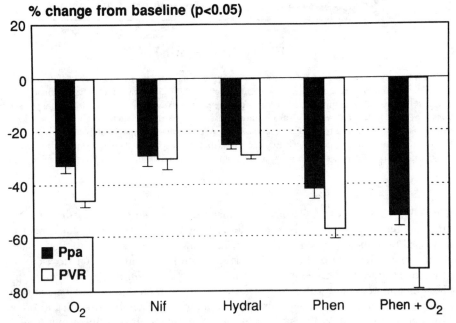

Figure 13.15. Effect of vasodilators upon the mean pulmonary artery pressure (Ppa) and pulmonary vascular resistance (PVR) in 16 patients with HAPE. The changes are indicated as a percentage decrease from the control level. Note that of the pharmacologic agents phentolamine resulted in the greatest decrease in pressure and resistance. O_2 = oxygen, Nif = nifedipine, Hydral = hydralazine, Phen = phentolamine. From Hackett, ref. 98.

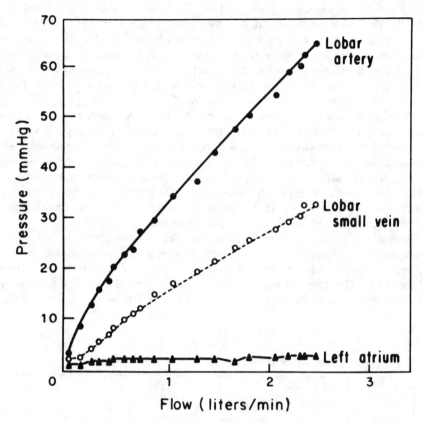

Figure 13.16. Vascular pressures during high flow through the left lower pulmonary lobe in six intact dogs. The maximum flow maintained by a perfusion pump was 2.5 L/min, which is approximately 5.4 times normal basal flow to this portion of the lung. Note progressive increase in lobar small vein pressure with increasing flow. This pressure was obtained by advancing a small catheter via a large pulmonary vein into a small vein. The high pressure in the lobar vein indicates an equally high capillary pressure. Left atrial pressure remains normal. One can conclude that with high flow the lobar small veins become an important site of the pressure fall from the lobar artery to the left atrium. From Hyman, ref. 99.

areas (Fig. 13.8 and 13.9). Cardiac pulmonary edema usually involves the lung in a diffuse, "butterfly" distribution of edema (Fig.13.7).[86] An important aspect of increased flow in nonconstricted areas of the lung is vasodilatation by flow-related shear stress where an endothelium derived factor in areas of high flow causes vascular dilatation. This does not occur if the endothelium is removed. If this phenomenon occurs in pulmonary arteries it would facilitate the transmission of high pressure and flow to the pulmonary capillaries.[87] The abnormalities in blood flow and ventilation (VQ mismatch) seen in patients with subclinical pulmonary edema also suggest inhomogeneous vascular changes.[70,71]

Sea level counterparts. Several sea level conditions illustrate that pulmonary edema may occur if portions of the pulmonary vascular bed are occluded while remaining portions of the lung are subjected to an increased blood flow.

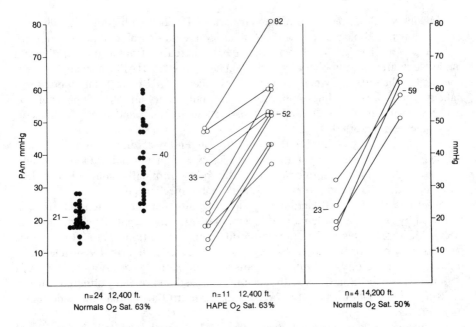

Figure 13.17. Response of the mean pulmonary (PA) pressure to acute hypoxia in eleven subjects with a previous history of HAPE (center panel) as compared with normal subjects (left panel) at this same altitude and with four subjects who had never had HAPE who were studied under similar conditions at a higher altitude (right panel). (All subjects were residents of the altitudes shown). These results indicate that not all subjects with a previous history of HAPE exhibit an abnormal rise in PA pressure when subjected to acute hypoxia of short (minutes') duration. From Hultgren, ref. 69.

1. Pulmonary embolism. In most cases of pulmonary embolism the amount of the pulmonary vascular bed that is obstructed is not sufficient to result in a significant rise in pulmonary artery pressure. In severe pulmonary embolism pulmonary edema has been observed in regions of the lung where the circulation was not occluded.[88,89] Surgical removal of occluding thrombi from branches of the pulmonary arteries has been accompanied by pulmonary edema in the reperfused segments.[90,91] An example of pulmonary edema associated with pulmonary embolism was reported by Combret.[96] A young woman developed an embolus obstructing a large portion of the main pulmonary trunk. Angiography indicated that perfusion was present only in the upper and middle lobes of the left lung. Pulmonary edema was present only in these areas. Hemodynamics studies revealed a pulmonary artery pressure of 45/19 mm Hg, a pulmonary artery wedge pressure of 9 mm, and a cardiac index of 1.9 L/min/m[2]. With an estimated mean pulmonary artery pressure of 37 mm the estimated pulmonary vascular resistance was 85 units (680 dyne/sec/cm[5]). This case represents the human analogy to the over perfusion canine studies reported in this chapter and indicates that at least 50-75 percent of the pulmonary vascular bed must be obstructed to permit overperfusion pulmonary edema.

2. Pulmonary edema has been observed following pneumonectomy.[92] The edema most frequently occurs following right pneumonectomy. The pulmonary artery wedge pressure is normal.[92]

3. Congenital absence of a pulmonary artery. Persons with congenital absence of the right pulmonary artery without other congenital cardiac abnormalities are susceptable to HAPE.[47] Such persons have an increased flow to one lung with a moderate degree of pulmonary hypertension at sea level.[93] HAPE in such persons is confined to the left lung where increased flow occurs. HAPE has been reported in a patient with a proximal interruption of the left pulmonary artery.[94] Kyphoscoliosis may be an analagous situation and two patients with HAPE and severe kyphoscoliosis have been reported.[25]

4. Correction of right-to-left shunts in congenital cardiac lesions has been followed in some cases by pulmonary edema with a normal wedge pressure. Increased flow into a pulmonary vascular bed chronically adapted to a low pulmonary flow has been proposed as the probable mechanism.[95]

5. Successful balloon dilatation of peripheral pulmonary artery stenosis has been followed by pulmonary edema in the portion of the lung supplied by the stenotic artery. Mean pressures in the artery after dilatation varied from 22 to 28 mm. Four patients with pulmonary edema had systemic pressures in the right ventricle, three had Fallot's Tetralogy, and one had transposition of the great arteries. In fifteen patients who had dilatations without pulmonary edema, mean pulmonary artery pressure after dilatation was below 20 mm Hg in all but one patient, who had a mean pressure of 22 mm.[97]

Centrogenic origin due to cerebral edema. It has long been recognized that head injury and cerebral edema may be accompanied by severe pulmonary edema even in the absence of pulmonary or cardiac disease.[98,99] This type of centrogenic pulmonary edema has been investigated experimentally. Usually, left ventricular filling pressures are raised as a consequence of central shifts in blood volume. Some observations indicate that left atrial pressure elevation may not always precede the onset of this type of pulmonary edema, and reflex constriction of small pulmonary veins may be an additional causative factor. Hypoxic stimulation of the vasomotor center may result in alpha adrenergic pulmonary vasoconstriction with pulmonary perfusion irregularities. Evidence for this possibility has been reported by Hackett and his workers, who found that phentolamine, an alpha antagonist, rapidly lowered pulmonary artery pressure and resistance in patients with HAPE (Fig. 13.15).[100] Cerebral edema does not appear to be a causative factor in HAPE.

Pulmonary venous constriction. The pulmonary veins may be involved in the genesis of HAPE by two possible mechanisms. In regions of high pulmonary flow, arterioles and capillaries may be dilated by the high pressure and the pulmonary veins may now become the site of the pressure drop across the vascular bed.[101,102] Hyman has obtained evidence from perfused dog lungs that indicates a progressive increase in lobar small vein pressure with increasing perfusion flow in the lung (Fig. 13.16).[103] Pulmonary veins may also constrict as a result of pulmonary arterial thromboses, particulate embolism, or release of serotonin from platelets.[104,105] Platelet aggregates are a common finding in fatal cases of HAPE. Welling and associates have shown that in the dog after prolonged alveolar hypoxia pulmonary capillary pressure is elevated due probably to pulmonary venous constriction. This was not observed with acute hypoxia.[106]

Protein content of edema fluid. Animal studies where the pulmonary vascular bed has been partially occluded by ligation and embolism have demonstrated an increased flow of lymph with a normal protein content.[76,77] Autopsy studies in

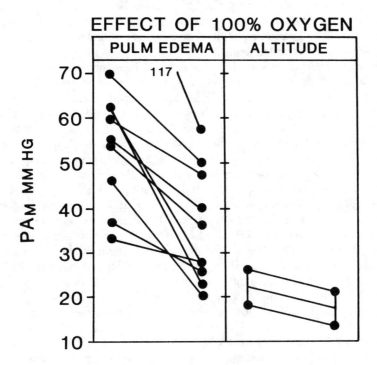

Figure 13.19. Effect of 100 percent oxygen breathing upon the mean pulmonary artery pressure in nine patients with HAPE. The pressure decreases in all patients, but a normal pressure is attained in only one. Data from normal subjects without HAPE at 12,400 feet (3,780 m) are shown in the right panel. All cases collected from the literature. Kobayashi and his colleagues made similar observations in five patients. From Hultgren, ref. 49.

HAPE, however, have indicated that the edema fluid is high in protein, there being alveolar hemorrhages, hyaline membranes and leucocyte infiltration. Schoene and his workers were able to recover lung lavage fluid from three patients with HAPE on Mount Denali and studies were also made on three controls.[107] The fluid exhibited a marked increase in high molecular weight proteins, erythrocytes, and leucocytes, most of which were alveolar macrophages. High protein content of edema fluid was also reported from two patients studied by Kobayashi and his colleagues.[35] The results indicated that HAPE is associated with increased vascular permeability or a "large pore" leak in the pulmonary circulation. This is very likely related to the excessive shear forces of the high flow through the microvascular circulation. In the studies of dog lung perfusion from our laboratory described earlier in this chapter, it was observed that the high flow through a single lobe of the lung was associated with a palpable thrill and a loud continuous bruit compatible with considerable turbulence. Increased permeability was considered to be due to the increased capillary pressure as well as capillary wall injury due to high shear forces. High pressure alone was not considered to be the major course of increased permeability since animal studies where the pulmonary vascular bed had been partially occluded by ligation and embolism have demonstrated an increased flow of lymph with a normal protein content.[77]

The role of increased permeability due to high shear forces was challenged by the work of West and his associates who demonstrated that the rapid elevation of capillary pressure without an increase in flow resulted in edema fluid with an increased protein content as well as electron microscopic evidence of disruption of the capillary endothelial layer, alveolar epithelial layer and sometimes all layers of the wall. In the rabbit model the pulmonary venous pressure and capillary pressure were raised by elevating the pulmonary venous reservoir to approximately 40-56 mm Hg. The flow through the system was low.[108,110] These results differ from those of Vriem who found that passive elevation of capillary pressure in the dog by pulmonary vein constriction resulted in edema fluid with a low protein content.[110]

Shear forces due to increased flow and elevation of capillary pressure may injure capillary walls and result in the release of cell derived factors from platelets, leucocytes, and other cells. These factors may play a role in the increase in permeability. For example, Richalet has reviewed the role of cellular derived vascular permeability factors in HAPE.[111] Further studies are clearly indicated to differentiate the role of high flow versus high pressure in increasing capillary permeability. Protein content of various types of pulmonary edema fluid is summarized in Table 13.24.

Mechanisms of Susceptibility to HAPE

It has been proposed that some persons who have had previous episodes of HAPE exhibit a more marked rise in pulmonary artery pressure and arteriolar resis-

Table 13.24
Pulmonary Edema Fluid Proteins

Type of fluid	Edema fluid protein gms/100 ml	Plasma protein gms/100 ml	Percent of Plasma protein	Reference
Cardiac failure				
8 patients	3.36	7.3	47	Sprung[140]
Cardiac pulmonary				
edema 9 dogs	1.29	2.65	49	Vreim[76]
HAPE				
3 patients	6.73	7.33*	92	Schoene[107]
2 patients	6.35	6.20	102	Kobayashi[35]
1 patient	4.3	7.0	61	Hultgren**
1 patient	5.6	5.9	95	Hackett[141]
Overperfusion				
model 8 dogs	4.8	5.9	81	Hultgren[44]
Non-cardiac PE				
12 patients	4.4	5.5	80	Sprung[140]

* Assumed normal value
** Pulmonary edema fluid drawn by Dr. Rod Wilson, Anchorage, AK.

tance than normal subjects during acute hypoxia.[49] The results are not convincing, however. Viswanathan and his workers, for example, studied 51 control subjects and 44 patients who had recovered from HAPE.[111] Studies were done at sea level under conditions of acute hypoxia. During hypoxia the HAPE subjects had a slightly higher rise in mean pulmonary artery pressure (15.3 mm to 24.8 mm) than controls (12.8 mm to 18.6 mm). Yet if one calculates the pulmonary arteriolar resistance, the increase in resistance in the HAPE subjects was the same as in the control group: 26 percent. The higher pressure in the HAPE cases was entirely due to a higher cardiac output.[112] Studies in Peru have not shown an increased response to hypoxia in subjects with a history of HAPE (Fig. 13.17). However, Fasules and his workers studied seven children after recovery from HAPE and reported that hypoxia induced a significantly higher mean pulmonary artery pressure (mean 56 mm ± 24) than in nonsusceptible children (mean 19 mm ± 4) $p<0.05$.[113] Recent studies by Yagi and his associates have shown that six of eight persons who had had an earlier episode of HAPE had a greater rise in pulmonary artery pressure and resistance during acute hypoxia than persons who had never had HAPE.[114] Pulmonary artery pressures were estimated by echo Doppler studies, and pressures and resistances were calculated by pulmonary artery catheterization. Resting pulmonary artery pressures were also higher in the subjects with previous episodes of HAPE.[114] The conflicting results of these studies make it doubtful that the magnitude of the rise in pulmonary artery pressure during *acute* hypoxia is a reliable method of predicting susceptibility to HAPE.[69] Nonetheless, the results do not conflict with the observation that *ascent to high altitude* may result in more severe pulmonary hypertension in susceptible subjects, as previously demonstrated.[70]

Hackett and his workers reported that patients with HAPE on Mount McKinley had a very low respiratory response to acute, induced hypoxia. The response was also low after recovery from HAPE, indicating that the abnormal response was not a temporary phenomenon. Patients with HAPE also had episodes of severe hypoxemia during sleep, along with frequent episodes of periodic breathing.[58] Matsuzawa and his colleagues found a blunted hypoxic ventilatory response (HVR) in eight of ten subjects who had experienced earlier episodes of HAPE.[115] Selland and his workers reported that not all cases of HAPE exhibited a low HVR when studied after recovery.[116] But low HVR has also been observed in world class climbers who have not had HAPE, so this cannot be used as a predictive test for HAPE. Marked arterial unsaturation during sleep indicates that acetazolamide and/or low flow oxygen may be effective in preventing HAPE or treating mild episodes. Selland and associates studied factors that may result in HAPE in seven susceptable subjects and nine controls in a hypobaric chamber.[116] They observed no signs of activated coagulation, excessive catecholamine release, or antidiuresis in the susceptible subjects; rather, the susceptible subjects showed exaggerated hypoxemia associated with relative hypoventilation and a widened alveolar arterial gas pressure difference. Hypoventilation especially during sleep as a possible factor in the development of HAPE is shown by the high prevalence of males in collected cases of HAPE. In 150 cases of HAPE seen at a Colorado ski resort 84 percent were males.[25] A similar male preponderance has been reported by Sophocles, Hochstrasser and Lobenhoffer.[52,34,31] Men are more likely to exhibit hypoventilation at high altitude than women.[117]

The higher susceptibility of children to HAPE compared with adults has not been explained or investigated. There is some evidence that children respond to high altitude with a higher pulmonary artery pressure than adults. Most cases of high altitude pulmonary hypertension have been observed in children or adolescents.[118] The lower susceptibility of women compared with men in developing HAPE is also of interest and requires study. It is possible that hormone levels in women are the cause of higher ventilation, especially during sleep, and that this may tend to reduce the possibility of HAPE. Women are far less likely than men to have sleep hypoxemia at sea level.[119]

Treatment

Early recognition of HAPE and prompt descent while the patient can still walk with assistance will save more lives than reliance on cumbersome oxygen equipment, pharmacological interventions, or aircraft evacuation. As previously pointed out, nearly all fatal cases of HAPE occur above 12,000 feet (3,660 m) in places where prompt access to definitive medical treatment is not available. At these altitudes HAPE may appear suddenly and death may occur within 24 to 48 hours after the onset of symptoms. Early recognition and a prompt decision to descend are essential. Weakness, fatigue, and an obvious decrease in physical performance associated with dyspnea, cough, headache, nausea, and vomiting are the most common initial symptoms that should never be overlooked by trip leaders and traveling companions.

Trip leaders should carefully evaluate party members in the evening after a day's trek or climb and in the morning before leaving camp, especially persons who are climbing slowly, refuse meals, and do not seem well. Simple physical signs should be determined, including the resting respiratory rate and heart rate. One should listen to the chest and mouth for evidence of fluid in the airways. These signs can frequently be detected without a stethoscope by placing one's ear to the naked back of the chest during deep breathing. The examination should be made after 10-15 minutes of supine rest. A resting respiratory rate $\geq$20/min and a resting heart rate $\geq$100/min should suggest the diagnosis of HAPE in someone who is not entirely well and fit.[45] Adults who normally have a slow heart rate may not have a heart rate $\geq$100/min in the presence of HAPE, and children will have faster respiratory rates and heart rates than adults. The symptoms, physical findings, and respiratory and heart rates should be recorded and any increase in these rates should be a reason for descent. The administration of acetazolamide and bed rest for two or three days are recommended for mild or suspected cases. Continued observations are necessary. Any deterioration requires an emergency descent regardless of weather or terrain.

Symptoms and signs of a grave prognosis are an indication for an emergency descent and include the following: (1) inability to walk without assistance more than 100 yards because of dyspnea or fatigue; (2) persisting cough productive of clear or blood-tinged fluid; (3) sounds of bubbling fluid in the airways with deep breathing; (4) severe cyanosis; (5) disturbances of mental acuity including irrational behavior, memory defects, somnolence, and delirium; obtundation or coma usually indicates death within a few hours and death may occur suddenly without warning; (6) urinary incontinence; (7) shock with a weak pulse and low blood pressure; (8) ataxia, including a staggering gait, inability to walk a straight line (heel-to-toe), and inability to turn around without staggering, all of which are signs of associated cerebral edema.

Atypical presentations of HAPE should be remembered. Patients may not complain of dyspnea. Respirations are shallow and inspection may not suggest that the patient is dyspneic. Confusion, obtundation and coma may occur especially during the night without the usual warning symptoms. Precordial pressure or pain may lead to the erroneous diagnosis of coronary artery disease. In children, nausea, vomiting, and weakness may erroneously suggest gastrointestinal disease. Orthopnea is absent in most cases of HAPE.

Descent. "Descend, descend, descend" is the most desirable yet most neglected form of treatment, as pointed out by Hackett.[120] Descent should be carried out with at least two persons assisting the victim in the event of deterioration en route; in mountainous terrain, where a litter descent is difficult, eight or more may be needed. A descent of only 1,000 to 2,000 feet may result in rapid improvement. In early Peruvian accounts of patients with HAPE who were brought to lower altitudes recovery was described as "por encanto" (as if by magic). On Mount Kilimanjaro a single-wheeled litter is employed to transport victims to a lower altitude (Fig. 13.18). Most cases of altitude illness occur at or above the Kibo Hut 15,425 feet (4,703 m), and many victims recover at the next lower hut, 12,200 feet (3,720 m); if the victim is still unconscious at that elevation the possibility of death is increased. The descent by litter requires four persons; descent by horse or mule can be made from the 12,200-foot hut, but at least two or three persons must

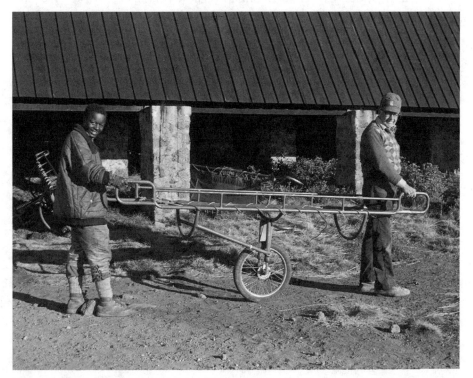

Figure 13.18. Single-wheeled litter used on Mount Kilimanjaro to take victims of altitude sickness from the Kibo Hut, 15,425 feet (4,703 m), down to lower elevations.

Table 13.25
Death from HAPE Among Patients Treated by Oxygen and Descent

Oxygen	Descent	Frequency Number of cases	%	Mortality Number of cases	%
Yes	Yes	39	24	1	3
Yes	No	62	37	3	5
No	Yes	42	25	5	12
No	No	23	14	10	44
	Totals	166	100	19	64

SOURCE: Lobenhoffer et al, ref. 31.

accompany the victim. One should not rely on aircraft assistance. Too often radio contact fails, aircraft are not available, weather and terrain may preclude landing, and the cost is high. If aircraft evacuation is to be performed the rescue vehicle must carry oxygen, which should be given to the patient en route or dropped, if a landing is not possible. The author has documented one patient with HAPE who died en route to a hospital probably because oxygen was not available in the aircraft.

Oxygen. High flow oxygen (6-12 L/min) via a well-fitting face mask is the most important method of therapy in the hospital setting. Within a few minutes symptoms disappear, heart and respiratory rate slow; and complete recovery will occur in 12-24 hours (Fig. 13.19).

In field conditions the situation is different. Few groups carry oxygen, because tanks are heavy and cumbersome to use, and furthermore, the average D tank contains only about 600-1,200 liters of oxygen, which is enough for only a few hours. Most failures of oxygen therapy in the field are probably due to the use of a low flow rate in an understandable effort to conserve the supply and extend its use. But with a rapid respiratory rate of up to 40/min, oxygen has to be administered at a higher flow rate in order to reach the alveoli; slow flow rates under such conditions only oxygenate the airways. Due to the lower barometric pressure oxygen at two liters per minute delivers less oxygen than at sea level. Most deaths in HAPE are due to failure to descend and the failure to use oxygen (Table 13.25).

Pharmacologic Agents

Nifedipine, a calcium channel blocker, has been used in the treatment of HAPE. Hackett gave 10-20 mg of nifedipine sublingually to six patients with HAPE at 14,100 feet (4,300 m) on Mount McKinley. Pulmonary artery pressure as estimated by echo-Doppler decreased and arterial oxygen saturation increased. Intravenous hydralazine was given to three patients with a similar effect but a longer duration of action.[121] Oelz gave nifedipine to six patients with HAPE at 14,950 feet (4,559 m) with similar results.[122] The subjects were able to continue exercise at the same altitude with continued improvement. Nifedipine was given as a slow-release preparation every six hours during the altitude stay. Control values were obtained in each patient after an eighteen-hour stay at the altitude station. No significant changes in systemic blood pressure or heart rate were observed. Oelz suggested that nifedipine

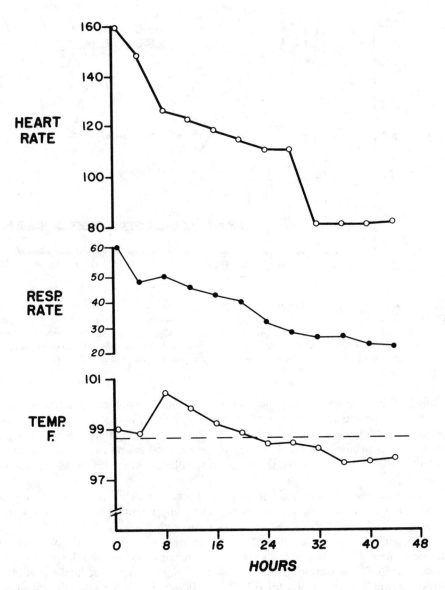

Figure 13.19. Effect of oxygen upon the heart rate and respiratory rate in a 14-year-old boy with HAPE. The initial rapid decrease is followed by a slower decrease as the edema clears. From Hultgren (personal observation).

should be used only to facilitate descent when oxygen is not available. His observations would have been strengthened if he had demonstrated sustained improvement in exercise capacity (by treadmill or cycle ergometry) during the study period.

Further evidence of the effectiveness of nifedipine in HAPE is the recent observation by Bärtsch and his associates that nifedipine given before and after ascent to 15,000 feet (4,590 m) in susceptible subjects prevented HAPE in 9 of 10 subjects,

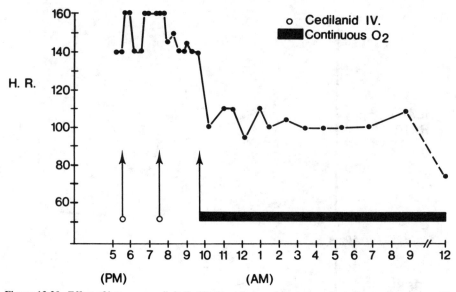

Figure 13.20. Effect of intravenous digitalis (Cedilanid) upon the heart rate in an 8-year-old patient with HAPE. Two injections of 0.6 mg of Cedilanid (Lanatoside C) were given at the arrows indicated by the open circles. No significant change in heart rate occurred. His clinical condition was worse. High-flow oxygen by tent (indicated by the black line) resulted in a rapid decrease in heart rate. The data suggest that left ventricular failure was not present. From Hultgren, personal observation.

while HAPE occurred in 7 of 11 subjects given a placebo. Subjects given nifedipine had a lower pulmonary artery systolic pressure, a lower alveolar-arterial pressure gradient, and a lower symptom score for AMS.[123] Nifedipine thus appears to be an exciting pharmacological breakthrough in the prevention and treatment of HAPE. Nifedipine is employed for the treatment of HAPE in several Rocky Mountain ski resorts.

Acetazolamide (Diamox) given orally or, if necessary, parenterally, especially in mild or moderate cases may result in sufficient improvement in ventilation to be beneficial. The usual dose is 250 mg every six to eight hours.

Morphine sulfate has been tested by Hackett, who observed that in patients who are very anxious and dyspneic, morphine may result in slower and deeper respirations and relief of anxiety.[57] The usual dose is 15 mg I.V. One anecdotal report by a physician who treated himself for HAPE at 11,000 feet (3,355 m) describes a worsening of symptoms induced by morphine. He described his symptoms as becoming a little worse each day and particularly so at night: "Very dyspneic, weak, confused, with headache and vomiting." He gave himself one-eighth of a grain of morphine, which made his symptoms worse, with obvious depression of respiration. He was assisted down to a nearby hospital where he recovered.[124]

Dexamethasone may be given if cerebral edema is suspected, but controlled studies in Peru have demonstrated no objective evidence of improvement in patients with uncomplicated HAPE.[125] The usual dose is 16 mg. I.V.

Medications of even more doubtful value and possible harmful side effects include furosemide, digoxin, and isoproterenol. Furosemide may seem to be a logical drug to use in HAPE because it is of clear value in the treatment of cardiac pulmonary edema. In HAPE, however, left ventricular failure is absent, circulating blood volume is already depleted, and blood pressure is low. If a large diuresis is induced by furosemide, the patient may develop severe orthostatic hypotension with the unfavorable effect of transforming an ambulatory patient into a litter case because of inability to stand. Digoxin is of no benefit since cardiac failure is absent and no objective effect has been demonstrated (Fig. 13.20).[44,125] Isoproterenol,too, may seem to be a logical drug to use because of its capacity to dilate constricted pulmonary arterioles and in that way lower pulmonary artery pressure. A controlled trial has demonstrated no benefit, and the hazard of inducing ventricular tachycardia is too great to use this drug in the field.[125] Other calcium channel blockers, such as diltiazam and verapamil may also cause pulmonary vasodilatation, but controlled trials have not been done. These drugs may further lower blood pressure. Nifedipine is useful in both treatment and prevention of HAPE. Chinese physicians have used aminophylline intravenously, but controlled studies have not been reported. Finally, although respiratory stimulants have not been evaluated in HAPE, it is doubtful that such agents would be of value since the respiratory control mechanisms are already maximally stimulated by hypoxia.

Methods to Improve Oxygenation

Hyperbaric therapy. Hackett employed hyperbaric therapy in the Himalayan Rescue Association hut at Pheriche in 1982 by utilizing two steel drums welded together with a tight fitting cover. A plastic window permitted visual access to the patient. A bicycle pump provided pressure. Subsequently, Igor Gamow developed a portable fabric cylinder pressurized by a foot pump. At 13,300 feet (4,056 m) inflation to a pressure of 100 mm Hg reduces the altitude to an equivalent of 8,400 feet (2,662 m). Several reports of field trials have been published.[126,127,128] Kasic and his associates compared the hyperbaric bag with supplementary oxygen in 32 patients with AMS or mild HAPE at an altitude of 9,300 feet (2,837 m). Bag therapy in 14 patients consisted of pressurizing the bag to 120 mm Hg above ambient pressure for two hours. Supplementary oxygen was given to 13 patients at a flow rate of 4 L/min for two hours. Mean arterial oxygen saturation increased 7 percent with pressurization and 9 percent with oxygen. Symptoms decreased as fast with pressurization as with oxygen. Symptomatic improvement was maintained in both groups one hour posttreatment.[129]

Advantages of the hyperbaric bag over oxygen stem from the compact size and low weight (13.5 to 17 pounds). It can be used many times to re-treat the victim or to treat others. Oxygen is more bulky, heavier, and cylinders run out. However, if relying on the bag, be sure to test it first before taking it along, as it can leak, and the pump can malfunction.

Someone with mild to moderate AMS might benefit from an hour or two in the bag. If the patient gets better, one should watch carefully to see if symptoms return. A placebo effect may be operating. If symptoms are only mild, the person can stay at that altitude, but if more severe symptoms intervene descent is appropriate.

Those with severe symptoms of AMS or symptoms of HAPE or HACE, who cannot be taken down should stay in the bag for four to six hours. If anything other than mild HAPE is suspected, and if the person improves, they should subsequently descend, and take medicines as outlined below.

Before putting the victim into the bag, read the instructions that come with it. Attend to urination and defecation before going inside. Explain to the subject the need to breathe normally, and to pop one's ears by swallowing as the bag is inflated. Tell the subject that if the bag should suddenly deflate, he should exhale. Before closing the zipper, ask the subject to use his arms and legs to increase the airspace inside the bag to save time and effort during inflation. Once inflated, about 10 to 20 pumps a minute are usually necessary.

Problems associated in using a hyperbaric bag include the victim feeling claustrophobic, and in having problems clearing one's ears and sinuses with increasing pressure. It is tiring for an operator to continue pumping air into the bag.

In all cases where the bag is used, an observer should be with the victim. Keep a written record of the person's symptoms, heart rate and breathing rate recorded every 30 minutes. Recognize that a considerable effort is involved in keeping someone in the bag and maintaining the pressure and air flow. While in certain circumstances it may be lifesaving in buying some time, it may only postpone the need to descend. Cases have occurred where individuals with severe AMS or HACE used the bag, improved, tried to avoid descent and then died.

The current models use a dry suit zipper as a seal, and their durability may limit the number of seasons they can remain functional. Valves are prone to breakdown as well. Prototypes are under development that will use commercial tube plastic and have a seal much like those used in rafting bag closures. Such models may be considerably cheaper than the current so-called Gamow Bag, named after its inventor.

Expiratory positive airway pressure (EPAP). This method commonly employs a Downs mask or a variation thereof consisting of a light, tightly fitting plastic mask providing positive expiratory pressure by a spring-loaded exhalation valve. Ambient air is breathed, but the unit can be employed with oxygen. The object is to increase alveolar pressure and facilitate oxygen transfer to the blood. Schoene and his colleagues studied the effect of EPAP using a Downs mask at 14,432 feet (4,400 m) in four climbers with HAPE and 13 healthy volunteers at rest and during exercise. Patients with HAPE exhibited an increase in arterial oxygen saturation, no change in heart rate and a decrease in respiratory rate. In healthy subjects arterial oxygen saturation increased and heart rate was higher. At 10 cm water pressure the increase in oxygen saturation in the HAPE patients was about 7 percent. The authors suggested that voluntary hyperventilation would be a better and safer method of increasing arterial oxygen saturation.[130] This method would seem to be superior to "grunt breathing", where forced expiration is performed via pursed lips or a narrow tube. This form of breathing, if performed too energetically, can cause a rupture of pulmonary blebs with a resulting pneumothorax.[131] Voluntary positive pressure breathing (VPPB) and pursed lip breathing (PLB) have been studied at actual and simulated altitudes. Both maneuvers resulted in a modest increase in arterial oxygen saturation.[132] These methods are not without hazard since EPAP may facilitate cerebral edema by venous congestion.[133] Two cases of mediastinal emphysema during the practice of "grunt breathing" on Mount Rainier have been reported.[134] EPAP may facilitate shunting via a patent foramen ovale and thus reduce arterial saturation.[135]

Other methods. Since patients with HAPE are essentially dying of asphyxia caused by fluid filling the airways, mechanical methods of fluid removal may be helpful. In one instance a patient kneeled in a head-down position and his companion stood over him astride and performed firm abdominal pressure while the patient coughed vigorously. This maneuver was effective in moving considerable fluid from the airways and resulted in a decrease in dyspnea for 20-30 minutes. The maneuver was repeated through the night and probably saved the patient's life.[136] An experienced physician who has the appropriate equipment may perform a tracheal intubation and suck out airway fluid with benefit to similar patients, although obviously this has not yet been tried in a controlled setting!

An example of appropriate management of HAPE under difficult conditions is summarized in the following report:

In April 1985 a five member Japanese party flew to 6,000 feet (1,830 m) to climb the West Buttress of Mount McKinley. Seven days later Y.S., age 37, developed HAPE during the ascent to a camp at 13,000 feet (3,965 m). The next morning Y.S. was worse and had difficulty in standing. He began coughing up bloody sputum. The party descended to 11,000 feet (3,355 m) and camped. An American party brought a CB radio, an bottle of oxygen and Diamox. Y.S. had a heart rate of 120/min and a respiratory rate of 28/min. Oxygen, 500 mg of Diamox and fluids were administered. The following day the condition of Y.S. had improved. His heart rate was 98/min. He was given more oxygen and Diamox and later was able to ski down to the Kahiltna Base Camp.[137]

The party should have descended to a lower altitude when Y.S. first became ill. The prompt adminstration of oxygen resulted in sufficient improvement so that the patient was able to descend unassisted. Diamox was probably also beneficial.

General care. Before descent or evacuation, the patient should be reassured and remain at rest with the head elevated (if this results in less dyspnea). If the bladder is distended urethral catheterization may be performed to avoid rupture of the bladder during descent or transport. An indwelling Foley catheter is rarely necessary. No sedatives except morphine (if necessary) should be given.

Emergency room management. Most mountain resort areas have ready access to emergency rooms, clinics or hospitals and some general guidelines for management of HAPE in such facilities are in order. A medical history and physical examination including vital signs should be obtained accompanied by pulse oximetry on entry. Oxygen should be administered via a plastic face mask at a flow rate of 4-6 liters per minute. Oxygen should not be delayed for chest x-rays or laboratory test. A PA and lateral chest x-ray should be performed even though the clinical diagnosis is evident since the amount of infiltrate will give some information regarding severity and other conditions may be detected such as lobar pneumonia or cardiac enlargement. Other laboratory studies should include a complete blood count, urinalysis, serum enzymes and an electrocardiogram. Nifedipine is commonly employed in many clinics now. Usually 30 mg of slow release capsules are given twice daily after an initial 10 mg sublingual dose. Aspirin, codeine or Tylenol may be used for headache. Morphine is rarely indicted except under conditions of anxiety, panic, or hyperventilation. Dehydration may be present due to anorexia, nausea, or vomiting and slow IV fluids may be necessary. While acetazolamide is of undetermined value in treatment, 250 mg twice daily may be used or 50 mg intravenously. Tracheal suction is rarely necessary unless copious amounts of fluid are present in the airways.

With bed rest and oxygen, improvement is rapid and complete symptomatic recovery may occur in 24-48 hours. Clearing of the pulmonary infiltrate in the chest x-ray may take 24-48 hours longer. In patients who have had HAPE for several days, recovery and clearing of the infiltrate may be slower. The course of recovery can be easily followed by charting the oxygen saturation, respiratory rate, and heart rate. Respiratory rate and heart rate should diminish rapidly after oxygen is started (Fig. 13.19).

After two to three hours of oxygen therapy, several choices are available regarding future management: severity can be assessed by symptoms, clinical findings, pulse oximetry, chest x-ray and response to therapy. In mild cases where improvement is rapid the patient may be allowed to return to the hotel room, condominium or home for 24 hours of bed rest and oxygen therapy. In most areas local hospital supply facilities will provide home oxygen via a concentrator or a tank and will instruct the patient in its use with nasal prongs. If the patient is essentially well on the following day an additional day of rest should be advised before returning to light activity. Severe cases should be hospitalized for observation and more intensive, supervised care. Descent by ambulance or helicopter to larger tertiary care hospitals is rarely necessary. The above guidelines permit the individual to remain in the resort area and avoid the abandonment of a family vacation. In 150 cases of HAPE seen at a Rocky Mountain ski resort only 17 percent had to be transported to a Denver hospital.[25]

In my opinion, certain treatment modalities are not indicated and may be dangerous. The administration of furosemide may lead to an unexpectedly large diuresis with postural hypotension. I am acquainted with one climber who developed HAPE at 12,000 feet (3,660 m) in a well known national park. He was transported to the local hosptial at 5,400 feet (1,647 m) where he rapidly improved for the first few hours and was capable of being discharged. Unfortunately he was given IV furosemide, had a profound diuresis, required IV fluids and his hospital stay was needlessly prolonged.

Intubation and assisted ventilation are not indicated in HAPE and may do harm or needlessly prolong hospitalization. Except for patients essentially moribund upon arrival at the hospital, all patients with HAPE can recover quickly without intubation or assisted ventilation. The duration of hospitalization was three days or less in 84 percent of cases treated without intubation by Lopez.[32]

A report of the treatment of two patients with uncomplicated HAPE described the use of intubation and IPPB using 100 percent oxygen. The duration of treatment and hospitalization were prolonged to four and eight days, respectively—longer than the usual duration of treatment and hospitalization for most cases of HAPE. The arterial PCO_2 was not elevated in either of the two reported cases.[138]

Complications. Complications of HAPE or coexisting conditions consist of pneumonia, pulmonary embolism or infarction, cerebral edema, cerebral thrombosis, acute myocarditis, and aspiration pneumonia. Appropriate laboratory studies may be necessary to establish the diagnosis. The presence of high fever and marked leucocytosis indicates the possibility of pneumonia, and if this complication is suspected, a broad spectrum antibiotic should be given. Aspiration pneumonitis should be suspected if there is a history of nausea, vomiting, or disturbances of consciousness. Adult patients with a heart rate of 140-160/min may have transient atrial flutter with 2:1 conduction. Usually this will revert spontaneously to sinus rhythm, but IV Digoxin should be administered to prevent the rare complication of 1:1 conduction with resulting circulatory collapse. Hemoptysis of bright red or dark clotted blood with pleurisy, fever, and a pleural rub or a pleural effusion should suggest pulmonary embolism and infarction. Chest films should be reviewed to look for unilateral pulmonary edema localized to the left lung, which will suggest the possibility of congenital absence of the right pulmonary artery. Shock, a very rapid heart rate, ventricular or atrial arrhythmias with cardiac enlargement should suggest the presence of an acute myocarditis or underlying cardiac disease.

Return to high altitude. After symptomatic recovery and clearing of the pulmonary infiltrates, at least one week of progressive exercise should be observed before returning to high altitude. Returning too early can lead to a recurrence of HAPE. Upon returning after a period of recovery and rehabilitation, one should climb slowly and record resting pulse and respiration rates daily. Acetazolamide 250 mg every eight or twelve hours before and during reascent is a wise precaution.

Prevention. Acclimatization, gradual ascent, and early recognition of symptoms remain the three major methods of prevention of HAPE. Above 12,000 feet (3,660 m) HAPE may progress rapidly and in 24-48 hours lead to complete incapacity or death. At most ski resorts between 8,000 and 9,000 feet (2,440-2,745 m), HAPE is less common and less serious and can be more rapidly treated, but it may ruin a carefully planned holiday. Even well-acclimatized individuals may develop HAPE if ascent to a higher altitude is too rapid or if unusually heavy work is performed. Descent to a lower elevation for two to four days rarely results in HAPE during reascent except in children. In adults, a stay of seven days or more is sufficient to result in HAPE upon reascent.

Travelers to the Andes of South America should plan to spend four to six days at an intermediate altitude for acclimatization. Bogota, Quito, Cuzco and Huaraz in Peru, and Mexico City are suitable locations for acclimatization. It is wise to rest the first day after arrival and then begin progressively longer walking trips into the environs to higher elevations. Travelers to Mount Kenya or Mount Kilmanjaro can find attractive hotels in the foothills at 5,000-7,000 feet (1,525-2,135 m) where they can gradually acclimatize for a few days. Unfortunately, most commercial tours and safaris advertise climbs on Kenya and Kilimanjaro with such a short time schedule that acclimatization is not possible. Persons who plan to climb these mountains should spend a week between 5,000 and 7,000 feet (1,525 m and 2,135 m) and then take two to three extra days of gradual ascent to the highest camps before attempting the summit. MacKinder's Camp on Mount Kenya is at 13,100 feet (3,993 m); the Kibo Hut on Mount Kilimanjaro is at 15,425 feet (4,703 m). In Nepal, Katmandu and neighboring villages offer similar opportunities. For travelers flying to Lukla, a few days spent in this area before going to higher elevations will be helpful.

General precautions for the avoidance and prevention of AMS are also applicable to the prevention of HAPE.

High risk individuals should take special precautions to prevent HAPE. These individuals include those who have had prior episodes of HAPE, persons who must ascend rapidly without acclimatization such as in a rescue mission, individuals with an absent pulmonary artery or with severe scoliosis.[25] In addition to acclimatization at an intermediate altitude the use of nifedipine 30 mg twice daily starting one day before ascent has been proven to be efficacious.[123] In one uncontrolled study acetazolamide has been shown to prevent reascent HAPE in persons residing in La Paz, Bolivia 12,730 feet (3,883 m).[139] Susceptible persons should be alert to early symptoms of HAPE so that prompt descent or medical therapy can be instituted.

References

1. GILBERT D. The first documented report of mountain sickness: The China or Headache Mountain story. *Respir. Physiol.* 1983; 52:315-26.
2. HAIDAR M. *The Tarikh-I-Rashida: A history of the Moghuls of Central Asia.* English verison by N. Elias, Lahore:Book Traders, 1896.
3. GOS C. *Alpine tragedy.* London: Allen and Unwin, 1908; 107-15.
4. MOSSO A. *Life of man on the high Alps,* ed. A Landon and T Fisher. London: Unwin, 1898.
5. RAVENHILL T. Some experiences of mountain sickness in the Andes. *J. Trop. Med. Hyg.* 1913; 20:313-20.
6. CRANE H. Soroche, mountain sickness, anoxemia. *Anales Fac. medicina,* 1927; 11:306-08.
7. HURTADO A. *Aspectos fisiológicos y patolóogicos la vida en la altura.* Lima: Im Rimac, 1937.
8. LUNDBERG E. Edema agudo del pulmón en el soroche. Conferencia sustentada en la asociación Médica de Yauli, La Oroya, 1952. Unpublished report.
9. LIZARRAGA L. Soroche, agudo, edema agudo de pulmón. *An. Facul. Med.,* Lima 1955: 38(2):244-74.
10. VEGA A. Algunos casos de edema pulmonar agudo por soroche grave. *An. Facul. Med.* Lima 1955; 38:233-40.
11. BARDALES A. Edema pulmonar agudo por soroche grave. *Rev. Peruana Cardiol.* 1957; 6(2): 115-20.
12. ALZAMORA-CASTRO V, GARRIDO-LECCA G, BATTILAN G. Pulmonary edema of high altitude. *Am. J. Cardiol.* 1961; 7:769-78.
13. GUZMAN A. Hypoxia aguda de altura y edema agudo pulmónar. *Rev. Acad. Pervana de Cirugia,* 1962; 15:20-46.
14. HULTGREN H, and SPICKARD W. Medical experiences in Peru. *Stanford Med. Bull.* 1960; 18:76-95.
15. HOUSTON C. Acute pulmonary edema of high altitude. *N. Engl. J. Med.,* 1960; 263:478-80.
16. HULTGREN H, SPICKARD W, HELLRIEGEL K, and HOUSTON C. High altitude pulmonary edema. *Medicine* 1961; 40:289-313.
17. PUGH L. Acute pulmonary edema and mountaineering. Notes and Queries. *Practitioner* 1955; 174:108-9.
18. SINGH I, KAPILA C, KHANNA P, NANDA R. and RAO B. High altitude pulmonary edema. *Lancet* 1965; Jan. 30:229-34.
19. MENON N. High altitude pulmonary edema. *N. Engl. J. Med.* 1965; 273:66-74.
20. MENON N. High altitude pulmonary edema. *Defense Science J* 1984; 34:317-27.
21. HOUSTON C. Personal communication.
22. CRAIG A, JR. Underwater swimming and loss of consciousness. *JAMA* 1961; 176:255-58.
23. LAKSHMINARAYAN S, and PIERSON D. Recurrent high altitude pulmonary edema with blunted chemosensitivity. *Am. Rev. Resp. Dis.* 1975; 111:869-72.
24. KAFER E, and LEIGH J. Recurrent respiratory failure associated with the absence of ventilatory response to hypercapnia and hypoxemia. *Am. Rev. Resp. Dis.* 1972; 106:100-15.
25. HULTGREN H, HONIGMAN B, THEIS K and NICHOLAS D. High altitude pulmonary edema in a ski resort. *West. J. Med.,* 1996; 164:222-27.
26. MAGGIORINI M, BÄRTSCH P, OEIZ O, et al. Elevated body temperature in severe acute mountain sickness (AMS). In *Hypoxia and mountain medicine,* ed. J Sutton, G Coates, and C Houston. Burlington, VT: Queen City Printers, 1992; 311. Abstract.
27. VOCK P, FRETZ C, FRANCIOLLI M, et al. High altitude pulmonary edema: Findings at high altitude chest radiography and physical examination. *Radiology* 1989; 170:661-66.
28. VOCK P, FISCHER H, and BÄRTSCH P. Radiomorphology of high altitude pulmonary edema: New views. In *Hypoxia and molecular medicine,* ed. J Sutton, G Coates and C Houston, Burlington, VT: Queen City Printers, 1993; 259-64.
29. BÄRTSCH P, MULLER A, HOFSTETTER D, et al. AMS and HAPE scoring in the Alps. In *Hypoxia and molecular medicine,* ed. J Sutton, G Coates. Burlington, VT: Queen City Printers, 1993: 265-71.
30. DICKINSON J, HEATH D, GASNEY I, and WILLIAMS D. Altitude-related deaths in seven trekkers in the Himalayas. *Thorax* 1983; 38:646-56.
31. LOBENHOFFER H, ZINK R, and BRENDEL W. High altitude pulmonary edema: Analysis of 166 cases. In *High altitude physiology and medicine,* ed. W Brendel and R Zink, New York: Springer Verlag, 1982.
32. LOPEZ C. Edema agudo pulmonar de altura in ninos. Doctoral thesis, Universidad Peruana Cayetano Heridia, Lima, Peru, 1971.

33. MARTICORENA E. Edema agudo pulmónar de altura. Doctoral thesis, Universidad Peruana Cayetano Heridia, Lima, Peru, 1971.
34. SOPHOCLES A. High altitude pulmonary edema in Vail, Colorado. *West. J. Med.* 1986; 144: 569-73.
35. KOBAYASHI T, KOYAMA S, LUBO K, et al. Clinical features of patients with high altitude pulmonary edema in Japan. *Chest* 1987; 92:814-21.
36. SOPHOCLES A, and BACHMAN J. High altitude pulmonary edema among visitors to Summit County, Colorado. *J. Fam. Pract.* 1983; 17:1015-17.
37. REINHART W, and BÄRTSCH P. Red cell morphology at high altitude. *Brit. Med. J.* 1986; 293:309-10.
38. REINHART W, KAYSER B, SINGH A, et al. Blood rheology in acute mountain sickness and pulmonary edema. *J. Appl. Physiol.* 1991; 71:934-38.
39. HULTGREN H, and WILSON R. Blood gas abnormalities and optimum therapy in high altitude pulmonary edema. *Clin. Res.* 1981; 29:99A. Abstract.
40. BÄRTSCH P, VOCK P, MAGGIORINI M, et al. Respiratory symptoms, radiographic, and physiologic correlations at high altitude. In *Hypoxia: The adaptations*, ed. J Sutton, G Coates, and J Remmers, Toronto, B.C.: Decker, 1990; 241-45.
41. FUKUSHIMA M, YOCHIMURA K, KUBOL K, et al. A case of high altitude pulmonary edema. *Jap. J. Thoracic Dis.* 1980; 18:753-57.
42. ANTEZANA G, LEGUIA G, GUZMAN A, et al. Hemodynamic study of high altitude pulmonary edema (12,200 ft). In *High altitude physiology and medicine*, eds, W Brendel, and R Zink, New York: Springer Verlag, 1982; 232-41.
43. LEVINE B, GRAYBURN P, VOYLES W, GREENE E, ROACH R, and HACKETT P. Intracardiac shunting across a patent foramen ovale may exacerbate hypoxemia in high-altitude pulmonary edema. *Ann Internal Med* 1991; 114:569-70.
44. HULTGREN H. High altitude pulmonary edema. In *Water and solute exchange*, ed. N Staub, New York: Marcel Dekker, 1978; 437-64.
45. GRAVELYN T, and WEG J. Respiratory rate as an indicator of acute respiratory dysfunction. *JAMA* 1980; 244:1123-25.
46. SCOGGIN C, HYERS T, REEVES J and GROVER R. High altitude pulmonary edema in the children and young adults of Leadville, Colorado. *N. Engl. J. Med.* 1977; 297:1269-72.
47. HACKETT P, CREAGH C, GROVER R, et al. High altitude pulmonary edema in persons without the right pulmonary artery. *N. Engl. J. Med.* 1980; 302:1070-73.
48. FRED H, SCHMIDT A, BATES T, and HECHT H. Acute pulmonary edema of high altitude: Clinical and physiologic observations. *Circulation* 1962; 1962; 25:929.
49. HULTGREN H, LOPEZ C, and LUNDBERG E. Physiologic studies of pulmonary edema at high altitude. *Circulation* 1964; 29:393-408.
50. PENALOZA D, and SIME D. Circulatory dynamics during high altitude pulmonary edema. *Am. J. Cardiol.* 1969; 23:369-78.
51. ROY S, GULERIA J, and KHANNA P. Hemodynamic studies in high altitude pulmonary edema. *Brit. Heart J.* 1969; 31:52-58.
52. HOCHSTRASSER J, NAZER A, and OELZ C. Altitude edema in the Swiss Alps: Observations on the incidence and clinical course in 50 patients. *Schweiz Med. Wochenschr.* 1986; 116:866-73.
53. RIOS B, DRISCOLL D, and MCNAMARA D. High altitude pulmonary edema with absent right pulmonary artery. *Pediatrics* 1985; 75:314-17.
54. SARNQUIST F. Physicians on Mt. Everest. *West. J. Med.* 1983; 139:480-85.
55. HORNBEIN T. Oxygen. In *Americans on Everest*, ed. J Ullman, Philadelphia: Lippincott, 1964; 351-58.
56. HULTGREN H, and MARTICORENA E. High altitude pulmonary edema: epidemiologic observations in Peru. *Chest* 1978; 74:372-76.
57. HACKETT P, and RENNIE D. The incidence, importance, and prophylaxis of acute mountain sickness. *Lancet*, 1976; 2:1149-54.
58. HACKETT P, ROACH R, et al. The Denali medical research project 1982-1985. *Am. Alpine J.* 1986; 28:129-37.
59. MAGGIORINI, M, BUHLER M, WAITER M, and OELZ O. Prevalence of acute mountain sickness in the Swiss Alps. *Brit. Med. J.* 1990; 301:853-55.
60. SNYDER P. Field aspects of experience, treatment, and prevention of altitude sickness on Mt. Kenya. *Proceedings*, Arctic Institute of North America, 1979; 44-48.
61. HULTGREN H, SPICKARD W, and LOPEZ D. Further studies of high altitude pulmonary edema. *Brit. Heart J.* 1962; 24:95-102.

318

62. ARIAS-STELLA J, and KRUGER H. Pathology of high altitude pulmonary edema. *Arch. Pathol.* 1963; 76:147-57.
63. NAYAK N. ROY S, and NARAYANAN T. Pathologic features of altitude sickness. *Am. J. Pathol.* 1964; 45:381-91.
64. KRITZLER R. Acute high altitude anoxia. Gross and histologic observations in twenty-seven cases. *War Medicine* 1944; 6:369-72.
65. NAKAGAWA S, KUBO K, KOIZUMI T et al. High altitude pulmonary edema with pulmonary thromboembolism. *Chest* 1993; 103:948-50.
66. HULTGREN H, ROBINSON M and WUERFLEIN. Overperfusion pulmonary edema. *Circulation* 1966; 33:132. Abstract.
67. HULTGREN H. High altitude pulmonary edema. In *Biomedicine of high terrestrial elevations*. A. Hegnauer, ed., Natick, Mass.: U.S. Army Research Institute of Environmental Medicine, 1969; 131-48
68. JOHANSSON B, STRANDGAARD S, and LASSEN N. On the pathogenesis of hypertensive encephalopathy: The hypertensive "breakthrough" of autoregulation of cerebral blood flow with forced vasodilatation, flow increase, and blood-brain-barrier damage. *Circ. Res.* 1974; 34-35, Suppl 1:167-71.
69. HULTGREN H. Pulmonary hypertension and pulmonary edema. In *Oxygen transport to human tissues*. J Loeppky and M Riedesel, eds., New York: Elsevier Biomedical, 1982; 243-54.
70. HULTGREN H, GROVER R, and HARTLEY L. Abnormal circulatory responses to high altitude in subjects with a previous history of high altitude pulmonary edema. *Circulation* 1971; 44:759-70.
71. HAAB P, HELD R, ERNEST E, and FARHI L. Ventilation-perfusion relationships during high altitude adaptation. *J. Appl. Physiol.* 1969; 26:77-81.
72. BÄRTSCH P, WABER U, HAEBERLI A, et al. Enhanced fibrin formation in high altitude pulmonary edema. *J. Appl. Physiol.* 1987; 63:752-57.
73. BÄRTSCH P, HAEBERLI N, NANCER A, et al. High altitude pulmonary edema: Blood coagulation. In *Hypoxia and molecular medicine*. J Sutton, G Coates, and C Houston, eds., Vt: Queen City Printers, 1993: 252-58.
74. SINGH I, CHOHAN I, and MAHEW N. Fibrinolytic activity in high altitude pulmonary edema. *Indian J. Med. Res.* 1969; 57:210-17.
75. GRAY G, BRYAN A, FREEDMAN M, et al. Effect of altitude exposure on platelets. *J. Appl. Physiol.* 1975; 39:648-51.
76. STAUB N. Mechanism of pulmonary edema following uneven pulmonary artery obstruction and its relationship to high altitude lung injury. In *High altitude physiology and medicine*. W Brendel and R Zink, eds, New York: Springer Verlag, 1982; 255-60.
77. LANDOLT C, MATTHAY M, ALBERTINE R, et al. Overperfusion, hypoxia, and increased pressure cause only hydrostatic pulmonary edema in anesthetized sheep. *Circ. Res.* 1983; 52:335-41.
78. GIBBON J, JR., and GIBBON M. Experimental pulmonary edema following lobectomy and plasma infusion. *Surgery* 1942; 12:694-704.
79. YOUNES M, and BSHOUTY Z. Effect of high blood flow, ventilation, breathing pattern, and alveolar hypoxia on lung fluid flux. In *Hypoxia: The adaptations*. J Sutton, G Coates, and J Remmers, eds., Toronto: B.C. Decker, 1990: 155-62.
80. FISHMAN A. Respiratory gases in the regulation of the pulmonary circulation. *Physiol. Rev.* 1961; 41:214-80.
81. LEHR D, TRILLER M, FISHER L, et al. Induced changes in the pattern of pulmonary blood flow in the rabbit. *Circ. Res.* 1963; 13:119-31.
82. FOWLER K, and READ J. Effect of alveolar hypoxia on zonal distribution of pulmonary blood flow. *J. Appl. Physiol.* 1963; 18:244-50.
83. DAWSON C, BRONIKOWSKI T, LINEHAN J, and HAKIM T. Hypoxic vasoconstriction can increase intraregional perfusion heterogeneity at a given perfusion level. *J. Appl. Physiol.* 1983; 54:654-60.
84. VISWANATHAN R, SUBRAMANIAN S and RADHA T. Effect of hypoxia on regional lung perfusion by scanning. *Resp.* 1979; 37:142-44.
85. SCHERRER U, VOLLENWEIDER L, DELABAYS A, et al. Inhaled nitric oxide for high altitude pulmonary edema. *N. Engl. J. Med* 1996; 334:624-9.
86. FLEISCHNER F. The butterfly pattern of acute pulmonary edema. *Am. J. Cardiol.* 1967; 20: 46-50.
87. SMIESKO V and JOHNSON P. The arterial lumen is controlled by flow-related shear stress. *The Physiologist* 1993; 8:34-36.

88. ALEXANDER J. Personal communication.
89. SINGER D, HESSER C, PICK R, and KATZ L. Diffuse bilateral pulmonary edema associated with unilobar miliary pulmonary embolism in the dog. *Circ. Res.*, 1958; 6:4-9.
90. MOSER K, DAILY P, PETERSON K, et al. Thromboendarterectomy for chronic, major-vessel thromboembolic pulmonary hypertension: Immediate and long-term results in 42 patients. *Ann. Int. Med.* 1987; 107:560-65.
91. LEVINSON R, SHURE D, and MOSER K. Reperfusion pulmonary edema after pulmonary artery thromboendarterectomy. *Am. Rev. Resp. Dis.* 1986; 139:1291-45.
92. ZELDIN R, NORMANDIN D, LANDTWING D, et al. Postpneumonectomy pulmonary edema. *J. Thorac. Cardiovasc. Surg.* 1984; 87:359-62.
93. POOL P, VOGEL J, and BLOUNT G, JR. Congenital unilateral absence of a pulmonary artery. *Am. J. Cardiol.* 1962; 10:706-32.
94. LEVINE S, WHITE D, and FELS A. An abnormal chest radiograph in a patient with recurring high altitude pulmonary edema. *Chest* 1988; 94:627-28.
95. VINCENT R, LANG P, ELIXSON E, et al. Extravascular lung water in children immediately after operative closure of either isolated atrial septal defect or ventricular septal defect. *Am. J. Cardiol.* 1985; 56:536-39.
96. COMBRET M, ROUBY J, SMIEGAN J, et al. Pulmonary edema during pulmonary embolism. *Brit. J. Dis. Chest* 1987; 81:407-11.
97. ARNOLD L, KEANE J, KAN J, et al. Transient unilateral pulmonary edema after successful balloon dilatation of peripheral pulmonary artery stenosis. *Am. J. Cardiol.* 1988; 62:327-30.
98. THEODORE J, and ROBIN E. Pathogenesis of neurogenic pulmonary edema. *Lancet* 1975; Oct. 18:749-51.
99. DRUCKER T. Increased intracranial pressure and pulmonary edema. *J. Neurosurg.* 1968; 28:112-17.
100. HACKETT P, ROACH R, HARTIG G, et al. The effect of vasodilators on pulmonary hemodynamics in high altitude pulmonary edema. *Int. J. Sports Med.* 1992; 13:568-71.
101. VISSCHER M. Basic factors in the genesis of pulmonary edema and a direct study of the effects of hypoxia upon edemogenesis. In *Biomedicine problems of high terrestrial elevations.* A Hegnauer, ed, Natick, Mass: U.S. Army Research Institute of Environmental Medicine, 1969; 90-93.
102. COURTICE R, and KORNER P. The effect of anoxia on pulmonary edema produced by massive intravenous infusions. *Australian J. Exp. Biol. Med. Sci.*, 1952; 30:511-26.
103. HYMAN A. Effects of large increases in pulmonary blood flow on pulmonary venous pressure. *J. Appl. Physiol.* 1961; 217:1177-78.
104. WEISBERG H, LOPEZ J, JURIA M, and KATZ L. Persistence of lung edema and arterial pressure rise in dogs after lung emboli. *Am. J. Physiol.* 1964; 207: 641-46.
105. DAICOFF G, CHAVEZ F, ANTON A, and SWENSON E. Serotonin-induced pulmonary venous hypertension in pulmonary embolism. *J. Thorac. Cardiovasc. Surg.* 1968; 56:810-15.
106. WELLING K, SANCHEZ R, RAVN J, et al. Effect of prolonged alveolar hypoxia on pulmonary artery pressure and segmental vascular resistance. *J. Appl. Physiol.* 1993; 75:1194-1200.
107. SCHOENE R, SWENSON E, PIZZO C, et al. The lung at high altitude: bronchoalveolar lavage in acute mountain sickness and pulmonary edema. *J. Appl. Physiol.* 1988; 64:2605-13.
108. WEST J, TSUKIMOTO K, MATHIEU-COSTELLO O, and PREDILETTO R. Stress failure in pulmonary capillaries. *J. Appl. Physiol.* 1991; 70:1731-42.
109. VRIEM C, SNASHALL P, and STAUB N. Protein composition of lung fluids in anesthetized dogs with cardiogenic pulmonary edema. *Am. J. Physiol.* 1976; 23:1466-69.
110. TSUKIMOTO K, YOSHIMURE N, ICHIOKA M, et al. Protein, cell and LTB4 concentrations of lung edema produced by high capilary pressures in rabbit. *J. Appl. Physiol.* 1994; 76:321-27.
111. RICHALET J-P. High altitude pulmonary oedema: still a place for controversy? *Thorax* 1995; 50:923-29.
112. VISWANATHAN R, JAIN S, and SUBRAMANIAN S. Pulmonary edema of high altitude: III. Pathogenesis. *Am. Rev. Resp. Dis.* 1969; 100:342-49.
113. FASULES J, WIGGINS J, and WOLFE R. Increased lung vasoreactivity in children from Leadville, Colorado, after recovery from high altitude pulmonary edema. *Circulation* 1985; 72:957-62.
114. YAGI H, YAMADA H, KOBAYASHI T, and SEKIGUCHI M. Doppler assessment of pulmonary hypertension induced by hypoxic breathing in subjects susceptible to high altitude pulmonary edema. *Am. Rev. Respir. Dis.* 1990; 142:796-801.
115. MATSUZAWA Y, FUJIMOTO K, KOBAYASHKI T, et al. Blunted hypoxic ventilatory drive in subjects susceptible to high altitude pulmonary edema. *J. Appl. Physiol.* 1989; 66:1152-57.

116. SELLAND M, STELZER T, STEVENS T et al. Pulmonary function and hypoxic ventilatory response in subjects susceptible to high altitude pulmonary edema. *Chest* 1993; 103:111-16.

117. HANNON JP. Comparative altitude adaptability of young men and women. *Environmental stress*, ed. LJ Folinsbee, et al., 1977; 335-50.

118. KHOURY G, and HAWES C. Primary pulmonary hypertension in children living at high altitude. *J. Pediat.* 1963; 62:177-85.

119. BLOCK A, BOYSEN P, WYNNE J, and HUNT I. Sleep apnea, hypopnea, and oxygen desaturation in normal subjects. *N. Engl. J. Med.* 1979; 300:513-17.

120. HACKETT P. Mountain sickness: Prevention, recognition, and treatment. American Alpine Club, New York: 1978.

121. HACKETT P, GREENE E, ROACH P, et al. Nifedipine and hydralazine for treatment of high altitude pulmonary edema. In *Hypoxia: The adaptations*. Sutton J, Coates G, and Remmers J, eds. Toronto, Philadelphia: B.C. Decker, 1990; pp. 219. Abstract.

122. OELZ O, MAGGIORINI M, RITTER M, et al. Nifedipine for high altitude pulmonary edema. *Lancet* 1989; 2:1241-44.

123. BÄRTSCH P, MAGGIORINI M, RITTER M, et al. Prevention of high altitude pulmonary edema by nifedipine. *N. Engl. J. Med.* 1991; 325:1284-89.

124. BATES T. Pulmonary edema of mountains. *Brit. Med. J.* 1972; 3:829. Letter to the Editor.

125. MARTICORENA E and HULTGREN H. Evaluation of therapeutic methods in high altitude pulmonary edema. *Am. J. Cardiol.* 1979; 43:307-12.

126. TABER R. A portable hyperbaric chamber for the treatment of high altitude disorders. *J. Wilderness Med.* 1990; 1:181-92.

127. HACKETT P. A portable, fabric hyperbaric chamber for the treatment of high altitude pulmonary edema. Abstract No. 65, 1989 Hypoxia Conference.

128. KING S, and GREENLEE R. Successful use of the Gamow hyperbaric bag in the treatment of altitude illness at Mount Everest. *J. Wilderness Med.* 1990; 1:193- 202.

129. KASIC J, YARON M, NICHOLAS R, LICKTEIG J, and ROACH R. Treatment of acute mountain sickness: Hyperbaric versus oxygen therapy. *Ann. Emerg. Med.* 1991; 20:1109-12.

130. SCHOENE R, ROACH R, HACKETT P, et al. High altitude pulmonary edema and exercise at 4,400 meters: Effect of expiratory positive airway pressure. *Chest* 1985; 87:330-33.

131. HOUSTON C, RENNIE D, and HULTGREN H. Barotrauma. *Off Belay* 1977; 2:23-25.

132. SAKAI A, YANAGIDAIRA Y, FUJIWARA T, et al. Relation between breathing pattern and SaO_2 at high altitude. In *High altitude medicine*, Matsumoto, Shinshu University, pp. 116-21.

133. OELZ O. High Altitude cerebral edema after positive airway pressure breathing at high altitude. *Lancet* 1983; 2:1148. Letter to the Editor.

134. VOSK A, and HOUSTON C. Mediastinal emphysema in mountain climbers. Report of two cases and review. *Heart and Lung* 1972; 6:799-805.

135. CUJEC B, POLASEK P, MAYERS E, and JOHNSON D. Positive and expiratory pressure increases the right to left shunt in mechanically ventilated patients with a patent foramen ovale. *Ann. Intern. Med.* 1993; 119:887-94.

136. HULTGREN H. Emergency maneuver in high altitude pulmonary edema. *JAMA* 1986; 255: 3245-46.

137. Accidents in North American mountaineering: Failure to descend. *Am. Alpine Club* 1986; 28: 18-19.

138. ZIMMERMAN G, and CRAPO R. Adult respiratory distress syndrome secondary to high altitude pulmonary edema. *West. J. Med.* 1980; 335-37.

139. SMITH L. High altitude illness. *JAMA* 1977; 237: 1199. Letter to the Editor.

CHAPTER 14

High Altitude Cerebral Edema

SUMMARY

High altitude cerebral edema (HACE) is a neurological syndrome manifested by symptoms and signs of central nervous system dysfunction and injury due to the hypoxia of high altitude. Common symptoms include ataxia, headache, lethargy, and irrational behavior, which may progress to unconsciousness. Common physical signs are truncal ataxia, papilledema, and abnormal reflexes. The incidence appears to be substantially less than pulmonary edema, and the altitude of occurrence is higher. Symptoms usually appear about five days after rapid ascent to an altitude over 9,000 feet (2,750 m). HACE is a common associated complication of HAPE. If the illness has been of short duration, descent may result in rapid improvement, but if descent or therapy is delayed, prolonged or persistent neurological sequelae may occur. Autopsy studies have revealed cerebral edema, petechial hemorrhages, focal tissue destruction, and spongiosis. Thrombosis of cerebral veins may be present. Although the exact etiology is unclear, severe hypoxia combined with an increase in cerebral blood flow and resulting capillary hemorrhages and edema are important factors. Steroids may be beneficial in some cases, but prompt descent is the most important therapeutic measure. Oxygen or a hyperbaric bag should be used if available.

• • •

High altitude cerebral edema (HACE) is a distinct clinical syndrome with symptoms and signs of diffuse and focal brain injury and dysfunction due to hypoxia. Symptoms consist of headache, vomiting, confusion, hallucinations, bizarre behavior, and incoordination. Neurological signs consist of ataxia, abnormal tendon reflexes, and often transient paralysis. Progression to obtundation, coma, and death occurs if prompt descent, oxygen administration or the use of a hyperbaric bag are not initiated.

Previous investigators have used other terms to designate this syndrome. Cerebral mountain sickness might be a more precise term, since HACE implies that cerebral edema is the cause of the various clinical features of acute mountain sickness but this has not been clearly established. Chiodi in 1960 used the term "mal de montaña" or "forma cerebral" or "mountain sickness, a cerebral form."[1] The inclusion of the term "mountain sickness" in the name is logical, because symptoms of severe acute mountain sickness and HACE may be very similar and manifestations of acute mountain sickness may have a similar etiology as HACE. Common usage is difficult to overcome, however, and for this reason, despite its etiologic implications, the term HACE will be used here.

Historical Aspects

Ravenhill, while serving as medical officer of a mining company in the Andes in 1913, described a "nervous form of mountain sickness: which was manifested primarily by symptoms and signs of cerebral dysfunction.[2] He differentiated this syndrome from acute mountain sickness and also recognized "a cardiac form of mountain sickness," which we now know as high altitude pulmonary edema or HAPE. Monge in 1937 described symptoms compatible with HACE.[3] Chiodi's clinical report of HACE in 1960 detailed the illness as he himself had experienced it.[1] In 1964 Fitch described the occurrence of cerebral symptoms in a young woman during a climb on Mount McKinley.[4] This woman, after climbing from 8,200 feet (2,500 m) to 16,400 feet (5,000 m), developed abdominal cramps, nausea, severe headaches, confusion, and incoherence, which progressed to stupor over a four day period. No specific neurological signs were present. She was evacuated by sled and aircraft, and at 10,000 feet (3,050 m) she regained consciousness. Examination in the hospital revealed no abnormal neurological signs or cognitive deficits except for a memory loss of her illness. There was no evidence of HAPE.

In 1965 Singh described severe neurological complications in 24 of 1,925 soldiers who ascended above 14,000 feet (4,270 m). In two patients who died, autopsy revealed diffuse cerebral edema. In two other patients a trephine operation was performed to relieve increased intracranial pressure, and cerebral edema was noted by inspection and subsequent histologic examination.[5] Since then, there have been numerous reports of cases of HACE, including an analysis of twelve cases by Houston and Dickinson in 1975. They suggested that the basic cause of the syndrome was cerebral edema.[6] Hansen had proposed this same concept in 1970 and suggested that many features of acute mountain sickness (AMS) and HACE including the headache and vomiting might be due to cytotoxic cellular edema of the brain secondary to hypoxia.[7] This concept was accepted by many investigators in the United States, and the term high altitude cerebral edema (HACE) was employed widely to identify the syndrome. Shortly after the Houston-Dickinson report, Lassen and Harper (1975) challenged the whole concept of cerebral edema and instead proposed a vasogenic etiology, suggesting that the clinical features were due primarily to the increase in cerebral blood flow with regional areas of capillary leakage of fluid.[8] If the fluid leaking into the interstitial space contained protein this would facilitate cerebral edema by the oncotic effect of the protein.

Clinical Features

The clinical characteristics of HACE are variable and can best be examined by a review of data from reported cases. Published reports and personal observations of 43 cases of HACE have been summarized in Tables 14.1A, 14.1B and 14.1C. Table 14.1A contains data from 19 cases where HACE was not complicated by other problems such as HAPE or bronchopneumonia. HACE may occur as a complication of other primary illnesses that result in severe hypoxia. The most common associated illness is HAPE which was present in 33 percent (13/43) of cases of HACE (Table 14.1B). Other illnesses associated with HACE include bronchopneumonia (4 cases), pulmonary embolism (4 cases), meningitis and myocarditis (one case of each); and these are summarized in Table 14.1C. Additional observations have been published by Dickinson.[9]

Symptoms and Signs

The five most common symptoms of HACE in order of frequency are; (1) semicoma or unconsciousness, (2) incoordination, (3) headache, (4) lethargy or

Table 14.1A
HACE Uncomplicated

No.	Age	Sex	Altitude (meters, feet)	Mode of travel	Days at altitude	Coma	Headache	Vomiting	Neurolgic signs symptoms	Papilledema	Retinal hemorrhages	Duration of illness	Death	Source of data
1	27	F	4,570 15,000	Air	5	0	+	+	0	0	+	17	0	(1) Houston, case 5
2	28	M	5,300 17,300	Air	1	+	+	0	0	+	+	5	0	(1) Houston, case 6
3	37	M	5,300 17,300	Air	1	0	+	0	Ataxia	+	0	6	0	(1) Houston, case 7
4	34	M	4,410 14,400	Air	5	0	0	0	Hallucinations Diplopia	?	?	3	0	(1) Houston, case 10
5	42	M	4,950 16,200	Walk	10	0	+	0	Ataxia Incoherent	?	?	2	0	(1) Houston, case 11
6	36	F	4,880 16,000	Air	?	0	+	0	Ataxia Diplopia	+	+	8	0	(1) Houston, case 12
7	33	F	5,080 16,400	Air	13	+	+	0	0	?	?	10	0	(2) Fitch
8	28	F	4,880 16,000	Air	9	+	0	+	Ataxia	?	?	10	0	(3) Shlim
9	24	F	4,070 16,000	Train	2	+	0	+	?	?	?	22	+	(4) Dalenz
10	?	M	12,500 ?	?	?	0	+	0	Hemiplegia	?	?	?	0	(5) Chiodi
11	29	M	5,200 17,000	Bus	6	+	0	0	Ataxia Aphasia	?	?	60	0	(6) Hultgren
12	21	M	5,200 17,100	Air	3	0	+	+	Ataxia	0	+	4	0	(6) Hultgren
13	30	M	4,000 13,000	Air	2	0	+	+	Ataxia Confusion	+	?	6	0	(7) Hultgren
14	40	M	5,200 17,000	?	5	+	+	0	?	?	?	2	+	(8) Clarke
15	32	M	7,800 25,700	Walk	"Weeks"	+	+	0	Transient blindness	?	?	2	+	(8) Clarke
16	48	F	5,360 17,500	?	?	0	0	0	0	?	?	5	0	(6) Hultgren
17	44	M	5,640 18,500	?	?	0	0	0	Ataxia, Transient blindness	+	+	10	0	(6) Hultgren
18	64	M	3,875 12,700	Air	3	0	0	0	Ataxia	+	?	8	0	(6) Hultgren
19	?	M	3,380 11,000	?	?	?	?	?	Ataxia	?	+	2	0	(6) Hultgren
Mean 35.1			4,655 16,144	12-T/2-W	5	7/19	11/19	5/19	13/17	6/8	5/6	10.1	3/19	
Range 21-64			3,380-7,800 11,000-18,500		1-13							2-60		

SOURCES: Listed with Table 14.1C

T = Transported by air, train or bus, W = Walked

Table 14.1B
HACE with HAPE

No.	Age	Sex	Altitude (meters, feet)	Mode of travel	Days at altitude	Coma	Headache	Vomiting	Neurolgic signs symptoms	Papilledema	Retinal hemorrhages	Duration of illness	Death	Source of data
1	39	F	3,500 11,400	Air	3	+	+	+	0	+	0	28	0	(1) Houston, case 1
2	28	M	4,880 16,000	Air	8	+	0	0	0	+	+	28	0	(1) Houston, case 2
3	41	M	4,270 14,000	Air	3	+	?	?	?	?	?	5	+	(1) Houston, case 4
4	36	M	3,200 10,500	Auto	2	+	+	0	Ataxia	+	0	6	0	(1) Houston, case 8
5	34	F	3,680 12,000	Train	2	+	0	+	Ataxia	?	?	22	0	(7) Hultgren
6	16	F	2,800 9,100	Auto	3	+	+	0	0	0	0	6	0	(9) Hultgren
7	22	M	4,100 13,400	Air	4	+	0	0	Ataxia	0	+	5	0	(10) Houston
8	38	F	4,400 14,300	Air	?	+	?	?	?	+	+	30	0	(7) Hultgren
9	44	M	4,200 13,800	Air	3	+	?	?	?	?	+	9	0	(7) Hultgren
10	41	M	4,260 14,000	Walk	?	+	0	0	?	?	?	?	+	(11) Dickinson, case 5
11	46	M	3,650 12,000	Walk	5	+	0	+	?	+	+	4	+	(11) Dickinson, case 6
12	26	F	4,300 14,000	Air	4	+	0	0	0	0	0	5	0	(7) Hultgren
13	?	M	4,000 13,000	Walk	7	+	0	0	?	0	+	17	0	(7) Hultgren
Mean 34.6			3,964 12,950	11-T/3-W	4	13/13	4/11	3/11	4/8	6/10	6/10	13.5	3/13	
Range 16-46			2,800-4,800 9,100-16,000		3-8							4-30		

SOURCES: Listed with Table 14.1C

T = Transported by air, train or auto, W = Walked

Table 14.1C
HACE Complicated

No.	Age	Sex	Altitude (meters / feet)	Mode of travel	Days at altitude	Coma	Head-ache	Vomiting	Neurologic signs / symptoms	Papill-edema	Retinal hemor-rhages	Duration of illness	WBC	Temp.	Heart rate	Death	Clinical diagnosis	Source of data
1	54	M	3,440 / 11,250	Walk	17	0	+	+	Collapse	+	0	9	27.2	101	160	+	Pneumonia	(11) Dickinson, case 1
2	54	M	3,400 / 11,250	Air	4	0	0	0	Somnolence	0	0	3	21.0	100	100	+	Pneumonia	(11) Dickinson, case 4
3	?	M	3,600 / 12,500	Walk	6	+	0	0	0	?	?	10	14.0	101	120	0	Pneumonia	(7) Hultgren
4	50	F	4,900 / 16,000	?	7	+	0	0	Ataxia	0	+	7	19.5	101	88	0	Pneumonia	(7) Hultgren
5	54	M	3,440 / 11,250	Walk	17	0	+	+	Collapse	+	?	11	27.2	101	160	+	Pneumonia myocarditis	(7) Hultgren
6	38	M	5,540 / 19,200	Air	5	+	0	+	Stupor	+	+	10	21.4	102	128	+	Pul. emb.	(11) Dickinson, case 2
7	27	M	5,180 / 17,000	Air	8	+	0	0	Ataxia	+	+	4	14.1	?	?	+	Pul. emb.	(11) Dickinson, case 3
8	38	M	5,490 / 18,000	Air	6	0	0	0	0	+	+	25	19.8	101	90	+	Pul. emb.	(1) Houston, case 3
9	22	M	6,100 / 20,000	Walk	12	+	0	0	Ataxia	?	?	20	?	?	?	0	Pul. emb.	(7) Hultgren
10	25	M	5,200 / 17,000	Walk	17	+	0	+	?	+	+	10	20.4	101	92	0	Meningitis	(1) Houston, case 9
Mean 16.2			4,629 / 15,345	4T	9.9	7/10	2/10	5/10	8	6/8	5/7	11	20.4	101	117	6/10		
Range 22-54			3,400-6,100	5W	4-17							3-25	14.1-27.2	100-102	88-160			

SOURCES to Tables 14.1A, 14.1B and 14.1C: (1) Houston C, and Dickinson J. Cerebral form of high altitude illness. *Lancet* 1975; Oct. 18: 758-76; (2) Fitch R. Mountain sickness: A cerebral form. *Ann. Int. Med.* 1964; 60:871-76; (3) Shlim D. A case of HACE. *Off Belay* June 1980; N51:9-12; (4) Dalenz J. El edema cerebral de altura. Inst. Boliviano Biol. Altura 1973; 21:29-31; (5) Chiodi H. Mal de montaña a forma cerebral: Posible mechanism etiopathogénico. Ann. Fac. Med. Lima 1960; 43(2):437; (6) Hultgren H. High altitude illness. In P Auerbach and E Geehr, eds., Management of wilderness and environmental emergencies. New York: Macmillan, 1983; (7) Hultgren H. Unpublished case report; (8) Clarke C. High altitude cerebral oedema. In High altitude deterioration, ed. J Rivolier, P Ceratelli, J Foray, and P Segantini. New York: S. Karger, 1984; (9) Hultgren H, Lopez C, Lundberg E, and Miller H. Physiologic studies of pulmonary edema at high altitude. Circulation 1964; 29:393-408; (10) Houston C. High altitude illness: Disease with protean manifestations. JAMA 1976; 236:2193-95; (11) Dickinson J, Heath D, Gosney J, and Williams D. Altitude-related deaths in seven trekkers in the Himalayas. Thorax 1983: 38:646-56.

T = Transported air, train or auto, W = Walked

Table 14.2
Symptoms of HACE in 42 Patients

Symptom	Number of occurrences
Unconsciousness, semicoma	28
Ataxia	25
Headache	17
Lethargy, weakness, fatigue	15
Vomiting	14
Dyspnea	8
Disorientation	7
Irrational behavior	3
Visual; auditory hallucinations	4
Blindness: transient, complete or partial, scotomata	3
Tinnitus	2
Vertigo	2
Diplopia	1

SOURCES: See Sources with Table 14.1C

weakness, and (5) vomiting. Other symptoms are disorientation, irrational behavior, and visual or auditory hallucinations. Diplopia is rare. A complete list of symptoms is summarized in Table 14.2. Symptoms usually appear fairly rapidly, often at night, such as loss of consciousness during sleep.[9] Prominent early warning symptoms are confusion or irrational behavior and incoordination. Most symptoms, especially disturbances of consciousness and ability to function mentally and physically, are progressive and can lead in a a few hours to a completely unconscious, helpless state.

The most common objective findings in addition to partial or complete loss of consciousness are ataxia (usually truncal), extensor plantar reflexes, stiff neck, and hyperreflexia including ankle clonus. One very simple but sensitive test for truncal ataxia is to have the subject walk on a two-by-four (flat side down), or walk in a straight line heel-to-toe and turn around quickly without losing of balance. A history from the patient and his colleagues as well as a simple neurological examination will usually be sufficient to make the diagnosis of mild HACE. This should not be ignored. Even mild cases should descend and be treated with oxygen or a hyperbaric bag without delay. (Physical findings are summarized in Tables 14.3 and 14.4.) Fundoscopic examination will reveal retinal hemorrhages, papilledema, or both in a substantial number of patients with HACE.[9] Fundoscopic examinations are reported in some of the 43 cases summarized in this chapter. Retinal hemorrhages were seen in 18/26 (69 percent), papilledema in 17/24 (71 percent), and both abnormalities were present in 9/24 (38 percent). Retinal hemorrhages may be an indication of petechial hemorrhages in the brain; which are common in HACE. Cerebral edema presenting as the acute onset of ataxia may occur. A 68-year old man in excellent physical condition was on the third day of a trek in the Himalayas when at the top of a pass at 17,000 feet (4,880 m) he suddenly became very ataxic, his affect diminished, and his mental acuity was impaired. He could not subtract seven from 100.

Table 14.3
Physical Findings in 44 Patients with HACE

Physical Sign	Number of occurrences
Disturbance of consciousness	31
Ataxia	27
Papilledema	23
Bladder dysfunction	21
Abnormal plantar reflexes	15
Abnormal limb tone or power	6
Abducens nerve palsy	2
Pupillary differences	2
Visual field defects	2
Speech difficulty	1
Hearing loss	1
Flapping tremor	1
Retinal hemorrhages	26

SOURCES: See Sources with Table 14.1C

Table 14.4
Objective Neurological Findings in HACE

Finding	Times Seen
Extensor plantar reflexes	14
Stiff neck	6
Ankle clonus	3
Hyperreflexia	2
Hemiplegia transient	3
Convulsive movements	3
Garbled speech	3
Urinary retention or anuria	4
Expressive aphasia	2
Positive Romberg	2
Decorticate posturing	2
Incontinence	2
Intention tremor	1
Nystagmus	1
Positive Kernig	1
Doll's eye ocular motion	1
Deafness 1	
Decerebrate rigidity	1
Dysdiadochokinesia	1
Apraxia	1

SOURCES: See Sources with Table 14.1C

During that day he had climbed to the pass from 14,500 feet (4,423 m) carrying a 35-pound pack. He was helped down to a camp at 13,000 feet (3,965 m) but fell repeatedly. He denied headache. Decadron was administered without improvement. After a day of rest, during which there was little improvement, he was assisted back across the pass and descended to 12,800 feet (3,904 m). He continued to be ataxic and again fell repeatedly. On arrival at the lower altitude his ataxia improved and quickly disappeared. He then developed an acute tracheitis with cough, chest pain, and a transient temperature elevation but no sputum. His chest was clear. It may be that this probable viral infection accentuated his ataxia.

Diagnosis and Evaluation

The Lake Louise Consensus Committee has proposed the following diagnostic criteria for HACE: "this illness can be considered an "end stage" of a severe form of AMS. In the setting of a recent gain in altitude, the presence of a change in mental status and/or ataxia in a person with AMS or the presence of both mental status change and ataxia in a person without AMS".[10] A self-assessment questionnaire (Table 14.5) has been developed by the author to evaluate the presence and nature of symptoms of HACE. It provides a useful check list for use in the field and can be completed by the patient. A clinical evaluation form (Table 14.6) has also been developed, which is designed to be completed by the physician after interviewing and examining the patient. The final functional score follows the guidelines of the Lake Louise Consensus Committee.

Laboratory Studies

Examination of the spinal fluid was made in 11 patients with HACE. Clear fluid was present in 8, and bloody fluid was noted in 2. One additional patient had an increase in cells and protein but this patient had meningitis. Spinal fluid pressure was reported in 7 patients (90 mm, 160 mm, 215 mm, 240 mm, 270 mm and 340 mm H_2O) and one report simply stated "spinal fluid dynamics were normal." One other patient had a pressure of 340 mm. On the fourth day after treatment his pressure was 85 mm.[11] The normal range of pressure in the recumbent position is 75-150 mm. In 34 patients with acute mountain sickness, most of whom had neurological symptoms and probably various degrees of HACE, Singh found cerebrospinal fluid pressure to be higher by 60-120 mm H_2O during the illness than upon recovery. Queckenstedt's tests were negative. Protein, sugar, and cell counts were normal. One patient had a CSF pressure of 410 mm H_2O which decreased during therapy over 15 days to 210 mm.[5] CPK levels are usually elevated with CPK-BB levels of one percent or more of total CPK indicating brain damage.[12]

Uncomplicated cases of HACE usually have a heart rate of <100 beats/min, slight or no elevation of temperature, and a normal or only slightly elevated white blood count. Cases complicated by HAPE will exhibit a substantially higher heart rate of usually >100/min, a high respiratory rate, normal or slight elevation of temperature, and a normal or slightly elevated white blood count. Cases complicated by pneumonia will usually exhibit a marked elevation of heart and respiratory rates, and also of temperature and white blood cell count (see Tables 14.1A-C).

Table 14.5
Self-Assessment Questionnaire for HACE

All responses should describe the most severe symptoms

Circle the appropriate descriptor.

1. MENTAL STATUS
   0-no problems
   1-a little confused and slow in
   thinking
   2-definitely confused, at times
   I can't concentrate, listless
   3-very confused, lethargic and
   had to be aroused at times
   4-I could not be awakened; I
   must have passed out

2. BALANCE, ATAXIA, STUMBLING
   0-no problem with balance
   1-some problem with balance,
   I occasionally feel unsteady
   2-definitely a problem keeping
   balance, very unsteady walking
   3-severe balance problems. I
   can hardly walk without help
   or I would fall
   4-very unsteady. I cannot
   stand without help

3. HEADACHE
   0-no headache at all
   1-mild headache, no problem
   2-very definite headache,
   unpleasant and bothersome
   3-a very bad headache, very
   unpleasant, can't do much
   4-terrible headache, the worst
   I have ever had

4. NAUSEA, NO APPETITE
   0-no nausea, good appetite
   1-definite mild nausea,
   appetite off
   2-quite nauseated, ate only a
   little
   3-severe nausea, cannot eat,
   limited activity
   4-terrible nausea, worst I have
   had, I can't do anything
   Did you vomit?
   (circle one) Yes No

5. HALLUCINATIONS, SEEING THINGS
   0-not at all
   1-occasional weired thoughts or
   imaginings
   2-very definite unpleasant dream-
   like thoughts, occasionally I
   see strange things
   3-very bad, I see and hear weird
   things, I can't go out
   4-I went berserk and had to be
   restrained

6. WEAKNESS, TIREDNESS, FATIGUE
   0-none at all
   1-a bit tired or weak
   2-definitely tired and weak, I
   can't do several things
   3-severely weak and tired, I
   can't do much or walk very far
   4-terrible, so weak and tired I
   can't do anything, incapacitated

7. SHORT OF BREATH, DYSPNEA
   0-none at all
   1-some trouble breathing, not bad
   2-definite shortness of breath,
   had to slow down
   3-very unpleasant shortness of
   breath even at rest, could
   not do much
   4-terrible trouble breathing,
   can't do anything at all
   Did you have to sit up to breathe?
   (circle one) Yes No

8. COUGH
   0-no cough at all
   1-some coughing off and on
   2-definitely a bothersome cough
   3-almost continuous coughing, very
   unpleasant, can't do much
   4-a terrible cough, it won't stop
   even at night
   Did you have a blood or pink sputum?
   (circle one) Yes No

Table 14.6
Clinical Evaluation of HACE

Responses to be obtained by interview

SEVERITY SCORE FOR EACH SYMPTOM

0-no symptoms
1-mild symptoms but no problem
2-moderately unpleasant
3-severely unpleasant
4-terrible worst I have had

SYMPTOMS SCORED BY NUMBERS ABOVE

1. MENTAL STATUS (circle one)
   0-normal
   1-lethargic lassitude slow
   2-confused disoriented
   3-semiconscious stupor
   4-unconscious coma

2. ATAXIA (circle one)
   0-none
   1-some trouble walking
   2-steps off line
   3-needs help to walk
   4-can't stand without assistance

3. HEADACHE   0 1 2 3 4

4. WEAK, FATIGUED   0 1 2 3 4

5. NAUSEA   0 1 2 3 4

6. VOMITING   0 1 2 3 4

7. INCONTINENT (circle one) Yes No

8. HALLUCINATIONS, BIZARRE BEHAVIOR
                  0 1 2 3 4

9. COUGH   0 1 2 3 4

FINAL FUNCTIONAL SCORE
Effect of symptoms upon activity level

0-no effect on any level of activity
1-minor effect heavy activity decreased
2-moderate effect only light activity
3-severe unable to do planned activity
4-very severe, totally incapacitated

PHYSICAL AND OBJECTIVE FINDINGS

1. DISTURBURED CONSCIOUSNESS
   0-none
   1-lethargy lassitude slow
   2-confused disoriented
   3-stupor semiconscious
   4-unconscious comatose

2. ATAXIA
   0-none
   1-balance maneuvers poor
   2-steps off line
   3-needs help to walk, falls often
   4-can't stand without assistance

3. RETINAL HEMORRHAGES
   Papilledema (circle one) Yes No

4. INCONTINENT
   (circle one)   Yes No

5. ABNORMAL PLANTAR REFLEXES
   (circle one)   Yes No

6. VITAL SIGNS
   Temp   H. Rate   Resp. Rate

   BP Vital Cap.___ %FEV$_1$___
   Predicted___ Predicted___

   Oxygen Sat.   PO$_2$

7. RALES   0 1 2 3 4

8. CHEST X-RAY (cirle one)
   Infiltrate   Yes No

9. LUMBAR PUNCTURE PRESSURE

Special Studies

Some case reports include data from special studies, which can be summarized as follows:

1. Mosso in 1898 and, more recently, Singh and his associates reported direct inspection of the brain via a hole in the skull. In one subject Mosso noted increased vascularity on the surface of the brain following ascent to 14,000 feet (4,270 m); a second subject showed no changes.[14] Singh's group placed burr holes in the skulls of two patients with HACE to exclude the possibility of a subdural hematoma. No hematoma was found, but the brain showed congestion and edema. A biopsy showed intercellular edema.[5]

2. Chiodi, after descent, measured his cerebral blood flow while breathing room air and during acute hypoxia induced by breathing 10 percent oxygen in nitrogen. There was no increase in blood flow during hypoxia, and he therefore concluded that his episode of HACE was due to a failure to increase cerebral blood flow with hypoxia.[1]

3. Brain CT scans were performed in nine cases of HAPE in Japan.[11] Eight showed cerebral edema with a decrease in the volume of the ventricles. Several weeks later repeat scans were normal. The report indicated that severe hypoxia in HAPE can result in cerebral edema. Similar results were obtained in twelve patients by Koyama, et al.[12]

4. MRI imaging was performed by Hackett and his associates in nine patients with HACE, eight of whom also had high altitude pulmonary edema (HAPE). The authors concluded that HACE is associated with a characteristic, reversible white matter edema, with a predilection for the splenium of the corpus callosum. The authors concluded that these observations clearly suggest a predominant vasogenic etiology of HACE.[13]

5. There have been some reports of brain damage in HACE. In 26 patients with HAPE studied in Japan the mean creatine phosphokinase was $1.023 \pm 1,363$ mIU. In two patients creatine kinase isoenzymes revealed a CK-BB level of one percent compatible with brain damage. Upon recovery the mean creatine phosphokinase level was 76 ± 60 mIU.[11] In a fatal case of HAPE with cerebral edema and petechial brain hemorrhages the total creatine kinase was 4,609 mIU with one percent CK-BB.[15] These levels of CK-BB are abnormal and indicate brain damage.

6. Cerebral venous thrombosis has been demonstrated in one patient by CT scan.[16]

Duration of HACE and Late Sequelae

The clinical course of HACE depends on the altitude, the duration of symptoms, and how expeditiously descent and/or treatment was begun. Prompt descent in patients with mild symptoms is usually followed by rapid recovery. Coma persisting for several days because of inability to descend is commonly associated with death or a prolonged recovery. The mean duration of illness from onset to clinical recovery in 34 surviving patients was 11.3 days (range 2-60 days). Duration of illness was similar in cases of pure HACE and in complicated cases.

Slow recovery ($\geq$10 days) occurred in 13/36 cases (37 percent). In 6/36 cases (17 percent) symptoms persisted for >10 days. Late sequelae in these 13 patients are summarized in Table 14.7. It is remarkable that permanent sequelae appear to be rare. One patient (Case 14.1A-11) still had mild truncal ataxia seven months after an

Table 14.7
Late Sequelae of HACE

Table & Patient No.	Diagnosis	Duration of Symptoms	Symptoms
14.1A - 8	HACE	"months:	Weakness
14.1A - 10	HACE	7 months	Ataxia
14.1A - 11	HACE	1.5 months	Ataxia
14.1A - 13	HACE	4 months	Loss of smell Poor memory Ataxia
14.1B - 1	HAPE-HACE	1 month	Weak-Difficulty with speech Emotionally labile
14.1B - 2	HACE-HAPE	2 weeks	Loss of speech
14.1B - 5	HACE-HAPE	2 weeks	Weak, ataxia
14.1B - 8	HACE-HAPE	2 weeks	Blunted memory
14.1B - 13	HACE-HAPE	10 days	Difficulty walking and speaking
14.1B - 4	HACE-HAPE	1.5 months	Weakness, fatigue
14.9 - D4	HACE-Pul. emb.	1 month	Ataxic, positive plantar reflexes

episode of HACE. One patient not listed in the table had a moderate depression for over one year after two days of unconsciousness due to HACE. Subsequently a complete functional recovery occurred. Of 44 patients reported by Dickinson, 10 recovered in two days and 32 in three to fourteen days; 2 patients were unconscious for more than two weeks.[9]

Epidemiology

Gender. Of the 43 cases of HACE reviewed in this chapter, 72 percent were males and 28 percent were females. The higher percentage of males probably does not indicate a gender difference for HACE but is rather simply a reflection of the fact that most climbing parties to very high altitudes consists largely of males.

Age. The mean age of the cases reviewed in this chapter was 33.6 years (range 16-64 years). Unlike HAPE, there are no case reports of HACE in children. The source of the cases in this chapter is, of course, largely an adult population going to very high altitudes where children rarely travel, yet in the Peruvian Andes I have been unable to find any reports of HACE in children except in cases of fatal or severe HAPE. This may be due in part to lower altitudes of exposure: in Peru the usual altitudes of exposure are from 12,000 feet (3,660 m) to 14,200 feet (4,330 m). Dickinson noted that most of the severe cases of HACE he observed were in obese males.[9]

Altitude of occurrence. The mean altitude of occurrence of uncomplicated cases of HACE reviewed in this chapter was 15,500 feet (4,728 m), in a range of 11,000 feet (3,355 m) to 25,700 feet (7,840 m). The mean altitude of occurrence of HACE complicated by HAPE was 12,850 feet (3,920 m), range 9,100-16,000 feet (2,776-

4,880 m). The significant difference in altitude (p <.05), which suggests that uncomplicated cases of HACE occur at a higher altitude than HAPE, would account for the low incidence of HACE in Peru and the continental United States.

In experimental animals and in a small number of human studies cerebral edema begins at a simulated altitude of 11,000 feet (3,880 m) and rapidly becomes more severe at higher altitudes.[17] Oxygen breathing rapidly reverses the edema. Cerebrospinal fluid pressure increases at similar altitudes, and at a simulated altitude of 17,000 feet (5,200 m) pressure may rise by as much as 150 mm Hg. Changes in cerebrospinal fluid pressure are less predictable than cerebral edema, because compensatory changes may occur, including increased absorption or decreased production of fluid. The threshold of altitude for cerebral edema may explain the rarity of occurrence of HACE below 11,000 feet (3,380 m).

Incidence. The incidence of HACE is difficult to ascertain because of the lack of a denominator. Singh reported an incidence of 1.25 percent in troops brought to 11,500 feet and 16,000 feet (3,507-4,880 m) in India.[5] The incidence of HAPE in the same population was 15.5 percent. In 40 accidents or deaths reported in 1976 from Mount McKinley, five cases of HAPE were reported, five cases of HAPE had HACE, and there was one case of apparently uncomplicated HACE.[18] In 278

Table 14.8
Epidemeological Features in 42 Cases of HACE

	HACE Uncomplicated (10 cases)	HACE + HAPE (13 cases)	HACE + Other Cond. (10 cases)	All Cases (42)
Mean	34.5	34.9	40.2	33.6
Range	21 - 64	16 - 46	22 - 54	16 - 64
Altitude (mean)				
	4,710 m = 15,500 ft	3.940 m = 12,850 ft	4,100 m = 13,500 ft	4,305 m = 14,100 ft
Range, m	3,380-7,800	2,800-4,880	3,440-6,100	2,800-7,800
Range, ft.	11,000-25,000	9,100-16,000	11,300-3,440	9,100-25,700
Mode of transport				
Air-Travel	13/15 (87%)	11/14 (78%)	4/9 (44%)	28/38 (73%)
Walked	2/15 (13%)	3/14 (22%)	5/9 (56%)	10/38 (27%)
Sex				
male	68%	65%	90%	72%
female	32%	35%	10%	28%
Days at altitude				
	5	3.8	9.9	8.8
Range - to onset of HAPE (weeks)				
	13	8	4-25	1-25
Duration of illness,				
days (m)	10.1	12.6	11.8	11.3
Range (days)	2-60	5-30	7-20	2-60
Number	19	13	10	42

trekkers at Pheriche in Nepal (14,245 feet/4,343 m), Hackett reported an incidence of HACE of 1.8 percent (five cases).[19] Details of epidemiological features are summarized in Table 14.8

Duration of altitude stay and mode of travel. The mean duration of altitude exposure before the onset of HACE in 35 cases was 9.9 days. In 20 cases the exposure was 5 days or less, in 9 cases 5-10 days, and in 6 cases greater than 10 days. (Five of the last group walked to high altitude, and the duration of altitude exposure before the onset of HACE is probably overestimated because it includes the travel time to high altitude.) In uncomplicated cases of HACE the mean duration of altitude exposure (with one exception of several weeks) was 5 days (range 1-13 days). HACE cases complicated by HAPE had a shorter duration of exposure of 3.8 days (range 1-8 days). These data suggest that uncomplicated HACE occurs at a higher altitude and after a longer period of exposure than when associated with HAPE. As might be expected, most of the cases of HACE followed a rapid transit to high altitude. In 36 cases where the mode of travel was specified, 26 traveled by air (22 cases) or bus-train (4 cases); only 10 walked most of the way.

Previous Episodes

Seven of the 43 cases reviewed in this chapter gave a history of previous, similar episodes at high altitude. Four of these patients had uncomplicated HACE. The incidence of previous episodes is probably underestimated, since details in many cases are missing. These observations suggest that there may be an individual susceptibility to HACE.

Associated Complications

It is evident from the review of reported cases that HACE is frequently precipitated by other medical problems, the most common being HAPE. Bronchopneumonia and pulmonary embolism also may precipitate HACE; all three conditions are associated with a decrease in arterial oxygen saturation. The reported cases also include one case of meningitis and one case of probable viral myocarditis. A clinical history of thrombophlebitis was reported in three cases. Four patients had pulmonary embolism and 3 of these patients died (Table 14.1C). One patient developed HACE at 20,000 feet (6,100 m) and nine days later while being carried down developed thrombophlebitis with subsequent pulmonary embolism.

Mortality

The mortality of HACE is difficult to determine. All reported deaths were preceded by coma. In 24 cases of HACE observed by Singh, 3 patients died: a mortality of 13 percent.[5]

Autopsy Studies

The results of autopsy studies are summarized in Tables 14.9. Cerebral edema was present in all but one of eleven autopsies. Case C-5 had only mild edema and degenerative changes in the cerebrum and brain stem. This patient had evidence of myocarditis with pneumonia, pulmonary edema, and small pulmonary artery thrombi with infarction. The diagnosis of myocarditis was supported by clinical observations of a high heart rate (160/min), a low blood pressure 60-90 mm Hg systolic), and an abnormal ECG (flat T waves). Case D-1 had no cerebral edema at

Table 14.9
Autopsy Studies in 11 Cases of HACE

Case no.[a]	Age	Sex	Brain			Lungs				Brain compression
			Edema	Hemorrhage	Thrombosis	Thrombosis	Infarction	Pneumonia	Edema	
A-9	24	F	+	+	0	0	0	0	0	+
B-3	41	M	+	+	0	0	0	+	+	not reported
B-10	41	M	+	+	0	0	0	0	+	+
B-11	46	M	+	0	0	0	0	+	+	+
C-1	54	M	+	0	0	+	0	+	+	not reported
C-2	54	M	+	0	0	+	+	+	0	not reported
C-5	54	N	+	0	0	+	+	+	+	not reported
D-1	38	M	0	+	+	+	+	+	+	0
D-2	27	M	+	+	+	+	+	+	0	+
D-3	38	M	+	+	0	+	+	+	0	0
D-4	22	M	+	+	0	+	0	0	+	not reported
			9/11	7/11	2/11	6/11	5/11	8/11	7/11	4/6

[a] Letters and case numbers refer to clinical Tables, 14.1.

autopsy, but cerebral vessels were congested and thrombi were present in the right parietal lobe with foci of degeneration in the adjacent brain tissue. Large pulmonary emboli were present, which showed early organization. Pulmonary infarction, edema, and bronchopneumonia were also present. The primary diagnosis in this case was probably pulmonary embolism. The other nine cases all had cerebral edema, with petechial hemorrhages, focal tissue destruction, and spongiosis. Two cases showed herniation of brain structures, which may have been the cause of death. In two autopsied cases reported by Singh, both cerebral and pulmonary edema were present; histologic studies were compatible with cerebral edema.[5] Additional autopsy studies have been reported by Dickinson.[9]

Etiology of HACE

There are several mechanisms of brain injury that should be considered in understanding the etiology of HACE:

Ischemic Injury. Ischemic injury, the most common and devastating type of brain injury, is usually due to arterial occlusion, arterial hemorrhage, shock, or cardiac arrest. Death of brain tissue occurs within four to six minutes of complete vascular occlusion, and permanent brain death usually follows after eight to twelve minutes of occlusion in normothermic man. Recovery from ischemic injury is frequently associated with permanent neurologic deficits.

Hypoxic injury with maintenance of arterial perfusion is the usual type of subtle brain dysfunction seen at high altitude. The influence of hypoxia upon brain edema has been reviewed by Baethman.[20] Although early concepts suggested that hypoxic brain edema occurred only when ischemia or hypercapnia was present, recently it has been shown that perfusion of the isolated dog or monkey brain with venous blood (PO_2 17-20 mmHg) results in marked brain edema.[21,22] The hypoxic threshold for brain edema has been shown to be at an arterial PO_2 of about 30 mmHg (see Fig. 14.1). This threshold value is in agreement with studies by Siesjo, who showed that energy-rich phosphates such as phosphocreatine begin to decline at almost the same time as the oxygen tension.[23] These data indicate that a determinant of cerebral edema in hypoxia is a failure of energy metabolism, which renders the tissues deficient in fuel for their active transport pumps (Fig. 14.2).[23,24] Focal metabolites are also released, including potassium, hydrogen ions, lactic acid, and adenosine, the most potent and rapidly acting vasodilator. Vasodilatation and an increase in vascular permeability can also result from hypoxic relaxation of vascular smooth muscle and a release of a vasodilator factor from vascular endothelial cells.[25] Studies by Brierly and his associates have shown selective vulnerability to injury in the hypoxic brain.[26] Animals subjected to severe hypobaric hypoxia equivalent to 37,500 feet (11,430 m) for ten to sixteen minutes showed selective damage to the precortical areas at the boundaries of the anterior and middle or middle and posterior cerebral arteries. In other animals, damage to the globis pallidus, putamen, and caudate nucleus was observed. Damage to these areas was thought to serve as a focus of vasogenic edema resulting from the breakdown of the blood brain barrier. Although cerebral blood flow is increased, severe cerebral dysfunction will occur if hypoxia is severe. This is usually manifested by disturbances of consciousness and ataxia. Despite considerable periods of hypoxic coma, complete recovery without permanent sequelae usually occurs.

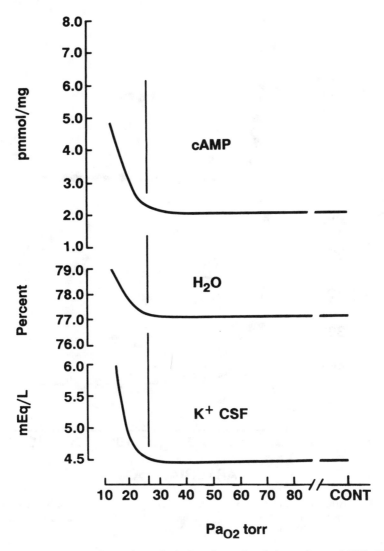

Figure 14.1. A. Formation of hypoxic cerebral edema in rats in relation to the arterial PO_2. Hypoxia was produced by inspired low oxygen gas mixtures. Note the increase in potassium loss (K) and water uptake by the cells (H_2O) at an arterial PO_2 of slightly less than 30 mm. The rise in cyclic AMP may have a role in edema formation. From Kogure K, Scheinberg P, Kishikawa H and Busto R. The role of monamines and cyclic AMP in ischemic brain edema. In eds H Pappius H and Feindel W., *Dynamics of brain edema*, New York: Springer, 1976; 203-14.

Anoxia with a circulatory deficit. Anoxia may be combined with a decreased cerebral blood flow such as hemorrhage or generalized circulatory failure. This is a common mode of death in acute, severe hypoxia or asphyxia. When cerebral hypoxia is extreme, the heart rate slows and a bradycardic arrest occurs as a consequence of failure of the medullary control centers.

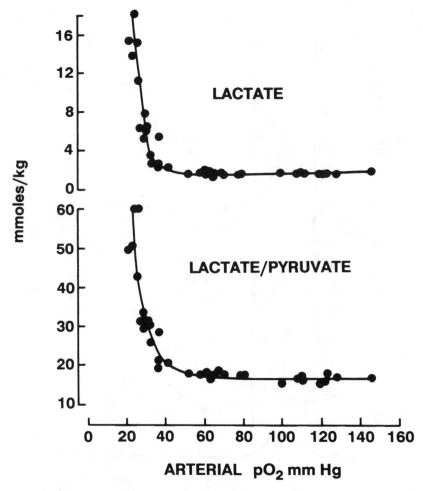

Figure 14.2. Tissue concentrations of cerebral lactate and lactate/pyruvate ratios in relaiton to arterial PO₂. The analyses were made of supratentorial rat brains, subjected to hypoxic air mixtures. Note the sharp increase at an arterial PO₂ of approximately 35 mm. From Siesjo, ref. 23.

Increased cerebral blood flow. Moderate decreases in arterial PO₂ result in only small increases in cerebral blood flow, which may be partly inhibited by the respiratory alkalosis during the first few days at high altitude. When arterial PO₂ decreases to levels below 30-50 mm Hg, however, there is a marked increase in cerebral blood flow, and with this degree of hypoxia local metabolites are released from brain tissue and result in vasodilatation.[23] An additional mechanism that results in arteriolar dilatation is an increased activity of the sympathetic nervous system, which takes place during the first weeks of exposure to high altitude. Sympathetic stimulation can cause cerebral arteriolar dilatation. Central neural pathways may be involved in selective regional vasodilation.[25] Systolic and mean blood pressures, too, are usually elevated during the first few days at high altitude. All these factors are probably involved in increasing cerebral blood flow. After several days cerebral blood flow decreases toward normal, sympathetic stimulation subsides, and systemic blood pressure decreases.

Although the mechanisms responsible for the clinical features of HACE are complicated and interlinked, three general hypotheses have been proposed. The first concept, the "bony box" theory, considers that hypoxia results in cytotoxic edema of the cells of the brain, an increase in brain volume, and a compression syndrome, which results in headache and interference with several neurological functions. The second theory (vasogenic theory) proposes that the clinical features of HACE are related to the increase in cerebral blood flow in such a way that arterial pressure transmitted to the capillaries results in localized areas of capillary damage, leakage of fluid and hemorrhages. A third concept suggests that both these factors are important.

1. The "bony box" theory. The "bony box" theory proposed that cellular, cytotoxic cerebral edema results from hypoxia-induced failure of the ATP dependent sodium pump. Hypoxia has a similar effect in many organs,[24] but the brain is especially vulnerable to an increase in volume. The brain can be compared to a single large cell without lymphatics enclosed in a rigid bony box. Approximately 80 percent of the gray matter and 70 percent of the white matter of the brain consist of water, 90 percent of which is intracellular and 10 percent extracellular. An increase in brain volume can compress vital centers and result in a variety of signs and symptoms.[7,27] Evidence to support the bony box theory can be summarized as follows:

a. In fatal cases of HACE, cerebral edema is always present at autopsy, commonly associated with local areas of hemorrhage, spongiosis (local areas of intercellular edema), and foci of necrosis, and occasionally also, venous thrombosis. Herniation of the cerebellar tonsils, unci, and cingulate gyri have been described.[6,9,28] (See Tables 14.1A-1C.)

b. In HAPE, cerebral edema has been demonstrated by computed tomography.[11]

c. Dilatation of the retinal vessels, retinal hemorrhage, and papilledema are commonly present in HACE, and being related to an increased blood flow probably also indicate the presence of increased intracranial pressure.

d. Several experimental studies in animals have clearly demonstrated the rapid development of cerebral edema upon ascent to high altitude. Kennedy and his associates exposed 24 cebus monkeys from sea level to an altitude of 14,100 feet (4,300 m). Studies made on the first, second, and third days of altitude exposure showed that both CSF pressure and SGOT levels increased; histologic evidence of brain edema was present primarily during the first day of exposure.[29]

e. Venous congestion: Oelz has reportd that possible occurrence of HACE after the use of positive expiratory pressure (PEEP) in the treatment of pulmonary edema. He postulated that PEEP raised cerebral venous pressure and thus facilitated brain edema. The positive pressure employed was 10 cm of water.[30]

f. Headache is a common symptom of HACE as well as of AMS. Many investigators have proposed that the mechanism of headache in both these conditions is brain compression resulting from cerebral edema.[5,6,27,28]

Arguments against the "bony box" theory. Several clinical observations do not support the above theory:

a. The rapid appearance and disappearance of neurological symptoms and signs are difficult to explain by cytotoxic cerebral edema alone, a process that may take several hours to develop or subside. Frequent observations have been made of helpless, semicomatose victims of HACE evacuated by air who were almost completely well and functional within an hour or two after arriving at the lower altitude.

b. The multitude of neurological signs and symptoms occurring in HACE (Tables 14.2-14.4) are not easily explained by cerebral edema alone but are more likely the result of localized areas of transient cerebral injury.

c. Headache is probably not due to cerebral edema. The relation between increased intracranial pressure and headache has been aptly summarized by Wolff: "The headache so often associated with increased intracranial pressure has generally been assumed but never proved, to be related to the increased pressure."[31] Wolff cites the following evidence: (1) elevation of intracranial pressure in normal human subjects to abnormally high levels does not cause headache; (2) in a series of 72 patients with a tumor of the brain, headache occurred almost as frequently with normal as with increased pressure; (3) headache homolateral to the lesion in a patient with a tumor of the brain was induced by lowering the intracranial pressure but could not be induced by elevation of the pressure to a high level of 550 mm. Gamache and Patterson have observed: "Simple elevation of intracranial pressure in an otherwise healthy patient does not produce headache. Headache is more commonly the reflection of traction on pain-sensitive structures in and around the base of the brain. Sudden shifts in intracranial homeostasis associated with marked rises and falls in intracranial pressure are more likely to produce headache than moderate changes or changes that develop slowly."[32]

For these reasons it is unlikely that cerebral edema is the sole cause of the many symptoms and neurological disturbances in HACE. It may be an important cause of death, however. When brain edema becomes severe and intracranial pressure rises above 400 mm of water, cerebral circulation decreases.[32,33,34] This decrease in blood flow associated with hypoxia can cause circulatory or respiratory arrest due to failure of central medullary control centers. This is a common mode of death in asphyxia. Herniation of brain structures may also be a contributing cause of death.

2. Vasogenic theory. The vasogenic theory proposes that a major abnormality in HACE is a marked increase in cerebral blood flow due to hypoxic vasodilatation. Vasoregulation, may break down in local areas of the brain and allow high flow and pressure to be transmitted to the capillary bed, and edema may result from the leakage of fluid from the capillaries and hemorrhages.[8,35] A similar mechanism has been proposed by Lassen and his coworkers to explain the clinical features of hypertensive encephalopathy.[36,37] In this situation systemic blood pressure overcomes the autoregulatory function of the cerebral circulation and high pressure is transmitted to the capillary bed (Fig. 14.3). At high altitude, physical exertion, coughing, and Valsalva maneuvers during heavy lifting may for a time further raise cerebral arterial pressure, possibly to the point of causing hemorrhages in the brain and retina. Brain volume is also increased by the increase in vascular volume due to the increase in blood flow. Several observations support the vasogenic theory.

a. Cerebral vasodilatation is a more logical mechanism of headache than cerebral edema. Many studies have demonstrated that in migraine, local cerebral vasoconstriction occurs during the aura but subsequent vasodilatation is accompanied by headache.[38] The administration of nitrates increases the severity of migraine headaches and in patients without migraine may even cause headaches. Nitrates are potent vasodilators. Animal studies have shown that nitrate administration results in an increase in carotid artery blood flow and an increase in intracranial pressure

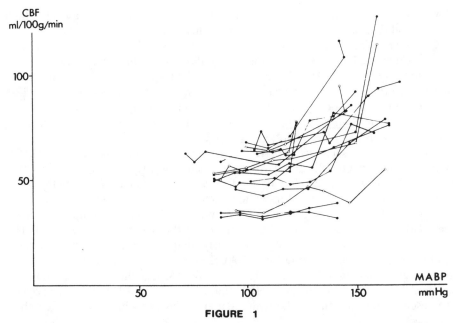

FIGURE 1

Figure 14.3. Autoregulation of cerebral blood flow in the baboon under angiotensin-induced hypertension. Curves from 16 hemispheres in 10 animals. Blood flow was measured by the intracarotid 133 Xenon injection method and blood pressure was increased gradually by angiotensin infusion. Blood flow is relatively constant from a resting mean blood pressure (MABP) of 75-100 mm Hg to MABP 120-150 mm Hg, where an abrupt increase occurs. This was observed in all animals but one. No animal showed a low cerebral blood flow at a high mean blood pressure. The limit of cerebral blood flow autoregulaiton was not changed by sympathetic denervation. The limit may be changed by hypoxic cerebral vasodilatation. From Johansson, Strandgaard, and Lassen, ref. 36.

despite a fall in systemic blood pressure.[39] Carbon dioxide is a potent vasodilator of the cerebral circulation and increases the severity of headache in AMS.[40] Low concentrations of carbon dioxide may relieve headache by increasing ventilation and arterial PO_2.[41] Nicotinic acid can produce headache although it does not increase cerebral blood flow.[42] Oxygen administration, which decreases cerebral hypoxia and cerebral blood flow promptly relieves headache in AMS. Ergotamine constricts cerebral vessels and can prevent the headache of migraine. It may also be effective in the relief of headache of AMS.[43,44]

b. It may be argued that marked increases in CBF do not occur until arterial PO_2 reaches very low levels (50-30 mm) and such degrees of hypoxia do not occur at the altitudes at which HACE occurs. This argument may be incorrect. HACE occurs at substantially higher altitudes than HAPE. In the case reports reviewed in this chapter the mean altitude of the occurrence of HACE was 15,500 feet (4,730 m), compared with 12,850 feet (3,920 m) for HACE associated with HAPE (p= 0.05). Moreover, HACE usually occurs at a lower altitude only in the presence of HAPE or bronchopneumonia, both of which are associated with a substantially lower arterial PO_2.

c. Cerebral blood flow has been shown to increase promptly with ascent to high altitude with a slow return to normal over five to twelve days.[5,45] Retinal blood flow increases in a similar manner and probably reflects the increase in cerebral blood flow.[46] Also, in the same way, sympathetic stimulation increases with ascent to high altitude and then subsides over several days. This is the time window during which HACE occurs. The mean duration of altitude exposure before the onset of HACE in the cases reviewed in this chapter was 9.9; 10 days or less in 83 percent.

d. Autopsy studies in HACE have consistently shown widespread petechial hemorrhages in the subarachnoid space as well as within the brain substance.[6,9,15,28] Retinal hemorrhages occur at similar altitudes and probably reflect what is occurring in the brain. Both types of hemorrhage could be due to high flow and pressure transmitted to the capillary bed.

e. Hackett and his associates performed MR imaging in nine patients with HACE eight of whom also had HAPE. Two patients had repeat studies after recovery. Six control subjects without HACE were studied. Seven of the nine patients with HACE showed an increased T_2 signal in white matter areas especially in the splenium of the corpus callosum but no gray matter abnormalities. All patients completely recovered and in two patients studied after recovery the MR changes resolved. The authors concluded that these studies clearly suggest a predominant vasogenic etiology in the initial abnormality in HACE.[47] Fukushima reported a decrease in ventricular volume by CT scans in eight cases of HAPE, indicating the presence of cerebral edema.[48] More recently, MRI studies in AMS and HAPE have revealed increased signal intensity in the white matter consistent with vasogenic cerebral edema.[49,50]

f. A possible argument against the vasogenic etiology of cerebral edema is the absence of protein elevation in the CSF. Increased capillary permeability usually results in an increase in protein content. A possible explanation is that in HACE capillary permeability is not increased until late in the course of the illness, and high pressure alone does not result in an increase in the protein concentration in edema fluid. Pulmonary edema fluid protein is not elevated in left ventricular heart failure, for example.

3. Multifactoral concept. A clinical syndrome such as HACE that has highly variable clinical presentations may not be due exclusively to one single mechanism, as in the two hypotheses just described. Not only cellular cytotoxic edema but increased blood flow with vascular damage and interstitial edema may be important, because the permeability of the blood brain barrier is increased by local factors and metabolites. Local areas of edema and hemorrhages combined with hypoxia may result in specific symptoms of considerable duration such as ataxia, but more transient, diverse symptoms could be related to local areas of spasm or vasoconstriction mediated by alkalosis. Similar episodes occur in migraine and have been related to local areas of vasoconstriction. Indeed, many symptoms of migraine and HACE are remarkably similar (See Chapter 28).

Severinghaus has reviewed the physiologic mechanisms in HACE. He dismisses the concept of failure of the sodium pump due to ATP depletion by pointing out that an ATP decrease occurs only after anoxia has silenced neuronal activity. He does not believe that increased cerebral blood flow is a viable hypothesis since prolonged hyperemia due to hypercapnia generates only minor transcapillary protein leakage localized to less hyperemic brain regions. Three alternate mechanisms are suggested: 1. Osmotic cell swelling even though small may be significant in a closed calvarium. 2. Focal ischemia resulting from intracranial hypertension from hyperemia and osmotic hypertension. 3. Cellular hypoxia activating macrophages and cytokines resulting in capillary wall damage and capillary leakage resulting in retinal hemorrhages and brain petechial hemorrhages.[51] The therapeutic effect of dexamethasone supports the third hypothesis, since it has been shown to reduce cerebral edema due to brain tumors or trauma by decreasing capillary permeability and improving blood-brain barrier integrity to decrease the edema formation.[52]

In summary, the etiology of HACE involves several circulatory disturbances that either locally or diffusely intensify the functional effects of hypoxia. The course of the illness with progression of initial symptoms of headache to ataxia and loss of consciousness probably involves a progressive development of several abnormalities: increased cerebral blood flow with capillary leakage of fluid and hemorrhages; cerebral edema, initially vasogenic but probably later cytotoxic in origin; transient local areas of vasoconstriction; and brain compression resulting from an increase in brain volume that puts pressure upon vital centers and impairs circulation. Any theory of the mechanisms involved in HACE must recognize the rapid recovery of many patients upon descent to a lower altitude as well as the relative rarity of permanent neurological sequelae. This leads to the speculation that in HACE the circulation is intact rather than being irreversibly damaged as it is in cerebral hemorrhage or thrombosis. Diffuse cerebral dysfunction due to hypoxia is a more tenable explanation of the unique features of HACE.

Individual susceptibility to HACE appears to occur just as it does in AMS and HAPE, and most victims have a history of similar episodes. Whether this susceptibility involves a diminished respiratory response to hypoxia or an unusual response of the cerebral circulation to hypoxia is unknown. These mechanisms of cerebral edema have recently been reviewed.[52,53,54,55]

Treatment

Field Treatment. An important part of any treatment program is the early detection of symptoms and signs of HACE and the triage of early, mild presentations versus acute emergencies. A general classification of severity of HACE is suggested as follows:

Class 1. Mild but definite symptoms and signs that permit normal activity but preclude climbing and load carrying. Headache, weakness, mild incoordination, and mental or emotional instability. Tests of ataxia slightly positive.
Class 2. Definite symptoms that permit ambulation but make strenuous activity impossible. Victim is still able to walk or descend with assistance.
Class 3. Symptoms and signs serious enough to disable the victim so that he is unable to walk or descend without assistance. May be confused or irrational but is still conscious.
Class 4. Loss of consciousness, unresponsive and unable to respond to commands or questions.

Class 1 and 2 victims should either descend with assistance or be given oxygen and bed rest if descent is difficult, dangerous, or not possible. Acetazolamide 250 mg b.i.d. and dexamethasone 4 gm q. 6 h. are indicated. Furosemide should not be given because an unexpected large diuresis may reduce plasma volume to such an extent that orthostatic hypotension and weakness may make it impossible for the victim to walk down with assistance. Plans for evacuation to a lower altitude should be developed. Class 3 and 4 victims are clearly acute emergencies and immediate descent is mandatory. Supportive measures that should be carried out before descent include: (1) bed rest; (2) high flow oxygen or the use of a hypobaric bag if available; (3) acetazolamide 250 mg t.i.d.; (4) dexamethasone 4 mg q. 6 h. or by slow IV drip; (5) a sitting position is preferable; (6) conscious patients should be encouraged to hyperventilate; (7) care should be taken to insure a patient airway especially if the patient is vomiting; (8) in cases of HAPE, expulsion of airway fluid by the head-down-buttocks-up position with assistance and deep coughing (the Bock maneuver) can be tried (see Chapter 13 "HAPE"); (9) clinical observations of heart rate, blood pressure, respiratory rate, and urine output should be made periodically and recorded. The chest should be examined for rales either with a stethoscope or the naked ear. If facilities are available a white blood count should be done. If facilities for determination of hematocrit are available the white count can be estimated by the thickness of the buffy coat. The recorded observations should be sent with the patient when descent is made. Such observations will provide prognostic and diagnostic information when definitive medical care can be provided. A high heart rate and respiratory rate, and rales will suggest HAPE. Fever and leucocytosis should suggest pneumonia. If pneumonia is suspected IV penicillin should be given. Chest pain, pleurisy, a pleural rub, and hemoptysis and edema of the legs should suggest the presence of pulmonary embolism and thrombophlebitis. If pulmonary embolism or thrombophlebitis are suspected anticoagulants should not be given in view of the danger of cerebral hemorrhage. Cardiac arrest may occur and CPR should be started promptly and continued until a definitive medical care facility is reached.

Hospital management. Depending upon the facilities available, victims of HACE who are hospitalized should be managed according to the following general guidelines. A chest film and basic laboratory studies should be performed on entry, and if clinical diagnosis so indicates, sputum smears, cultures, and blood cultures should be obtained. In view of the danger of medullary compression, lumbar puncture should not be performed unless meningitis is suspected. CT scans are useful but probably will not be available except in tertiary care hospitals. Lung scans and peripheral venograms are indicated if thrombophlebitis or pulmonary embolism are suspected. Management in an intensive care unit is important and the usual general ICU care and precautions should be observed. Treatment measures fall into two general categories: well-accepted physiological measures, and methods of doubtful value. Certainly high-flow oxygen by a well fitting face mask is an accepted high-priority treatment method that should be started immediately upon hospital entry. Strategically located hospitals in areas where victims of HACE and HAPE are frequently seen should have adequate supplies of oxygen. In patients with HAPE, bronchial drainage of airway fluid may be helpful. General therapeutic measures have been discussed by several investigators.[44,54-57] The physician should be aware of the possibility that patients showing symptoms and signs attributed to HACE may have other conditions such as meningitis, encephalitis, neoplasms, cerebrovascular accidents, or head injuries. These conditions should be excluded by appropriate studies. Because slow recovery or failure to improve is rare in the typical case of HACE, such a clinical course should suggest other diagnostic possibilities.

Experimental studies of vasogenic cerebral edema produced by local applications of cold metal to the brains of cats have shown that certain drugs — dexamethasone, acetazolamdie, and furosemide — will greatly shorten the recovery time of the cerebral edema. When these drugs are used in combination, edema cleared more rapidly than with any of the drugs alone. Massive doses of steroids had no advantage over standard doses.[55] Controlled field studies by Hackett and his associates have indicated that dexamethasone 2 mg q. 6 h. started before rapid ascent was of little value in preventing symptoms of AMS, including mild-to-moderate episodes of HACE: two subjects with HACE improved rapidly after being given 4 mg of dexamethasone every six hours.[56] Hackett recommends treating HACE with prompt descent and dexamethasone (4-8 mg) IV, IM or by mouth followed by 4 mg every six hours plus oxygen administration (2-4 L/min). Abrupt discontinuation of dexamethasone may result in a return of symptoms.[56,58]

The mechanisms of action of steroids is unknown. No significant changes in physiological variables, including ventilation or arterial blood gases, have been demonstrated. Steroids do not increase cerebral blood flow.[57] Steroids should be used with caution, since in some types of cerebral edema such as that associated with malaria, dexamethasone may be harmful.[59] Fishman has cautioned against the use of steroids in cerebral edema due to hypoxia or ischemia. His view is based on the harmful effect of steroids in cerebral malaria and the fact that steroids have not been shown to be therapeutically useful in brain edema due to hypoxia or ischemia.[60] Although both dexamethasone and furosemide have been used in the hospital treatment of HACE without clear evidence of either benefit or harm,[28] Acetazolamide has apparently not been used in this setting. The above observations suggest that a trial of a combination of these three drugs may be indicated in the hospital management of HACE. Lassen has stated that acetazolamide should not be used in the treatment of HACE.[61] It should be pointed out that steroids are of doubtful value in the treatment of other varieties of cerebral edema.[60] If steroids are used and bronchopneumonia is suspected, antibiotics should be administered at the same time. Other treatment measures, including the use of intravenous mannitol, drugs to lower blood pressure, water, and salt restriction, are of doubtful value, but clinical trials of additional therapeutic measures in HACE are clearly indicated.

Prevention

Persons who have already experienced episodes of HACE should probably not go to altitudes exceeding 14,000 feet (4,270 m) unless they observe several precautions. These include: (1) adequate acclimatization at an intermediate altitude; (2) use of acetazolamide 250 mg b.i.d. during the first week above 14,000 feet (4,270 m); (3) use of acetazolamide, dexamethasone, and prompt descent after the first symptoms or signs of HACE; (4) avoidance of trekking to areas where prompt descent is not possible. Not to observe these precautions would be foolhardy and a disservice to fellow climbers. Even climbers who have never experienced HACE should still observe sensible precautions of gradual ascent and an awareness of early symptoms so that descent can be carried out before the victim becomes a litter case. Prophylactic acetazolamide and dexamethasone should not be given routinely, however, but should be used only for persons who have a history of HACE.

References

1. CHIODI H, Mal de montaña a forma cerebral: Possible mechanismo etipathogénico. *Ann. Fac. Med.* Lima 1960; 43(2):437.
2. RAVENHILL T. Some experiences of mountain sickness in the Andes. *J. Trop. Med. & Hyg.* 1913; 20:313-20.

3. MONGE M. High altitude disease. *Arch. Int. Med.* 1937; 59:32-40.
4. FITCH R. Mountain sickness: A cerebral form. *Ann. Intern. Med.* 1964; 60:871-76.
5. SINGH I, KHANNA P, SRIVASTAVA M, et al. Acute mountain sickness. *N. Engl. J. Med.* 1969; 280: 175-84.
6. HOUSTON C, and DICKINSON J. Cerebral form of high altitude illness. *Lancet* 1975; Oct. 18:758-61.
7. HANSEN J, and EVANS W. A hypothesis regarding the pathophysiology of acute mountain sickness. *Arch. Environ. Health.* 1970; 21:666-69.
8. LASSEN N, and HARPER A. High altitude cerebral edema. *Lancet,* 1975; 2:1154. Letter to the Editor.
9. DICKINSON J. Cerebral acute mountain sickness. *Sem. Resp. Med.* 1983; 5:151-58.
10. HACKETT P, and OELZ O. The Lake Louise Consensus on the definition and quantification of altitude illness. In *Hypoxia and Mountain Medicine,* eds., J Sutton, G Coates, and C Houston. Burlington, VT: Queen City Printers, 1992: 327-30.
11. KOBAYASHI T, KOYAMA S. KUBO K, et al. Clinical features of patients with high altitude pulmonary edema in Japan. *Chest* 1987; 92:814-21.
12. KOYAMA S, KOBAYASHI S, KUBO K, et al. The increased sympathoadrenal activity in patients with high altitude pulmonary edema is centrally mediated. *Jap. J. Med.* 1988; 27:10-16.
13. HACKETT P. High altitude cerebral edema with MR imaging. *JAMA* In press.
14. MOSSO A. *Life of man on the high Alps.* Ed. A. Landon and T Fischer. London: Unwin, 1898.
15. FUKUSHIMA M, YOSHIMURA K, KUBO K, et al. A case of high altitude pulmonary edema. *Jap. J. Thor. Dis.* 1980; 18:753-57.
16. ASAJI T, SAKURAI E, TANIZAKI Y, et al. Report on medical aspects of Mt. Lhotse, an Everest expedition, in 1983: With special reference to a case of cerebral venous thrombosis in the altitude. *Jap. J. Mount. Med.* 1984; 4:98.
17. PETERSON E, BARNSTEIN M, and JASPER H. Cerebrospinal fluid pressure under conditions existing at high altitude. *Arch. Neurol. Psych.* 1944; 52:400-08.
18. WILSON R. Acute high-altitude illness in mountaineers and problems of rescue. *Ann. Int. Med.* 1973; 78:421-28.
19. HACKETT P, RENNIE D, and LEVINE H. The incidence, importance, and prophylaxis of acute mountain sickness. *Lancet* 1976; 2:1149-54.
20. BAETHMAN A. Cerebral edema: The influence of hypoxia and impaired microcirculation. In W. Brendel and K. Zink, eds., *High altitude physiology and medicine.* New York: Springer Verlag, 1982: 99-208.
21. GILBOE P, DREWES L, and KINTNER D. Edema formation in the isolated canine brain: Anoxia vs. ischemia. In H. Pappius and W. Feindal, eds., *Dynamics of brain edema.* New York: Springer Verlag, 1976; 228:35.
22. SIESJO M, MEYERS R, and HOLSTEIN S. Unilateral asphyxial brain damage produced by venous perfusion of one carotid artery. *Neurology* 1973; 23:150.
23. SEISJO B, MILSSON J, ROKEACH M, and ZWETNOW. Energy metabolism of the brain at reduced cerebral perfusion pressures and in arterial hypoxia. In J Brierly and B Meldrum, eds., *Brain hypoxia: Clinics in developmental medicine.* London: Heineman, 1971: 79-93.
24. JAMISON R. The role of cellular swelling in the pathogenesis of organ ischemia. *West. J. Med.* 1974; 120:205-18.
25. FARACI F, MAYHAN W, and HEISTAD D. Cerebral circulation during hypoxia. In *Hypoxia: The tolerable limits,* ed. J Sutton, C Houston, and G Coates. Indianapolis: Benchmarck Press, 1988: 169-80.
26. BRIERLY J. The neuropathological sequelae of profound hypoxia. In *Hypoxia: The tolerable limits,* ed. J Sutton, C Houston, and G Coates. Indianapolis: Benchmarck Press, 1988:147-51.
27. RENNIE D. High altitude edema: Cerebral and pulmonary. In *Mountain medicine and physiology.* London: Alpine Club, 1975: 85-98.
28. DICKINSON J, HEATH D, GOSNEY J, and WILLIAMS D. Altitude-related deaths in seven trekkers in the Himalayas. *Thorax* 1983; 38:646-56.
29. KENNEDY G, BUCCI T, et al. Effects of altitude on the cebus monkey with emphasis on the central nervous system. *Fed. Proc.* 1970; 29:591. Abstract.
30. OELZ O. High altitude cerebral oedema after positive airway pressure breathing at high altitude. *Lancet* 1983; 2:1148. Letter to the Editor.
31. WOLFF H. *Headache and other head pain.* New York: Oxford University Press, 1950.
32. GAMACHE F, JR., and PATTERSON J, JR. Headache associated with alterations in intracranial pressure. In *Wolff's headache and other head pain,* ed. Dalssio. New York: Oxford University Press, 1987: 352-56.

33. KETY S, SHENKIN H, and SCHMIDT C. The effects of increased intracranial pressure on cerebral circulatory funcitons in man. *J. Clin. Invest.* 1948; 27:493-99.
34. SHULMAN K, and VERDIER G. Cerebral vascular resistance changes in response to cerebrospinal fluid pressure. *Am. J. Physiol.* 1967; 213:1084-88.
35. SUTTON J, and LASSEN N. Pathophysiology of acute mountain sickness and high altitude pulmonary edema: An hypothesis. *Bull. Europ. Physiopath. Resp.* (Nancy) 1979; 15:1045-52.
36. JOHANSSON B, STRANDGARD S, and LASSEN N. On the pathogenesis of hypertensive encephalopathy: The hypertensive "breakthrough" of autoregulation of cerebral blood flow with forced vasodilatation, flow increase, and blood-brain barrier damage. *Circ. Res.* 1974; 34-35 (Suppl. 1):167-71.
37. LASSEN N, and AGNOLI A. The upper limit of autoregulaiton of cerebral blood flow on the pathogenesis of hypertensive encephalopathy. *Scand. J. Clin. Invest.* 1972; 30:113.
38. MEYER J, et al. migraine and cluster headache treatment with calcium antagonists supports a vascular hypothesis. *Headache* 1985; 25:358-67.
39. ROGERS M, TRAYSTMAN R, and EPSTEIN M. Nitroglycerine effects on intracranial pressure. *Am. J. Cardiol.* 1979; 43:342. (Abstract).
40. MAHER J, CYMERMAN A, REEVES J, et al. Acute mountain sickness: Increased severity in eucapnic hypoxia. *Aviat. Space Environ. Med.* 1975; 46:826-29.
41. HARVEY T, WINTERBORN M, LASSEN N, et al. Effect of carbon dioxide in acute mountain sickness: A rediscovery. *Lancet* 1988; Oct. 17:639-41.
42. SCHEINBERG P. Effect of nicotinic acid on cerebral circulation with observations on extracerebral contamination of cerebral venous blood in nitrous oxide procedure for cerebral blood flow. *Circulation* 1950; 1:1148-54.
43. DALESSIO D. High altitude headache. *JAMA* 1983; 249:1770. Letter to the Editor.
44. CARSON R, EVANS W, SHIELDS J, and HANNON J. Symptomatology, pathophysiology, and treatment of acute mountain sickness. *Fed. Proc.* 1969; 28:1085-91.
45. SEVERINGHAUS J, CHIODI H, EGER I, et al. Cerebral blood flow in man at high altitude. *Circ. Res.* 1966; 19:274-82.
46. FRAYSER R, GRAY G, and HOUSTON C. Control of the retinal circulation at altitude. *J. Appl. Physiol.* 1974; 37:302-4.
47. HACKETT P, YARNELL P, and HILL R. MRI in high altitude cerebral edema: Evidence of vasogenic edema. Abstract in *Proceedings, Sixth Hypoxia Symposium*, 1989.
48. FUKUSHIMA M, KOBAYASHI T, KUBO K, et al. A case of high altitude pulmonary edema followed by brain computerized tomography and electroencephalogram. *Aviat. Space Environ. Med.* 1988; 59:1076-79.
49. MATSUZAWA Y, KOBAYASHI T, KUJIMOTO K, et al. Cerebral edema in acute mountain sickness. In *High altitude medicine*, G Ueda, J Reeves, and M Segiguchi. Matsumoto, Japan: Shinshu University, 1992: 300-4.
50. YAMAGUCHI S, KOBAYASHI T, MATSUZAWA Y, et al. MRI findings in patients with high altitude pulmonary edema. In *High altitude medicine*, G Ueda, J Reeves, and M Segiguchi. Matsumoto, Japan: Shinshu University, 1992: 305-8.
51. SEVERINGHAUS J. Hypothetical roles of angiogenesis, osmotic swelling and ischemia in high-altitude cerebal edema. *J. Appl. Physiol.* 1995; 79:375-79.
52. FISHMAN R. Brain edema. *N. Engl. J. Med.* 1973; 293:706-11.
53. DE VLIEGER M, DE LANGE S, and J BEKS, eds., *Brain Edema*. New York: Wiley and Sons, 1981.
54. HAMILTON A, CYMERMAN A, and BLACK M. High altitude cerebral edema. *Neurosurg.* 1986; 19:841-49.
55. LONG D, MAXWELL R, and CHOI K. A new therapy regimen for brain edema. *Proc. Int. Soc. Brain Edema*, ed. H Revlen. New York: Springer-Verlag, 1987; 293-300.
56. HACKETT P, and ROACH R. Medical therapy of altitude illness. *Ann. Emerg. Med.* 1987; 16:980-86.
57. SHENKIN H, and BOUZARTH W. Clinical methods of reducing intracranial pressure: Role of the cerebral circulation. *N. Engl. J. Med.* 1970; 282:1465-71.
58. HACKETT P, ROACH R, and SUTTON J. High altitude medicine. In P Auerback and E Geehr, eds., *Management of wilderness and environmental emergencies*. St. Louis: C.V. Mosby, 1989.
59. WARRELL D, LOOAREESUWAN S, WARRELL M, et al. Dexamethasone proves deleterious in cerebral malaria: A double-blind trial in 100 patients. *N. Engl. J. Med.* 1982; 306:313-19.
60. FISHMAN R. Steroids in the treatment of brain edema. *N. Engl. J. Med.* 1982: 306:359-60.
61. LASSEN N. Personal communication.

CHAPTER 15

Chronic Mountain Sickness

SUMMARY

Chronic mountain sickness (CMS) is a rare form of altitude illness that occurs after months to years of continued residence at elevations usually in excess of 10,000 feet (3,050 m). Symptoms consist of progressive weakness, fatigue, and dyspnea as well as impairment of intellect and higher mental functions. Marked polycythemia, arterial unsaturation, and pulmonary hypertension are diagnostic findings. Complete recovery occurs upon descent to a lower altitude, but a return to high altitude usually results in a recurrence. Care must be taken to differentiate CMS from various forms of cyanotic pulmonary disease as well as from asymptomatic high altitude polycythemia. The cause of CMS is not clear, but the most plausible hypothesis is an insensitivity to hypoxia and possibly also to carbon dioxide, which develops in susceptible persons during prolonged exposure to high altitude.

• • •

Chronic mountain sickness (CMS) is also known in Peru as soroche chronico, or Monge's Disease. It affects a small percentage of the long-term residents of high altitude by the gradual development of progressive polycythemia, pulmonary hypertension, and hypoxemia. The main symptoms are weakness, fatigue, somnolence, and slowed mental functioning, which may progress to complete incapacity. (The term "slow man" has been applied to such patients.) Symptoms are relieved by descent to sea level. The probable etiology is a decreasing respiratory sensitivity to hypoxia, and probably also to carbon dioxide, with resulting hypoventilation and chronic severe hypoxia and marked polycythemia.

Historical Aspects

In 1925, Monge presented to the National Academy of Medicine in Lima a report entitled "On a Case of Vasquez Disease (Erythremia Syndrome of High Altitude)." The patient was a 38-year-old engineer who worked in Cerro de Pasco, 14,200 feet (4,330 m). He noted one year after arrival an inability to sleep, mental confusion, and marked cyanosis. He also had severe pain in his back and extremities and required two canes when walking. His red cell count was 8.6 million/mm³, leucocytes 10,000/mm³, and hemoglobin 21 gms/100 ml. All his symptoms disappeared when he descended to sea level, but reappeared when he returned to high altitude. An English translation of Monge's original case report has been published.[1] Much of the work on CMS has been done by physicians working in Peru. In 1928, Monge described 24 high altitude natives of the Peruvian Andes who showed clinical symptoms associated with cyanosis and marked polycythemia.[2] He recognized the clinical presentation as a unique entity related to altitude exposure and applied the term "la enfermedad de los Andes" to this form of altitude illness, which was later to be referred to as "chronic mountain sickness" or CMS. Talbott and Dill referred to CMS in 1936,[3] and in 1937 Monge published additional observations.[4] In 1942, Hurtado described eight cases[5] and in 1942-43 Monge added further data in three reports.[6,7,8] After a lapse of some years, Rotta in 1956 reported the first hemodynamic studies in CMS.[9] Banchero in 1966 reported on physiological data,[10] and Penaloza in 1974 reported on ten cases in which he had carried out systematic physiologic studies.[11] Lopez described additional cases from Peru.[12] There have also been reports of CMS occurring in the United States.[13-16] Additional historical aspects of CMS have been described by Winslow and Monge.[1]

Clinical Features

Symptoms. Characteristically, CMS occurs in adult male residents of the Andes who have lived continously above 10,000 feet (3,050 m) for many months to years. Fatigue, weakness, and a decrease in exercise tolerance to the point of being unable to perform any physical labor are the most common symptoms. Slowed mental function, a decrease in memory, confusion, headaches, dizziness, and somnolence also occur. Despite the presence of marked pulmonary hypertension and polycythemia, evidence of heart failure in the form of edema, ascites, or dyspnea is rare. The fact that symptoms usually progress slowly over a course of months or years facilitates recognition and treatment.

Physical signs. Marked cyanosis of the lips, nose, ears, fingers, and cheeks is characteristic. The cyanosis, which may result in an almost purple or black color in the involved areas, is the result of the combination of marked polycythemia and hypoxemia. There also may be clubbing of the digits, but this is rarely marked. Splinter hemorrhages under the nails may be present, although these may also occur in manual laborers who do not have CMS.[17] Signs of right heart failure, such as an elevated jugular venous pressure, hepatomegaly, ascites, or peripheral edema, are rare. This is confirmed by hemodynamic studies showing normal resting right atrial pressures.[11] Physical examination may reveal a right parasternal heave of a dilated, hypertrophied right ventricle and a loud, often palpable pulmonic closure sound of marked pulmonary hypertension. A short, early, or mid-systolic murmur may be present at the pulmonic area. Wide splitting of the second sound should suggest a right bundle branch block. An atrial gallop of right ventricular origin may be present along the lower left sternal border. The fundi show tortuosity and dilatation of retinal vessels. The blood pressure is usually low, with a narrow pulse pressure. Diastolic blood pressure may be elevated. The heart rate is moderately elevated in most patients, but rarely exceeds 100/min. In most instances the clinical features and symptoms require many years to develop. Since most patients descend to a lower altitude, deaths are rare. The mechanism of death in a few instances appears to be due to pulmonary embolism, cerebral thrombosis, or congestive (right heart) failure.

Radiological Studies

Chest roentgenograms reveal cardiac enlargement, prominence of the main pulmonary artery and its proximal branches, and an increase in pulmonary vascular markings. The right atrial contour may be enlarged (Fig. 15.1). The cardiac enlargement is due to enlargement of the right ventricle and right atrium. Cardiac volumes determined from chest roentgenograms in 8 patients with CMS were 672 ml/M^2 ± 75 ml, compared with 485 ml/M^2 in 12 normal high altitude residents.[11] Left

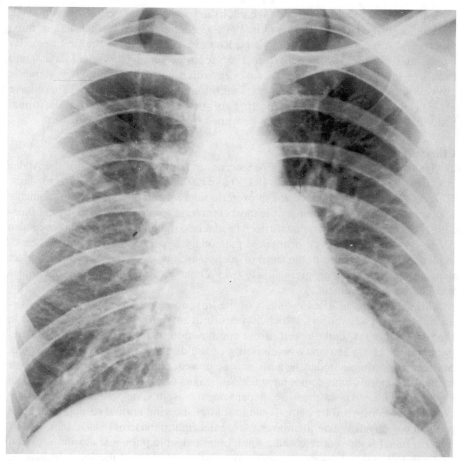

Figure 15.1. Typical chest roentgenogram of a patient with CMS, showing cardiac enlargement, prominent central pulmonary artery branches, and increased vascularity.

ventricular angiograms revealed a small left ventricle with enroachment of the chamber by the dilated right ventricle. Echocardiographic studies have confirmed these observations.[18]

The Electrocardiogram

The electrocardiogram reveals changes compatible with right ventricular and right atrial hypertrophy (Fig.15.2). Common findings are right axis deviation, prominent peaked P waves in the right precordial leads, S waves extending across the precordium to V_6 and right precordial T wave inversion. Tall R waves in V_1 - V_2 are often present. Deep S waves in V_2 - V_3 may suggest left ventricular hypertrophy, but this is probably a positional effect or the result of septal hypertrophy, because in CMS there is no evidence of hypertrophy of the free wall of the left ventricle. The frontal plane QRS vector is shifted rightward and superiorly. In 8 patients with CMS the mean frontal plane axis was + 152 degree +/- 14, compared with + 95 degree +/- in 12 normal residents.[11]

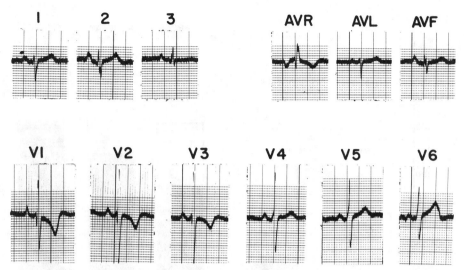

Figure 15.2. Electrocardiogram of a patient with CMS, showing a pattern of right ventricular hypertrophy.

Laboratory Data

A striking feature of CMS is the marked elevation of the hemoglobin and hematocrit. The mean hemoglobin in 8 patients with CMS reported by Penaloza and his associates was 24.8 gms/100 ml compared with 20.1 gms in 12 normal high altitude residents. The mean hematocrit was 79.3 percent in these patients and 59.4 percent in the normal residents.[11]

Velarde more recently reported on 72 patients with CMS studied in Puno, Peru at 11,800 feet (3,850 m). The mean hemoglobin was 23.5 percent and the mean hematocrit was 71 percent. Serum uric acid levels were elevated in 38 percent, probably owing to increased red cell production and turnover.[19] Both the morphology of the red cells and the number of leucocytes were normal. Hurtado reported leucocyte counts of 3,800 ml to 7,200 ml.[5] The differential count was normal.[5] The total blood volume is increased, with a marked increase in red cell volume, but plasma volume is decreased (Fig. 15.3). Arterial oxygen saturation is decreased. In 8 patients with CMS the mean arterial saturation was 69.6 percent ± 4.9, compared with a saturation of 81.1 percent ± 4.6 in normal high altitude residents.[11] The arterial PCO_2 is slightly higher than that normally present in the native population.[20]

Hemodynamics

Penaloza and his associates performed hemodynamic studies in 8 patients with CMS and compared the results with data from 12 normal residents living at the same altitude of 14,200 feet (4,330 m).[11] Pulmonary artery mean pressure was elevated in all cases, with a mean value of 47 mm ± 18 mm Hg. One patient had a mean pressure of 85 mm. In the 12 normal residents the mean pulmonary artery pressure was 23 mm ± 5 mm. Right atrial and pulmonary artery wedge pressures were normal. The cardiac output was slightly elevated to 4.0 L/min/M ± 0.9, compared with normal residents, 3.8 L/min/M ± 1.0. This difference is not significant. Additional data from published reports of CMS are summarized in Table 15.1.

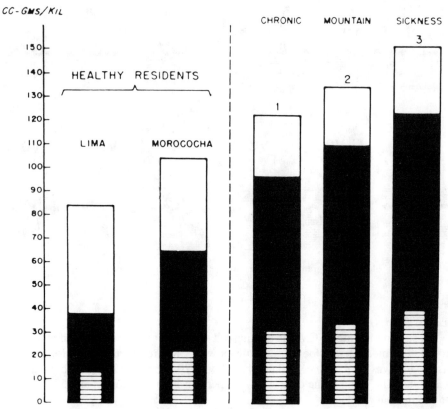

Figure 15.3. Total mean blood volumes determined by Evans blue dye in 20 healthy residents of Lima, 20 healthy natives living in Morococha at 14,900 feet (4,545 m), and 3 patients with CMS from Morococha. White areas = plasma volume; black areas = red cell volume; horizontal bars = hemoglobin. From Hurtado, ref. 5.

Pulmonary Function

Little published information is available regarding pulmonary function studies in CMS. The two patients described in the case reports below had normal vital capacities and normal maximal breathing capacities. The patient described by Hecht had a normal vital capacity.[13] The patient described by Gronbeck had a decreased vital capacity (59 percent of normal) but a normal FEV_1.[14] None of these four patients, therefore, had evidence of significant obstructive pulmonary disease.

Diagnosis

The diagnosis of CMS is based upon four essential findings: (1) characteristic symptoms, (2) clinical evidence of severe cyanosis and pulmonary hypertension, (3) laboratory demonstration of marked polycythemia, an abnormally low arterial oxygen saturation, and (4) exclusion of other causes of cyanosis and polycythemia including chronic pulmonary disease, polycythemia vera, and congenital heart disease. Insufficient data are available to indicate whether an abnormal elevation of

Table 15.1
Hemodynamic Features of CMS in 16 Patients with CMS

Case No.	Altitude (Feet,	Meters)	Sex	Age	PCV %	Hb gm%	SaO_2 %	$\overline{P_{RA}}$ mmHg	$\overline{P_{PA}}$ mmHg	$\overline{P_w}$ mmHg	Q 1/min/m²	PVR[g]	P_{BA} S	mmHg D	$\overline{P_{BA}}$	SVR[b]
1[a]	13,200	4,026	F	35	72	23.2	63	5	38	6	2.1	800	-	-	-	-
2[b]	14,200	4,331	M	-	86	23.2	66	6	62	6	5.5	450	-	-	-	-
3[c]	14,900	4,331	M	43	72	-	-	7	39	7	-	-	95	70	78	-
4[c]	14,200	4,331	M	-	-	-	67	-	33	-	-	-	120	95	102	-
5[c]	14,200	4,331	M	-	-	-	67	-	53	-	-	-	140	110	118	-
6[c]	12,200	4,331	M	23	85	26.0	81	-	34	-	-	-	120	80	95	-
7[d]	14,200	4,331	M	27	73	24.2	78	1	34	3	2.8	517	125	75	88	140
8[d]	14,200	4,331	M	35	79	26.0	70	5	31	6	2.7	501	132	75	88	176
9[d]	14,200	4,331	M	22	80	26.2	68	3	32	-	5.4	-	162	92	120	113
10[d]	14,200	4,331	M	38	83	2701	75	5	55	7	2.9	905	123	85	100	188
11[d]	14,200	4,331	M	40	84	27.3	66	2	53	-	5.0	-	118	107	110	109
12[d]	14,200	4,331	M	38	86	23.2	67	6	62	6	4.7	599	120	87	100	107
13[d]	14,200	4,331	M	35	75	20.5	71	2	33	3	4.2	361	95	70	80	96
14[d]	14,200	4,331	M	41	78	25.6	76	6	33	9	4.5	279	155	100	128	143
15[d]	14,200	4,331	M	51	80	26.2	61	5	85	-	4.1	-	172	112	133	161
16[d]	9,950	3,035	M	30	81	22.0	73	-	27	-	2.7	370	-	-	-	-
Mean	13,790	4,206		35.2	79.6	26.4	69.9	4.4	44.7	5.9	3.9	531	129	89	103	127
S.D.	± 286			2.3	1.3	0.6	1.5	0.6	4.2	0.6	0.4	69	6.5	4.1	4.9	11.0
Normal values[f] (n=35)	14,900	4,545		22	59	19.4	78.4	3	29	5	4.0	330	119	73		

SOURCES: [a]Hultgren, personal observations; [b]Monge, ref. 7; [c]Marticorena, ref. 18; [d]Penaloza, ref. 11; [e]Hecht, ref. 13; [f]Banchero, ref. 10.

SVR = systemic vascular resistance
PVR = pulmonary vascular resistance
Dynes = sec – cm²
$\overline{P}$ = mean pressure
Q = cardiac output
PBA = brachial artery pressure
S = systolic
D = diastolic

arterial PCO_2 is of diagnostic value. CMS must be differentiated from chronic mountain polycythemia, which may be accompanied by similar elevations of hemoglobin and hematocrit,[21,22] but which is not accompanied by the usual symptoms of CMS, most notably those of impaired physical and mental incapacity.[1,23]

Case Reports

The following two case reports illustrate most of the essential features of CMS.

Case 1. D.R. is a 43-year-old English mining engineer who had been in Peru for ten months working in Morococha, 14,900 feet (4,540 m). After six months he began noticing gradually increasing headache, weakness, anorexia, and insomnia, which interfered with his capacity to work. He was referred to the Chulec General Hospital, 12,230 feet (3,730 m), for evaluation. Physical examination revealed a blood pressure of 100/80 mm Hg, heart rate 60/min, and marked cyanosis. Slight clubbing of the digits was present. The pulmonic second sound was loud. Venous pressure was normal. The chest was clear. Cardiac findings were normal. Abdomen was normal.

Laboratory tests: hematocrit 72 percent, WBC 8,000, Bilirubin 1.4 mg, total proteins 6.5 gms/100 ml, urinalysis normal. The maximum breathing capacity was 142 L/min. An electrocardiogram revealed a pattern of right ventricular hypertrophy (Fig. 15.2). A chest x-ray revealed normal lung fields and prominence of the pulmonary artery and its branches. The right ventricle and right atrium were moderately enlarged (Fig. 15.1). A right heart catheterization revealed a pulmonary artery pressure of 52/26 mm Hg (mean 40 mm), a PA wedge pressure of 8 mm Hg, and a right atrial pressure of 7 mm. The cardiac output was not measured.

The patient was advised to return to sea level. He left Peru and returned to England where he became symptom-free.

Comment. There were no signs of pulmonary disease in this patient and the maximum breathing capacity was normal. Recovery was prompt upon return to sea level.

Case 2. J de P is a 52-year-old Peruvian housewife who had lived in Morococha 14,900 feet (4,540 m) for 25 years. She was born in the Andes at 9,840 feet (3,000 m). She had previously been well and had raised four children. For the past four years she had become increasingly cyanotic and had suffered progressive fatigue, weakness and exercise intolerance. She denied headache, anorexia, and weight loss. She never had a cough, sputum production, or any symptoms of pulmonary disease. Physical examination revealed marked cyanosis, clubbing, slightly increased venous pressure, a slight right ventricular heave, and a loud pulmonic second sound. The lungs were clear. The heart was normal. The blood pressure was 182/115 mm Hg and the heart rate 105/min. The vital capacity was 4.5 liters and the maximum breathing capacity was 90 L/min. A right heart catheterization revealed a pulmonary artery pressure of 62/36 mm Hg (mean 50 mm) and a right atrial pressure of 9 mm Hg. Voluntary hyperventilation and 100 percent oxygen breathing lowered the pulmonary artery pressure to 42/19 mm Hg, 30 mm mean. The hematocrit was 70 percent. A chest X-ray revealed clear lungs with moderate enlargement of the right atrium, right ventricle, pulmonary artery, and central branches of the pulmonary artery.

Comment. This patient had no clinical evidence of lung disease. The vital capacity and maximum breathing capacity were normal. The cause of the hypertension was not investigated.

Certain types of lung disease may simulate CMS at high altitude, as illustrated by the following case report.

M de N is a 40-year-old Peruvian woman living at 15,200 feet (4,636 m) in the Andes. Eight months earlier she began noticing progressive exertional dyspnea and right upper abdominal pain and tenderness, which was more severe after meals. For six months she noted right chest pain made worse by motion, coughing, or deep breathing. Occipital headaches began at that time. For two months she had a nonproductive persistent cough. She had no fever and no hemoptyses. She had previously been well and had cared for her eight children.

Physical examination revealed marked cyanosis. The blood pressure was 130/100 mm Hg; heart rate 100/min. Marked clubbing was present as well as moderate venous distention. A right ventricular parasternal heave and a loud P_2 were present. A grade 3/6 murmur of tricuspid regurgitation was present along the lower sternum. Persistent crepitant rales were present over both posterior lung fields and over the right lung posteriorly. The hematocrit was 62 percent, Hg 19.0 gms; white cell count 8,200; sputum negative for acid fast bacilli. Chest X-ray revealed moderate enlargement of the right ventricle, right atrium, and central pulmonary artery branches. Streaky densities were present in the lower lung fields. Right heart catheterization revealed a pulmonary artery pressure of 115/75 mm Hg with a mean pressure of 90 mm. The mean right atrial pressure was elevated to 18 mm Hg. The brachial blood pressure was 150/90 mm Hg. The arteriovenous difference was 4.3 ml/100 ml. The arterial oxygen saturation was 71 percent and it rose to 95 percent on 100 percent oxygen. An open lung biopsy was performed. The lung was stiff and fibrotic. Microscopic examination revealed cystic lung disease with fibrosis.

Comment. This patient with pulmonary fibrosis presented some of the essential features of CMS. The presence of lung disease was suggested by the history of pleurisy, the finding of persistent pulmonary rales, and the X-ray demonstration of basal infiltrates. Right ventricular failure with tricuspid regurgitation and a large tender liver are rare in CMS. Unfortunately pulmonary function studies were not performed. It is evident that the diagnosis of CMS can only be made if preexisting pulmonary disease is excluded.

Epidemiology and Prevalence

Most reports of CMS have been made by Peruvian investigators, but cases have also been reported from Tibet, India, and China. Chinese investigators have used a hemoglobin of >20 gms percent and a red cell count of >6.5 million as a diagnostic criteria in persons living above 13,120 feet (4,000 m). In Lhasa, 11,700 feet (3,568 m), no cases of high altitude polycythemia were seen in 160 females, in comparison with 42 cases in 579 males (7.3 percent).[24] Few cases of CMS have been reported in Nepalese Sherpas, probably because Sherpas and yak herders do not live continuously above 12,000 feet (3,660 m) but ascend to altitudes over 14,000 feet (4,270 m) only periodically.

Twenty-seven cases of CMS have been reported from the western Himalayas by Nath.[25] All were males, with a mean age of 36 years (25 to 48). Twenty-six cases occurred above 13,000 feet (3,965 m) after a mean duration of stay of seven years (1.2-15.3 yrs). With a few exceptions, clinical and laboratory features were similar to cases reported from Peru. Cardiorespiratory symptoms were more common, but clubbing of the digits and somnolence were not seen. Only 15 cases of the 27 had evidence of right ventricular enlargement by electrocardiography. Four had polycythemia only and therefore were probably not typical cases of CMS but represented chronic mountain polycythemia. In all 27 cases, resolution of the syndrome occurred upon descent. Relapse occurred in the one patient who returned to high altitude. In 12 cases of CMS in the western Himalayas described by Nath in another publication, a trial of aspirin, acetazolamide, and yogic breathing exercises at high altitude resulted in clinical and objective improvement.[26] Wu and his associates have described 26 patients with CMS living between 12,070 feet (3,680 m) and 13,707 feet (4,179 m) in the northeast section of Qinghai-Tibet. All had been born at altitude and none had ever visited sea level. Twenty-two were men and four were women. The mean age was 44.6 years (± 7.8). Clinical features were similar to cases described in Peru. Hemodynamic and echocardiographic studies were performed. Data were compared with healthy Tibetans living at the same altitude. Seven patients moved to a lower altitude, 7,418 feet (2,261 m) and experienced slow improvement but symptoms returned when they moved to a higher altitude. Phlebotomy and oxygen breathing resulted in modest transient improvement especially in mental symptoms.[27]

Two possible cases of CMS have been reported from the United States, one from 10,000 feet (3,050 m) in Colorado,[13] and one from 6,500 feet (1,982 m) in California.[14] In both cases pulmonary function studies were essentially normal; arterial PCO_2 levels were slightly elevated. Improvement occurred with descent and symptoms returned three to four weeks after reascent. The results are summarized in Table 15.2. These two patients do not resemble the cases of CMS reported from Peru or the Himalayas since there was little or no evidence of significant pulmonary hypertension.

Klepper and his associates described a case of possible chronic mountain sickness in a 64-year-old man who was a lifetime resident of Mexico City, 7,500 feet (2,300 m). Clinical manifestations included exertional dyspnea, pedal edema, hypersomnolence, loud snoring during sleep with frequent arousals, and deep cyanosis. Sleep was interrupted by nine arousals per hour. The hemoglobin was 21.4 gms/100 ml and the packed cell volume was 76 percent The arterial pH was 7.27, PO_2 47 mm Hg, O_2 saturation 75 percent, and PCO_2 66 mm Hg. Evidence of pulmonary hypertension was present in the chest roentgenogram and the electrocardiogram. Echo-Doppler studies indicated a pulmonary artery systolic pressure of 50-55 mm Hg. The patient was six feet one inch tall and weighed 274 pounds.[15] In view of the obesity, the sleep disorder, and the relatively low altitude this patient probably represented the sleep apnea syndrome rather than true chronic mountain sickness. The common factor is probably a low HVR, hypoventilation becoming more severe during sleep. In a survey of 600 men in La Paz, Bolivia, 12,730 feet (3,883 m), 42 (7 percent) had a hemoglobin of >22.7 gms/100 ml. Most of these men were elderly and obese which may be a factor in excessive polycythemia and possibly CMS.[16]

CMS usually requires years of residence at high altitude to develop, although actual incidence is unknown because once symptoms appear the patient may move to a lower elevation. Also, some cases of asymptomatic chronic mountain polycythemia are often reported as cases of CMS. The low incidence of symptomatic cases is reflected by the small number of reported cases in the literature.

Table 15.2
Data from Two Reports of CMS in the United States

	Gronbeck	Hecht	Comments G	H
Sex	Female	Male		
Age	67	28		
Duration at altitude	7 years	lifetime		
Altitude	6,500 ft (2,000 m)	9,950 ft (3,015 m)		
Symptoms	fatigue - dyspnea wt. gain, edema	fatigue - dyspnea		
Duration symptoms	6 months	3 months		
Hgb	19.1 gms	22 gms		
Hcrt	60.2%	81%		
PO_2	60 mm	73% sat.	X	SLC
PCO_2	49 mm	39 mm	X	SLC
ECG	normal	mild RVH		
Chest film	upper normal	normal size		
Vital cap.	1.52 L 59%	4.5 L n = 4,300		
FEV_1	1.45 L 80%	not done		
BP	160/95	normal		
Venous admixture	nd	17% n = L6 x		X
A-V diff.	nd	4.7 n = 3.9		SLC
Cardiac index	nd	2.7 n = 2-4		SLC
PA mean pressure	nd	27 n = 15		SLC
Sleep study	no apnea	nd		
RV ejection fraction	38%	nd		
LV ejection fraction	78%	nd		
Recovery upon descent	+	+		
Return of symptoms on return to HA	+	+		
Duration of alt. exposure	3 weeks	1 month		

SOURCES: Gronbeck, ref. 14; Hecht, ref. 13.

NOTES: All studies on Gronbeck's patient were done at sea level. All studies on Hecht's patient were done at SLC except pulmonary studies, which were done at sea level. Both patients experienced a remission of symptoms upon descent to sea level and a reappearance of symptoms upon returning to altitude. The altitudes involved are relatively low compared with CMS reported from Peru.

X = sea level studies.

Pathology

Little information is available on the pathology of CMS. Only three reports of autopsy studies in four patients have been published,[28,29,30] and they probably did not have typical CMS. Two had obesity and two had kyphoscoliosis. All four deaths were due to cardiac insufficiency. Arias-Stella and his associates reviewed three previously reported autopsies and added a report of a 48-year-old woman who was born and raised in Cerro de Pasco, altitude 14,200 feet (4,330 m).[30] Major clinical symptoms were progressive dyspnea, edema, and cough with hemoptysis. Major findings at autopsy included generalized edema and marked cyanosis, pronounced dorsal kyphoscoliosis, and hypertrophy and dilatation of the right ventricle and right atrium; the heart weighed 320 gms. (The patient weighed 47 kg/103 lbs.) The weight of the right ventricle was approximately 67 percent of the total ventricular weight (normal = 30 percent). Severe atheromas were present in the pulmonary artery and its branches, and muscularization of the peripheral pulmonary arteries was present with some intimal fibrosis. Fresh and partially organized thrombi were found in the large, medium, and small pulmonary arteries. Pleural effusions, ascites, and congestion of the liver confirmed the presence of right heart failure. This case, like the other three, is not typical of CMS and probably represents a case of cor pulmonale with right ventricular failure due to kyphoscoliosis aggravated by high altitude. Recurrent pulmonary emboli occurred before death.

Clearly, one of the problems in the recognition and study of "pure" cases of CMS is the possible presence of other disease conditions that predispose patients to arterial unsaturation and pulmonary hypertension at high altitude, including kyphoscoliosis, emphysema, pulmonary fibrosis, and obesity. Heath has taken the position that CMS is not "a distinct pathological entity,"[28] and in terms of a diagnostic anatomic entity, he is, of course, correct. But CMS is certainly a well-defined functional disorder, and in that sense it is a distinct pathophysiologic entity. Hurtado's sage reply to Heath's denial of CMS as a distinct pathologic entity was that a similar argument could be made to deny the existence of some mental diseases!

Physiological Aspects of CMS

Polycythemia. A constant finding in CMS is a marked increase in red cell volume, hematocrit, hemoglobin, and blood viscosity. Chronic hypoxemia probably related to hypoventilation and a decrease in the hypoxic ventilatory response (HVR) is the likely cause; however, an increase in hematocrit or hemoglobin above arbitrary limits is not a diagnostic criterion of CMS, since there is a considerable overlap of these values with asymptomatic individuals. There appears to be no relation between arterial oxygen saturation at rest and the hematocrit (See Fig. 15.4.)

Winslow examined the effect of reducing the hematocrit in three patients with CMS by phlebotomy.[31] In one patient, reduction of hematocrit from 67 percent to 46 percent increased exercise capacity, reduced the oxygen consumption at a given workload, increased the anaerobic threshold, and resulted in less fatigue during exertion. Winslow and Monge obtained similar results in eight patients with CMS who had hematocrits reduced by phlebotomy or phlebotomy and a saline infusion.[1] Exercise capacity and maximum heart rate were increased. Pulmonary artery pressure decreased and resting arterial oxygen saturation increased. Improvement was variable, being marked in some patients but very slight in others. In two patients symptoms of CMS were markedly improved. Cardiac output was increased to maintain normal tissue oxygen delivery (Table 15.3).[31] The severity of CMS was probably mild, since all subjects had nearly normal working capacities. Improvement in gas exchange by reduction in hematocrit has been reported by Cruz.[20] The

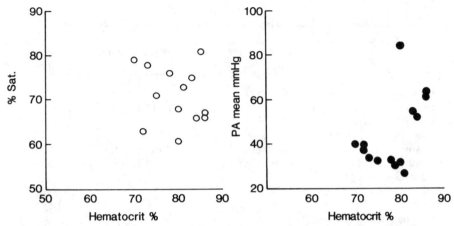

Figure 15.4. *Left panel:* Relation between hematocrit and arterial oxygen saturation in 13 patients with CMS. No correlation is evident. *Right panel:* Relation between hematocrit and mean pulmonary artery pressure in 14 patients with CMS. Little correlation is evident except that when the hematocrit is above 80 percent a higher PA mean pressure may be present. Studies performed during exercise may have resulted in a better correlation. Data from published literature and personal observations.

beneficial results of phlebotomy are not unexpected: since similar results have followed phlebotomy in sea-level patients with polycythemia due to pulmonary disease[32] or congenital heart disease.[33,34]

Hypoventilation. Several studies have shown that natives born at high altitude or persons who have lived at high altitude for a long time exhibit a decreased ventilatory response to hypoxia (HVR).[21,22,35-37] The insensitivity to hypoxia appears in those born at sea level only after many months or years of exposure to altitude.[38] It is possible that this phenomenon represents medullary respiratory center depression by chronic hypoxia.[21,22] Arterial PCO_2 is slightly elevated.

Lozano studied six high altitude residents with marked polycythemia (mean hematocrit 75 percent). The arterial PCO_2 was 34.8 mm compared with 31.9 mm in six normal subjects living at the same altitude.[39] Symptoms were mild or absent and all were able to work. Cruz has reported a mean arterial PCO_2 in 22 patients of 38.1 mm ± 2.9 compared with 32.5 mm ± 2.5 in normal residents.[40] Values for arterial PCO_2 in normal residents and pH in high altitude residents are 32 mm and 7.43, respectively.[21] Collected data are shown in Figure 15.5.

Studies in the United States have confirmed these observations. Weil reported that long-term residents of Leadville, Colorado, 10,150 feet (3,100 m) had a diminished HVR compared with residents of Denver, Colorado, 5,400 feet (1,635 m).[38] A lesser degree of blunted HVR was seen in non-native residents of Leadville (Fig.15.6). The blunted response was related to the length of time spent at altitude; after 25 years the response was similar to that of native residents. Depression of the response to CO_2 was also present in the Leadville residents. Exercise ventilation was not diminished, however. The hypoventilation syndrome at sea level has many of the features of CMS, including polycythemia and pulmonary hypertension.[41,42]

Thus an important feature of patients with CMS is a reduced HVR, a diminished respiratory response to CO_2, and a slight increase in arterial PCO_2 compatible with

Table 15.3
Changes Induced by Decreasing the Hematocrit in Eight Patients with CMS

	Control	Posthemodilution	Percent Change
Hematocrit	67%	49%	-27%
Maximum work	475 Kpm	638 Kpm	+ 34%
Maximum heart rate	138/min	162/min	+ 17%
Maximum ventilation	53 L/min	52 L/min	no change
PA pressure	40/30 mm Hg	23/15 mm Hg	-43/50%
Ventilatory threshold	0.793 L/min	1.005 L/min	+27%
O_2 saturation			
rest	80%	85%	+ 6%
exercise	71%	70%	no change
Cardiac output[a]			
rest	4.1 L/min	5.4 L/min	+32%
exercise	4.6 L/min	9.6 L/min	+109%
Heart rate[b]			
rest	93/min	109/min	+17%
exercise	106/min	132/min	+25%
A-V difference			
rest	15.0 ml/100 ml	9.0 ml/100 ml	-40%
exercise	17.9 ml/100 ml	11.3 ml/100 ml	-37%

SOURCE: Winslow et al., ref. 31.

NOTES: These data indicate that hemodilution in patients with CMS is accompanied by an increase in maximum work capacity and a decrease in pulmonary artery pressure. The improvement in cardiac performance is indicated by the higher cardiac output and lower A-V difference both at rest and during exercise. These results suggest that right ventricular failure had been present prior to hemodilution. Right ventricular filling pressures were not reported.

[a] Data from Winslow and Monge, ref. 1.
[b] Measurements made in one subject at a constant exercise workload of 300 K pm/min.

the hypoventilation that is an important cause of the low arterial oxygen saturation in these patients. Native life-long residents in the Peruvian Andes have little or no increase in ventilation with hypoxia compared to acclimatized newcomers (Fig. 15.7).

Hypoxemia. A marked decrease in arterial oxygen saturation is present in all patients with CMS. Hypoventilation is an important cause, but other factors are also present, such as abnormal lung function, an increased A-a gradient and sleep hypoxemia. The mechanism of the effect of polycythemia upon pulmonary gas exchange is unknown, but arterial oxygen saturations are increased by a reduction in hematocrit. Animal studies by West and his associates have shown that acute polycythemia had no deleterious effects upon acute pulmonary gas exchange in dogs within the hematocrit range of 36-76 percent.[43] Some patients exhibit a significant right-to-left shunt not corrected by 100 percent oxygen. Shunting via a patent foramen ovale may occur, but this has not been investigated. Kreuzer and Tenney reported an increased A-a gradient in patients with CMS.[44]

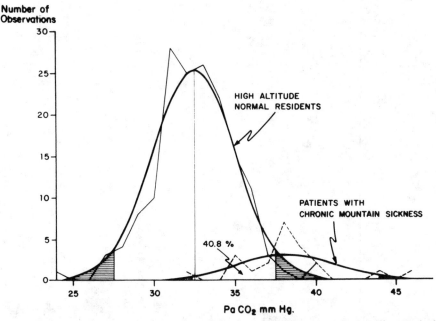

Figure 15.5. Arterial PCO_2 in normal high altitude residents and patients with CMS. Differences in the height of the curves represent different numbers of subjects and patients studied. Mean and standard deviation of 159 normals and 22 CMS patients were 32.5 ± 2.5 mm and 38.1 ± 2.9 mm, respectively. The best Gaussian curves have been fitted using the normal equation. From Cruz and Recavarren, ref. 20.

Kryger and Grover studied 20 men in Leadville with hematocrits exceeding 58 percent and 10 men with normal hematocrits for that altitude.[45,46] Ten of the study group had some abnormalities of lung function detected by spirometry while the other 10 had normal pulmonary functions. The results are shown in Table 15.4. A-a gradients were higher in the study group (18.0 mm and 10.1 mm) compared with 8.3 mm in the controls. Administration of 100 percent oxygen resulted in an increase in ventilation in the study group but not in the control group. Study patients had a higher respiratory rate, a smaller tidal volume, and a greater dead space ventilation than controls. Arterial saturations were lower in study patients during the day and markedly lower during sleep (Fig. 15.8). Mean arterial PCO_2 levels were higher in the study subjects (33.3 mm) compared with normal controls (31 mm), indicating hypoventilation. Isocapnic ventilatory drive was not abnormal, however, compared with control subjects. These results indicate several mechanisms resulting in increased hypoxemia in patients with polycythemia, including VA/Q abnormalities, a depressed respiratory center response to hypoxia, abnormal breathing mechanics, and sleep hypoxemia.[47]

Manier and associates examined pulmonary gas exchange in eight Andean natives with excessive polycythemia (hematocrit 65.1 ± 6.6 percent and arterial PO_2 45.6 ± 5.6 mm Hg) at an altitude of 12,000 feet (3,650 m). The hypoxemia was attributed to an increased blood flow to poorly ventilated areas of the lung but without a true intrapulmonary shunt. Hypoventilation as well as a low venous PO_2 may

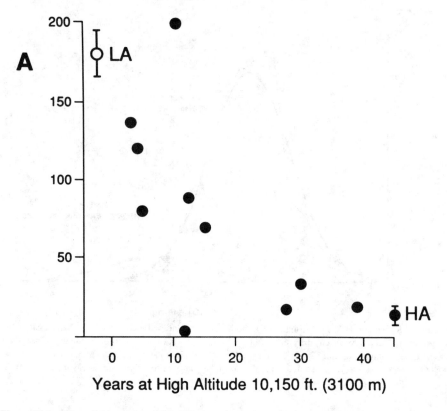

Figure 15.6. Effect of time spent at high altitude on hypoxic ventilatory drive (HVR). LA = low altitude residents; HA = high altitude residents. "A" describes the shape of the relation between ventilation and inspired oxygen tension over a wide range of alveolar oxygen tensions and is therefore a measure of ventilatory drive. From Weil, ref. 38.

also have been present. Six of the natives had an arterial PCO_2 above the mean for normal high altitude residents of 30.5 ± .8 mm Hg. Hemodilution had little effect on arterial PO_2 but ventilation increased and V_A Q mismatching fell slightly.[48]

Pulmonary hypertension. Marked pulmonary hypertension with a normal or low cardiac output is present in most cases of CMS. An important cause is hypoxic vasoconstriction, since the pulmonary artery pressure is rapidly lowered by oxygen breathing. Since oxygen does not lower the pressure to normal levels, a fixed or anatomic increase in pulmonary vascular resistance is probably also present. Thromboses in small branches of the pulmonary arterial tree may be one cause of this fixed arterial resistance. Increased blood viscosity alone does not appear to raise pulmonary artery pressure (Fig. 15.4).

Gender and age. CMS occurs largely in males. In 98 reported cases 79 were males and 19 were females. Nearly all cases have been from 22 to 51 years old. In Lhasa, high altitude polycythemia was present only in males.[24] The 27 cases reported from the western Himalayas were all males.[25] Several factors may be responsible for this sex difference. Males are more susceptible than women to sleep

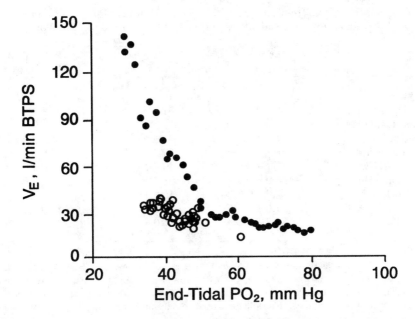

Figure 15.7. The ventilatory response to hypoxia (HVR) in an acclimatized low lander (solid circles) and a lifelong native of Cerro de Pasco (open circles), 14,200 feet (4,331 m). Note that in the native there is no significant increase in ventilation (V_E) with hypoxia. Redrawn from Winslow, ref. 1.

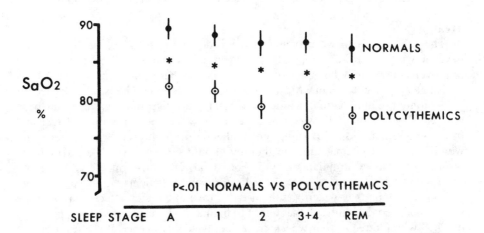

Figure 15.8. Arterial oxygen saturation SaO_2 in long-term high altitude residents while awake (A) and during stages of sleep (1-REM) at 10,160 feet (3,100 m). During sleep hypoxemia occurs in polycythemics but not in normals. Ear oximeter data. From Kryger and Grover, ref. 46.

Table 15.4
Laboratory Data from Patients with Chronic Mountain Polycythemia and
Normal Subjects, Leadville, Colorado (altitude 10,150 feet/3,100 m)

	Normal controls	Polycythemia normal lungs	Polycythemia lung disease
Number	10	10	10
Age - years	49 ± 2.6	31 ± 5.9	45 ± 6.0
Years at altitude			
>300 m	41 ± 4.0	31 ± 5.9	44.7 ± 6.0
Hematocrit %	48 ± 1.3	59.3 ± 1.7	62.0 ± 2.4
Hgb gm/100 ml	17.1 ± 0.5	19.7 ± 0.7	19.0 ± 0.8
$PaCO_2$ mm Hg	30.9 ± 0.9	33.5 ± 1.0	33.2 ± 0.9
(A-a) PO_2 mm Hg	8.3 ± 1.4	10.1 ± 1.9	18.0 ± 1.0
O_2 Sat %	91.6 ± 0.6	86.2 ± 1.1	81.0 ± 1.4
VD/VT %	35.7 ± 1.6	40.0 ± 1.7	46.0 ± 2.3

SOURCE: Kryger and Grover, ref. 49.

NOTES: $PaCO_2$ and PaO_2 = arterial PCO_2 and PO_2 respectively; (A-a) PO_2 = alveolar-arterial PO_2 difference; SaO_2 = arterial O_2 saturation; VD/VT = ratio of dead space to tidal volume. These data indicate that high altitude polycythemia is similar in many respects to the polycythemia of chronic lung disease. Note that arterial PCO_2 is higher in these conditions than in normal subjects at the same altitude, indicating the presence of some degree of hypoventilation.

hypoxemia.[47] Also, in premenopausal women menstrual blood loss and dietary iron deficiency may prevent marked polycythemia. Hematocrits in normal women at high altitude are lower than in men. Hormonal differences may also be responsible. CMS occurs in older persons. Velarde reported a mean age of 62 years in 72 patients.[19] In normal sea level subjects, arterial PO_2 decreases slightly with advancing age owing to changes in pulmonary function and a decrease in the HVR.[1]

Treatment

The most satisfactory treatment of CMS is descent to sea level. Studies in Peru, have shown that bed rest, continuous oxygen, and venesection will also result in improvement and may be employed in severe cases before descent. Improved gas exchange by phlebotomy in CMS has been reported.[1,20,31,40] The benefical effect of phlebotomy in adults with cyanotic congenital heart disease at sea level has been reviewed by Perloff.[34] Reversal of inverted T waves occurs with bed rest and oxygen administration.[18] If right ventricular failure is present, as evidenced by weight gain and edema, diuretic therapy should be employed. Acetazolamide or other respiratory stimulants may be beneficial for short-term use, although no controlled trials of acetazolamide have been reported. Patients with sleep hypoxia and polycythemia may benefit by the use of Provera, but side effects may limit its use.[49] Published data indicate that return to high altitude results in the reappearance of CMS within three to four weeks, hence permanent residence at sea level or at a much lower altitude is indicated.

Little information is available regarding the management of patients with CMS who must remain at high altitude for economic, family, or other reasons. In Peru, workers in mines at altitudes of around 14,000 feet (4,270 m) work five days a week and return to lower elevations on weekends. Some of the better-off workers may even live in Lima and return to work for five days after a weekend at home. Lopez has used periodic sojourns at a lower altitude to obtain a remission of CMS. Patients with CMS in Cuzco, Peru, are advised to make three sojourns a year, each of not less than 70 days at an elevation of 2,000 feet (600 m) to relieve symptoms and obtain a reversal of physiological abnormalities to normal.[50] Venesection, low flow oxygen at night, and the administration of Provera will be beneficial in most patients. Provera (medroxyprogesterone acetate) has been used successfully for over five years in some patients.[49] The usual dose is 20-60 mg per day. Provera has side effects, however, including impotence and cannot be tolerated by all patients.

In summary, CMS is a rare condition confined largely to persons who reside for years at altitudes exceeding 10,000 ft (3,030 m). Major presentations are fatigue, somnolence, and mental confusion. Marked polycythemia and cyanosis are present. The prevalence increases with advancing age. Descent is essential for improvement, but for those who cannot descend, continuous oxygen therapy and phlebotomy will provide improvement. CMS should be differentiated from asymptomatic mountain polycythemia, which in most instances does not require treatment.

References

1. WINSLOW R, and MONGE C. Hypoxia, polycythemia, and chronic mountain sickness. Baltimore, Md: Johns Hopkin's University Press, 1987.
2. MONGE C. La enfermedad de los Andes (sindromes eritremicos). *Anal. Facult. Med. Lima*, 1928; 11. (1):309-14.
3. TALBOTT J, and DILL D. Clinical observations at high altitude: Observations on six healthy persons living at 17,500 ft. and report of one case of chronic mountain sickness. *Am. J. Med. Sci.* 1936; 192:626-29.
4. MONGE C. High altitude disease. *Arch. Int. Med.* 1937; 59:32-40.
5. HURTADO A. Chronic mountain sickness. *JAMA* 1942; 120:1278-82.
6. MONGE C. Life in the Andes and chronic mountain sickness. *Science* 1942; 95:79-84.
7. MONGE C. Chronic mountain sickness. *Physiol. Rev.* 1943; 23:166-84.
8. MONGE M, and MONGE C. High altitude disease: Mechanism and management. Springfield, Ill: C. Thomas, 1966.
9. ROTTA A, CANEPA A, HURTADO A, VELASQUEZ T, and CHAVEZ R. Pulmonary circulation at sea level and high altitude. *J. Appl. Physiol.* 1956; 9:328-36.
10. BANCHERO N, SIME F. PENALOZA D, et al. Pulmonary pressure, cardiac output, and arterial oxygen saturation during exercise at high altitude and at sea level. *Circulation* 1966; 33:249-62.
11. PENALOZA D, and SIME F. Chronic cor pulmonale due to loss of altitude acclimatization (chronic mountain sickness). *Am. J. Med.* 1974; 50:728-43.
12. LOPEZ C. Soroche cronico. *Rev. Peruana Card.* 1969; 55:45-52.
13. HECHT H, and MCCLEMENT J. A case of chronic mountain sickness in the United States. *Am. J. Med.* 1958; 25:470-77.
14. GRONBECK C. Chronic mountain sickness at an elevation of 2,000 m. *Chest* 1984; 85:577-78.
15. KLEPPER M. BARNARD P, and ESCHENBACHER W. A case of chronic mountain sickness diagnosed by routine pulmonary function tests. *Chest* 1991; 100:823-25.
16. TUFTS D, HAAS J, BEARD J, and SPILVOGEL H. Distribution of hemoglobin and functional consequences of anemia in adult males at high altitude. *Am. J. Clin. Nutr.* 1985; 42:1-11.
17. RENNIE D. Splinter hemorrhages at high altitude. *JAMA* 1974; 288:974-75.
18. MARTICORENA E. Personal communication.

19. VELARDE O. Monge's disease. Paper presented at the First National Congress of High Altitude Medicine, La Oroya, Peru, 1981.
20. CRUZ A, and RECAVARREN S. Chronic mountain sickness: A pulmonary vascular disease. In W Brendel and R Zink, eds., *High altitude physiology and medicine*, New York: Springer Verlag, 1982, pp 271-77.
21. SEVERINGHAUS J, and CARCELEN A. Cerebrospinal fluid in man native to high altitude. *J. Appl. Physiol.* 1964; 19:319-21.
22. SEVERINGHAUS J, BAINTON D, and CARCELEN A. Respiratory insensitivity to hypoxia in chronically hypoxic man. *Resp. Physiol.* 1966; 1:308-34.
23. REATEGUI-LOPEZ. Soroche cronico: observaciones realizadas en el Cuzco en 30 casos. *Rev. Peruana Cardiol.* 1969; 15:45-52.
24. HU S, Hypoxia in China: An overview. In *Hypoxia, exercise, and altitude*, eds. J Sutton, C Houston, and N Jones. New York: A.R. Liss, 1983; 157-82.
25. NATH C, KASHYAP S, and SUBRAMANIAN A. Chronic mountain sickness-probrang type. *Defense Sci. J.* 1984; 34:443-50.
26. NATH C, KASHYAP S, and SUBRAMANIAN A. Chronic mountain sickness. Probrang type. *Armed Forces Med. J. India*, 1983; 39:131-40.
27. WU T, ZHANG Q, JIN B, et al. Chronic mountain sickness (Monge's disease): An observation in Quinghai-Tibet plateau. In *High altitude medicine*, ed. G Ueda, J Reeves, and M. Segiguchi. Matsumoto, Japan: Shinshu University, 1992: 314-24.
28. HEATH D, and WILLIAMS D. *Man at high altitude*. Edinburgh: Churchill, Livingstone, 1977: 137-51.
29. FERNAN-ZEGARRA L, and LAZO TOBOADA F. Man de montaña cronico: Consideraciónes anatómopatológicas y referencias clinicas de un caso. *Rev. Peruana Patol.* 1961; 6:49-55.
30. ARIAS-STELLA A, KRUGER H, and RACAVARREN S. Pathology of chronic mountain sickness. *Thorax* 1973; 28:701-08.
31. WINSLOW R, STATHAM N, GIBSON C, et al. Improved oxygen delivery in polycythemic natives of high altitude. *Blood* 1979; 54; Suppl 61A. Abstract.
32. RAKITA L, GILLESPIE D, and SANCETTA S. The acute and chronic effects of phlebotomy on general hemodynamics and pulmonary functions of patients with secondary polycythemia, associated with pulmonary emphysema. *Am. Heart J.* 1965; 70:466-75.
33. ROSENTHAL A, NATHAN D, MARTY A, et al. Acute hemodynamic effects of red cell volume reduction in polycythemia of congenital heart disease. *Circulation* 1970; 42:297-307.
34. PERLOFF J, ROSOVE M, CHILD J, and WRIGHT G. Adults with cyanotic congenital heart disease: Hematologic management. *Ann. Int. Med.* 1988; 109:406-13.
35. CHIODI H. Respiratory adaptations to chronic high altitude hypoxia. *J. Appl. Physiol.* 1957; 10: 81- 87.
36. SORENSEN S, and SEVERINGHAUS J. Irreversible respiratory insensitivity to acute hypoxia in man born at high altitude. *J. Appl. Physiol.* 1968; 25:217-20.
37. SEVERINGHAUS J. Hypoxic respiratory drive and its loss during chronic hypoxia. *Clin. Physiol.* 1972; 2:57-79.
38. WEIL J, BYRNE-QUINN E, SODAL I, et al. Acquired attenuation of chemoreceptor function in chronically hypoxic man at high altitude. *J. Clin. Invest.* 1971; 50:186-95.
39. LOZANO R, and MONGE C. Renal function in high altitude natives and in natives with chronic mountain sickness. *J. Appl. Physiol.* 1965; 20: 1026-27.
40. CRUZ J, DIAZ C, MARTICORENA J, and HILARIO V. Phlebotomy improves gas exchange in chronic mountain polycythemia. *Respiration* 1979; 38:305- 13.
41. VOGEL J, HARTLEY H, JAMIESON G, and GROVER R. Impairment of ventilatory response to hypoxia in individuals with obesity and hypoventilation: A concept of the Pickwickian syndrome. *Circulation* 1967; 36;Suppl 2:258. Abstract.
42. BERGOFSKY E. Cor pulmonale in the syndrome of alveolar hypoventilation. *Prog. in CV Dis.* 1967; 9:414.
43. WEST J, BALGOS A, and WILFORD D. Does polycythemia impair pulmonary gas exchange? *Physiologist* 1988; 31:121-22. Abstract.
44. KRUEZER F, TENNEY S, MITHOEFER J, and REMMERS J. Alveolar-arterial oxygen gradient in Andean natives at high altitude. *J. Appl. Physiol.* 1964; 19:13-16.
45. KRYGER M, MCCULLOUGH R, DOCKEL R, et al. Excessive polycythemia of high altitude: Role of ventilatory drive and lung disease. *Am. Rev. Respir. Dis.* 1978; 118:659-66.
46. KRYGER M, and GROVER R. Chronic mountain sickness. *Sem. Respir. Med.* 1983; 5:164-68.

47. BLOCK A, BOYSEN P, WYNNE J, and HUNT L. Sleep apnea, hypopnea, and oxygen desaturation in normal subjects: A strong male predominance. *N. Engl. J. Med.* 1979; 300:513-17.

48. MANIER G, GUENARD H, GASTAING Y, et al. Pulmonary gas exchange in Andean natives with excessive polycythemia - effect of hemodilution. *J. Appl Physiol.* 1988; 65:2107-17.

49. KRYGER M, MCCULLOUGH R, et al. Treatment of excessive polycythemia of high altitude with respiratory stimulant drugs. *Am. Rev. Resp. Dis.* 1978; 117:455-64.

50. LOPEZ L. Mal de montaña chronico: Tratamiento y prevención. *Primeras J. Med. y Cir. de Altura.* La Oroya, Peru, 1978.

CHAPTER 16

Sleep

SUMMARY

Disturbance of sound sleep characterized by frequent arousals, periodic breathing, shortness of breath and many dreams is the most common discomfort experienced at high altitude. Periodic breathing consists of three to four deep breaths, followed by a complete cessation of breathing for eight to twelve seconds for a total cycle length of eighteen to twenty seconds. During sleep both at sea level and high altitude ventilation is depressed and there is a resulting fall in arterial oxygen saturation. At sea level the resulting fall in arterial saturation is slight, but at high altitude the shape of the O_2 dissociation curve results in substantial falls in arterial saturation. There is considerable individual variation in the degree of sleep hypoxemia: at 17,500 feet (5,337 m), some arterial saturations fall to as low as 40 percent for most of the night. Periodic breathing and sleep hypoxemia tend to diminish with acclimatization and both may be abolished by acetazolamide.

• • •

The inability to obtain sound and restful sleep is one of the most common discomforts experienced by the visitor to high altitude. Disturbed sleep tends to diminish after the first week or two after arrival, but in some persons the inability to sleep may persist for months and may require descent.

Typically the newcomer to high altitude experiences the following general symptoms during sleeping hours: frequent arousals, periodic breathing, shortness of breath, frequent dreams, and headache. Headache and symptoms of AMS may be severe in the morning after arising and diminish during the day. Studies of newcomers brought to 10,000 feet (3,050 m) and 12,470 feet (3,815 m) revealed an incidence of disturbed sleep of 83 percent compared with symptoms of headache (33 percent) and anorexia (25 percent). Hackett and his associates noted periodic breathing in 22 percent of climbers at 14,000 feet (4,270 m) on Mount McKinley.[2]

Sleep stages may be roughly classified into three general levels: light sleep (Stages 1 and 2), deep sleep (Stages 3 and 4), and rapid eye movement (REM) sleep, which occurs at repetitive intervals during the sleep period and is usually associated with dreaming. (Table 16.1 shows the classification sequence). During REM sleep, bursts of rapid eye movement can be detected by small electrodes attached to the skin of the scalp. REM sleep occurs approximately every 90 minutes and with each occurrence lasts longer. During REM sleep respiratory rate, heart rate, and blood pressure exhibit fluctuations that do not usually occur in light or deep sleep stages.[3] As sleep progresses from Stage 1 to Stage 4, respiratory rate, heart rate, and blood pressure progressively decrease.

Frequent Arousals

Anholm and his associates studied five subjects exposed to a progressive increase in simulated altitude for six weeks (Operation Everest II).[4] Nighttime awak-

Table 16.1
Classification of Sleep Stages

Stage	Activity pattern
Sleep onset	Periodic breathing may occur. Frequent arousals.
Non-rapid eye movement sleep, Stages 1-2, light sleep	Respiration may be irregular with some apneas or decreased breathing. Heart rate decreases. Blood pressure decreases slightly.
Stages 3-4, deep sleep	Regular respiration, rare apneas. Heart rate slower. Blood pressure falls further.
Rapid eye movement sleep	Respiration may be regular or irregular. Apneas more common with REM sleep than with non-REM sleep. Heart rate fluctuates. Blood pressure fluctuates.

SOURCE: Martin, ref. 3.

enings occurred 37 times per subject at 21,400 feet (7,620 m) with 15 awakenings on return to sea level (p <0.05). Total sleep time decreased from 337 minutes at sea level to 167 minutes. REM sleep decreased from 18 percent of sleep time at sea level to four percent. Brief arousals increased from 22 to 161 per hours. At 21,400 feet (7,620 m) sleep arterial oxygen saturation was 52 percent. All of the subjects exhibited periodic breathing during most of the sleep period. Symptoms and periodic breathing were as frequent at 16,000 feet (4,880 m) as at 26,500 feet (8,050 m). Frequent arousals may result in a modified sleep deprivation state with fatigue and sleepiness during the day.

Periodic Breathing

In 1886 Mosso noted a curious pattern of breathing in his brother during altitude studies in the Alps at elevations of 11,877 feet (3,620 m) and 14,961 feet (4,5605 m).[5] The pattern consisted of three to four deep breaths followed by a cessation of breathing for approximately ten seconds. This alternation occurred over long periods of time during sleep. A reconstructed drawing of the breathing pattern in Mosso's brother is shown in Figure 16.1. (The original recording was made by Mosso on a smoked revolving drum.) Mosso also observed other patterns of abnormal breathing during his studies, including cycles of deep breathing alternating with periods of shallow breathing without cessation of respiration. A typical pattern of periodic breathing at 12,500 feet (3,815 m) in a young physician is shown in Figure 16.2. The total cycle length consisting of two or three deep breaths, followed by apnea is approximately 18-20 seconds. Periodic breathing occurs in nearly every person at some time during sleep at altitudes greater than 10,000 feet (3,050 m). It is not uncommon at Aspen, Colorado (8,000 feet/2,440 m). Occasionally periodic breathing may occur at rest during the awake state. It is less common in women than in men.[6] The urge to take a few deep breaths is uncomfortable and is associated

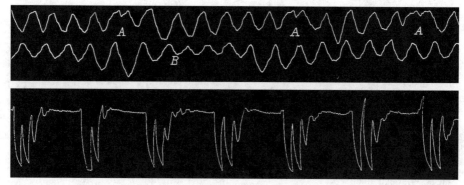

Fig. 16.1. Periodic breathing patterns recorded in 1886 by Angelo Mosso on his brother, Ugolino, during sleep at the Regina Margherita Hut at 3,620 m (upper panel) and at 4,560 m (lower panel). In the lower panel, the periods of apnea (arrest of breathing) are 12 seconds in duration. From Mosso, ref. 5.

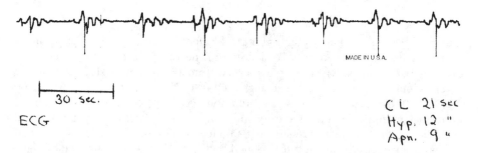

Figure 16.2. Periodic breathing in a young physician at 12,470 feet (3,800 m) during sleep. Note one deep breath followed by two or three smaller breaths and apnea for 9 seconds. Total cycle length, approximately 21 seconds. From Malconian et al., ref. 25.

with frequent arousals caused by the sensation of shortness of breath. During the apneic phase (absence of breathing activity) in the awake state the urge to breathe disappears. Persons who snore during periodic breathing can make companions miserable! Periodic breathing does not appear to become more frequent with increasing altitudes above 10,000 feet (3,050 m). Most episodes of periodic breathing occur during non-REM quiet sleep. Oxygen inhalation will eliminate periodic breathing.[6,7] (See Fig. 16.3).

Masuyama and his associates studied periodic breathing at an altitude of 17,580 feet (5,360 m) in nine climbers.[8,9] The climbers with a high HVR (hypoxic ventilatory responses) had the most frequent and longest periods of periodic breathing at altitude. It was also observed that the longer the periodic breathing, the higher was the sleep arterial oxygen saturation. The authors concluded that periodic breathing improves arterial oxygenation, because the mean arterial oxygen saturation during periodic breathing was significantly higher than the saturation before the onset of

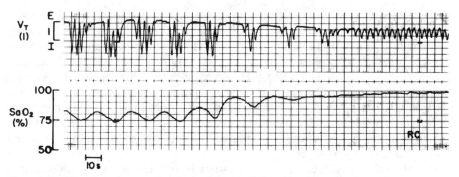

Figure 16.3. The effect of oxygen breathing upon periodic breathing (above) and arterial oxygen saturation (below) during sleep at 17,700 feet (5,400 m). Periodic breathing is replaced by shallow, continuous breathing as arterial oxygen saturation is increased. From Lahiri et al., ref. 21.

periodic breathing. Periodic breathing therefore appears to be physiologically advantageous for the healthy sojourner from the lowland. White and his associates have reported similar observations.[10]

Cyclic variations in heart rate and rhythm accompany periodic breathing, with a rapid rate during deep breathing and a slow rate during apnea. Periodic breathing is a harmless phenomenon and should not be considered a symptom of AMS. Frequent arousals and severe sleep disturbance, however, are usually considered to be symptoms of AMS. Periodic breathing is the appropriate term for this phenomenon occurring in normal persons. Cheyne-Stokes breathing (first described by John Cheyne and William Stokes over 150 years ago)[11] is a similar alternation of deep breathing (hyperpnea) and cessation of breathing (apnea) occurring in patients with heart failure. The cycle length is longer, with a duration of up to 40 seconds depending upon the degree of heart failure, and there are hyperpneic periods and apneic periods of approximately similar duration. Periodic breathing is associated with cyclic variations in arterial PO_2 and PCO_2. Cheyne-Stokes breathing in patients with heart failure exhibits a similar cyclic change in arterial PO_2 despite the longer cycles. It should be noted that in both types of periodic breathing the arterial PO_2 is lowest when breathing is occurring and highest when breathing has ceased. This is an example of the delay in the circulation time and in the response of the carotid bodies to a change in PO_2. Periodic breathing at altitudes has been reviewed by Strohl and Fouke.[12]

Nocturnal Dyspnea. Awakenings with a sensation of shortness of breath are common during sleep at high altitude. Although they are most commonly associated with periodic breathing, they may also be accompanied by a severe, prolonged sensation of not being able to take a full, deep satisfying breath and a sensation of a tight constricting band around the chest. Unlike dyspnea due to heart failure, the sensation is not relieved by sitting up or walking about. It may last for hours or even throughout the night, and there may be an accompanying feeling of panic and fear. The symptom usually disappears after arising and becoming active. A possible explanation is that the symptom is due to mild HAPE caused by sleep hypoxemia. It is well known that symptoms of HAPE may worsen during nighttime hours. This explanation is speculative, since no studies have been made of this phenomenon.

Sleep hypoxemia. During sleep in normal persons, central nervous system activity is diminished, as evidenced by the loss of temperature control, muscle flaccidity, and increased pain threshold and a decrease in respiratory rate, heart rate and blood pressure.[13,14,15] The decrease in respiratory activity results in a slight increase in arterial PCO_2 with a corresponding slight decrease in PO_2 that can only be detected by careful monitoring. Patients with obesity, pulmonary disease, or obstructive airway disease may experience severe degrees of hypoxemia during sleep.[16] Sleep hypoxemia has also been observed in normal persons during sleep at sea level.[17] At high altitude most normal persons exhibit significant hypoxemia during sleep, and in some cases it may be severe.

In the study by Anholm described earlier in this chapter five subjects in a hypobaric chamber exhibited a mean arterial oxygen saturation of 41 percent during sleep at a simulated altitude of 26,500 feet (8,050 m) compared with a mean saturation of 58 percent when awake.[4] The results at three altitudes are summarized in Table 16.2. In a study of five normal subjects on Mount Logan by Sutton and associates, all subjects experienced marked sleep hypoxemia at 11,000 feet (3,355 m). Three subjects at 17,500 feet (5,340 m) over an eight day period had even greater degrees of hypoxemia.[18] Changes in arterial oxygen saturation in two subjects are illustrated in Figure 16.4. One of the two subjects spent half of the night with an arterial oxygen saturation of approximately 40 percent. Short-term acclimatization over a period of eight to eleven days improved arterial saturation during sleep from a mean initial value of 63 percent ± 10 increasing to 73 percent ± 5. Acclimatization over a longer period of time does not appear to reduce sleep hypoxemia. In another study, Powles and Sutton observed twenty subjects at one week and after six weeks of exposure to 17,500 feet (5,340 m) on Mount Logan. They found that awake arterial oxygen saturations were the same at one week and six weeks, that is, 96 percent and 73 percent. Hypoxemia during sleep was also similar at one and six weeks: 67 percent and 61 percent. Periodic breathing was not associated with a greater degree of sleep hypoxemia although variations in O_2 saturation were greater.[19] At sea level, sleep hypoxemia could not be predicted by ventilatory responses either to hypercapnia or to isocapnic hypoxia. Hypoxemia during sleep was less severe in two women than in three men. Sleep hypoxemia may result in frequent awakenings caused by headache and/or shortness of breath, and it is probably the basis for the increasing severity of symptoms of AMS, HAPE, and HACE during the night and

Table 16.2
Sleep Hypoxemia at Three Simulated Altitudes

Altitude		Bar. press	Percent of Arterial O_2 saturation	
feet	meters	mm Hg	Whole night	Awake
16,000	4,527	429	78.6	81.0
21,400	6,100	347	66.1	69.4
26,500	7,620	282	52.2	53.7

SOURCE: Anholm et al., ref. 4.

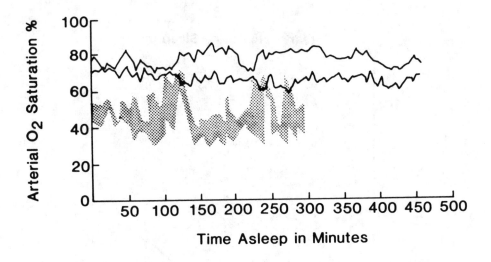

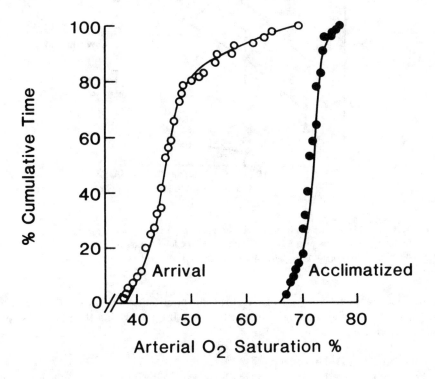

Figure 16.4. The upper figure shows arterial oxygen satuation in a normal subject who was airlifted to 17,500 feet (5,340 m) and studied three nights after arrival and eleven days later. The shaded area indicates the arterial saturation during the first study and the lines indicate the range of arterial saturation during the second study. The improvement in saturation is probably due to acclimatization, since no medications were administered. The panel below, from the same subject, indicates the arterial oxygen satuation against the percent of sumulative sleep time. The shift of the curve to the right indicates the effect of acclimatization. From Sutton et al., ref. 18.

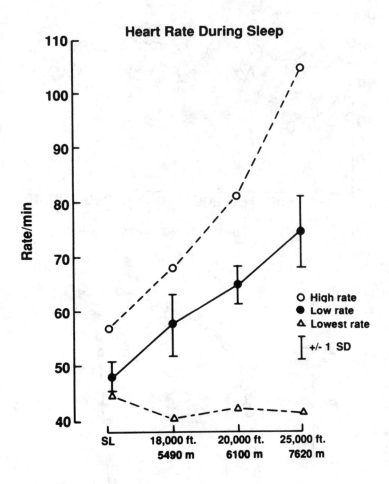

Figure 16.5. Mean heart rates in eight subjects during sleep at sea level and at three altitudes. The high and low rates represent rates over a one-minute period. The lowest rates are the lowest transient rates observed during sinus arrhythmia. From Malconian et al., ref. 25.

in the first few hours after arising. Hemoconcentration occurs during the night, as evidenced by a higher hemoglobin and hematocrit upon arising than before sleep. (See Chapter 6.)

Cardiac Rhythm During Sleep

Few studies have been made of the heart rate and rhythm during sleep at high altitude. Cummings recorded his own electrocardiogram during sleep at 16,500 feet (5,033 m) and noted a pronounced sinus arrhythmia with heart rates as low as 33 beats per minute. Atrial premature beats and junctional escape beats were present.[20]

Lahiri reported studies on eight acclimatized lowlanders during sleep at 20,800 feet (6,300 m). Periodic breathing was present from 56-90 percent of the study period. The mean cycle length was 20 ± 2 seconds with an apneic duration of 8 ± 1 second. Cycling of the heart rate occurred, with the highest rate at the end of the period of hyperventilation.[7,21,22] At 25,000 feet (7,620 m) studies in four subjects revealed sinus arrhythmia in three, atrial premature beats in two, and ventricular premature beats in one subject.[4]

Twenty-four-hour ambulatory ECGs were recorded on fourteen climbers at altitudes of 14,430 feet (4,400 m), 25,600 feet (7,800 m), and 18,730 feet (5,710 m) during expeditionary climbs by Horii and his associates.[23] The mean heart rate at these altitudes when awake was 94/min ± 4.9 and 75/min ± 6.7 when asleep. The lowest mean heart rate when asleep was 62/min ± 5.0. In some climbers the normal circadian rhythm at sea level almost completely disappeared, with mean heart rates being similar when awake and during sleep. Prolongation of the QT interval was noted especially during sleep. Arrhythmias were not described. Karliner and his associates reported similar findings on Mount Everest.[24]

More complete data were obtained in seven subjects during a simulated ascent of Mount Everest in a hypobaric chamber (OEII).[25] All were studied at sea level and 18,000 feet (5,490 m); six were also studied at 20,000 feet (6,100 m), and four at 25,000 feet (7,625 m). Heart rates (over a 60-second period) varied from sinus bradycardia to sinus tachycardia. At each altitude the lowest rates were similar (41/min), but the fastest rates were higher at each altitude, being 105/min at 25,000 feet (7,625 m) (see Fig. 16.5). Rapid cycling of the heart rate presumably related to periodic breathing occurred at each altitude. Each cycle consisted of six beats at a slow rate (mean 40/min) followed by an abrupt increase in rate of sixteen beats at 120/min (Fig. 16.6 and 16.7). Cycle lengths were shorter at higher altitudes. Cycling was not observed during sleep at sea level. Periodic breathing and cycling of the heart rate were observed during sleep at 12,500 feet (3,813 m), but the magnitude of the change in heart rate was less.[25]

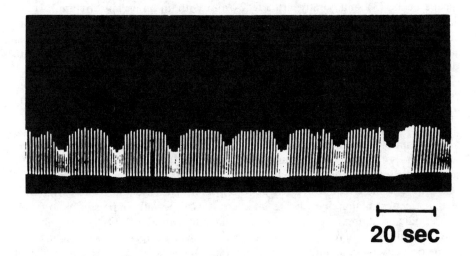

20 sec

Figure 16.6. Cycling of the heart rate at 347 mm Hg (6,100 m) in one subject. This recording of an ambulatory monitoring tape shows fast rate (shorter vertical lines) and the slow rate (taller vertical lines). The cycle length is 17.5 seconds. From Malconian et al., ref. 25.

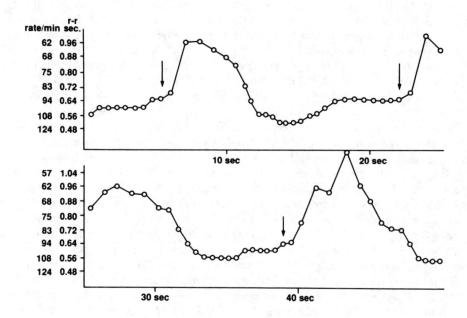

Figure 16.7. Changes in beat to beat r-r intervals and heart rate during three respiratory cycles at 282 mm Hg (7,620 m). Onset of apneas indicated by vertical arrows. From Malconian et al., ref. 25.

Bradyarrhythmias were common during sleep at each altitude, but not at sea level.[25] Arrhythmias recorded were: (1) blocked P waves without a preceding P-R prolongation, (2) sinus arrest or marked bradycardia with junctional or ventricular escape beats, (3) sinus bradycardia to 24/min without an escape rhythm, (4) AV dissociation with a junctional rhythm, and (5) idioventricular rhythm. The mechanism of these arrhythmias at high altitude remains to be explained. Since similar arrhythmias with cyclic variations in heart rate have been reported in patients with sleep apnea at sea level, hypoxemia is probably an important causative factor. In such patients atropine blocked the cyclic arrhythmia by eliminating the bradycardia, but 100 percent oxygen only moderately blunted the changes in the heart rates, indicating that the arrhythmias were primarily mediated by vagal effects upon the sinus node.[26]

Mechanism of Sleep Disorders

The basis for frequent arousals during sleep at high altitude is poorly understood. Clearly, some arousals are caused by periodic breathing, shortness of breath, headache, and the effect of hypoxia upon central nervous system function. Intermittent airway obstruction may also result in arousals, especially in persons who snore.

Periodic breathing is related to hypoxemia, a low arterial PCO_2, and an inherent normal rhythmicity in respiration, which increases and decreases in a cyclic manner. The periodicity is present during sleep but not in the awake state.[13,14,15] At sea level the central control of respiration is finely tuned to very slight changes in arterial PCO_2, with an increase in PCO_2 stimulating breathing and a decrease inhibiting respiration. The system is very rapidly responsive. At high altitude, especially during the first week or two after arrival, respiration is largely controlled by the peripheral chemoreceptors, which are responsive to changes in arterial PO_2. Arterial PCO_2 is decreased owing to hypoxic hyperventilation and thus exerts less control over breathing. Because the peripheral chemoreceptors respond more slowly to changes in arterial PO_2, the normal cyclical changes in respiration are exaggerated: a decrease in breathing will cause a rise in arterial PCO_2 and stimulate breathing. The increased breathing then lowers arterial PCO_2 and elevates PO_2, but the carotid bodies will not stimulate respiration as much, and thus a cyclical pattern results. The apneic cycles during periodic breathing are not caused by airway obstruction but rather are due to failure of the stimuli to reach a threshold of stimulation, since during apnea there is no activity of the respiratory muscles, diaphragm, or abdomen. A very crude analogy of the CO_2 and O_2 control systems is the driver of an automobile on a freeway with a companion. The driver uses his speedometer to arrive at and maintain a steady rate of speed with only slight variations. This is the CO_2 control system. Suppose the speedometer is no longer operative and the driver's companion now controls the rate of speed by estimating the velocity and ordering the driver to speed up or slow down. Greater variations in speed will occur. This represents the O_2-CO_2 control system. After one to two weeks at high altitude the initial respiratory alkalosis is compensated for by the excretion of bicarbonate, and the tendency for periodic breathing is diminished; PCO_2 levels remain low, however, and in many persons periodic breathing may persist throughout the altitude stay. Acclimatized native residents of high altitude do not exhibit periodic breathing. Lahiri and his associates have shown that whereas high altitude Sherpas do not exhibit periodic breathing, low altitude Sherpas do.[6]

The basis of sleep hypoxemia is probably the depression of central respiratory control mechanisms by alkalosis and by damping of ventilation by the low arterial PO_2—a self-reenforcing feedback loop. During sleep even at sea level, central nervous system functions are "turned down," with a resulting decrease in ventilation. The magnitude of the decrease in ventilation at high altitude during sleep is probably similar to the magnitude of the decrease at sea level, but because of the shape of the O_2 dissociation curve, the fall in arterial oxygen saturation is greater (Fig. 16.8). In some persons hypoxic respiratory depression may occur. Animal studies have demonstrated that respiration may be depressed by severe hypoxia.[27] In cases of severe HAPE where severe hypoxemia is present, the administration of oxygen may paradoxically increase ventilation, suggesting the presence of hypoxic respiratory center depression.[19,28,29] An additional factor that may depress the respiratory center may be a marked decrease in cerebral blood flow due to bradyarrhythmias. Heart rates as low as 30/min and cardiac standstill for several seconds may occur. Clearly these rhythms may result in marked decreases in cardiac output and cerebral blood flow, which may also depress respiratory center activity and ventilation.

Prevention and Treatment

Several interventions will prevent or minimize sleep disturbances at high altitude. Acetazolamide has been found to be effective in reducing the magnitude of sleep hypoxemia, as shown in Figure 16.9. Mean arterial oxygen saturations of 60 percent are increased to 72 percent by the use of acetazolamide, which also prevents transient episodes of more severe hypoxemia.[30] Acetazolamide can diminish

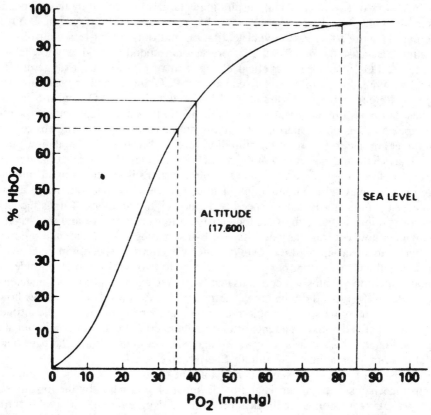

Figure 16.8. Sleep at sea level has a nominal effect upon arterial oxygen saturation and content; at high altitude the effect is greater. If sleep results in a fall in arterial oxygen tension of 5 mm at sea level the effect upon arterial saturation is slight. At 17,000 feet (5,785 m) the same fall in oxygen tension will result in an 8 percent decrease in saturation.

periodic breathing as well as ameliorate symptoms of acute mountain sickness. The action of acetazolamide is to increase ventilation by producing a metabolic acidosis. Bradyarrhythmias during sleep are also diminished secondary to the increase in ventilation, because acetazolamide has no significant direct effect on cardiac rhythm.

Nighttime administration of low-flow oxygen improves sleep and alleviates shortness of breath and headache by increasing the arterial PO_2. Oxygen will initially increase the duration of apneic pauses during periodic breathing, but after a few minutes periodic breathing may resume.[6] Carbon dioxide inhalation eliminates apneic pauses but cycling of deep and shallow breaths usually continues.[6,7,21] Studies on Mount Logan indicate that sleep hypoxemia becomes less severe after a few days at high altitude. The effect of drugs such as progesterone, protriptyline, aminophylline and almitrine is unknown, but studies of such interventions are clearly indicated. Almitrine is less effective than acetazolamide in ameliorating periodic breathing at high altitude.[31]

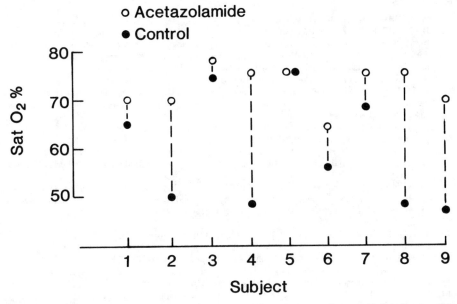

Figure 16.9. Effect of acetazolamide on the lowest arterial oxygen saturation recorded during the night in nine subjects at 17,500 feet (5,340 m). From Sutton et al., ref. 30.

Sedatives such as barbiturates, codeine and diazepam (Valium) depress respiration at sea level.[32] At high altitude, owing to the shape of the O_2 dissociation curve, a similar degree of depression will result in more severe hypoxemia.

Further studies are clearly needed to evaluate methods of improving sleep at high altitude and reducing the severity of sleep hypoxemia, since these two problems are common effects of high altitude exposure that can make nights miserable and reduce physical and mental efficiency during daytime hours.

Sleepiness at High Altitude

A minor aspect of sleep is the tendency to develop sleepiness during the first few hours of altitude exposure. Frequent yawning and drowsiness may be followed by falling easily into a deep sleep during a rest stop. On a climb of Mount Shasta, California, one climber was noted to be trailing behind the rest of the party by a considerable distance at 9,500 feet (2,900 m). Finally he was no longer seen and a pair of climbers descended to find him fast asleep under a large boulder. After arrival at camp he did not come to supper and was found asleep again behind a boulder. He was moderately cyanotic and when awakened was confused and disoriented for a few minutes. His cyanosis and confusion were probably related to sleep hypoxemia.[2] Climbers and trip leaders should be aware of this phenomenon, which can result in party members getting lost or becoming severely hypoxemic and disoriented. Mosso (pp. 252-53) described several instances of sleepiness at high altitude, including a man who became so sleepy at an altitude of 11,155 feet (3,400 m) on the Col Du Géant that despite the danger, he had to stop and sleep on the snow a short walk from the Col.[5]

References

1. HULTGREN H. Personal Observations.
2. HACKETT P. The Denali Medical Research Project, 1982-1985. *Amer. Alpine J.* 1986; 28:129-37.
3. MARTIN R. *Cardiorespiratory disorders during sleep.* New York: Futura, 1984:1-13.
4. ANHOLM J, POWLES R, DOWNEY C. Operation Everest II. Arterial oxygen saturation and sleep at extreme simulated altitude. *Am. Rev. Resp. Dis.* 1992; 145: 817-26.
5. MOSSO A. *Life of man on the high Alps.* London: Fisher Unwin, 1989:44.
6. LAHIRI S, and BARNARD P. Role of arterial chemoreflex in breathing during sleep at high altitude. In *Hypoxia, exercise, and altitude,* ed. J Sutton, C Houston, and N Jones. New York: A. R. Liss, 1983: 75-85.
7. WEST J, PETERS R, AKNES G, et al. Nocturnal periodic breathing at altitudes of 6,300 m and 8,050 m. *J. Appl. Physiol.* 1986; 61:280-87.
8. MASUYAMA S, KOHCHIYAMA S, OKITA S, et al. Relationship between disodered breathing during sleep at high altitude and ventilatory chemosensitivities to hypoxia and hypercapnia. *Am. Rev. Resp. Dis.* 1987; 135:A184,.
9. MASUYAMA S, HASAKO K, KOHCHIYAMA S, et al. Periodic breathing during sleep at high altitude and ventilatory chemosensitivities to hypoxia and hypercapnia. In *High altitude medical science,* ed. G. Ueda, S Kusama, and N Voelkel. Matsumoto, Japan: Shinshu University, 1988: 229-33.
10. WHITE D, GLEESON K, PICKETT C, et al. Altitude acclimatization: Influence on periodic breathing and chemoresponsiveness during sleep. *J. Appl. Physiol.* 1987; 63:401-12.
11. FISHBERG A. *Heart failure.* Philadelphia: Lea and Febiger, 1940:159-74.
12. STROHL K, and FOUKE J. Periodic breathing at altitude. *Sem. Resp. Med.* 1983; 5:169-74.
13. HARPER R. Neurophysiology of sleep. *Sem. Resp. Med.* 1983; 5:65-73.
14. ELDRIDGE F, and MILLHORN D. Oscillation, gating, and memory in the respiratory control system. In *Handbook of physiology, Respiratory II*: 93-114.
15. GOTHE B, MANTEY P, GOLDMAN M, and CHERNIAK N. Periodic breathing in normal humans during quiet sleep. In *Hypoxia: Man at altitude,* ed. J Sutton, N Jones, and C Houston. New York: Thieme-Stratton, 1982:202. Abstract.
16. TRASK C, and CREE E. Oximeter studies on patients with chronic obstructive emphysema, awake and during sleep. *N. Engl. J. Med.* 1962; 266:639-42.
17. BLOCK P, BOYSEN P, WYNNE J, and HUNT L. Sleep apnea, hypopnea, and oxygen saturation in normal subjects: A strong male predominance. *N. Engl. J. Med.* 1979; 300:513-17.
18. SUTTON J, GRAY G, HOUSTON C, and POWLES P. Effects of acclimatization on sleep hypoxemia at altitude. In J West and S Lahiri, eds., *High altitude and man.* Bethesda, Md.: American Physiological Society, 1984:141-46.
19. POWLES P, and SUTTON J. Sleep at altitude. *Sem. Resp. Med.* 1983; 5:178-80.
20. CUMMINGS P, and LYSGAARD M. Cardiac arrhythmia at high altitude. *West. J. Med.* 1981; 135:66-68.
21. LAHIRI S, MARET K, SHERPA M, and PETERS R, JR. Sleep and periodic breathing at high altitude: Sherpa natives vs. sojourners. In J West and S Lahiri, eds., *High altitude and man.* Bethesda, Md.: American Physiological Society, 1984:73-90.
22. WARD M, MILLEDGE J, and WEST J. *High altitude medicine and physiology.* Philadelphia: University of Pennsylvania Press, 1985:263-81.
23. HORII M. TAKASAKI K, OHTSUKA K, et al. Changes in heart rate and QT interval at high altitude in Alpinists: Analysis by Holter ambulatory monitoring. *Clin. Cardiol.* 1987; 10:238-42.
24. KARLINER J, SARNQUIST F, GRABER D, et al. The electrocardiogram at extreme altitude: Experience on Mt. Everest. *Am. Heart J.* 1985; 109:505-13.
25. MALCONIAN M, HULTGREN H, NITTA M, et al. The sleep electrocardiogram at extreme altitudes (Operation Everest II). *Am. J. Cardiol.* 1989; 65:1014-20.
26. GUILLEMINAULT C, CONNELLEY S, WINKLE R, et al. Cyclical variation of the heart rate in sleep apnea syndrome: Mechanisms and usefulness of 24-hour electrocardiography as a screening technique. *Lancet* 1984; 1:126-31.
27. MILLHORN D, ELDRIDGE F, KILEY J, and WALDROP T. Prolonged inhibition of respiration following acute hypoxia in glomectomized cats. *Respir. Physiol.* 1984; 57:331-40.
28. MARTICORENA E. Personal communication.
29. HACKETT P. Personal communication.
30. SUTTON J, HOUSTON C, MANSELL A, et al. Effect of acetazolamide on hypoxemia during sleep at high altitude. *N. Engl. J. Med.* 1979; 301:1329-31.

31. HACKETT P, ROACH R, HARRISON G, et al. Respiratory stimulants and sleep periodic breathing at high altitude: Almitrine versus acetazolamide. *Am. Rev. Resp. Dis.* 1987; 135:896-98.
32. ROEGGLA G, ROEGGLA M, WAGNER A, et al. Effect of low dose sedation with diazepam on ventilatory sedation response at moderate altitude. *Wien. Klin. Wochenshr.* 1994; 106:649-51.

CHAPTER 17

High Altitude Systemic Edema

SUMMARY

Edema of the face, hands and feet associated with an increase in weight occurs in 10-20 percent of persons who ascend to high altitude. It is more common in women than in men. It is not related to symptoms of mountain sickness. Upon descent a spontaneous diuresis occurs and the edema disappears. Recurrent episodes in the same person are common. Salt and water retention with edema has also been observed in long treks at lower elevations. Studies of Japanese women with systemic edema at moderate altitudes revealed a decrease in hemoglobin, hematocrit, and serum albumen compatible with an increase in plasma volume. Extracellular fluid volume was increased. A decrease in serum potassium suggested an elevation in serum aldosterone. Furosemide usually results in a prompt diuresis with loss of edema. If symptoms of acute mountain sickness are present acetazolamide should be used.

• • •

Asymptomatic edema of the face, hands and feet may occur during exposure to high altitude. Women are more commonly affected than men. Edema may occur only during the first week or two after arrival, but in some persons it may persist throughout the altitude stay. Edema of the face is occasionally severe enough to nearly close the eyelids (moon facies), and is most commonly observed in the morning upon arising. Edema of the legs and feet may cause fatigue and a heavy clumsy sensation in the lower extremities that impairs walking. Edema of the fingers may result in inability to remove rings. Symptoms of acute mountain sickness may also be present. In some cases exertional dyspnea, fatigue and pulmonary rales may be noted, suggesting the presence of high altitude pulmonary edema. Other cases may exhibit retinal hemorrhages, papilledema or symptoms suggesting cerebral edema, including ataxia.[1,2] Upon return to sea level a spontaneous diuresis occurs, followed by a loss of weight and disappearance of the edema. Physical examination is unremarkable aside from the presence of edema and the occasional occurrence of pulmonary rales. Diastolic blood pressure may be elevated. Urine output is decreased. Signs of pulmonary edema, ataxia or retinal hemorrhages are coincidental and are not an essential part of the syndrome.

Sheridan described peripheral edema in all six members of a group climbing in Borneo.[3] On the sixth day of the climb at 13,120 feet (4,000 m) all members of the party (one woman and five men) had edema, which was most evident on the face, back of the hands, and ankles. Ankle circumference was increased. Edema continued to increase until the tenth day. Descent was accompanied by a diuresis in all members of the party. The average decrease in ankle circumference was 5 cm. Hackett and Rennie described peripheral edema in ten trekkers at Pheriche 14,245 feet (4,343 m), on the route to Mount Everest.[2] Seven of the cases were women. The edema was largely facial and peri-orbital, but there was also edema of the hands and legs. Pulmonary rales were present in five of the women and the three men. Two of the cases had retinal hemorrhages and papilledema. Proteinuria was not noted.

Incidence

The actual incidence of HASE is unknown owning to the lack of planned, systematic studies. Hackett and Rennie noted the presence of systemic edema in 18 percent of 200 trekkers at 14,000 feet (4,243 m). Edema was twice as common in females.[1-2] Of 12 trekkers with edema in multiple areas, 9 were women. Mountain sickness was slightly more common in those with systemic edema (61 percent) compared to those without systemic edema (43 percent). The presence of edema in women did not appear to be related to the menstrual cycle or to the use of birth control pills, and edema may occur in postmenopausal women who are not on estrogen replacement therapy. Singh noted the occurrence of edema of the legs and feet in some of his reported cases of men with acute mountain sickness (AMS).[4]

Etiology

There are several possible mechanisms involved in the retention of salt and water at high altitude that could result in systemic edema.

1. Activation of the renin-angiotensin-aldosterone system. This would be accompanied by a rise in aldosterone. Most studies have shown, however, that aldosterone is decreased at high altitude.[5]

2. Increase in anti-diuretic hormone (ADH). This system is sensitive to plasma osmolality. A decrease in plasma volume because of dehydration would increase ADH secretion with retention of salt and water. ADH levels have not been correlated with fluid retention and systemic edema at high altitude.[6] In intact dogs hemorrhage is accompanied by an increase in ADH secretion.[7]

3. Atrial natriuretic peptide (ANP) is secreted primarily by the right atrium when right atrial volume is increased.[8] Secretion of ANP results in an increased exertion of sodium and water, and this may be the mechanism of the diuresis some persons experience upon ascent to high altitude (hohendiuresis). ANP has also been shown to decrease plasma volume by a direct effect upon capillaries.[8] If the decrease in plasma volume is severe, this could by way of a feedback mechanism shut down the release of ANP and result in retention of salt and water with edema formation. Hypoxia has been shown to be accompanied by a release of ANP that presumably acts independently from changes in right atrial diameter.[8]

There have been only a few investigations of high altitude systemic edema. Japanese physicians studied female mountain guides in the Hida range at an altitude of 8,200-10,000 feet (2,500-3,000 m) during the first month following ascent from sea level.[9,10] Systemic and facial edema were common during the first two weeks after ascent. Major findings were: (1) a decrease in erythrocytes, hemoglobin, and serum proteins persisting for at least twelve days after ascent (Fig. 17.1), (2) a decrease in serum potassium (Fig. 17.2), (3) an initial decrease in serum sodium followed by an increase after the sixth day and a high level the rest of the stay, (4) an increase in extracellular fluid, (5) a decrease in eosinophils and an increase secretion of 17-ketosteroids, (6) a decrease in sodium clearance with no significant change in renal function, (7) moderate cardiac enlargement, (8) occasional increases in diastolic blood pressure. Cardiac enlargement was detected by measurement of

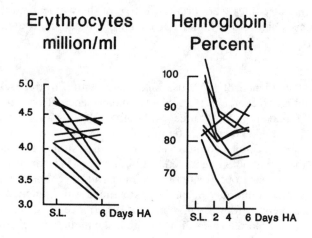

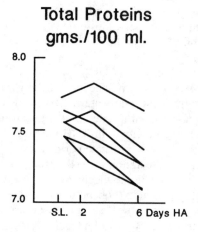

Figure 17.1. Erythrocyte counts, hemoglobin, and serum proteins in Japanese women exposed to high altitude. The decrease in these three values is compatible with an increase in plasma volume. From Sumiyoshi et al., refs. 9 and 10.

serial chest films. Patients with "idiopathic" systemic edema have been shown to have a modest increase in pulmonary artery pressure and pulmonary artery wedge pressure, which could be accompanied by an increase in heart size.[11] There may also be an increase in pericardial fluid, which would result in an apparent increase in heart size. This should be confirmed by echocardiographic studies under similar conditions.

The significant data from these studies are a decrease in red cell count, hemoglobin, and serum proteins suggesting an *increase* in plasma volume—quite the opposite to the usual effect of high altitude, which is an increase in red cell count

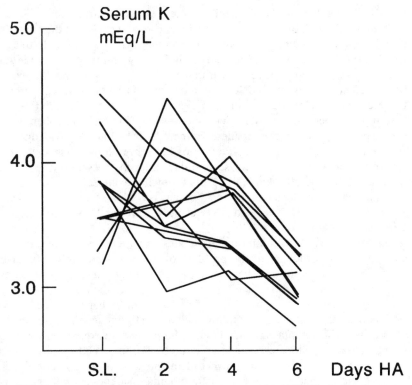

Figure 17.2. Serum potassium levels in Japanese women exposed to high altitude. The decrease reaches a maximum by day 6 after ascent. From Sumiyoshi et al., refs. 9 and 10.

and hemoglobin compatible with a *decrease* in plasma volume. Also, serum potassium was decreased, whereas in some studies altitude exposure has been shown to be associated with an increase in serum potassium.[12] Evidence of salt and water retention was shown by an increase in extracellular fluid, a decrease in sodium clearance and an increase in heart size by chest x-ray. In normal subjects, echocardiographic studies have shown a decrease in left ventricular and left atrial dimensions upon ascent to high altitude.[13,14] These data suggest that the increase in heart size was related either to hypervolemia or pericardial fluid. One can only speculate about the mechanism of the edema in these Japanese women. The decrease in serum potassium and the sodium retention suggests that an elevated aldosterone contributed to the retention of sodium and water.[15] Aldosterone levels were not measured, however. The Japanese investigators made their measurements beginning on the second day after arrival and the maximum decrease in hemoglobin was present from day 2 to day 6 (Fig. 17.1). An additional factor that should be considered is the high salt diet of the Japanese, especially in the huts of the Japanese Alps. I encountered a severe case of persistent systemic edema in a young American woman that began a few days after she started a trek in the Japanese Alps. She had done hiking and climbing at similar altitudes in the Sierra Nevada range of California without experiencing edema, but on the Japanese trek she was consuming a traditional Japanese diet high in salt.

It should be pointed out that systemic edema may occur during long treks at sea level. At high altitude, however, systemic edema can occur without the stimulus of exercise. I have observed this phenomenon in women who were brought to 12,500 feet (3,775 m) by auto and performed only light activity during their altitude stay.

Williams and Milledge have shown that five days of strenuous hill-walking resulted in retention of water and sodium, a decrease in hematocrit, an increase in leg volume, and an elevation of plasma aldosterone and plasma ANP.[16,17] The decrease in hematocrit is consistent with the decrease in hematocrit, hemoglobin, and serum proteins seen in the Japanese women described above. Milledge attributed the retention of sodium to activation of the renin-aldosterone system. The elevated levels of ANP persisted for several days after the cessation of exercise. It was speculated that the elevated ANP levels following exercise were acting on the kidneys and that the renal sensitivity to ANP that was blunted during exercise was not restored to normal. The elevated ANP resulted from atrial distention secondary to the increase in blood volume.[18]

Recent studies by Bärtsch and his associates in patients with acute mountain sickness (AMS) are relevant to the problem of salt and water retention at high altitude.[19] These studies showed that ascent to high altitude was accompanied by an increase in renin, aldosterone, atrial natriuretic factor, and antidiuretic hormone. Plasma levels of all four hormones were elevated, with higher levels occurring in patients who developed acute mountain sickness. Higher levels were observed during exercise. The authors concluded that sodium and water retention was largely due to the increase in aldosterone and antidiuretic hormone and that the effect of these two hormones overcame any effect of the atrial natriuretic factor. Previous studies have shown that patients with acute mountain sickness commonly experience fluid retention, weight gain, and occasionally systemic edema.[20]

Planned studies of women with a history of systemic edema who are brought to high altitude must be carried out to establish the mechanism of edema formation. In particular, studies should test the observations of a decrease in red cell count and hemoglobin in the Japenese women, since these observations are clearly at odds with observations made in normal subjects. The decrease in potassium suggests the appearance of transient aldosteronism.

Prevention and Treatment

Because systemic edema afflicts only a small percentage of people who travel to high altitude, preventive measures should be recommended to those who have experienced earlier episodes that resulted in discomfort. Persons who do not experience symptoms of AMS associated with edema may prevent fluid retention by small daily doses of furosemide (20 mg) and by observing a low salt diet. Nutritional potassium intake should be increased in the form of fruit, fruit juices, soups and nuts. Dyazide, a potassium-sparing diuretic, may also help to prevent a depletion of body potassium and resulting muscular weakness.

For someone who experiences symptoms of AMS associated with systemic edema, acetazolamide should be used instead of furosemide, although side effects of acetazolamide such as tingling of the fingertips, numbness of the lips, and myopia may limit the duration of the use of this drug. If edema persists after acetazolamide is stopped because of side effects, furosemide or Dyazide may be started.

I have observed one patient who experienced symptoms of moderate acute mountain sickness, weight gain, and troublesome systemic edema during annual treks in the Sierra Nevada Mountains between 8,000 feet and 12,000 feet (2,400-3,600 m). Acetazolamide 250 mg twice daily resulted in a prompt disappearance of the symptoms of mountain sickness. The medication was discontinued after five days because of mild side effects. When systemic edema reappeared two days later, furosemide 40 mg per day was started and there was a prompt diuresis and disappearance of the edema. Again, when the medication was discontinued edema reappeared two days later. On subsequent trips acetazolamide alone prevented symptoms of mountain sickness as well as systemic edema. These results indicated that acetazolamide is effective in the prevention and treatment of mountain sickness and systemic edema, but discontinuation of acetazolamide may result in a return of edema, which can then be controlled by furosemide. As shown in patients with "idiopathic" edema, discontinuation of a diuretic may result in a rapid return of systemic edema.[21]

References

1. HACKETT P, and RENNIE, D. Acute mountain sickness. *Lancet*, 1977; 1:1492. Letter to the Editor.
2. HACKETT P, and RENNIE D. Rales, peripheral edema, retinal hemorrhage, and acute mountain sickness. *Am. J. Med.*, 1979; 67:214-218.
3. SHERIDAN J, and SHERIDAN, R. Tropical high altitude peripheral edema. *Lancet*, 1970; 1:242. Letter to the Editor.
4. SINGH I, KHANNA P, SRIVASTAVA M, et al. Acute mountain sickness. *N. Engl. J. Med.*, 1969; 280:175-84.
5. MILLEDGE J. Renin-Aldosterone System. In J West and S Lahri, eds., *High altitude and man*. Bethesda, Md.: American Physiological Society, 1984:47-57.
6. HACKETT P, FORSLING M, MILLEDGE J, et al. Release of vasopressin in man at altitude. *Horm. Metab. Res.*, 1978; 10:571.
7. SHARE L. Control of plasma ADH titer in hemorrhage: Role of atrial and arterial receptors. *Am. J. Physiol.*, 1968; 215:1384-89.
8. CODY R, ATLAS S, LARAGH J, et al. Atrial natriuretic factor in normal subjects and heart failure patients. Plasma levels and renal, hormonal and hemodynamic responses to peptide infusion. *J. Clin. Invest.*, 1986; 78:1362-74.
9. SUMIYOSHI K, SUMIYOSHI M, YAMADA K, et al. Changes of blood elements and the circulatory system in climbing. *Jap. Circ. J.*, 1962; 26:535-47.
10. SUMIYOSHI K, SUMIYOSHI M, OTANI N, and KURONO, T. Changes of blood elements and the circulatory system in climbing. Report II. *Jap. Circ. J.*, 1964; 28:661-75.
11. OBEID A, STREETEN D, EICH R, and SMULYAN H. Cardiac function in idiopathic edema. *Arch. Int. Med.*, 1974; 134:253-58.
12. JANOSKI A, WHITTEN B, SHIELDS J, and HANNON J. Electrolyte patterns and regulation in man during acute exposure to high altitude. *Fed. Proc.*, 1969; 28:1185-89.
13. HULTGREN H, and FOWLES R. Left ventricular function at high altitude examined by systolic time intervals and M-mode echocardiography. *Am. J. Cardiol.*, 1982; 52:862-66.
14. SUAREZ J, ALEXANDER J, and HOUSTON, C. Enhanced L. left ventricular performance at high altitude during Operation Everest II. *Am. J. Cardiol.*, 1987, 60:137-42.
15. LEUTSCHER J, JR., and LEIBERMAN A. Idiopathic edema with increased aldosterone output. *Trans. Assn. Am. Physicians*, 1957; 70:158-64.
16. WILLIAMS E, WARD M, MILLEDGE J, WITHEY E, et al. Effect of the exercise of seven consecutive days of hill-walking on fluid homeostasis. *Clin. Sci.*, 1979; 56:305-16.
17. MILLEDGE J, BRYSON E, CATLEY D, et al. Sodium balance, fluid homeostasis, and the renin aldosterone system during the prolonged exercise of hill walking. *Clin. Sci.*, 1982; 62:595-604.
18. MILLEDGE J, MCARTHUR S, MORICE A, et al. Atrial natriuretic peptide and exercise-induced fluid retention in man. *J. Wilderness Med.*, 1991; 2:94-101.

19. BÄRTSCH P, MAGGIORINI M, SCHOBERSBERGER W, et al. Enhanced exercise-induced rise of aldosterone and vasopressin preceding mountain sickness. *J. Appl. Physiol.* 1991; 71:136-43.
20. HACKETT P, RENNIE D, HOFMEISTER S, et al. Fluid retention and relative hypoventilation in acute mountain sickness. *Respiration* 1982; 43:321-29.
21. MACGREGOR G, ROULSTON J, MARKANDU N, et al. Is "idiopathic" edema idiopathic? *Lancet*, 1979; 1:397-400.

CHAPTER 18

Thromboembolism

SUMMARY

Thromboembolism is a recognized problem in treks and expeditionary climbs to very high and extreme altitudes. Only rare episodes have been reported below 14,000 feet (4,550 m). The following clinical conditions may occur: venous thrombosis, pulmonary embolism, strokes, transient ischemic attacks, and thrombosis in the pulmonary circulation. Polycythemia, hemoconcentration, dehydration, and periods of immobility in a tent during a storm are causative factors. Cerebral episodes may be due to vascular spasm, arterial thrombosis, cerebral venous thrombosis, or in rare instances, embolism. Strokes may occur as a primary event or as a complication of pulmonary or cerebral edema.

Early recognition, oxygen and prompt descent are important methods of management. Low-dose subcutaneous heparin, intravenous heparin, or warfarin anticoagulation should not be used in the field.

• • •

Thromboembolism has occurred in many climbers and travelers to high altitude, as evidenced by frequent descriptions of these events in the mountaineering literature. Thromboembolic episodes at high altitude consist of the following: venous thrombosis, pulmonary embolism, strokes, transient ischemic attacks, and thrombosis in small pulmonary arteries, arterioles, and capillaries.

Venous Thrombosis

The incidence of peripheral venous thrombosis at high altitude is unknown. Most episodes of pulmonary embolism are probably preceded by venous thrombosis. Steele described a case of calf pain and phlebitis on Mount Everest at 21,000 feet (6,400 m).[1] The patient had the highest hematocrit of any of the expedition members—a 36 percent increase over his sea-level value compared to an increase of 23 percent for the other members. Leg edema was not present. He was assisted down to base camp where he recovered.

Pulmonary Embolism

Pulmonary embolism has occurred in several mountaineers. A particularly dramatic case occurred on K₂ in 1954, when a 24-year-old climber spent five nights stormbound in a tent at 24,500 feet (7,465 m). After two days he developed thrombophlebitis with leg edema, and two days later he began to cough up bloody sputum. A diagnosis of pulmonary embolism was made by an experienced physician and descent was started. Unfortunately the group was overtaken in an avalanche and the patient perished.[2] Restricted motion in the tent, a limited fluid intake with hemoconcentration, and an increased hematocrit were probable causative factors.

Another case of pulmonary embolism occurred on K₂ in 1978. J.W., an experienced climber, had to bivouac at 27,500 feet (8,390 m) after a successful climb to the summit. The following day during the descent from a camp at 25,300 feet (7,716 m) he began to suffer chest pain and a persistent cough. There were signs of fluid and consolidation in the left chest. Five days later hemoptysis occurred and signs of pulmonary infarction were now present in the right lung. The diagnosis of pulmonary embolism was confirmed by a lung scan after returning to the United States. Surgery was later necessary to remove a thick fibrous peel over most of the left lung. The patient recovered and two years later resumed climbing.[3] He indicated that he was severely dehydrated at the time of the bivouac, having had nothing to drink for over 30 hours at 26,000 feet (8,000 m).

Thrombophlebitis and pulmonary embolism can occur as a complication of other high altitude problems. M.W. is a young climber who developed cerebral edema and coma on Makalu II at 21,000 feet (6,400 m). Over a four-day period he was carried to a lower altitude where he regained consciousness. At 13,750 feet (4,500 m) he tried to stand but was unable to do so because of pain from a cold injury to his feet and a left leg that was swollen with thrombophlebitis. Over the next few days while being transported to Katmandu he experienced repeated pulmonary embolism. Residual neurologic dysfunction persisted for several months, but there were no pulmonary complications. Immobility and dehydration during the four days of loss of consciousness were contributing factors to the occurrence of thrombophlebitis and pulmonary embolism. Three years later M.W. returned to Mount Everest and developed thrombophlebitis of his right leg, which was painful and swollen. He subsequently developed pleuritic chest pain and hemoptysis. He was evacuated to a hospital in Katmandu and treated with heparin and warfarin. He recovered without complications. It would appear that once a person has experienced thrombophlebitis and pulmonary embolism recurrent episodes are likely.[4]

Houston and Dickson described a 38-year-old man who developed high altitude cerebral edema (HACE) with coma at 17,900 feet (5,460 m) in the Himalayas. He was hospitalized and died suddenly on the sixth day of hospitalization. Autopsy examination revealed multiple bilateral pulmonary emboli and pulmonary infarction with thrombosis of deep pelvic veins. Multiple intracerebral and subarachnoid hemorrhages were present.[5]

Ward described five cases of pulmonary embolism that occurred between 24,500 feet (7,500 m) and 27,400 feet (8,360 m) in the Himalayas.[6] In one patient a bronchopleural fistula and empyema developed. Dickinson and his colleagues in 1983 described seven cases of altitude-related deaths seen in Katmandu.[7] Pulmonary artery thrombosis without pulmonary infarction was present at autopsy in two cases and thrombosis with infarction was present in three. Deep vein thrombosis was noted in only one of these cases. The underlying disease in these cases consisted of bronchopneumonia, high altitude pulmonary edema (HAPE), and HACE. Oelz described the occurrence of a pulmonary embolus preceded by HAPE and HACE. Dehydration was present and was probably aggravated by the administration of furosemide.[8] Pulmonary artery thrombosis and embolism may therefore be complications of these problems and not a primary process. Reported cases of pulmonary embolism, pulmonary infarction, and pulmonary artery thrombosis are summarized in Table 18.1.

It is evident that many episodes of pulmonary embolism occur in the setting of prolonged recumbency in a tent owing to bad weather, accompanied by an increased hematocrit, dehydration, and hemoconcentration. Deep vein thrombosis and throm-

Table 18.1
Pulmonary Embolism, Infarction and
Gross Pulmonary Artery Thrombosis at High Altitude

Ref	No	Age	Altitude feet	Altitude meters	Condition	Associated Condition
7	1	24	24,500	7,465	Pul embolus & infarction	Thrombophlebitis
3	2		25,300	7,700	Pul embolus infarction	None Late empyema
4	3		14,750	4,500	Pul embolus	Cerebral edema
5	4	38	17,200	5,490	Pul embolism & infarction	Cerebral edema Died
6	5	38	17,250	5,540	Pul embolism & infarction	Cerebral edema - died Bronchopneumonia - died
6	6	27	16,900	5,180	Pul embolism & infarction	Cerebral edema Died
6	7	54	11,200	3,440	Pul embolism & infarction	Bronchopneumonia - died Deep vein thrombosis - died
6	8	62	13,000	3,880	Pul thrombosis	Bronchopneumonia - died Pulmonary edema
7	9	32	27,400	8,382	Pul embolism & infarction	None Late empyema
7	10	23	24,500	7,465	Pul embolism	?
7	11	32	26,000	7,925	Pul embolism & infarction	?

NOTES: All patients were males. Seven patients died. Reported episodes of pulmonary embolism, infarction and thrombosis at high altitude.

bophlebitis are common precursors. Other episodes occur in the presence of altitude illness, including HAPE, HACE, and bronchopneumonia, which may also be associated with dehydration and immobility. Such illness may also stimulate clotting factors, producing a disseminated intravascular coagulation. The role of polycythemia as an additional aggravating factor in intravascular thrombosis must be considered. Prolonged inactivity in a sitting position with compression of the veins of the legs while viewing television and during long aircraft flights is a well-known cause of pulmonary embolism.

Cruickshank and his associates reported six subjects who developed deep vein thrombosis and pulmonary emboli following long aircraft flights (the economy class syndrome). The embolic events occurred from two to ten days after the flight and were usually precipitated by sudden movement but were not always preceded by calf pain. A study of sudden deaths during aircraft flights at Heathrow airport, London, revealed that 18 percent were due to pulmonary embolism. Women over the age of forty years with a history of venous thromboses were at high risk, but men in their forties with no prior history were also at risk.[9]

Pulmonary embolism occurring after a long automobile drive and an aircraft flight is illustrated by a case in which a 68-year-old retired professor of surgery was evaluated for the recent onset of dyspnea and chest pain. After a one-month stay in Italy, where he did a lot of driving, the professor made a long drive to Vienna,

Innsbruck, and Munich. At Innsbruck he noted for the first time shortness of breath, orthopnea, and cough. On one occasion he coughed up some blood. He flew back to the United States, where he was hospitalized. On hospital entry he noted right-sided, pleuritic chest pain. A chest x-ray revealed an infiltrate in the right lung, initially considered to be a pneumonitis. An ultrasound venous scan revealed a thrombosis of the right popliteal vein, and a lung scan revealed a wedge-shaped perfusion defect in the right lung, compatible with a pulmonary embolus. Anticoagulants were started and continued for two months. Recovery was uneventful. The patient had never had any previous similar episodes. He had not sustained any trauma to his leg, nor had he noted any edema or symptoms in his leg. During long hours of driving, he did not periodically stop and walk about. Pulmonary symptoms following long periods of immobility in an auto or aircraft should raise the possibility of pulmonary embolism. Venous thrombosis may be present without symptoms or edema. It is possible that the patient had a second pulmonary embolus during the aircraft trip.

An additional factor that may contribute to venous thrombosis is vein-wall injury due to trauma, which is the third contributing factor of Virchow's triad of stasis, hypercoagulability and injury. Untreated deep vein thrombosis is a serious problem, and before the use of anticoagulants as many as 20 percent of patients developed pulmonary embolism. Spontaneous resolution requires four to eight weeks.[10]

Strokes. Strokes occurring at high altitude have frequently resulted in hemiplegia and have been ascribed to cerebral thrombosis. Of interest is the finding of thrombosis in the venous system of the brain in several instances of high altitude strokes. Song and his associates reported one case of cerebral venous thrombosis and the summary findings in three other cases.[11] In the first case, the patient was a 27-year-old man who climbed Lhotse, 27,924 feet (8,511 m), and returned to base camp at 17,400 feet (5,350 m). Here he developed severe headache, drowsiness, and partial loss of consciousness. There was no evidence of pulmonary edema. He returned to Japan, where he exhibited time disorientation, ptosis on the left, and slightly ataxic gait. Disc margins were blurred. A CT scan revealed a high density lesion on the left temporal subcortical area. The lateral ventricles were compressed to the right. Because of the possibility of a tumor, a craniotomy was done that revealed a hemorrhagic infarct of the cerebrum due to thrombosis of the vein of Labbe. The patient and the three others had been at an elevation above 16,250 feet (5,000 m) for 2-43 days. Although the patient described above had a hemoglobin of 21.5 grams, hemoconcentration was not present in the other climbers. Other cases of cerebral venous thromboses have been reported.[12,13,14]

Several reports describe cases in which cerebral thrombosis occurred as a complication of HAPE. In one case, M.E., a 30-year-old American tourist who had trekked over a two-week period to 18,100 feet (5,520 m) in Nepal, developed symptoms of HAPE.[4] During the next three days he descended with assistance to 12,800 feet (3,900 m); acetazolamide and dexamethasone were given during the descent. Although he seemed to feel better, on the morning of the fourth day he awoke with numbness and weakness of the right leg, and four hours later he had a right hemiparesis with incontinence and aphasia. He was treated with oxygen, dexamethasone, and IV fluids. On the next day he was flown to Katmandu and hospitalized. A complete right hemiplegia was present with an expressive aphasia and a right facial paralysis. He was evacuated by plane to Bangkok and later to a hospital in the United States. At the Bangkok hospital, an M-mode and two-dimensional echocardiogram revealed a possible mild to moderate mitral valve prolapse. The patient's past history was negative for any cardiovascular disease, heart murmur or hypertension. After the patient was evacuated to a hospital in the United States, a CT scan revealed a 4 cm^2 middle cerebral infarct. The diagnosis of mitral valve prolapse was not confirmed. His hospital course was uneventful with only a slow, partial recovery.[4] The altitude at which the stroke occurred, 12,800 feet (3,900 m), is lower than the altitude of occurrence of most reported cases. In this case, HAPE may have been a contributing factor, but a cerebral embolus via a patent foramen ovale cannot be excluded. Patency of the foramen ovale and possible left-to-right shunting of blood from the right to the left atrium have been reported in cases of HAPE by Levine and his associates.[15] Although mitral valve prolapse is occasionally associated with cerebral embolism,[16] this possibility is unlikely in view of the negative studies in the United States.

Hackett and his associates described two cases of stroke at high altitude. The first patient also developed a stroke as a complication of HAPE. A previously healthy man developed HAPE at 19,030 feet (5,800 m) in the Himalayas. He recovered upon descent, but three days later while descending at 13,124 feet (4,000 m) he developed a severe right hemiplegia, aphasia, and diminished consciousness. Descent by helicopter was not accompanied by improvement and a CT scan a week later revealed a large left hemispheric infarct. This episode was compatible with a cerebral thrombosis. The other patient was a 42-year-old climber on a Mount Everest expedition who awoke with a complete paralysis of the right arm and right leg weakness. He descended from 26,248 feet (8,000 m) to base camp at 16,400 feet (5,000 m) where the paresis cleared, but severe weakness, ataxia, and vertigo appeared. Upon return to the United States a clinical diagnosis of multiple cerebral infarcts was made. A CT scan of the brain was normal. His hematocrit three weeks after descent was 70 percent. Over the next four years symptoms improved, but mild ataxia, nystagmus, and dyslexia persisted.[17] Multiple infarcts are highly suggestive of an embolic origin rather than a discrete cerebral thrombosis. The use of furosemide may facilitate pulmonary embolism.[18]

There is increasing evidence that patency of the foramen ovale may be involved in the mechanism of strokes at high altitude. The hypothesis is that venous thrombosis, thrombophlebitis, and pulmonary embolism are not uncommon in climbers at extreme altitudes. Under these conditions pulmonary hypertension may increase right atrial pressure sufficiently to permit a right-to-left shunt and to provide a route for paradoxical embolism. Coughing and heavy physical effort may facilitate the right-to-left shunt. Several observations support this hypothesis. (1) Autopsy studies in unselected cases have demonstrated patency of the foramen ovale in approximately 20 to 35 percent of cases.[18] (2) With the advent of contrast echocardiography, patency of the foramen ovale can be detected noninvasively. Using a cough or a Valsalva maneuver, the prevalence of patency of the foramen ovale observed at autopsy has been confirmed by these noninvasive methods.[19] (3) Strokes or cerebral infarcts are relatively rare in persons under 40 years of age, and in almost half of these cases no cause is found. The possibility that some of these episodes were due to paradoxical embolism was investigated by Webster and his colleagues using contrast echocardiography.[20] The subjects were forty patients under 40 years of age who had experienced a nonhemorrhagic cerebral infarction or a transient ischemic attack. Each was paired with an age and sex-matched normal control. A patient foramen ovale was present in 30 percent of the stroke patients at rest and in 50 percent during a Valsalva maneuver. In the control group a patent foramen ovale at rest was present in only 7.5 percent and in 15 percent during a Valsalva maneuver.

Similar observations have been reported by Lechat and his associates.[21] These authors suggested that paradoxical embolism may be a more common cause of stroke than previously believed.[4] Although most strokes occur in persons over 40 years of age, strokes at high altitude are more common in younger persons and the altitude of occurrence is much higher than the altitude range of more common altitude illnesses such as acute mountain sickness or pulmonary edema. For example, in 24 instances of pulmonary embolism, strokes, or transient ischemic attacks at high altitude, the mean age was 31 years (23-54 years). The mean altitude of occurrence was 18,300 feet (5,580 m), range 12,800-27,400 feet (3,900-8,360 m). (See Tables 18.1-18.3). For these reasons it is recommended that any person who has had a stroke or a transient ischemic attack at high altitude should have an contrast echocardiogram to determine whether or not a patent foramen ovale is present. Ideally, studies should include contrast echocardiography with appropriate maneuvers, including deep breathing, Valsalva's maneuvers, and positional changes. Transesophageal studies should be reserved for doubtful cases.[22] Another rare cause of strokes in younger individuals is a dissection of a carotid artery.[23]

Transient ischemic attacks. A transient ischemic attack consists of a focal cerebrovascular event from which the patient recovers completely in less than 24 hours. Common symptoms are vertigo, ataxia, dysarthria, facial numbness, hemianopia, ataxic hemiparesis, clumsy hand, and amaurosis fugax (transient unilateral blind-

Table 18.2
Cerebrovascular Thrombosis at High Altitude

Ref	No	Age	Altitude feet	Altitude meters	Pathology Clinical Diagnosis	Course Complications
6	1	38	18,200	5,540	Subarachnoid veins	Pul. embolism- Pul. infarction Bronchopneumonia Cerebral edema
6	2	27	16,800	5,180	Veins and venous sinuses	Cerebral edema
7	3	<40	14,000	4,267	Hemiplegia	?
7	4	<40	20,000	6,096	Hemiplegia	Death (Sherpa)
7	5	<40	>21,000	6,401	Hemiplegia	(Sherpa)
7	6	41	>19,000	5,791	Hemiplegia	?
4	7	64F	17,500	5,300	CVA-possible hemorrhage	Patient had migraine Death
14	10	38	>14,000	4,250	Cortical venous thrombosis	
9	11	31	?		Possible cortical venous thrombosis	
4	12	30	12,800		Hemiplegia Aphasia	Onset 4 days after developing HAPE

Reported instances of cerebrovascular thrombosis at high altitude.

Table 18.3
High Altitude Transient Ischemic Attacks

Ref	No	Age	Altitude feet	Altitude meters	Condition	Duration Days	Course
13	1	32	26,000	8,100	Left hemiparesis Right hemiparesis 2 days later	2 ?	Recovered
7	2	Hillary	18,820	5,790	Hemiplegia Dysphasia	3 ?	Recovered repeat episode years later
7	3	?	21,000	6,400	Dysphasia Severe headache	?	Patient had migraine
14	4	?	13,500	4,100	Mild right Hemiparesis	?	Recovered
1	5	Shipton Everest 1933	?	?	Dysphasia	?	Temporary
18	6	33	19,600	5,980	Visual field defect Incoordination	1	Recovered
18	7	46	18,000	5,490	Headache Blurred vision Numbness Left arm hand Incoordination	1	Recovery
18	8	29	13,500	4,118	Headache Dizzyness, dysarthria Focal numbness	1	Recovery Two similar subsequent episodes

Reported instances of transient ischemic attacks at high altitude.

ness). Transient ischemic attacks may be due to thrombosis with subsequent clot lysis, but the possibility of vascular spasm cannot be excluded.[24,25,26] One patient had a history of migraine (Case 3, Table 18.3) and one patient who had a fatal cerebrovascular accident (Case 7, Table 18.2) also had a history of migraine. Migraine may be exacerbated by ascent to high altitude and hemiplegia or transient ischemic attacks may occur during episodes of migraine, presumably due to vascular spasm.

Atrial fibrillation. Atrial fibrillation is associated with a risk of embolism resulting in a stroke or a transient ischemic attack. Individuals with a history of atrial fibrillation should consult their physician before going to high altitude regarding the need for anticoagulation either with warfarin or aspirin.

Thrombosis in small pulmonary vessels. In fatal cases of HAPE, thromboses have been described in small pulmonary arteries, arterioles and capillaries. In many cases, masses of platelets occluding pulmonary capillaries have been described. Such lesions may obstruct the pulmonary circulation and contribute to the development of HAPE, as described in Chapter 14. The possibility that such occlusions are preterminal and not an etiologic factor should also be considered. The thromboses and platelet accumulations may be a result of the vascular damage that occurs in

HAPE, which is evident by intra-alveolar hemorrhage and the high protein content of the edema fluid.

Prevention and Treatment

Methods of preventing pulmonary embolism are evident from the above discussion. Adequate hydration and maintenance of regular leg exercise even in a confined environment should be observed. If thrombophlebitis, deep vein thrombosis, or pulmonary embolism are diagnosed, evacuation to a lower altitude and an appropriate medical facility is indicated. Low-dose subcutaneous heparin, intravenous heparin, or warfarin should not be given in the field. Persons with a history of cerebrovascular episodes at high altitude should not return to high altitude, since there is no method of prevention, including acclimatization. Patients with HAPE, HACE, or pneumonia who are hospitalized and do not promptly respond to conventional therapy should be evaluated for possible pulmonary embolism or a cerebrovascular accident. Pulmonary angiography, head CT scans, or brain NMR studies are acceptable methods of diagnosis of these conditions. Treatment with anticoagulants, TPA or streptokinase should depend upon the individual circumstances and the possible risks of provoking serious hemorrhage. Anticoagulants should not be used for cerebrovascular accidents because they may cause cerebral bleeding.[27] Following a transient ischemic attack aspirin 325 mg twice daily should be started.[27,28] Gastrointestional hemorrhage is the most frequent complication, and because of gastrointestinal distress many patients cannot tolerate this dose. Patients allergic to aspirin may use ticlopidine hydrochloride 250 mg twice daily.[29] Recent studies have indicated that 30 mg of aspirin daily may be almost as effective as the larger dose and will have fewer adverse effects.[30] The addition of other antiplatelet drugs, such as dipyridamole or sulfinpyrazone is not indicated.[31] Low molecular weight heparin may provide anticoagulation under field conditions since it has several advantages over warfarin. It is long acting so only two injections per day are necessary. It has a predictable action so daily blood tests are not needed. It does not result in thrombocytopenia. It results in less bleeding.[32,33] Protamine sulfate should be available since it can rapidly reverse the anticoagulant effect of heparin in the event of hemorrhagic complications. Patients with a history of recurrent thrombotic episodes should be investigated for factors which are associated with hypercoagubility such as the anticoagulant response to activated protein C (APC).[33] APC resistance occurs in 20 percent of unselected consecutive patients with deep-venous thrombosis and in three percent of healthy individuals.[34] Other factors which may enhance thromboses are antithrombin III deficiency, protein C deficiency, and protein 5 deficiency.[35] A referral to an experienced hematologist is indicated in patients with more than one thrombotic episode.

References

1. STEELE P. *Doctor on Everest.* Readers Union Newton Abbot, 1973, pp. 163-65.
2. HOUSTON C, and BATES R, eds. *K² the savage mountain.* Seattle: The Mountaineers, 1979.
3. WICKWIRE J. Pulmonary embolus and/or pneumonia on K-2. In Hypoxia: *Man at altitude,* ed. J Sutton, N Jones, and C Houston. New York: Thieme-Stratton, 1982:173-76.
4. HULTGREN H. Personal observations.
5. HOUSTON C, and DICKINSON J. Cerebral form of high altitude illness. *Lancet* 1975; 2:758-761.
6. WARD M. *Mountain medicine,* London: Crosby, Lockwood, Staples, 1975: 289-92.

7. DICKINSON J, HEATH D, GOSNEY J, and WILLIAMS D. Altitude-related deaths in seven trekkers in the Himalayas. *Thorax* 1983; 38:646-656.
8. OELZ O. High altitude cerebral edema after positive airway pressure breathing at high altitude. *Lancet* 1983; 2:1148.
9. CRUICKSHANK J, GORLIN R, and JENNETT B. Air travel and thrombotic episodes. The economy class syndrome. *Lancet* 1988; 2:497-98.
10. CLARK C. Cerebral infarction at extreme altitude. In Hypoxia: *Exercise and altitude*, ed. J Sutton, C Houston, and N Jones N. New York: A. R. Liss, 1983: 453-454.
11. SONG S, ASAJI T, TANIZAKI Y, et al. Cerebral thrombosis at altitude: Its pathogenesis and the problems of prevention and treatment. *Aviat. Space Enviorn. Med.* 1986; 57:71-76.
12. FUKIMAKI T, MATSUTANI T, ASAI A, et al. Cerebral venous thrombosis due to high altitude polycythemia: Case report. *J. Neurosurg.* 1986; 65: 148-50.
13. AOKI T, TSUDA T, ONIZUKA T, et al. A case of high altitude illness with pulmonary and cerebral infarction. *Jap. J. Thor. Dis.* 1983; 21:770-74.
14. HACKETT P.: Cerebral venous thrombosis at altitude. *J. Wilderness Med.* 1987; 5:9-10.
15. LEVINE B, GRAYBURN P, VOYLES W, et al. Intracardiac shunting across a patent foramen ovale may exacerbate hypoxemia in high altitude pulmonary edema. *Ann. Int. Med.* 1991; 114: 569-70.
16. BARNETT H, BOUGHNER D, TAYLOR D, et al. Further evidence relating mitral valve prolapse to cerebral ischemic events. *N. Engl. J. Med.* 1980; 302:139-44.
17. HACKETT P, ROACH R, and SUTTON J. High altitude medicine. In P Auerbach and E Geehr, ed., *Management of wilderness and environmental emergencies*. Toronto: C.V. Mosby, 1989: 1-34.
18. CROYL P, PLACE R, HILGENBERG A. Massive pulmonary embolism in a high school wrestler. *JAMA*. 1979; 241:827-28.
19. DUBOURG O, BOURDARIAS J, FARCOT J, et al. Contrast echocardiographic visualization of cough-induced right to left shunt through a patent foramen ovale. *J. Am. Coll. Card.* 1984; 4: 587-94.
20. WEBSTER M, SMITH H, SHARPE D, et al. Patent foramen ovale in young stroke patients. *Lancet* 1988; 1:11-12.
21. LECHAT P, MAS J, LASCAULT G, et al. Prevalence of foramen ovale in patients with stroke. *N. Engl. J. Med.* 1988; 318:1148-52.
22. BRICKNER M, GRAYBURN P, FADEL B, et al. Detection of patent foramen ovale by Doppler color flow mapping in patients undergoing cardiac catheterization. *Am. J. Cardiol.* 1991; 68: 125-28.
23. HART P, EASTON J. Dissection of cervical and cerebral arteries. *Neurologic Clinics*. 1983; 1: 155-81.
24. SCHULTS W, and SWAN K. High-altitude retinopathy in mountain climbers. *Arch. Ophthalmol.* 1975; 93:404-08.
25. MOHR J. Cryptogenic stroke. *N. Engl. J. Med.* 1988; 318:1197-98.
26. WOHNS R. Transient ischemic attacks at high altitude. *Crit. Care Med.* 1986; 14:517-18.
27. MARCUS A. Aspirin as an antithrombotic medication. *N. Engl. J. Med.,* 309:1515-1516, 1983.
28. CANDELISE L, LANDI G, PERRONE P, et al. A randomized trial of aspirin and sulfinpyrazone in patients with TIA. *Stroke* 1982; 12:175-79.
29. ROTHROCK J and HART R. Ticlopidine hydrochloride use and threatened stroke. *West. J. Med.* 1994; 160:43-47.
30. Dutch TIA Trial Study Group. A comparison of two doses of aspirin (30 mg vs. 293 mg a day) in patients after transient ischemic attack or minor ischemic stroke. *N. Engl. J. Med.* 1991; 325: 1261- 66.
31. LEWIS H. Aspirin porphylaxis for thrombosis. *JAMA* 1988; 259:587-588. Questions and Answers.
32. LEVINE M, GENT M, HIRSH J, et al. A comparison of low-molecular-weight heparin administered primarily at home with unfractionated heparin administered in the hospital for proximal deep-vein thrombosis. N. Engl. J. Med. 1996; 334:677-81.
33. BAUER K. Hypercoagulability - a new cofactor in the protein C anticoagulant pathway. *N. Engl. J. Med.* 1994; 330:566-67.
34. ROSENDAAL F, FOSTER T, VANDERBROUKE J, et al. High risk of thrombosis in patients homozygous for Factor V Leiden (Activated protein C resistance). *Blood* 1995; 85:1504-08.
35. *Hemostasis and thrombosis: Basic principles and clinical practice*. R. Colman ed. Philadelphia, Lippincott, 1994.

CHAPTER 19

Headache

SUMMARY

Headache is the most common symptom associated with ascent to high altitude. Headache is rarely experienced below 8,000 feet (2,440 m), but ascent to 12,000 feet (3,660 m) results in headache in most persons. About 20 percent of visitors to ski areas in the Rocky Mountains will experience headache. Headache begins a few hours after ascent and diminishes over the next two or three days. Altitude headache is usually diffuse and steady and often has a throbbing character. It is usually worse in the morning and following heavy activity. The mechanism of high altitude headache is unknown, but hypoxic dilatation of cerebral vessels with stretching of pain-sensitive structures is a likely possibility. Nitroglycerine-induced headache may have a similar mechanism. Inhalation of carbon dioxide causes cerebral vasodilatation and intensifies altitude headache. Headache is relieved by oxygen, descent, or a hyperbaric bag. Headache is prevented by gradual ascent, rest upon arrival, and the use of acetazolamide before and following ascent.

• • •

Clinical Features

Headache is the most common symptom of acute mountain sickness (AMS) and may occur as the only symptom associated with ascent to high altitude. Hackett and Rennie reported headache to be the most common symptom in 200 trekkers interviewed at Pheriche in Nepal, 13,900 feet (4,243 m), where 69 percent experienced this symptom.[1]

For many centuries headache has been associated with high altitudes. The Chinese in 37 and 32 B.C. referred to mountain passes on the western border of China as Great Headache Mountain and Little Headache Mountain.[2] Altitude headache was aptly described in diary notes recorded by a member of Barcroft's expedition to the Peruvian Andes as the group traveled by train from Lima to La Oroya in 1924:

Dec. 24	Casapalca 13,606 feet (4,150 m). Two hours from Lima.
3:10 p.m.	Drowsiness, headache, malaise.
4:00 p.m.	Ticlio 15,585 feet (4,845 m). Severe frontal and parietal headache. Feel rotten—lying down.
4:20 p.m.	Vomited.
5:30 p.m.	La Oroya 12,400 feet (3,782 m). Able to walk from train to auto. Very dizzy. Splitting headache. Taken directly to hospital and put to bed.
Dec. 21-24	In bed with severe headache which prevented sleep.
Dec. 25	Out of bed. No headache.[3]

Headache is usually frontal, occasionally bitemporal or parietal, and rarely occipital. About 25 percent are unilateral. The discomfort has a steady component with occasionally a throbbing sensation related to the pulse rate.[4] Acute mountain sickness usually begins with a headache that grows worse and worse, pounding "like a devil's anvil," aggravated by straining, coughing, or lifting and little improved by aspirin or similar remedies. Some describe it as a tight band compressing the skull: others feel as if their head were about to burst. It is as bad lying down as standing but is slightly improved by mild exercise. It is the most common and most unpleasant altitude symptom, and it lasts for several days before gradually going away unless the victim persists in going higher.[5] In my observations headache is worse in the morning soon after arrival and tends to become less severe during daily activity. Headache along with drowsiness is usually the first symptom experienced at high altitude. It may be so severe that any physical activity is impossible.[6] Clinical features of high altitude headache are summarized in Table 19.1.

Severity of headache may be described by the patient in three categories: 0–None at all; 1–Mild, no problem; 2–Very definite, somewhat unpleasant and bothersome; 3–Severe, very unpleasant, can't do anything but rest in bed. Clinical grading of the degree of incapacity of headache usually employs the following classifications: 0–No effect on any level of activity; 1–Minor effect, only heavy activity decreased; 2–Moderate effect, can perform light activity only; 3–Severe, unable to do light or any planned activity; 4–Very severe, totally incapacitated, bed rest needed. Commonly associated symptoms with altitude headache are nausea, vomiting, and, occasionally, visual disturbances. Altitude headache may occasionally present itself in unusual ways, as illustrated by the following two case reports.

Case 1. A patient with a form of headache precipitated by exposure to moderate and high altitude was recently seen by me in consultation. This 41-year-old secretary experienced severe headaches upon exposure to even moderate altitudes below 5,000 feet (1,525 m), and during aircraft flights of more than three hours duration.

Table 19.1
Clinical Features of High Altitude Headache

Onset of few hours after ascent
Maximum severity first and second day
Usually gone by the fifth day
Throbbing
Frontal or generalized, rarely occipital
Steady
Worse in morning hours
Worse with CO_2 inhalation
Relief with oxygen
Prevention by acetazolamide
Worse with increased hypoxia
Worse with straining, coughing, or lifting
Little relief with aspirin, Tylenol, or codeine
Not improved by lying down or standing
Improved by walking about and exercising
Associated symptoms of anorexia, nausea, vomiting, dizziness, malaise

She first noticed headaches at the age of nine during a trip to Echo Lake, California, 7,200 feet (2,200 m), and she has had headaches during nearly every altitude exposure since that time. After two or three hours of exposure a diffuse severe (grade 8/10) headache usually begins, and continues until descent. The headaches were steady, all over her head, and rarely only frontal. They were worse in the morning hours. Vomiting accompanied her severe headaches and usually occurred suddenly with only slight nausea. Recently during a long flight from Nairobi, she again experienced severe headache which was accompanied by repeated vomiting but without nausea or any phenomena that would suggest migraine, such as flashes of light, scotomata, photophobia or vertigo. Her past medical history was negative. A physical examination including a neurological examination was normal. A chest X-ray, electrocardiogram, and laboratory studies were normal.

A careful study of the patient's response to isocapnic hypoxia revealed a normal hypoxic respiratory response (HVR).* With 20 minutes of hypoxia the HVR decreased in a normal manner to about 50 percent. Oxygen saturation was only slightly lower than predicted, indicating no significant pulmonary failure of oxygen transport. No symptoms were noted during the test. It is possible that this patient has an uncommon form of migraine. It was been estimated that 10 to 15 percent of patients with migraine experience only headache. Acetazolamide, 125 mg twice daily on the day of ascent and continued for three days after ascent, completely prevented headache in this patient on the last two ascents to altitudes above 8,000 feet (2,440 m).

Case 2. A young female physician successfully completed a 175-mile trek from Katmandu, 4,500 feet (1,375 m), to the Everest Base Camp at 17,500 feet (5,400 m) in 21 days without any significant symptoms of AMS. She then climbed to the summit of a nearby peak at 19,000 feet (5,795 m). On the ascent she developed a severe headache not relieved by descent to her camp at 17,000 feet (5,185 m). Despite codeine and acetazolamide the headache continued, accompanied by nausea, vomiting, weakness, and dehydration. Symptoms progressed to incapacitation (Class 4). Oxygen at 4 L/min somewhat relieved the headache, and she was then able to walk down 2,000 feet (610 m) where three hours later she recovered spontaneously.[6] It is of interest that she had no altitude symptoms until the ascent from base camp to 19,000 feet (5,795 m). It is likely that the added exertion of the climb was a contributing factor. Although high altitude cerebral edema (HACE) cannot be excluded, there was no ataxia, nor were there neurological symptoms or signs.

Complications and Associated Symptoms

Severe headache associated with mental changes, ataxia, or neurological signs is a serious medical emergency, and usually an indication of HACE. Oxygen and/or prompt descent is indicated. Severe dyspnea, cough, a sense of suffocation or chest pressure, and severe weakness or fatigue may suggest the presence of high altitude pulmonary edema (HAPE). Clinical features commonly associated with AMS are usually present also in HAPE—headache, anorexia, nausea, vomiting, fatigue, weakness, insomnia, weight gain, and edema.

---

* Dr. John Severinghaus kindly performed the hypoxia studies.

Incidence

The incidence of altitude headache and the conditions determining the incidence are similar to those that affect the incidence of AMS. These include speed of ascent, the altitude attained, previous acclimatization, the amount of physical exertion upon arrival, and a history of altitude headache. Nearly everyone who ascends rapidly to 17,500 feet (5,400 m) will suffer a severe headache.[7] In visitors to the intermediate altitudes of Rocky Mountain resort areas the incidence of headache is about 25 percent, but headache of sufficient severity to limit activity occurs in only some 12 percent of visitors. Women appear to be affected as commonly as men and there appears to be no age predilection.[8,9]

Diagnosis

The diagnosis of high altitude headache depends on the history. Care must be taken to exclude the possibility of HACE and HAPE. In rare instances persons with brain tumor or other neurological diseases may exhibit their first symptoms as a high altitude headache.[10] Shlim reported the sudden manifestation of brain tumors in three apparently normal subjects going to high altitude. Hypoxia may have resulted in swelling in an already compromised intracranial volume because of increased capillary permeability.[11] In most patients, oxygen or the use of a hyperbaric bag (Gamow bag) will usually relieve the headache in 15 to 20 minutes. Physical signs commonly seen in AMS include cyanosis, edema, pallor, dehydration, and occasionally rales.

Etiology

Several factors may be involved in the etiology of high altitude headache. Ward has described three important causative mechanisms: (1) increased cerebral blood flow with increased tension on arterial walls, (2) dilatation of extracerebral arteries with increased wall tension, and (3) cerebral edema with distortion of pain sensitive cerebral structures.[12] The first of these is a conceptually reasonable theory, in that headache follows a similar course to that of cerebral blood flow, increasing during the first few days at high altitude and diminishing over five to six days. Retinal vein blood flow, which probably reflects cerebral blood flow, is also increased. Carbon dioxide inhalation results in an increase in cerebral blood flow and increases the severity of headache. Hypobaric chamber studies have shown normocapnia to be associated with more severe symptoms of acute mountain sickness and headache than hypocapnia.[13] Harvey and his associates reported that the inhalation of 3 percent CO_2 improved symptoms of AMS.[14] Subsequent studies by Bärtsch and his colleagues reported that 3 percent CO_2 was no more effective than a placebo in the treatment of AMS, whereas oxygen resulted in a marked rise in arterial oxygen saturation, a decrease in cerebral blood flow, and clearly improved symptoms in all patients with AMS.[15] Oxygen inhalation in all studies decreased cerebral blood flow and relieved high altitude headache. Baumgartner and his colleagues reviewed studies of the role of cerebral blood flow in acute mountain sickness and concluded that a causal relation between changes in CBF and the pathogenesis of AMS has not yet been shown.[16]

King and Robinson carried out studies of high altitude headache in 30 men exposed to a simulated altitude of 14,000 feet (4,270 m) for 30 hours.[4] Digital compression of the superficial temporal arteries resulted in disappearance of the headache in a majority of the subjects. The performance of a Valsalva maneuver reduced the amplitude of the temporal arterial pulsations and diminished the headache. These observations suggest that altitude headache may be related to vascular dilatation and not to cerebral edema. If the headache were related to cerebral edema it should have become worse during the Valsalva maneuver, which increases cerebrospinal fluid pressure. Nitroglycerine is a potent vasodilator and its most common side effect is headache.

Other studies have cast doubt upon the causative effect of increased cerebral blood flow in headache. Reeves and his associates have shown that the presence and severity of high altitude headache is not related to internal carotid arterial blood velocity.[17] Bailliart and his colleagues found that exposure to an altitude of 12,464 feet (3,800 m) increases common carotid blood flow, and they speculated that a rapid change in blood flow in the meningeal arteries might stretch the arterial walls and thus result in headache.[18]

Although it has been postulated that high altitude headache may have a similar mechanism to that of migraine headaches, which can be precipitated by exposure to high altitude, this theory seems unlikely. In particular, it is often mentioned that ergotamine may relieve high altitude headache and that this may support the migraine-like mechanism of the headache. However, in the original study of ergotamine carried out by Carson and his associates, the results were inconclusive. Ergotamine was given intravenously to twelve subjects with headache on Pikes Peak, and control saline injections were given in a double-blind study; in four subjects ergotamine relieved headache and in three subjects saline had a similar effect.[19] Hackett and Hartig studied headache in three volunteers at 16,400 feet (5,000 m) in a hypobaric chamber with measurements of cerebral blood flow by transcranial Doppler velocity and cerebrospinal fluid pressure by lumbar catheters. Headache was very closely related to arterial oxygen saturation but not directly related to cerebral blood flow or cerebrospinal fluid pressure. Oxygen breathing and hyperventilation reduced headache, cerebral blood flow, and cerebrospinal fluid pressure; hypoxia had the reverse effect. The authors concluded that the changes in intracranial pressure as estimated by cerebrospinal fluid pressure correlated best with headache, and they indicated that a change in brain compliance consistent with cerebral edema may be responsible for the headache.[20] Gamache and Patterson reviewed the role of changes in intracranial pressure and headache and concluded: "Simple elevation of intracranial pressure in an otherwise healthy patient does not produce headache. Headache is more commonly the reflection of traction on pain sensitive structures in and around the base of the brain such as large arteries and veins which surround and anchor the brain." The authors then offered this caveat: "Sudden shifts in intracranial homeostasis associated with marked rises or falls in intracranial pressure are more likely to produce headache than moderate changes in the intracranial environment or changes that develop slowly.[21]

Treatment

General measures of treatment for altitude headache are rest, a high fluid intake, a light, high carbohydrate diet, and avoidance of smoking, alcohol, and sedative drugs. Light outdoor physical activity with intermittent episodes of voluntary hyperventilation are probably preferable to bed rest and sleep, which can bring on hypoventilation and aggravate symptoms. Low-flow oxygen, 1-2 L/min via a plastic face mask or a nasal cannula, is the most immediately effective method of relieving headache, although in some instances only partial relief occurs. Portable oxygen tanks are available in most high altitude hotels and resorts. Acetazolamide, 125-250 mg twice daily, may relieve headache and promote restful sleep. Dexamethasone may be used if other measures fail; the usual dose is 4 mg by mouth or intramuscularly every four hours. An initial dose of 8 mg may be given. However, because of possible side effects and recurrence of symptoms as well as depression if the medication is stopped, dexamethasone should only be used in severe cases, and usually only as a preparation for descent.[22] Descent is nearly always effective in severe cases of headache even if the descent is only 2,000-3,000 feet (610-915 m) lower. Hyperbaric bag therapy was compared with the use of dexamethasone in 31 climbers with AMS. One hour of bag therapy was comparable to the use of dexamethasone in relief of symptoms. Dexamethasone had a more sustained effect.[23]

Symptomatic therapy includes aspirin 325 mg four times daily or acetaminophen 650 mg four times daily. Prochlorperazine (Compazine), 5-10 mg intramuscularly can be given for nausea and vomiting. Prochlorperazine edisylate (Compazine Edisylate) given intravenously has been shown in a double-blind trial to relieve severe headaches at sea level. Eighty-two adult patients with vascular or tension-type headaches were studied. The treatment group received 10 mg of the drug intravenously and the control group received intravenous saline.[24] Within 60 minutes after injection 74 percent (31/42) of the treatment group had complete relief of the headache compared with only 14 percent (6/42) of the control group. There were few adverse effects. One patient experienced asymptomatic orthostatic hypotension. Codeine may be necessary but should be avoided before bedtime because of its respiratory depression effect.[25] Migraine may simulate high altitude headache, and if the usual measures outlined above are ineffective, beta blockers or calcium channel blockers may be tried, as described in Chapter 28. I have seen one patient who had severe headache without other symptoms of AMS upon repeated exposures to altitude. Acetazolamide was of no value in prevention, but propranolol 20 mg twice daily completely prevented the headaches. It is possible that this patient had migraine headaches, although none of the other usual symptoms of migraine was present. Broome and associates evaluated the use of 400 mg of ibuprofen once daily in the treatment of high altitude headache in a field study. Twenty-one subjects were studied and a placebo control was employed. Eight of eleven subjects preferred ibuprofen to placebo and fewer subjects (14 percent) given ibuprofen required other medications compared to those who received a placebo (83 percent). It was speculated that ibuprofen impaired a prostaglandin mediated increase in cerebrovascular permeability. Further studies are clearly indicated.[26] Sumatriptan may relieve altitude headache. Bärtsch and his associates gave 100 mg to nine subjects with headache and obtained relief in five.[27] This medication has been successful in the relief of migraine headache when 6 mg was given subcutaneously.[28] Since it is a vasoconstrictor its effect adds support to the concept that altitude headache is caused by cerebral vasodilatation.[26] More studies are clearly indicated.

Burtscher and his colleagues compared ibuprofen and sumatriptan in the treatment of high altitude headache. Ibuprofen was effective in relieving the headache in seven subjects while sumatriptan was not. Those given the latter had headache relief when ibuprofen was substituted.[29] These results clearly contradict those of Bärtsch described above.

Prevention

Preventive measures are clearly indicated in persons who have experienced headache during previous visits to high altitude. These measures should include spending one or two days at an intermediate altitude before going to a higher elevation. Honigman and his associates have shown that visitors of Keystone, Colorado, 9,600 feet (2,928 m), who spend one or two days in Denver (5,400 feet/1,635 m) before ascent have fewer symptoms of AMS than visitors who go from lower altitudes to Keystone in one day.[9] They suggest that a high fluid intake and abstinence from alcohol the first day after arrival will also diminish symptoms. Acetazolamide 125 to 250 mg twice daily starting on the day of ascent and continuing for three to four days after arrival is an effective method of preventing or reducing symptoms of AMS, including headache. In some persons, codeine and ephedrine are effective.[18] Diuretics such as furosemide are not indicated. Nifedipine may prevent HAPE, but there is no evidence that it prevents AMS. After arrival the usual measures to alleviate symptoms as outlined under Treatment should be observed.

First-time visitors to high altitude usually do not need to use acetazolamide prophylactically, although they may carry acetazolamide in case of the onset of a severe headache. In any case, acclimatization is recommended. Persons who have tolerated altitude before without adverse symptoms ordinarily do not need to take any medications as a preventive measure unless they are going to a substantially higher altitude, in which case they should carry acetazolamide to be started if headache is severe.

The exact mechanism of high altitude headache is still not clear. The incidence and severity of headache can be greatly reduced by observing simple preventive measures, including the use of acetazolamide in those who are headache-prone. Severe headache refractory to the usual methods of therapy is usually relieved by oxygen or descent. Headache persisting after descent requires medical investigation to rule out neurological disease.

References

1. HACKETT P, and RENNIE D. The incidence, importance, and prophylaxis of acute mountain sickness. *Lancet* 1976; 2:1149-54.
2. GILBERT D. The first documented report of mountain sickness: The China or Headache Mountain story. *Respir. Physiol.* 1983; 52:315-26.
3. BARCROFT J. *Respiratory function of the blood. Part I: Lessons from high altitude.* Cambridge: Cambridge University Press, 1925.
4. KING A, and ROBINSON S. Vascular headache of acute mountain sickness. *Aero. Med.* 1972; 43:849-54.
5. HOUSTON C. *Going higher: The story of man and altitude.* Boston: Little, Brown, 1987: 136-38.
6. NICELY P, and CHILDERS J. Mt. Everest reveals its secrets to medicine and science. *J. Indiana State Med. Ass.* 1982; 75:704-8.
7. HOUSTON C. The Arctic Institute of North America high altitude physiology study, 1967-1979. *Sem. Resp. Med.* 1983; 5:122-25.
8. MONTGOMERY A, MILLS J, and LUCE J. Incidence of acute mountain sickness at intermediate altitude. *JAMA* 1989; 261:732-34.
9. HONIGMAN B, THEIS K, KOZIOL-McLAIN J, et al. Acute mountain sickness in a general tourist population at moderate altitude. *Ann. Int. Med.* 1993; 118:587-92.
10. SHLIM D, and COHEN M. Guillain-Barre syndrome presenting as high altitude cerebral edema. *N. Engl. J. Med.* 1989; 321:545. Letter to the Editor.
11. SHLIM D, NEPAL K, and MEIJER H. Sudden symptomatic brain tumors at altitude. *Ann. Emerg. Med.* 1991; 20:315-16.

12. WARD M. *Mountain medicine*. London: Crosby, Lockwood, Staples, 1975: 262-63.
13. MAHER J, CYMERMAN A, REEVES J, et al. Acute mountain sickness: Increased severity in eucapneic hypoxia. *Aviat. Space Environ. Med.* 1975; 46:826-29.
14. HARVEY T, RAICHLE M, WINTERBORN M, et al. Effect of carbon dioxide in acute mountain sickness: A rediscovery. *Lancet* 1988; 2:639-41.
15. BÄRTSCH P, BAUMGARTNER R, WABER U, et al. Comparison of carbon dioxide enriched, oxygen enriched, and normal air in treatment of acute mountain sickness. *Lancet* 1990; 336: 772-75.
16. BAUMGARTNER R, BÄRTSCH P, MAGGIORINI M, et al. The role of cerebral blood flow in acute mountain sickness. In *Hypoxia and mountain medicine*, ed. J Sutton, G Coates, and C Houston. Burlington, Vt: Queen City Printers, 1992: 327-30.
17. REEVES J, MOORE L, MCCULLOUGH R, et al. Headache at high altitude is not related to internal carotid arterial blood velocity. *J. Appl. Physiol.* 1985; 59:909-15.
18. BAILLIART O, BONNIN P, NORMAND H, et al. Distribution of common carotid blood flow, measured by Doppler, in men at high altitude. *Aviat. Space Environ. Med.* 1990; 61:1102-6.
19. CARSON R, EVANS W, SHIELDS J, et al. Symptomatology, pathophysiology, and treatment of acute mountain sickness. *Fed. Proc.* 1969; 28:1085-91.
20. HACKETT P, and HARTIG G. Cerebral blood velocity and cerebral spinal fluid pressure in acute mountain sickness. In *Hypoxia and mountain medicine*, ed. J Sutton, G Coates, and C Houston. Burlington, Vt: Queen City Printers, 1992: 304. Abstract.
21. GAMACHE F, JR., and PATTERSON R, JR. Headache associated with alterations in intracranial pressure. *Wolff's headache and other head pain*, ed. D Dalessio. New York: Oxford University Press, 1987: 352-56.
22. RABOLD M. Dexamethasone for prophylaxis and treatment of acute mountain sickness. *J.Wilderness Med.* 1992; 3:54-60.
23. KELLER H, MAGGIORINI M, BÄRTSCH P, and OELZ O. Simulated descent and dexamethasone in treatment of acute mountain sickness. *Brit. Med. J.* 1995; 310:1232-34.
24. JONES J, SKLAR D, DOUGHERTY J, and WHITE E. Randomized double-blind trail or intravenous prochlorperazine for the treatment of acute headache. *JAMA* 1989; 261:1174-76.
25. HACKETT P. High altitude medicine. In *Management of wilderness and environmental emergencies*, ed. P Auerbach and E Geehr. St. Louis: C. V. Mosby, 1989: 14.
26. BROOME JR, STONEHAM MD, BEELEY JM, et al. High altitude headache - treatment with ibuprofen. *Aviat. Space Environ. Med.* 1994; 65:19-20.
27. BÄRTSCH P, MAGGI S, KLEGER G, et al. Sumatriptan for high altitude headache. *Lancet* 1994; 344:1445. (Letter)
28. CADY R, WEND T, KIRCHNER J, et al. Treatment of acute migraine with subcutaneous sumatriptan. *JAMA* 1991; 265:2831-35.
29. BURTSCHER M, LIKAR W, NACHBAUER W, et al. Ibuprofen versus sumatriptan for high altitude headaches. *Lancet* 1995; 346:254-55. (Letter)

CHAPTER 20

High Altitude Pulmonary Hypertension

SUMMARY

A moderate degree of pulmonary hypertension is present in all high altitude residents and its presence is of little clinical significance despite considerable individual variations in pressure. In some children and young adults marked pulmonary hypertension may be present with pulmonary artery pressures approaching systemic levels. Most of these patients are asymptomatic despite clinical, X-ray, and ECG evidence of considerable right ventricular hypertrophy. The pulmonary artery pressure decreases with descent to sea level. This condition is best defined as "high altitude pulmonary hypertension." It should not be confused with primary pulmonary hypertension, which has a poor prognosis and rarely occurs at high altitude. In rare instances, children who rapidly ascend to altitudes exceeding 12,000 feet (3,660 m) and adults who move to altitudes exceeding 19,000 feet (5,800 m) may develop severe pulmonary hypertension, right ventricular failure, ascites and edema. Death may occur unless descent is carried out.

• • •

Clinical Features

A moderate degree of pulmonary hypertension due to an increased pulmonary vascular resistance is present in all high altitude residents. In most instances the hypertension is mild and of no clinical importance. In some persons, especially children or young adults, a marked elevation of pulmonary artery pressure may be present without clinical symptoms.[1,2] The term high altitude pulmonary hypertension should not be confused with primary pulmonary hypertension, which is a serious progressive disease that has increasing complications and a poor prognosis once symptoms appear. There is no clear evidence that primary pulmonary hypertension is more common at high altitude compared with sea level.

The following case descriptions are illustrative of high altitude pulmonary hypertension:

M.S. is an American boy who was born in La Oroya, Peru, 12,230 feet (3,730 m). When he was four years old an electrocardiogram revealed a pattern compatible with right ventricular hypertrophy. He continued to live in La Oroya, where he attended school. He descended to sea level on vacations annually, usually for a two week stay. At the age of eight, after ascending from a fifteen day stay in Lima, he developed high altitude pulmonary edema of moderate severity (grade 2) and was hospitalized. Physical examination revealed a cyanotic boy with a heart rate of 110/min and a respiratory rate of 34/min. Rales were present at both lung bases. A grade 3/6 midsystolic murmur was present at the pulmonic area. A slight right ventricular heave was present and the pulmonic second sound was load and palpable. The electrocardiogram was compatible with right ventricular hypertrophy (Fig. 20.1). The chest film revealed bilateral pulmonary infiltrates, a prominent pulmonary artery, and a rounded cardiac apex compatible with right ventricular hypertrophy (Fig. 20.2). A cardiac catheterization study was done on the day of hospital entry (Table 20.1). The striking finding was a pulmonary artery pressure of 144/104 mm Hg (mean 117 mm) with a normal pulmonary artery wedge pressure of 4 mm Hg. Breathing 100 percent O_2 for fifteen minutes resulted in a decrease in the pulmonary artery pressure to 76/36 mm Hg (57 mm mean). Treatment by bed rest and oxygen brought clinical recovery, and the patient was discharged two days after entry.

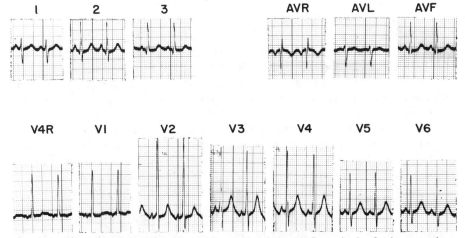

Figure 20.1. Electrocardiogram of patient M.S. recorded during his first episode of pulmonary edema. Right axis deviation, prominent R waves in the right precordial leads, abnormal P waves and a rapid heart rate are compatible with right ventricular hypertrophy and pulmonary edema.

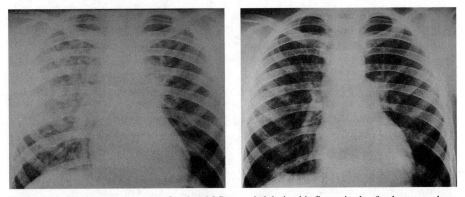

Figure 20.2. Chest roentgenogram of patient M.S. recorded during his first episode of pulmonary edema (left). There is an infiltrate in the right lung field. The roentgenogram on the right Fig. 17E.2B was recorded eleven days after recovery. The infiltrate is no longer present. Prominence of the pulmonary artery and the rounded cardiac apex are compatible with pulmonary hypertension. The cardiothoracic ratio is 50 percent.

Table 20.1
Cardiac Catheterization Data in Patient M.S.

Findings	HAPE		Recovery (18 days later)			After 3 months at sea level		
	Rest	O_2	Rest	O_2	Hyp	Rest	O_2	Hyp
PA S/D mm Hg	144/104	76/36	56/33	50/20	94/64	47/9	40/8	55/10
PA mean mm Hg	117	57	47	35	82	22	18	25
Heart rate/min	129	84	88	72	138	68	70	95
Arterial O_2 %	76	100	89	100	65	97	100	78

O_2 = oxygen breathing.
Hyp. = induced hypoxia.

Because the pulmonary artery pressure was unusually high for altitude pulmonary edema, a second cardiac catheterization was performed eighteen days later. (The results are summarized in Table 20.1). The pulmonary artery pressure was 56/33 mm Hg (47 mm mean). Little change occurred with 100 percent oxygen, but induced hypoxia was accompanied by a marked rise in pressure to 94/64 mm Hg (82 mm mean).

The patient continued to live in La Oroya and carried out normal activities without symptoms. One year after his hospital entry he went on a long vacation to sea level. After three months residence at sea level he had another cardiac catheterization. (The results are shown in Table 20.1). Pulmonary hypertension of a similar degree was still present along with a similar response to oxygen and induced hypoxia. An additional finding was the presence of a mild degree of infundibular pulmonic stenosis with a small pressure gradient. No gradient had been demonstrated by pullout tracings during the two previous catheterization studies. The electrocardiogram was unchanged.

The patient returned to La Oroya where he again developed moderate pulmonary edema upon ascent. He had a prompt response to therapy with oxygen and bed rest. He remained asymptomatic on normal activity and continued to live in La Oroya until the age of sixteen, when he moved to sea level. Details of this case have been published.[3]

This patient is an example of severe high altitude pulmonary hypertension who was asymptomatic on normal activity at high altitude. During his residence at high altitude he did not experience any complications of his pulmonary hypertension except occasional episodes of high altitude pulmonary edema.

A second example of severe high altitude pulmonary hypertension has been reported from Leadville, Colorado.[4] The patient is a girl born at that altitude (10,150 feet/3,100 m). At the age of fifteen she was first studied as part of a survey for pulmonary hypertension. She was asymptomatic and very active in sports (the ski champion of her high school). Physical examination revealed a slight right ventricular lift, a prominent pulmonic second sound, and a short, faint pulmonic systolic murmur. The electrocardiogram showed a right axis deviation and changes compatible with right ventricular hypertrophy. A chest film was normal. Cardiac catheterization was performed with the demonstration of marked pulmonary hypertension. The pulmonary artery pressure was 67/27 mm Hg (44 mm Hg). The pulmonary artery wedge pressure was 8 mm Hg. During supine cycle ergometer exercise the pulmonary artery pressure rose to 144/85 mm Hg (109 mm mean). Breathing 100 percent oxygen was accompanied by a decrease in pulmonary artery pressure to 37/21 mm Hg. The patient moved to sea level, and after eleven months a repeat catheterization was performed. The pulmonary artery pressure was 33/8 mm Hg (17 mm mean); during exercise the pressure rose to 70/23 mm Hg (38 mm mean), hypoxia (13 percent oxygen) caused a rise in pressure to 63/23 mm Hg (35 mm mean). Seven months after the sea level study the patient returned to Leadville. Clinical signs of pulmonary hypertension appeared. A cardiac catheterization six months after the patient's return to Leadville revealed the recurrence of her pulmonary hypertension. She was advised to move to a lower altitude. The patient has continued to remain asymptomatic at sea level and has experienced no complications of her pulmonary hypertension.[4] (Details are summarized in Table 20.2.)

These two patients are examples of severe asymptomatic high altitude pulmonary hypertension. Induced hypoxia and exercise result in a marked rise in pressure. After descent to sea level the pulmonary artery pressure is decreased substantially, but not to normal levels, and hypoxia and exercise still cause a rise in pressure. Long-term follow-up at sea level has not shown any evidence of progression of pulmonary hypertension or associated complications.

Khoury and Hawes have reported severe pulmonary hypertension in eleven young children born in the Leadville-Climax area of Colorado, elevation 11,200-10,200 feet (3,390-3,360 m).[5] The age range was 6 to 23 months. Presenting symptoms were cough, cyanosis, and dyspnea. Two patients had syncope. Physical findings consisted of a loud pulmonic closure sound, a systolic murmur, liver enlargement, and edema. The electrocardiograms were compatible with right ventricular hypertrophy. Chest X-rays revealed cardiomegaly. Hemoglobins ranged from 6.5 to 15 gm/100 ml. Five patients had hemodynamic studies. Pulmonary hypertension was present in all, with pressures ranging from 45/16 mm Hg to 115/75 mm Hg. Two children died suddenly. At autopsy in one case the right atrium and right ventricle were dilated and right ventricular hypertrophy was present. Central pulmonary arteries were thick-walled and pulmonary arterioles exhibited marked medial hypertrophy. The remaining patients remained well after moving to a lower altitude. All studies were apparently done at Denver, Colorado, altitude 5,200 feet

Table 20.2
Cardiac Catheterization Data in a Young Girl from Leadville, Colorado

Findings	Altitude 1			Sea level			Altitude 2		
	Rest	Ex	O_2	Rest	Ex.	Hyp	Rest	Ex	O_2
PA S/D mm Hg	67/27		37/21	33/8	70/23	63/23	70/32	86/53	40/13
PA mean mm Hg	44	109		27	38	35	49	72	25

NOTES: Studies were done at high altitude (Altitude 1), after 11 months at sea level (Sea level), and six months after returning to Leadville (Altitude 2).

Ex = exercise.

O_2 = oxygen breathing.

Hyp = Induced hypoxia.

(1,515 m). The surviving children probably represented severe high altitude pulmonary hypertension rather than instances of primary pulmonary hypertension, because recovery occurred with descent to a lower altitude.

Clinical Complications

Two clinical complications related to the development of severe pulmonary hypertension upon ascent to high altitude have recently been reported.

Sui and his colleagues reported fifteen cases of severe pulmonary hypertension in Han Chinese infants who were brought to Lhasa, 13,000 feet (3,600 m) from lower altitudes.[6] All had marked right ventricular hypertrophy at autopsy with an increase in right ventricular weight of about four times normal. The ratio of right ventricular weight to left ventricular weight varied between 80 percent and 160 percent (normal values are 20-30 percent; (mean, 24 percent). Histologic studies revealed marked medial hypertrophy of pulmonary arteries, arterioles, and venules. Some degree of venous obstruction was also observed, and could be the cause of pulmonary hemorrhages, since pulmonary hemosiderosis was present in some of the cases. Collateral vessels in the bronchial mucosa could also have caused hemorrhages. All children except one were of Han ancestry, and thirteen were born at low altitude; the age was 3-16 months (mean, 9 months). The mean duration of altitude exposure was 2.1 months. Clinical symptoms consisted of dyspnea, cough, irritability, and sleeplessness. Physical findings included a rapid heart rate, rapid respiratory rate, cyanosis, edema of the face, liver enlargement, and rales. Chest X-rays revealed cardiac enlargement, probably caused by right ventricular dilatation. There were no additional laboratory and hemodynamic studies. The authors referred to this syndrome as "subacute infantile mountain sickness," but "accelerated pulmonary hypertension of high altitude" might be a more accurate term, since it is likely that the syndrome is not confined to infants, but can occur in older children as well. Although the syndrome is rare, parents who move to high altitude with infants should be aware of this problem. No reports of a similar syndrome have been made in the United States. Over the last fifteen years at Chulec General Hospital in Peru, 12,230 feet (3,730 m), Marticorena has seen only three cases of severe pulmonary hypertension. All were studied by echocardiography and cardiac catheterization. The findings were compatible with high altitude pulmonary hypertension. There was no evidence of valvular disease. All the patients did well after returning to sea level.[7]

Anand and his colleagues reported the occurrence of pulmonary hypertension with congestive failure in 21 men during a stay of seventeen and a half weeks at extreme altitude.[8] Their mean age was 22.2 ± 1.8 years. Edema and ascites appeared after spending 10.5 ± 5.7 weeks at 19,000-22,000 feet (5,800-6,700 m). Studies were done at sea level. The hemoglobin was 18.5 ± 2.0 gms/100 ml; hematocrit was 61.2 ± 5.7 percent. The ECG showed right axis deviation, QRS axis 131 ± 25 degrees and T wave inversion in all precordial leads. The R/S ration in V was >100 percent in 10 cases. Cardiac enlargement by chest X-ray occurred in 20. Echocardiographic studies revealed right ventricular enlargement (2.5 ± 0.5 cm) in all cases. Pericardial effusions were present in 17. The mean right atrial pressure was 8.2 ± 4 mm Hg, mean pulmonary artery pressure 26.0 ± 4.5 mm Hg, and pulmonary wedge pressure 11.4 ± 2 mm Hg. Pulmonary vascular resistance was increased (273 ± 197 dynes/sec/cm). Cardiac output was normal 3.2 ± 0.6 L/min/m².

Mild supine exercise and oxygen inhalation had no effect on the pulmonary vascular resistance. The effect of induced hypoxia apparently was not determined. Right ventricular enlargement and cardiomegaly regressed over eight to twelve weeks.

Because the studies were done at sea level, one can speculate that at altitude pulmonary artery pressures were substantially higher and the red cell mass probably was higher. The authors did not state how soon after descent the studies were done, but hemoglobin decreases rapidly following descent.[9] Also, clinical symptoms and signs at altitude were not described. Anand employed the term "adult subacute mountain sickness" for this syndrome.

The remarkable similarity of this syndrome to that of the Han children described by Sui leads one to speculate that the important causative factor was the appearances of marked pulmonary hypertension with resulting congestive failure. However, in view of the severe degree of polycythemia, the extreme altitude, and the appearance of congestive failure, the clinical picture may have been that of rapidly appearing chronic mountain sickness. Further studies of this unusual syndrome are clearly indicated. It should be noted that Anand's term "adult subacute mountain sickness" to describe his patients is not appropriate: Monge described subacute mountain sickness, a different condition, in 1937.[10,11] (See Chapter 16.) A more appropriate term would be "pulmonary hypertension of high altitude with congestive failure."

An additional cause of severe pulmonary hypertension during temporary residence at altitude is pulmonary artery thrombosis. Singh and Chohan described the necropsy findings in a man who developed pulmonary hypertension at high altitude. His condition was not reversed by descent to sea level, but gradually worsened over 35 months. At autopsy there was extensive occlusive thrombosis of the pulmonary trunk extending from near the pulmonary valve to the hila of the lungs. Although it was not possible to exclude the possibility of pulmonary embolism, thrombotic occlusion seems most likely.[12]

Diagnosis

In asymptomatic patients the diagnosis of high altitude pulmonary hypertension is usually made fortuitously when a patient has a routine physical examination, chest X-ray, or electrocardiogram. The following abnormalities will usually be present: clinical signs of a right ventricular parasternal heave, a loud pulmonic closure sound, and a prominent a-wave in the jugular venous pulse; a pulmonic systolic or diastolic murmur; a chest X-ray that reveals prominence of the right atrium, right ventricle, and central pulmonary arteries; electrocardiographic signs of right ventricular hypertrophy; echocardiography showing a paradoxical systolic motion of the interventricular septum as well as dilatation of the right ventricle. Echo-Doppler studies can provide an approximate estimate of the pulmonary artery systolic pressure.[13] Although these noninvasive studies may make right heart cardiac catheterization unnecessary, in doubtful cases this procedure is still of great value in providing precise information. Angiography is seldom necessary, because pulmonary embolism or pulmonary artery thromboses can usually be ruled out by a normal nuclear lung scan. A positive scan may require angiographic confirmation.

In conclusion, it is evident that all high altitude residents have some degree of pulmonary hypertension. Young persons may occasionally have severe pulmonary hypertension, but there are usually no symptoms, and signs of pulmonary hypertension are only evident on physical examination, the electrocardiogram, and chest X-ray. Unless symptoms appear, descent is not indicated. The pulmonary artery pressure decreases upon descent. Two rare conditions may be due to the development of severe pulmonary hypertension following ascent to high altitude. Han infants brought to Lhasa, 13,000 feet (3,940 m), may develop right ventricular failure, severe polycythemia, and probably severe pulmonary hypertension after spending five to fifteen weeks above 19,000 feet (5,800 m). Usually, slow recovery occurs upon descent. Adults who spend many weeks at altitudes of 19,000-20,000 feet (5,800-6,700 m) may also develop pulmonary hypertension and right ventricular failure. Descent results in improvement.

References

1. VOGEL J, PRYOR R, and BLOUNT S, JR. The cardiovascular system in children from high altitude. *J. Pediatr.* 1964; 64:315-22.
2. HULTGREN H, KELLY J, and MILLER H. Pulmonary circulation in acclimatized man at high altitude. *J. Appl. Physiol.* 1965; 20:233-38.
3. HULTGREN H, LOPEZ C, LUNDBERG E, and MILLER H. Physiologic studies of pulmonary edema at high altitude. *Circulation* 1964; 29:393-408.
4. GROVER R, VOGEL J, VOIGT G, and BLOUNT S, JR. Reversal of high altitude pulmonary hypertension. *Am. J. Cardiol.* 1966; 18:928-32.
5. KHOURY G, and HAWES C. Primary pulmonary hypertension in children living at high altitude. *J. Pediatr.* 1963; 62:177-85.
6. SUI G, LIU Y, ANAND I, et al. Subacute infantile mountain sickness. *J. Pathol.* 1988; 155:161-70.
7. MARTICORENA E. Personal communication.
8. ANAND I, MALHOTRA R, CHANDERSHEKHAR Y, et al. Adult subacute mountain sickness: A syndrome of congestive failure in men at very high altitude. *Lancet* 1990; 335:561-65.
9. GROVER R. Return to low altitude sickness. *JAMA* 1989; 262:2926. Questions & Answers.
10. MONGE M, and MONGE C. Historical confirmation. *High altitude disease: Mechanism and management.* Springfield, IL: Charles C Thomas, 1966: 71-76.
11. MONGE C. High altitude disease. *Arch. Int. Med.* 1937; 59:32-40.
12. SINGH I, and CHOHAN I. Blood coagulation changes at high altitude predisposing to pulmonary hypertension. *Brit. Heart J.* 1972; 34:611-17.
13. CHAN K, CURRIE P, SEWARD J, et al: Comparison of three Doppler ultrasound methods in the prediction of pulmonary artery pressure. *J. Am. Coll. Cardiol.* 1987; 9:549-54.

CHAPTER 21

Retinal Hemorrhages

SUMMARY

Retinal hemorrhages occur in active climbers and trekkers at altitudes above 14,000 feet (4,270 m) and with an increasing prevalence at higher altitudes. Probably all persons at 25,000 feet (7,625 m) will have hemorrhages. The hemorrhages only rarely affect vision and usually resolve within a few days or weeks after descent. Hemorrhages are probably related to an increased blood flow and dilatation of retinal vessels. Other factors involved are rapid ascent, extreme altitudes, heavy physical activity, coughing, and straining (Valsalva maneuvers). There appears to be no demonstrable effective therapy except descent. If visual acuity is impaired and hemorrhages are severe, descent should be advised. The affected persons should be told about the presence of hemorrhages so that they can make an informed choice about descent.

• • •

High altitude retinal hemorrahges (HARH) occur in active mountaineers and trekkers above 14,000 feet (4,270 m) and with an increasing incidence at higher altitudes. Although they are usually asymptomatic, if they are severe they may result in blurred vision. The hemorrhages subside with descent and rarely cause permanent visual deficits.

Historical Notes

The first description of retinal hemorrhages at high altitude in the American literature was published by Frayser and her associates.[1] The study was initiated by observations in July 1968 of two persons who were working at 17,500 feet (5,340 m) on Mount Logan, Yukon Territory. Dr. Charles Houston observed numerous small retinal hemorrhages in both cases and initiated further studies of this phenomenon. In 1969 Singh and his associates observed retinal hemorrhages in soldiers with acute mountain sickness in the Himalaya.[2] In May 1968 Dr. Rodman Wilson described a climber on Mount McKinley who turned back at 14,000 feet (4,270 m) because of blurred vision and symptoms of HAPE. Upon arrival at Anchorage, Alaska, he was found to have "many retinal petechial hemorrhages" with a slow resolution of his visual defect.[3] Following the report by Frayser and Houston, several studies of this phenomenon have been published.

Clinical Features

Retinal hemorrhages are usually asymptomatic and can be detected only by a careful ophthalmoscopic examination via dilated pupils. Although hemorrhages are painless, in severe cases they may cause blurred vision, and field defects can be demonstrated. The incidence of hemorrhages may be as high as 56 percent in persons at 17,500 feet (5,340 m).[4] Hemorrhages are more common in active persons and usually appear after a few days of altitude exposure. They may diminish after acclimatization but increase with rapid ascent and heavy effort. They do not seem to be related to symptoms of AMS, although some observations suggest that they may be more common in persons with severe headache.

Physical Findings

Increased size and tortuosity of retinal vessels as well as hyperemia of the discs are normal responses to hypoxia, which results in increased retinal blood flow. Hemorrhages are peripapillary throughout the fundus and rarely involve the macula. They are variable in appearance and may be diffuse or punctate, confluent or flame-shaped. They are most commonly preretinal but in the more severe cases may extend into the vitreous. Common types are "dot and blot," "pool," or "preretinal hemorrhages." Macular hemorrhages may be solitary, or they occur with diffuse posterior pole hemorrhages. In these cases, fluorescein angiography indicates no leakage and complete blocking of underlying fluorescence. Hemorrhages near the fovea may cause a paracentral scotoma. In rare cases "cotton-wool spots" may be present. Injection of fluorescein is followed by leakage of the dye in areas of hemorrhage.[5-8] Papilledema is not a common feature of retinal hemorrhages and when present should suggest the presence of cerebral edema. Wiedman has described a systemic classification of retinal pathology at high altitude and recommends systemic funduscopic examinations to predict high altitude illness.[9] Such examinations seem well advised above 15,000 feet (4,575 m).

Hemorrhages are resorbed after descent. In a few persons field defects may be detected up to one year later, but usually there are no residual defects in visual acuity.

Incidence and Epidemiology

The incidence of retinal hemorrhages is variable and depends in part upon systematic ophthalmoscopic examinations of all susceptible subjects. A summary of various reports is presented in Table 21.1. At altitudes above 17,000 feet (5,200 m) the incidence of retinal hemorrhages is approximately 36-56 percent. The incidence of macular hemorrhages with associated scotomota is about 5 percent. Cotton-wool spots are less frequent and occur in 1-2 percent of cases.[9] Sutton has noted that retinal hemorrhages are rare at 14,000 feet (4,270 m) but common at 17,500 feet (5,340 m).[10]

Factors that appear to be associated with a higher incidence of hemorrhages are rapid ascent, altitudes above 15,000 feet (4,500 m), heavy physical effort soon after

Table 21.1
Incidence of High Altitude Retinal Hemorrhage

Ref.	Case no.	Location	Incidence	Percent	Altitude feet	Altitude meters
2	1	Himalaya	24/1,925	1.3%	≥11,400	≥3,477
1	2	Logan	9/25	36	17,500	5,340
24	3	Everest	1/31	3	>17,500	5,340
6	4	Dhaulagiri	5/15	33	19,300	5,890
7	5	Aconcagua	4/6	66	22,835	6,965
5	6	Everest	1/20	0.5	≥16,000	≥4,880
4	7	Logan	22/39	56	17,500	5,340
8	8	Aconcagua	14/39	36	>14,200	>4,330

arrival, and coughing, straining, and repeated Valsalva maneuvers of the sort that accompany heavy lifting. There may be a weak relationship with severe headache and severe sleep hypoxemia. There may be a history of migraine,[8] with males and females equally affected, but there are no data on age predisposition. Hemorrhages may disappear after a prolonged stay at high altitude. Retinal hemorrhages are rare in Sherpas.[6] It is not known whether persons with disease states usually associated with retinal hemorrhages are more susceptible than others to altitude-induced hemorrhages, although one report suggests that this may be possible.[11] Males and females appear to be equally affected.[4]

A controlled study of retinal hemorrhages was carried out in eight men subjected to a progressive increase in altitude in a hypobaric chamber over 40 days (Operation Everest II). Retinal photographs were taken at sea level and at four altitudes, including 25,000 feet (7,625 m). No abnormalities were seen at sea level or at 10,000 feet (3,050 m), but at 17,000 feet (5,185 m), seven of the subjects showed obvious dilatation of retinal vessels. At 23,000 feet (7,015 m) four of seven subjects had retinal hemorrhages, and all eight subjects had retinal hemorrhages at 25,000 feet (7,625 m). After descent, resolution of the hemorrhages was observed at 72 hours; in one subject with severe hemorrhages complete resolution had occurred within ten days.[12] Nakashima and his workers studied the incidence of retinal hemorrhages in 35 climbers at base camp, 16,465 feet (5,020 m), in Tibet. They found a higher incidence of hemorrhages in newcomers to altitude, 8 of 11 (73 percent), compared with experienced high altitude climbers, 9 of 24 (37 percent). All the newcomers had binocular hemorrhages compared with only half of the experienced climbers. None had any impairment of vision.[13] Butler made a systematic study in 14 members of the 1989 American Mount Everest expedition who spent six weeks between 17,400 and 27,000 feet (5,300-8,200 m). Four of five climbers had retinal hemorrhages, one of whom had a central retinal vein occlusion with vitreous hemorrhages that reduced vision to counting fingers. Risk factors appeared to be the baseline intraocular pressure, the use of non-steroidal anti-inflammatory drugs, and coughing but not the use of aspirin.[14]

Etiology

The underlying mechanism of retinal hemorrhages at high altitude is related to increased flow, pressure, and permeability of the delicate retinal vessels. The increase in flow is due to hypoxia, which also increases cerebral blood flow. The retinal vessels do not autoregulate, that is, they cannot constrict to maintain a steady flow and pressure, but must accept the increased flow and surges of pressure that may result from exercise, coughing, and Valsalva maneuvers. Increased flow has been demonstrated by Frayser, who found that retinal blood flow was approximately doubled at 17,500 feet (5,360 m) compared with sea level. Arterial oxygen saturation at that altitude was approximately 70 percent. Oxygen breathing decreased retinal blood flow to approximately sea-level values. Retinal flow was decreased nine days after arrival compared with five days.[15]

Hypocapnia without hypoxia significantly reduces retinal blood flow.[16] Retinal hemorrhages associated with bilateral papilledema may be associated with high altitude cerebral edema. Compression of the retinochoroidal anastomosis can result in retinal venous hypertension and hemorrhage.[17] A raised intraocular pressure does not appear to be related to retinal hemorrhages. Measurements of intraocular pressure in climbers up to an elevation of 19,800 feet (6,000 m) revealed no increase in pressure.[18]

Rennie and Morrissey noted an increase in the diameter of retinal veins and arteries of about 24 percent at 19,300 feet (5,883 m).[6] Leakage of fluorescein and hemorrhages indicate increased capillary permeability and capillary rupture. It is more likely that high intravascular pressure is the cause of increased permeability rather than the direct effect of hypoxia upon the vascular wall. Thus the process may be analogous to the increased capillary leakage of protein and red cells in HAPE, where high pressure is transmitted to the pulmonary capillary bed.

The macular region of the fundus may be less susceptible to hemorrhages, since the transit time of the retinal circulation is fastest in this area and slower in the periphery. Vessels are more likely to leak under a given intravascular pressure when flow is slow.

There is one reported autopsy study of retinal hemorrhages in a physician who died of pulmonary and cerebral edema in Nepal. Histologic studies revealed hemorrhages from veins and capillaries but not from arteries. The hemorrhages were similar to those found in the brain.[19]

It is possible that microembolization occurs as a result of platelet clumping and causes vascular occlusion, cotton-wool spots, or pale centers. It should be noted that retinal hemorrhages have been found in cases of carbon monoxide poisoning at sea level, presumably the result of a similar effect on the retinal circulation. Some of the hemorrhages had white centers. Most of the patients had been exposed to carbon monoxide for more than twelve hours.[20] Carbon monoxide poisoning should be considered as a possible causative or aggravating factor or retinal hemorrhages at high altitude.[21]

McFadden and his workers have demonstrated that heavy exercise increased fluorescein leakage and retinal hemorrhages.[4] It has also been suggested that Valsalva maneuvers performed while lifting or carrying heavy loads or straining may increase hemorrhage. Repeated coughing will probably have a similar effect. During heavy exercise blood pressure will rise and hypoxemia will become more intense. Valsalva maneuvers or isometric exercise will increase venous pressure during the period of strain, and the blood pressure will rise above normal after strain ceases.[22-23] Coughing, especially if prolonged, will result in large pulses of high arterial pressure as well as increases in venous pressure. Vomiting will have a similar hemodynamic effect. The high transient arterial and venous pressures generated during these maneuvers will be transmitted to the retinal circulation and could clearly increase vascular leakage. Retinal hemorrhages during coughing and the Valsalva maneuver at sea level have been reported.[24,25,26] Coughing at high altitude may be severe enough to fracture ribs.[27] It is not known whether aspirin will increase the incidence of retinal hemorrhages. Aspirin does not increase the progression of age-related macular degeneration or diabetic retinopathy.[28,29]

Prevention and Management

Gradual ascent and acclimatization will probably reduce the incidence of retinal hemorrhages, and avoidance of heavy physical effort and control of coughing during the first week of arrival at high altitude are also probably of value. Acetazolamide and furosemide appear to offer no protective effect, but low-flow oxygen during sleep may be useful. Antiplatelet medications have not been systematically investigated. Visual acuity should be systematically evaluated at altitudes greater than 14,000 feet (4,300 m). Trip physicians should include an ophthalmoscope in their medical kits. Descent is advisable if visual acuity is impaired or extensive retinal hemorrhages are present. The presence of a few hemorrhages should not make descent mandatory, but the patient should be informed of the problem so that an informed decision can be made. Prophylactic measures such as a few days of rest, descent to a lower camp, or low-flow sleeping oxygen may be advisable. Repeated examinations of the fundus and tests of visual acuity should be performed. Progression of hemorrhages or visual defects are an indication for descent. After returning to a lower elevation, anyone who has had retinal hemorrhages should have periodic examinations by a qualified opthalmologist for residual field defects or persistent scotomata. Hemorrhages have usually resorbed after one to two months without residual signs.

References

1. FRAYSER R, HOUSTON C, BRYAN A, et al. Retinal hemorrhage at high altitude. *N. Engl. J. Med.* 1970; 272:1183-84.
2. SINGH I, KHANNA P, SRIVASTAVA M, et al. Acute mountain sickness. *N. Engl. J. Med.* 1969; 280: 175-84.
3. WILSON R. Personal communication.
4. MCFADDEN D, HOUSTON C, SUTTON J, et al. High altitude retinopathy. *JAMA* 1981; 245: 581-86.
5. WIEDMAN M. High altitude retinal hemorrhage. *Arch. Ophthalmol.* 1975; 93:401-3.
6. RENNIE D, and MORRISSEY J. Retinal changes in Himalayan climbers. *Arch. Ophthalmol.* 1975; 93:395-400.
7. SHULTZ W, and SWAN K. High altitude retinopathy in mountain climbers. *Arch. Ophthalmol.* 1975; 93:404-8.
8. SCHUMACHER G, and PETAJAN J. High altitude stress and retinal hemorrhage. *Arch. Environ. Health* 1975; 30:217-21.
9. WIEDMAN M, and TABIN G. High altitude retinal hemorrhage as a prognostic indicator in altitude illness. *Int. Ophthalmol. Clin.* 1986; 26:175-86.
10. SUTTON J, GRAY G, MCFADDEN M, et al. Retinal hemorrhage at altitude. *Am. Alpine J.* 1980; 22:513-18.
11. HACKETT P, and RENNIE D. Cotton-wool spots: A new addition to high altitude retinopathy. In W Brendel and R Zink, eds., *High altitude physiology and medicine.* New York: Springer Verlag, 1982: 215-16.
12. ROCK P, MEEHAN R, MALCONIAN M, et al. Operation Everest II: Incidence of retinal pathology during a simulated ascent of Mt. Everest. *Fed. Proc.* 1986; 45:1030.
13. NAKASHIMA M, SAITO A, ENDO K, et al. The incidence of high altitude retinal hemorrhage (HARH). In G Ueda, J Reeves, and M Segiguchi, eds., *High altitude medicine.* Matsumoto, Japan: Shinshu University, 1992:275-78.
14. BUTLER F, HARRIS D, and REYNOLDS R. Altitude retinopathy on Mount Everest. *Opthalmology* 1989; 99:739-46.
15. FRAYSER R, GRAY G, and HOUSTON C. Control of the retinal circulation at altitude. *J. Appl. Physiol.* 1974; 37:302-4.
16. HICKAM J, and FRAYSER R. Studies of the retinal circulation in man. *Circulation* 1966; 33: 302-16.
17. MULLER P, and DECK J. Intraocular and optic nerve sheath hemorrhage in cases of sudden intracranial hypertension. *J. Neurosurg.* 1974; 41:160-66.
18. CLARKE C, and DUFF J. Mountain sickness, retinal hemorrhages, and acclimatization on Mount Everest in 1975. *Brit. Med. J.* 1976; 2:495-97.
19. LUBIN J, RENNIE D, HACKETT P, et al. High altitude retinal hemorrhage: Clinical and pathological case report. *Ann. Ophthalmol.* 1982; 14:1071- 76.
20. KELLEY J, and SOPHOCLES G. Retinal hemorrhages in subacute carbon monoxide poisoning. *JAMA* 1978; 239:1515-17.
21. HANSON D, and GETTINGAN M. Near death on Mt. McKinley. *Summit* 1985; July-Aug:18-20.

22. COMPTON D, HILL P, and SINCLAIR J. Weightlifters' blackout. *Lancet* 1956; 2:1234-37.
23. SHARPEY-SCHAFER E. The mechanism of syncope after coughing. *Brit. Med. J.* 1953; 2:860-63.
24. DUKE-ELDER S, and MACFAUL P. Diseases of the retina. In *A system of ophthalmology*, vol. 10. St. Louis: C. V. Mosby, 1972.
25. DUANE T. Valsalva retinopathy. *Am. J. Ophthalmol.* 1973; 75:637-42.
26. MARR W, and MARR E. Some observations on Purtscher's disease: Traumatic retinal angiopathy. *Am. J. Ophthalmol.* 1962; 54:693-705.
27. STEELE P. Medicine on Mt. Everest. *Lancet* 1971; 2:32-39.
28. KLEIN M. Macular degeneration: Is aspirin a risk for progressive disease? *JAMA* 1991; 260:2279. Questions and Answers.
29. Early Treatment Diabetic Retinopathy Study Research Group. Effects of aspirin treatment on diabetic retinopathy. *ETDRS report No. 8.* 1991; 98:757-65.

CHAPTER 22

Syncope

SUMMARY

Syncope or near syncope may occur at high altitude under several conditions. Most commonly it is seen in persons within 24 hours of rapid ascent to an altitude exceeding 8,000 feet (2,440 m). It often occurs while standing, after eating, or after drinking alcoholic beverages. Clinical findings are usually negative except for a slow heart rate in some patients. The mechanism is probably a vasovagal faint precipitated by a decrease in plasma volume, a decrease in cardiac volume, and orthostasis. Syncope has also been observed in acclimatized individuals at very high altitudes where hypoxemia may be causative. In rare instances exertional syncope may occur, but its mechanism is unknown.

• • •

Recent Arrivals

Syncope or near syncope is occasionally seen at high altitude. It is more common in recent arrivals but it may occur in persons who are acclimatized.

At Keystone, Colorado, 9,300 feet (2,840 m), 59 persons with syncope were seen in an emergency room over a twelve-month period.[1] Nearly all had experienced a true loss of consciousness. Most episodes occurred within 24 hours after arriving from a low altitude. A typical scenario is someone 30-40 years of age who flies to Denver, Colorado, and drives to Keystone in the afternoon. That evening while the person is standing in a bar or restaurant syncope occurs. (Table 22.1 shows the incidence of various activities.) Examination in an emergency room reveals no abnormalities except for occasionally a sinus bradycardia. Only one of the patients in this study had experienced a previous syncopal episode, and since none had any evidence of a casual mechanism for syncope, most episodes were considered to be of vasovagal origin. The mean age of the patients with syncope was 34 years. Thirty-seven of the 59 patients were interviewed by telephone after they had returned to their residences at a lower altitude. Only one had experienced a subsequent syncopal episode. The relation of syncope to recent arrival at altitude

Table 22.1
Activity of Time of Syncope in 59 Patients

Standing in restaurant or bar	15
Standing in other locations (kitchen, elevator, grocery, emergency room, ski shop, ski lift line)	15
Awakened and in bathroom	9
Following exertion	8
Unknown locations	12

was further established by a review of 18 residents of the Keystone area who experienced syncope. Six (33 percent) had a readily identifiable cause of syncope, including pain, seizure, hypoglycemia, and smoke inhalation. Seventeen Colorado residents living at 3,280 feet to 6,560 feet (1,000-2,000 m) who had episodes of syncope were also evaluated. Four (24 percent) had an identifiable cause for syncope.

Etiology

Most episodes in the patients who arrived from low altitude were considered to be of vasovagal origin. This diagnosis was based upon the setting of the episode and the absence of any other cause of syncope. Several factors related to the altitude could be involved. A prompt decrease in plasma volume occurs upon ascent to high altitude.[2] Left ventricular dimensions decrease, as demonstrated by echocardiography.[2,3] This would facilitate the Bezold-Jarisch reflex in which mechanoreceptors in the heart (left ventricle) respond to hypercontraction by activating the cholinergic (vagal) pathways that cause both vasodilatation and bradycardia.[4-7] Syncope has been shown by echocardiography to be associated with a decrease in left ventricular volume.[7,8] When the left ventricular volume is small, the sensitivity of the Bezold-Jarisch reflex is enhanced.[7] Beta-adrenergic stimulation may also play a role. The increase in heart rate upon ascent to altitude is due primarily to beta stimulation, and in sensitive persons beta adrenergic stimulation by isoproterenol can accentuate the hypotensive response to a tilt test.[8] Hyperventilation and alkalosis may reduce cerebral blood flow and may result in symptoms. Many of the episodes occurred after eating or drinking, which are known precipitating factors in syncope. Grubb and his associates have demonstrated that cerebral vasoconstriction occurs during head-upright tilt-induced vasovagal syncope in patients with a history of recurrent syncope.[9] This may be facilitated by the respiratory alkalosis that is present during the initial exposure to high altitude.

Another altitude-related factor in syncope was reported by Sagawa and Shiraki. They studied the response to head-up tilt in eleven subjects at 12,140 feet (3,700 m) after a similar study at sea level. At sea level head-up tilt was accompanied by an increase in systemic vascular resistance,which was nearly absent at altitude, and the resulting fall in blood pressure was greater. The authors concluded that hypoxia attenuates the baroreflex response to head-up tilt. The major result is a marked reduction in the peripheral resistance during tilt.[10]

Syncope during hypoxia induced by breathing a low oxygen mixture was studied by Henderson and his associates in 1917.[11] Syncope was associated with a sudden rapid drop in diastolic blood pressure followed by a fall in systolic pressure and a decrease in heart rate. Individual susceptibility to syncope was variable and some individuals collapsed while breathing 13-14 percent oxygen or an altitude equivalent to 10,400 and 12,200 feet (3,172-3,721 m). Recovery of pre-syncopal values was slow occasionally requiring one to two hours of recumbency. Anderson and his colleagues induced syncope in volunteers by using 9.8 percent oxygen. The syncope induced was a typical vasovagal faint characterized by a decrease in blood pressure from 164/83 mm Hg to 85/75 mm Hg and a decrease in heart rate from 120/min to 56/min. Forearm blood flow increased from 3.1 ml/100 ml per arm volume/min to 13 ml indicating peripheral vasodilatation.[12] Typical findings are shown in Figure 22.1.

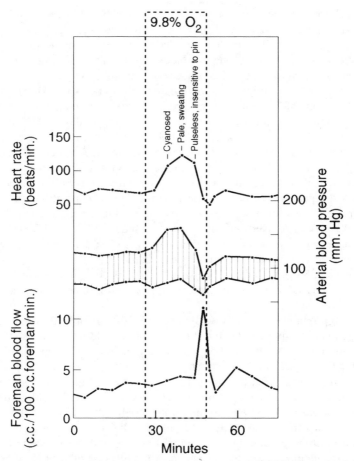

Figure 22.1. Symptoms and typical changes in heart rate (top), arterial blood pressure (middle), and forearm blood flow (bottom) while breathing 9.8 percent oxygen. The increase in forearm blood flow indicates peripheral vasodilatation. From Anderson, ref. 12.

Acclimatized Persons

Syncope during or following exertion has been observed in acclimatized persons at high altitude. A typical example occurred in a 42-year-old physically fit marathon runner who participated in two Mount Everest expeditions.[13] One year earlier while running at 18,000 feet (5,490 m) he blacked out. He returned to Mount Everest the following year and camped at 17,500 feet (5,338 m). Three days after arriving, while standing in a tent, he had a brief episode of syncope. He recovered in one or two minutes; his heart rate was then 40/min, and his blood pressure 128/85 mm Hg. A few days later while carrying a load to 19,700 feet (6,000 m) he blacked out twice without warning and sustained a laceration of his head. Over the next few days he had several similar episodes, and a few times he was able to avert syncope by sitting down. Recovery was facilitated by a supine-legs elevated position. After these episodes his heart rate was 40-50/min; his blood pressure was normal. He returned to the United States for an evaluation. Various studies including a physical examination, ECG, treadmill test, ambulatory monitoring, echocardiogram, and a chest X-ray were all normal. He continued running and had one syncopal episode during a run, but an eight-year follow-up has revealed no symptoms on normal activity and he continues to run regularly. The mechanism of the patient's exertional syncope remains unknown. Studies at high altitude would be informative.

Another example of high altitude syncope in a climber is illustrated by an episode that occurred in one of a group of thirteen mountaineers who went to Mexico to climb the volcanoes. After one night and one day in Mexico City the group went to the Tlamacas Lodge at 13,000 feet (3,965 m). The next morning at 3:15 a.m. they started the climb of Popocatepetl. Above 14,300 feet (4,362 m) during a rest break one of the climbers fainted and fell backward off the rock on which he was sitting. Unable to arrest, he slid, rolled, and tumbled down the snowfield until his fall was stopped by a climber 150 feet below. He was not badly hurt, but he was cut and bruised. Some members of the party escorted him back to a hut.[14]

Several episodes of exertional syncope at altitudes of 9,000-14,000 feet (2,745-4,270 m) have been reported to the author. One episode in the Himalayas resulted in a fall and a fractured spine.[15] Pugh has described a climber at Everest base camp, 17,500 feet (5,338 m), who ran a race with one of his companions. Near the end of the race he collapsed and was unconscious for several minutes. The mechanism of his syncope was not clear.[16]

Severe hypoxia may precipitate syncope. A 28-year old experienced woman climber ascended from an 8,000-foot (2,440 m) roadhead to a camp at 16,500 feet (5,032 m) in three days. The third day involved nine hours of steep climbing with a load up 4,000 feet (1,220 m). An advance group had made camp, set up a tent, and begun cooking a meal. After the woman climber arrived at the tent she dozed off on her sleeping bag. Within several minutes she became cyanotic and obtunded and could not be aroused. Two companion climbers helped her to her feet and walked her up and down the windy snowfield outside. She was encouraged to breathe deeply. She soon became quite alert and was able to walk unassisted. She had no memory of the incident in the tent.[13] The most likely cause of her loss of consciousness was hypoventilation during sleep with resultant severe hypoxia.

In Operation Everest II one subject experienced transient syncope. This young man had spent 40 days in the chamber with a gradual ascent to the equivalent of 23,000 feet (7,015 m). At 11:30 p.m. he began to feel ill, had a very severe headache, and collapsed. Oxygen was administered and he improved, but he became confused again when oxygen was stopped. After further oxygen administration he recovered and his headache disappeared. A physical examination including a neurological examination was normal. He was removed from the chamber and had no further symptoms. According to Dr. Houston, this episode is very similar to the episodes of collapse and syncope observed in hypobaric chamber training runs during World War II.[17]

Syncope related to exertion at sea level is not uncommon especially after a competitive distance race. In this situation vascular pooling in the legs may result in othostasis and a vasovagal faint. Cardiac arrhythmias may also occur.[18] In one report a 45-year-old man lost consciousness as the result of atrial standstill one minute after a maximum treadmill test. He was successfully resuscitated. A repeat exercise test was terminated when his heart rate suddenly slowed and was replaced by a slow, ectopic atrial rhythm.[19] A similar case of asystole after exercise in a 34-year-old healthy man was reported by Osswald.[20] With avoidance of strenuous exercise no further episodes occurred.

It is evident that syncope at high altitude may occur under various circumstances, although it is most commonly seen in recent arrivals who have ascended rapidly. A vasovagal mechanism is likely. Syncope may also occur under conditions of severe hypoxia and during exertion. The mechanism of these episodes remains to be evaluated.

Referemces

1. NICHOLAS R, MEARA P, and CALONGE N. Is syncope related to acute high altitude exposure? *JAMA*, 1992; 268:904-6.
2. HULTGREN H, BILISOLY J, FAILS H, et al. Plasma volume changes during acute exposure to high altitude. *Clin. Res.* 1973; 21:224. Abstract.
3. FOWLES R, and HULTGREN H. Left ventricular function at high altitude examined by systolic time intervals and M-mode echocardiography. *Am. J. Cardiol.* 1983; 52:862-60.
4. HANCOCK E. Syncope. In *Scientific American medicine*, Cardiovascular Medicine, Sect. IV:105. New York: Scientific American, 1986.
5. SHALEY Y, GAL R, TCHOU P, et al. Echocardiographic demonstration of decreased left ventricular dimensions and vigorous myocardial contraction during syncope induced by head-up tilt. *J. Amer. Coll. Cardiol.* 1991; 18:746-51.
6. CASTELLO R, JANOSIK D, MEHDIRAD A, et al. Mechanisms underlying head-up tilt-induced syncope: An echocardiographic study. *Circulation* 1991; Suppl 2:162. Abstract.
7. ABBOUD F. Ventricular syncope: Is the heart a sensory organ? *N. Engl. J. Med.* 1989; 32:390. Editorial.
8. ALMQUIST A, GOLDENBERG I, MILSTEIN, S, et al. Provocation of bradycardia and hypotension by isoproterenol and upright posture in patients with unexplained syncope. *N. Engl. J. Med.* 1989; 320:346.
9. GRUBB B, GERARD G, ROUSH K, et al. Cerebral vasoconstriction during head-upright tilt-induced vasovagal syncope. *Circulation* 1991; 84:1157-64.
10. SAGAWA S, and SHIRAKI K. Changes in cardiovascular responses to orthostasis in human at a simulated altitude of 3,700 m. In G Ueda, J Reeves, and M Segiguchi, eds., *High altitude medicine*. Matsumoto, Japan: Shinshu University, 1992; 35-39.
11. HENDERSON Y, and SEIBERT E. Medical studies in aviation. *JAMA* 1918; 71:1382-01.
12. ANDERSON D, ALLEN W, BARCROF H, et al. Circulatory changes during fainting and coma caused by oxygen lack. *J. Physiol.* 1946; 104:426-34.
13. HULTGREN H. Personal observations.
14. FOX J. Mexico, Popocatepetl, Ixtacihuatl, Orizaba. In *The Mountaineer*. Seattle: The Mountaineers, 1975: 97.
15. SHLIM D. Personal communication.
16. PUGH L. Physiological and medical aspects of the Himalayan Scientific and Mountaineering Expedition, 1960-61. *Brit. Med. J.* 1962; 2:621-27.
17. HOUSTON C, SUTTON J, CYMERMAN A, and REEVES J. Operation Everest II: Man at extreme altitude. *J. Appl. Physiol.* 1987; 63:877-82.
18. HUYCKE E, CARD H, SOBEL S, et al. Postexercise cardiac asystole in a young man without organic heart disease. *Ann. Int. Med.* 1987; 106:844-45.
19. TAMURA Y, ORODERA O, KODERA K, et al. Atrial standstill after treadmill exercise test and unique response to isoproterenol infusion in recurrent postexercise syncope. *Am. J. Cardiol.* 1990; 65:533-36.
20. OSSWALD S, BROOKS R, O'NUNAIN S, et al. Asystole after exercise in healthy persons. *Ann. Int. Med.* 1994; 120:1008-11.

CHAPTER 23

Coronary Artery Disease

SUMMARY

Patients with symptomatic coronary artery disease (angina pectoris or left ventricular failure) will usually experience a moderate increase in symptoms during the first few days of altitude exposure. This is due to an increase in cardiac work largely mediated by increased sympathetic activity. The heart rate, blood pressure, and cardiac output are increased. Alkalosis may favor coronary vasoconstriction. Symptoms usually subside after seven to ten days. Contrary to popular opinion, high altitude does not put an added burden on the heart after one has become acclimatized; on the contrary, cardiac work is less than at sea level. Except for the higher heart rate, most other factors determining cardiac work are decreased. Left ventricular dimensions are decreased. Blood pressure is lowered. Maximum exercise is less than at sea level and is now limited by other factors and not by the cardiovascular pump. During maximum exercise at high altitude the double product (systolic blood pressure x heart rate), which is an estimate of cardiac work, is less than during maximum exercise at sea level. Myocardial infarction is rare in mountaineers and high altitude residents. Patients with known or suspected coronary disease who plan to go trekking at high altitude should consult their physician for an estimate of the risk of a coronary event. A medical history, physical examination, and an exercise test or an exercise thallium scan will provide the necessary prognostic information. Low-risk patients in good physical condition who can acclimatize adequately probably have no greater risk of complications at high altitude than at sea level. In remote areas, however, the lack of rapid access to medical care should be considered, and all patients should be cautioned that during the first few days of high altitude exposure symptoms may be increased. Moderate restriction of activity and an increase in medication during this period are advisable. High-risk coronary patients should not go to high altitude. Their risk status may be improved by coronary bypass surgery or angioplasty after which a high altitude visit may be tolerated.

$$\bullet \; \bullet \; \bullet$$

Acute Effects of High Altitude

Patients with coronary artery disease may experience an increase in symptoms and a reduction in exercise capacity during the first week after arrival at high altitude. Rest angina, nocturnal angina, and paroxysmal nocturnal dyspnea may become more severe or appear for the first time. After seven to ten days symptoms usually subside to the level present before ascent.

In the unacclimatized person with coronary disease, rapid ascent to high altitude may increase symptoms by increasing cardiac work and possibly by facilitating coronary vasoconstriction. The increase in cardiac work is the result of several factors. Increased sympathetic nervous system stimulation due to hypoxemia will increase heart rate, blood pressure, cardiac output, and velocity of cardiac contraction as discussed in the Chapter 3, "Systemic Circulation." Another minor effect is a small increase in the work of breathing.

The respiratory alkalosis during the first few days of altitude exposure may facilitate coronary artery constriction. Respiratory alkalosis produced by voluntary hyperventilation has been shown to interfere with myocardial oxygen supply by coronary vasoconstriction and the increased oxygen affinity for blood.[1,2] Voluntary hyperventilation has been shown to produce coronary spasm in patients with variant angina; the effect is due to the hypocapneic alkalosis, since hyperventilation while breathing CO_2 does not result in coronary spasm.[3]

The effect of high altitude upon the coronary circulation is thus primarily related to the initial increase in cardiac work and possibly coronary vasoconstriction rather than to an impairment of oxygen delivery to the myocardium due to the decrease in arterial oxygen saturation. Oxygen delivery to the myocardium is adjusted to compensate for hypoxemia by an increase in coronary blood flow, which has a large reserve capacity. For example, at sea-level hyperoxia resulting from breathing 100 percent oxygen does not significantly augment myocardial oxygen availability or relieve chronic myocardial ischemia despite a great increase in arterial oxygen saturation.[4] Coronary flow reserve is sufficient to prevent myocardial ischemia in normal subjects performing maximum exercise at extreme altitudes, as discussed in Chapter 3.

Physiological Effects

The effect of exercise on patients with coronary disease at altitude does not appear to result in a greater degree of myocardial ischemia than the same level of exercise at sea level. Grover studied 149 men by ECG telemetry while they were skiing in the Rockies above 10,150 feet (3,100 m). Half of the men developed near maximum heart rates of 150/min or more and 25 percent had heart rates above 160/min. Five men, all over 40 years, developed abnormal ST depression (≥ 1 mm) during or immediately after exercise. Thus in the population of 90 men over 40 years the incidence of ST depression was 5.6 percent.[5] This is not greater than the incidence of ST depression in normal men in the same age group at sea level. Froelicher reported an incidence of ST depression of 8.6 percent in 451 men age 40 to 54 years exercising at sea level. The incidence in 563 men age 30-39 years was 5.5 percent.[6] Cumming reported an incidence of 7.7 percent in 314 subjects age 40 to 50 years.[7]

Exercise

Additional exercise studies were conducted by Brammell and Morgan.[8,9] In these studies, nine men who had exercise-induced angina and/or ST segment depression performed treadmill exercise at 5,280 feet (6,100 m) and during acute exposure to 10,150 feet (3,100 m). Mean maximum oxygen uptake was reduced by 11 percent at altitude. Ventilation, heart rate, and systolic blood pressure at submaximum workloads were increased, but maximum values were unchanged. Angina and/or ST segment depression occurred at the same heart rate systolic pressure product but at lower workloads. These results indicate that the mild hypoxemia at 10,150 feet (3,050 m) had little direct effect upon myocardial ischemia. Instead, the effect of hypoxemia was largely due indirectly to a higher blood presure and heart rate during exercise. If, for example, myocardial oxygen delivery had been impaired by hypoxemia or coronary arteriolar constriction, the double product at which angina and/or ST depression appeared would be expected to be decreased (Fig. 23.1). These data suggest that the decrease in arterial oxygen saturation and alkalosis played only a minor role if any, in the decrease in myocardial oxygen delivery in these patients.

Similar data have been obtained from studies at sea level. The Levy hypoxemia test was once used to identify patients with coronary disease and to estimate the severity of ischemia. The test consisted of breathing 10 percent oxygen in nitrogen for twenty minutes. The appearance of angina and ST segment depression indicated the presence of ischemia. When the test is done at sea level, the hypoxemia produced was equivalent to an altitude of 16,000-20,000 feet (4,880-6,100 m) with arterial saturations varying between 70 to 85 percent. In several thousand tests no deaths or serious cardiac effects occurred.[10] Some patients however became hypotensive or developed a severe bradycardia. In a comparison of the hypoxemia test with the

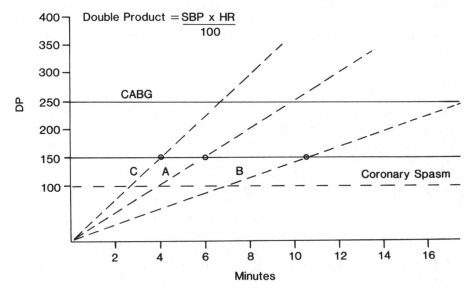

Figure 23.1. The double product is a rough estimate of cardiac work. It is calculated by multiplying the heart rate by the systolic blood pressure. For convenience, the result is usually divided by 100. The lower solid horizontal line indicates a double product of 150 that could result from an exercise heart rate of 100/min with a systolic blood pressure of 150 mm. Slope A indicates that the patient with coronary disease will experience angina and stop exercise when this double product is reached after six minutes of treadmill exercise. Slope B illustrates the beneficial effect of nitroglycerine and a beta-blocking drug, both of which decrease heart rate and blood pressure during exercise. The patient now can walk for ten minutes before chest pain, but chest pain occurs at the same double product. Slope C indicates the effect of acute high altitude exposure. The double product of 150 is now reached after only four minutes of exercise, since at high altitude heart rate and blood pressure are higher than at sea level. The horizontal line labeled CABG shows the increase in double product resulting from coronary bypass surgery. This enables patients to walk longer before the higher double product that produces chest pain is reached. The lower broken line labeled Coronary Spasm indicates that constriction or obstruction of the coronary arteries will lower the double product at which chest pain occurs, resulting in a shorter exercise time.

exercise test (supine cycle ergometry) by Kasselbaum and his associates, the hypoxemia test produced significant (≥0.5 mm) ST depression in 26 percent of 39 patients with coronary disease. The exercise test produced more depression (≥1.0 mm) in 18 percent of the same 39 patients with a maximum mean heart rate of 114/min.[11] This level of moderate exercise therefore produced more ischemic changes in the electrocardiogram than did the relatively severe degree of induced hypoxemia. The exercise was approximately equivalent to walking on a treadmill at three miles per hour up a 12.5 percent grade, (Bruce Stage 3), or equivalent to walking up a hill.

Although one cannot accurately compare these results with exposure to high altitude, one can speculate that if a patient with coronary disease can reach Stage 3 of the Bruce treadmill protocol (≥6 minutes) without discomfort, the patient may also be able to tolerate an altitude of approximately 14,000 feet (4,270 m) without discomfort. These studies also indicate that the acute effects of high altitude are primarily due to a transient increase in cardiac work of a moderate degree and do not appear to be directly related to myocardial hypoxia. The acute effect of high altitude upon patients with angina pectoris is illustrated by the following case descriptions.

Case 1. A 70-year-old physician had stable angina manifested by one to three attacks of effort angina daily, usually occurring after meals. The pain subsided rapidly upon resting and taking a nitroglycerine tablet. His daily medication consisted of isosorbide 40 mg orally, twice daily, nifedipine 20 mg twice daily and propranolol 40 mg twice daily. His normal activity was limited to level walking and sedentary work. He attended a one-week medical meeting in Aspen, Colorado (altitude 8,000 feet/2,440 m). He had no problems on the flights to Denver and to Aspen. On the evening of his arrival at Aspen he had a large dinner and while walking back to his lodging, he developed repeated episodes of angina requiring intermittent rest stops and nitroglycerine. He had to stop after about ten steps and it took him about one and a half hours to walk three blocks. He had omitted his evening medication, which he took when he finally reached his room. He had nearly continuous angina during the night while sitting in a chair. He denied dyspnea. He finally slept about two hours in the morning. He felt better the following day but could only walk short distances and rested most of the day. He continued his medication without increasing the daily dosages. On the third night he slept well and after six days had no more angina or limitation of activity than he had experienced at sea level. He did not see a physician during his stay in Aspen. Upon returning from his trip his electrocardiogram was unchanged. He subsequently had coronary bypass surgery and is now free of angina.

Comment. (1) One can speculate that the increased cardiac work induced by hypoxia possibly intensified his symptoms. (2) Proper management would have consisted of increasing his medication, eating lightly, resting, and using oxygen the first few days at altitude. (3) He should have consulted a physician, since he could have been experiencing an acute infarction. (4) Spending a few days in Denver or Colorado Springs might have provided sufficient acclimatization to minimize his discomfort. One can also speculate that acetazolamide taken prophylactically might have been helpful. (5) His symptoms subsided as sympathetic stimulation became less intense.

Case 2. Another example of angina becoming worse by exposure to high altitude is represented by a 70-year-old businessman who has had angina pectoris since a myocardial infarct 22 years earlier. His angina had progressed slowly to the point where he experienced chest pain with slight physical effort. By limiting his activity he was able to carry on a sedentary existence with one or two episodes of chest pain a day. Occasionally he has nocturnal angina. His medications include nitroglycerine prn, aspirin 325 mg/ day, propranolol 40 mg t.i.d., and diltiazem 60 mg t.i.d. He has never had hypertension. He has had frequent treadmill tests in which he stops after one or two minutes because of chest pain. He has not had coronary arteriography or coronary bypass surgery. Recently he and his wife traveled to Denver, Colorado, (5,400 feet/1,647 m), where they spent the night. At that altitude he did not notice any increase in symptoms, but the following day driving to Vail, crossing Loveland Pass, altitude 11,992 feet (3,658 m), the patient began to experience frequent episodes of angina and dyspnea relieved by nitroglycerine. His wife noted he was quite blue and clearly in distress. After they reached Vail (8,200 feet/2,500 m) his anginal attacks continued but he was able to sleep moderately well. The following day repeated episodes of chest pain and dyspnea were so severe they they returned to Denver. Once over Loveland Pass at an altitude of about 6,000 feet (1,830 m), the patient felt very much better and upon return to sea level his original attacks returned to the pre-ascent frequency.

Comment. This patient who had such severe angina and limitation of effort at sea level, should not have gone to Vail, and when his angina became worse at Vail he should have called a physician. Quite possibly low-flow oxygen might substantially have relieved his symptoms. It is of interest that he did not experience any increase in symptoms at Denver.

Practical experience indicated only slight and rarely severe adverse effects of altitude upon patients with coronary disease. Shlim and Houston made a survey of 148,000 persons who obtained trekking permits in Nepal from 1984 to 1987 at altitudes of 9,000 to 17,000 feet (2,745-5,185 m). Death occurred in 23 persons, and 111 were rescued by helicopter. The most frequent cause of death was trauma (11 persons), followed by illness (8 persons), and acute mountain sickness (3 persons). No cardiac deaths occurred. Among the evacuations for cardiac problems were two men in their late fifties who had severe coronary disease and had been advised not to trek. One 27-year-old man had persistent ectopic beats, which persisted after descent. Three other men, aged 39, 41, and 45, were evacuated for undiagnosed "cardiac pain." About 10 percent of the trekkers were 50 years or older.[12] Sudden cardiac deaths among skiers and hikers at moderate altitudes are rare and occur approximately once for every 1,630,000 hours of skiing. Most deaths occur in men over 40 years. The incidence is slightly greater than at sea level but no greater in physically fit individuals.[13]

Each year hundreds of visitors and workers go from Lima, Peru, near sea level to Cerro de Pasco at 14,200 feet (4,300 m) or La Oroya, 12,230 feet (3,730 m). Some stay for several days and others remain as employees or visitors for longer periods. The ascent from Lima is rapid and requires three to five hours. Dr. Emilio Marticorena, chief of the Medical Service at Chulec General Hospital in La Oroya for over 25 years, says he has "never seen an acute myocardial infarct, unstable angina, or sudden death in a previously known coronary patient within two weeks of arrival at La Oroya."[14] He is currently supervising a rehabilitation project for patients with coronary disease who have come from Lima to La Oroya.[15]

Elderly subjects with a high prevalence of coronary artery disease

Coronary events and electrocardiographic signs of myocardial ischemia are rare in elderly individuals who travel from sea level to moderate altitudes. Yaron and his associates recorded electrocardiograms in 97 elderly persons (mean age 69.9 + 4.4 years) who visited Vail, Colorado for a reunion meeting at an altitude of 8,200 feet (2,484 m). At sea level thirty-eight percent had abnormal resting electrocardiograms and 21 percent had some clinical evidence of coronary artery disease. A moderate increase in systolic blood pressure occurred upon arrival. No acute changes compatible with myocardial ischemia were observed in recordings made for five consecutive days. No symptoms of myocardial ischemia occurred.[16,17]

Surveys of elderly men have shown a 20-25 percent prevalence of coronary artery disease and about 33 percent will have an abnormal resting electrocardiogram.[18]

Cardiac Arrhythmias

Cardiac arrhythmias may be precipitated by acute altitude exposure as a consequence of the increased activity of the sympathetic nervous system and possible alkalosis with a resulting decrease in serum potassium. At Keystone, Colorado, 9,600 feet (2,928 m), I have observed several persons who have experienced the onset of atrial fibrillation, atrial flutter, or atrial tachycardia during the first 48 hours after arrival. About 30 percent of these patients have had similar arrhythmias at sea level.[18] Some persons may experience an increase in premature beats, as illustrated by a case in which a 75-year-old business executive with known coronary disease went hunting at elevations of 8,000-9,000 feet (2,440-2,745 m). He had had coronary bypass surgery and a subsequent angioplasty and was free of angina. He brought a bottle of oxygen with him on the trip. He developed bigeminy due to ventricular premature beats with a drop in his palpable pulse from 80 to 40/min and a pounding in his chest and neck. During previous similar episodes, his bigeminy had been documented by an electrocardiogram. After taking oxygen via a plastic face mask his rhythm returned to normal. Extrasystoles during a climb of Kilimanjaro, 19,335 feet (5,895 m) have been reported by a physician who had no evidence of cardiac disease.[19] Thus cardiac arrhythmias do not necessarily indicate underlying heart disease.

Sudden Death

Sudden death due to coronary artery disease is rare in young persons. Between 1965 and 1985, sudden cardiac death at sea level related to a 42-week period of basic training occurred in only 19 of 1.6 million Air Force recruits, aged 17-28 years. Nearly half of these deaths (8 of 19) were due to myocarditis, and six were due to congenital abnormalities, coronary abnormalities, hypertropic cardiomyopathy, or mitral valve prolapse; only two deaths were associated with coronary arteriosclerosis. In 17 of the 19 cases death was associated with strenuous physical exertion.[20] These data indicate that young men undergoing regular heavy exercise have a very low incidence of sudden death and that arteriosclerotic coronary disease is a rare cause. Myocarditis and congenital defects are more common. In middle-aged physically-conditioned men sudden death is most commonly due to coronary artery disease. An analysis of such cases reveals in many some previous clinical

Table 23.1
Prodromal Symptoms Reported by 45 Subjects Within One
Week of Sudden Cardiac Death Related to Exercise

Symptom	Number
Chest pain/angina	15
Increasing fatigue	12
Indigestion, heartburn	10
Excessive dyspnea	6
Ear or neck pain	5
Malaise	5
Upper respiratory tract infection	4
Dizziness, palpitation	3
Headache	2

SOURCE: Friedewald and Spence, ref. 21.

symptoms or signs suggesting the possibility of coronary disease. In 45 instances of sudden cardiac death during exercise, more than one symptom was experienced by 16 of the 45 subjects. Only 9 of the 45 subjects with prodromal symptoms consulted a physician (Table 23.1).[21] In such men a medical history of heart disease, a physical examination, an electrocardiogram and an exercise test would usually have indicated the correct diagnosis.[22]

Prolonged Altitude Exposure

Prolonged exposure to high altitude for months or years have been shown to result in a lower blood pressure, a lower prevalence of hypertension, and a reported low incidence of acute myocardial infarction.[23,24] The mortality from coronary artery disease in high altitude residents has been reported to be lower than in persons living at a lower altitude.[25,26] This could be a selection process, however, because it may be that persons who experience the onset of symptoms move to a lower altitude.

The amelioration of angina with prolonged altitude exposure is due to a diminution of the acute effects of ascent with a resulting decrease in cardiac work. These changes include decreased sympathetic nervous system stimulation, decreased heart rate, cardiac output, and blood pressure, and a decreased blood volume with resulting smaller left ventricular dimensions. Respiratory alkalosis also diminishes, and thus coronary constriction is less likely to occur.

Cardiac Function in Normal Persons

There is no evidence that very high or extreme altitudes have a deleterious effect upon cardiac function in normal persons.[26] In Operation Everest II maximum cycle ergometer exercise was performed by normal subjects at simulated altitudes of 25,000 feet (7,670 m) and 29,000 feet (8,840 m) after spending 40 days in a hypobaric chamber. Despite severe hypoxemia and a respiratory alkalosis, no ST-T wave changes occurred that could be attributed to ischemia or myocardial dysfunction.[27] Cardiac function remained normal.[28] Guenter studied 16 normal subjects during maximum exercise at sea level while breathing 10 percent oxygen. Despite a mean arterial PO_2 of 31 mm, no electrocardiographic evidence of ischemia was observed.[29]

Exposure to very high or extreme altitudes does not have an adverse effect upon cardiac function. High altitude climbing to maximum effort requires less cardiac work than maximum effort at sea level. This is related to the inability of the respiratory system to maintain arterial oxygen tension rather than to the circulatory system's ability to maintain tissue oxygen delivery (see Chapter 10). The double product (systolic blood pressure multiplied by the heart rate) is a simple measure of cardiac work. At sea level during maximum effort a heart rate of 200/min and a systolic blood pressure of 180 mm Hg may be attained by normal persons for a double product of 36,000. At 20,000 feet (6,100 m) maximum effort may be accompanied by a heart rate of only 150/min and a systolic pressure of 150 mm, for a double product of 22,500, which means a decrease in cardiac work of approximately 35 percent.[30] A prolonged stay at high altitude is accompanied by the previously mentioned changes in the circulation, which result in less cardiac work and a lower myocardial oxygen demand. Experienced mountaineers usually maintain physical fitness by regular, vigorous exercise and frequent climbs. If symptoms of coronary disease appeared, climbing would be discontinued and, one assumes, a medical evaluation would be sought.

The Physician's Role

Persons over the age of 50 who are perfectly healthy and physically active and have none of the risk factors for coronary artery disease may still be required by some trekking companies to have an electrocardiogram recorded as a screening test. The value of the electrocardiogram in such persons has been questioned.[31] However, as a baseline test for possible subsequent episodes that might indicate symptoms of coronary disease, the electrocardiogram may have some value.

Persons with known or suspected coronary disease should consult their physician before undertaking a trek or trip to a high altitude area. The physician should evaluate the physical fitness of the patient, estimate the potential risks, recommend precautions, and prescribe an appropriate regimen of medications.[32] Warning symptoms of unstable angina, heart failure, myocardial infarction, or cardiac arrhythmias should be described so that the patient can take appropriate action if any of these events occur.

All patients with coronary disease should have a careful estimate of the chance of a cardiac event or sudden death. This is evaluated by a medical history, physical examination, chest X-ray, and electrocardiogram. Exercise tests or nuclear studies provide important noninvasive safe methods of further determining prognosis. There is little indication for hypoxemia tests in current practice.[10,33] Exercise tests will, in most instances, identify low- and high-risk patients with acceptable accuracy. Low-risk patients are those who can walk on a treadmill (Bruce protocol) for nine minutes or more without chest pain and with less than one mm ST depression in the exercise or postexercise electrocardiogram. No significant ventricular arrhythmias occur, and there is a normal increase in blood pressure. This group has a five-year predicted survival of approximately 95 percent and a low incidence of future cardiac events.[34] They can carry out moderate to heavy exertion without danger and can engage in occupations associated with considerable mental or emotional stress.[35] They may go to high altitude and participate in trekking with a minimum of risk of a coronary event. Guidelines and indications for exercise testing have been published.[36]

Patients with a less favorable prognosis, who are at a higher risk for a coronary event, exhibit one or more of the following abnormalities on exercise testing: (1) ≥2 mm ST depression at a heart rate of <130/min; (2) cannot walk more than six minutes; (3) exercise is limited by chest pain; (4) multiple extra systoles and/or an inadequate rise in blood pressure during exercise occur. Patients in this category should be offered coronary arteriography to define their risk status further. Over 50 percent of such patients will have arteriographic evidence of high-risk coronary disease, including left main coronary disease or triple vessel disease with some abnormality of left ventricular function. In such patients, coronary bypass surgery or coronary angioplasty will usually be recommended not only to relieve symptoms and increase exercise capacity but also to increase survival.[34] Following bypass surgery or angioplasty the patient's risk status should be evaluated by exercise testing or nuclear angiography.[37] Low-risk patients with slight or no symptoms on moderate to severe physical activity after surgery may participate in a high altitude trek with little risk.

In some patients exercise test results may be inconclusive for various reasons. Nuclear studies are then indicated.[37,38,39] Patients may be unable to exercise because of orthopedic problems. In such instances an oral persantine thallium scan will usually identify patients with significant areas of ischemic myocardium that will indicate the need for coronary arteriography.[38]

Patients with significant ischemia demonstrated by nuclear studies should have coronary arteriography to detect lesions that may require coronary bypass surgery or angioplasty. Patients who have had coronary bypass surgery usually become asymptomatic and can carry out exercise programs without the need of medications. In such patients exercise testing or nuclear studies usually indicate a low-risk status that would not be a contraindication to a visit to a high altitude area. Some physicians disagree with this viewpoint, believing that even after a successful bypass operation residual disease is probably present and that going to an altitude of 18,900 feet (5,765 m) would entail such a degree of risk that it would be unwise to undertake such a trip.[40] This and the contrary point of view have been discussed.[41,42]

Patients with severe coronary disease, congestive failure, or cardiac arrhythmias who are capable of only limited activity should not visit high altitude areas, since they are at high risk of cardiac events during the first week or two after ascent. If travel to a moderate altitude or travel by air is necessary, oxygen and a increase in medications may be necessary to control symptoms.

Exercise testing is usually not indicated in persons who have no symptoms or evidence of coronary disease. The number of positive tests in such persons is low (5-10 percent) and about half of the apparent positive tests are "false positives", as judged by nuclear studies being normal. Finally, in the small number of persons with true positive tests, coronary arteriography usually shows only mild disease with a favorable prognosis. A possible indication for exercise testing in asymptomatic persons over the age of 50 may be the presence of multiple-risk factors for the possible presence of coronary disease or the fact that such a person will be spending long periods of time in an area where there are no medical facilities. Risk factors for the possible presence of coronary disease are: (1) sudden death or coronary disease in family members under the age of 50, (2) history of hypertension, (3) ST depression of any magnitude in the resting ECG, (4) any previous episode of chest pain, (5) a history of smoking, (6) diabetes, (7) obesity, and (8) abnormal serum lipids.[35,36]

For patients with coronary disease who are going to high altitude the physician should describe the symptoms of ischemic events as well as medications to be used and methods of management. The necessity of rest, the use of oxygen, and prompt evacuation to a hospital facility should be emphasized. The trip physician should be supplied with all necessary clinical information regarding the patient's cardiac status. The patient should consider the availability of medical facilities and means of rapid transport should a cardiac event occur; it may be unwise to travel to a remote area where medical facilities are not available. Adequate acclimatization at a moderate altitude should be experienced before going higher. The patient must be physically fit before going on a walking trek. Hill walking with a light pack is an excellent method of conditioning: if one can walk for twelve miles without difficulty on a trail over hilly terrain, one ought to be fit enough for nearly any trek. The patient himself, however, must make the final decision, based upon the information he receives from his physician.

References

1. NEIL W, and HALLENHAUER M. Impairment of myocardial supply due to hyperventilation. *Circulation* 1975; 52:854-58.
2. RASMUSSEN K, JUUL S, BAGGER J, and HENNINGSEN P. Usefulness of ST deviation induced by prolonged hyperventilation as a predictor of cardiac death in angina pectoris. *Am. J. Cardiol.* 1987; 59: 763-68.
3. ARDISSIMO D, DESERVI S, FALCONE C, et al. Role of hypocapnic alkalosis in hyperventilation: Induced coronary artery spasm in variant angina. *Am. J. Cardiol.* 1987; 59:707-09.
4. NEILL W. Effects of arterial hypoxemia and hyperoxia on oxygen availability for myocardial metabolism. *Am. J. Cardiol.* 1969; 24:166-77.
5. GROVER R, TUCKER C, MCGROARITY R, and TRAVIS R. The coronary stress of skiing at high altitude. *Arch. Int. Med.* 1990; 150:1205-08.
6. FROELICHER V, THOMAS M, PILLOW C, et al. Epidemiologic study of asymptomatic men screened by maximal treadmill testing for latent coronary artery disease. *Am. J. Cardiol.* 1974; 34:770-76.
7. CUMMING G. Yield of ischaemic exercise electrocardiograms in relation to exercise intensity in a normal population. *Br. Heart J.* 1972; 34:919- 23.
8. BRAMMELL H, MORGAN B, NICOLI S, and ALEXANDER J. Exercise tolerance is reduced at altitude in patients with coronary artery disease. *J. Wilderness Med.* 1990; 1:147-53.
9. MORGAN B, ALEXANDER J, NICOLI S, and BRAMMELL H. The patient with coronary heart disease at altitude: Observations during acute exposure to 3,100 meters. *J. Wilderness Med.* 1990; 1:147-53.
10. BURCHELL H, PRUITT R, and BARNES A. The stress and the electrocardiogram in the induced hypoxemia test for coronary insufficiency. *Am. Heart J.* 1948; 36:373-80.
11. KASSELBAUM D, SUTHERLAND K, and JUDKINS M. A comparison of hypoxemia and exercise electrocardiography in coronary artery disease. *Am. Heart J.* 1968; 75:759-76.
12. SHLIM D, and HOUSTON R. Helicopter rescues and deaths among trekkers in Nepal. *JAMA* 1989; 261: 1017-19.
13. BURTSCHER M, PHILADELPHY M, and LIKAR R. Sudden cardiac death during mountain hiking and skiing. *N. Engl. J. Med.* 1993; 329:1738-39. Letters to the Editor.
14. MARTICORENA E. Personal communication.
15. MARTICORENA E, MARTICORENA J, et al. Neuva technica en rehabilitación cardiac y prevention primaria coronaria: Utilización de las grandes alturas. *Arch. Biolog. Andina*, 1984-85, 13:18.
16. YARON M, ALEXANDER J, and HULTGREN H. Low risk of myocardial ischemia in the elderly at moderate altitude. *J. Wilderness Med.* 1995; 6:20-28.
17. ROACH R, HOUSTON C, HONIGMAN B, et al. How well do older persons tolerate moderate altitude? *West. J. Med.* 1995; 162:32-36.
18. FURBERG C, MANOLIO T, PSATY B, et al. Major electrocardiographic abnormalities in persons aged 65 years and older (the Cardiovascular Health Study). *Am. J. Cardiol.* 1992; 69:1329-35.

19. ALEXANDER J. Age, altitude and arrhythmia. *Texas Heart Inst. J.* 1995; 22:308-16.
20. PHILLIPS M, ROBINOWITZ M, HIGGINS J, et al. Sudden cardiac death in Air Force recruits. *JAMA* 1986; 256:2696-99.
21. FRIEDEWALD V, and SPENCE D. Sudden cardiac death associated with exercise: The risk-benefit ratio. *Am. J. Cardiol.* 1990; 66:183-88.
22. WALLER B. Sudden death in middle-aged conditioned subjects: Coronary atherosclerosis is the culprit. *Mayo Clin. Proc.* 1987; 62:634-35. Editorial.
23. HULTGREN H, et al. Reduction of systemic arterial blood pressure at high altitude. *Adv. Cardiol.* 1970; 5:49-50.
24. MORTIMER E, JR., MONSON R, and MACMAHON B. Reduction in mortality from coronary heart disease in men residing at high altitude. *N. Engl. J. Med.* 1977; 296:581-85.
25. VOORS A, and JOHNSON W. Altitude and arteriosclerotic heart disease mortality in white residents of 99 of the 100 largest cities in the United States. *J. Chronic Dis.* 1979; 32:157-62.
26. HULTGREN H. Coronary heart disease and trekking. *J. Wilderness Med.* 1990; 1:154-61.
27. MALCONIAN M, ROCK P, HULTGREN H, et al. Operation Everest II: The electrocardiogram at rest and exercise during a stimulated ascent of Mt. Everest. *Am. J. Cardiol.* 1990; 65:1475-80.
28. SUAREZ J, ALEXANDER J, and HOUSTON C. Enhanced left ventricular systolic performance at high altitude during Operation Everest II. *Am. J. Cardiol.* 1987; 60:137-42.
29. GUENTER C. Effects of severe arterial hypoxemia on electrocardiogram during exercise. *Chest* 1975; 68:149-54.
30. WEST J, BOYER S, GRABER D, et al. Maximal exercise at extreme altitudes on Mount Everest. *J. Appl. Physiol.* 1983; 55:678-87.
31. SOX H. The baseline electrocardiogram. *Am. J. Med.* 1991; 91:573-75. Editorial.
32. RENNIE D. Will mountain trekkers have heart attacks? *JAMA* 1989; 261:1045-46. Editorial.
33. KHANNA P, DHAM S, and HOON R. Exercise in hypoxic environment as screening test for ischemic heart disease. *Aviat. Space Environ. Med.* 1976; 47:1114-17.
34. Veterans Administration Cooperative Study of Medical Versus Surgical Treatment for Stable Angina: Progress report, H Hultgren, ed., *Prog. in Cardiovasc. Dis.* 1985-86; 28:213-401.
35. BRUCE R, and FISHER L. Strategies for risk evaluation of sudden cardiac incapacitation in men in occupations affecting public safety. *J. Occup. Med.* 1989; 31:124-33.
36. Guidelines for exercise testing: American College of Cardiology/American Heart Association Task Force on Assessment of Cardiovascular Procedures (Subcommittee on Exercise Testing). *J. Am. Coll. Cardiol.* 1986; 8:725-38.
37. BORER J, BACHARACH S, GREEN M, et al. Real-time radionuclide cineangiography in the noninvasive evaluation of global and regional left ventricular function at rest and during exercise in patients with coronary artery disease. *N. Engl. J. Med.* 1977; 296:839-44.
38. HENDEL R, LAYDEN J, and LEPPO J. Prognostic value of dipyridamole thallium scintigraphy for evaluation of ischemic heart disease. *J. Am. Coll. Cardiol.* 1990; 15:109-16.
39. FLEG J, GERSTENBLITH G, ZONDERMAN A, et al. Prevalence and prognostic significance of exercise-induced silent ischemia detected by thallium scintigraphy and electrocardiography in asymptomatic volunteers. *Circulation* 1990; 81:428-36.
40. Trekking in Nepal: Safety after coronary artery bypass. *JAMA* 1988; 259:3184. Questions and Answers.
41. HULTGREN H. The safety of trekking at high altitude after coronary bypass surgery. *JAMA* 1988; 260:2218.
42. WEST J. The safety of trekking at high altitude after coronary bypass surgery. *JAMA* 1988; 260: 2218-19.

CHAPTER 24

Congenital and Valvular Heart Disease

SUMMARY

Residents of high altitude areas who have certain types of congenital heart disease have been shown to have a higher pulmonary artery pressure and resistance than sea-level dwellers. Ventricular septal defects and atrial septal defects are the most common varieties affected. It is also likely that at high altitude pulmonary hypertension is more prevalent and severe in some types of acquired heart disease such as mitral stenosis. Sea-level residents who have these varieties of heart disease and go to high altitude may experience an increase in symptoms as a result of hypoxic pulmonary vasoconstriction. Moderate restriction of physical activity and an increase in medication may be required. Cyanosis may increase in patients with right-to-left shunts. Persons so affected who contemplate a permanent move to high altitude should take up temporary residence in the area to determine the effect upon symptoms. Patients with moderate to severe pulmonary hypertension at high altitude usually fare better at sea level.

• • •

Congenital Heart Disease

Patients with certain forms of congenital and valvular heart disease may be adversely affected by high altitude, primarily owing to hypoxic pulmonary vasoconstriction.

Although many patients with congenital heart disease and valvular heart disease have had correction of the abnormality by open heart surgery, there are some patients who, for various reasons, may not have had surgery. Eisenmenger's syndrome can only be corrected by heart-lung transplantation, for example, and in other patients residual pulmonary hypertension persists even after surgical intervention.

Atrial Septal Defects

The effects of high altitude upon the pulmonary arteriolar resistance and pulmonary hypertension in congenital heart disease have been examined by several investigators. In 1962, Dalen and his associates reviewed the records of patients with secundum atrial septal defects living at low elevations (less than 2,000 feet/ 610 m) and at moderate elevations of more than 4,000 feet (1,220 m).[1] Pulmonary hypertension, defined as a mean pulmonary artery (PA) pressure exceeding 35 mm Hg, was present in only 3 of 49 patients (6 percent) from low elevations and in 11 of 53 patients (21 percent) from high elevations. All these patients were less than 20 years of age. It was concluded that residence at even moderate altitudes is associated with earlier development of pulmonary hypertension in patients with this abnormality as compared with patients living at low elevations.

Ventricular Septal Defects

Studies of infants with ventricular septal defects showed that pulmonary vascular resistance was twice as high in infants living in Denver as compared with infants at sea level.[2,3,4] A descent to a lower altitude by patients with these defects will result in a decrease in pulmonary artery pressure and an improvement in symptoms. Willerson and his associates described a two-year-old boy with altitude dependent pulmonary hypertension. The boy had a ventricular septal defect with a mean pulmonary artery pressure of 60 mm Hg. The administration of 100 percent oxygen reduced the pressure to 30 mm Hg. The pulmonary systemic flow ratio was 1.5/1.0. The child moved to sea level and at five years had a second study. The pulmonary artery mean pressure had decreased to 20 mm Hg with a similar pulmonary systemic flow ratio of 1.6/1.0.[5]

Primary Pulmonary Hypertension

Patients with primary pulmonary hypertension may also experience a decrease in pulmonary artery pressure and pulmonary vascular resistance upon descent to a lower altitude. Symptoms may be markedly improved, as shown by a case reported by Shettigar and associates.[6] A 27-year-old Hispanic man was born and lived at 4,700 feet (1,434 m) in Colorado. At 19 he developed progressive exertional dyspnea with chest pain and exertional syncope. His activity became limited to only a sedentary life-style. Physical examination revealed a prominent jugular a wave, a right ventricular lift, and a loud P_2. An ECG was compatible with right ventricular hypertrophy. A chest film showed clear lung fields, prominent central pulmonary arteries, and right ventricular enlargement. A treadmill test (Bruce) resulted in syncope after four minutes. His mean PA pressure was 45 mm Hg, PAW 5 mm, and pulmonary resistance 9 Wood units. He was advised to move to sea level, which he did, with a moderate improvement in symptoms. Infusions of Tolazoline and of isoproterenol reduced the PA mean pressure to 22 and 20 mm, respectively. Pulmonary vascular resistance was reduced to 2.8 and 2.1 Wood units. Premedication PA pressure was 43 mm and resistance was 6.8 Wood units, a moderate decrease from the altitude values. Sublingual isoproterenol glossets 20 mg every two hours improved walking distance and prevented exertional syncope. Improvement persisted for three years when symptoms again became severe. Pulmonary vascular resistance had increased to 14.5 Wood units with a mean PA pressure elevated to 67 mm Hg. The patient was lost to follow-up. Primary pulmonary hypertension may be more common at high altitude, and symptomatic patients should be encouraged to move to a lower altitude.[7,8]

Patients with pulmonary hypertension should not go to high altitude for a prolonged stay, especially if symptoms appear or become worse during a temporary visit to high altitude. If such patients must move to a higher altitude for economic or personal reasons, a trial stay of two to four weeks is recommended before they make a permanent decision. These considerations are more important in infants and children than in adults, since in these patients the pulmonary vascular bed is probably more reactive and thus more responsive to changes in altitude Cardiac catheterization studies of the effect of hyperoxia and hypoxia upon the pulmonary vascular resistance are useful in determining whether or not hypoxia significantly increases pulmonary artery pressure, since such patients are more likely to tolerate high altitude poorly.[4] The effect of calcium channel blockers can also be evaluated to determine whether or not such preparations would be useful in lowering pulmonary artery pressure. The development of noninvasive methods of estimating pulmonary artery systolic pressure by echo-Doppler methods has obviated the need for cardiac catheterization in many of these patients.[9]

Valvular Heart Disease

Patients with valvular heart disease living at high altitude also appear to have a higher pulmonary artery pressure and resistance than do similar patients at sea level. It has been estimated that in the Peruvian Andes the prevalence of pulmonary hypertension in rheumatic mitral regurgitation is 20 percent and in mitral stenosis 70 percent compared with sea-level prevalences of 1 and 10 percent, respectively.[10] Pulmonary artery pressure in such patients may decrease upon descent to a lower altitude. Similarly, patients with mitral stenosis who go to high altitude may exhibit an increase in dyspnea owing to a decrease in diastolic filling time by tachycardia and, in some instances, an increase in pulmonary vascular resistance.

In patients with mitral stenosis, Yu and his associates noted an increase in pulmonary artery pressure and pulmonary vascular resistance in 11 of 13 patients breathing 12 percent oxygen for fifteen minutes.[11] Idiopathic hypertrophic subaortic stenosis (IHSS) may be aggravated by ascent to high altitude In one instance a patient with IHSS traveled to a Rocky Mountain resort at 8,200 feet (2,500 m). While skiing, the patient collapsed and developed pulmonary edema and a shock-like state. Furosemide was given without effect. The patient recovered upon descent to Denver. The diagnosis was established by echocardiography, and beta-blocker therapy was started.[12] It is likely that the combined effect of the decrease in left ventricular volume, a diuretic and the sympathetic nervous system activity induced by hypoxemia increased the degree of aortic stenosis, with nearly disastrous results.

Pulmonary Artery Abnormalities

Congenital absence of the right pulmonary artery is now well recognized as a risk factor for HAPE.[13] This abnormality may result in HAPE occurring at an altitude of less than 8,000 feet (2,440 m). Right pulmonary artery hypoplasia may also increase the risk of HAPE.[14] Other conditions which restrict the pulmonary circulation and may increase the risk of HAPE are proximal interruption of the left pulmonary artery,[15] congenital or acquired spinal scoliosis[16] and partial anomalous pulmonary venous connection with an intact atrial septum, in which the veins from the right upper and middle lobe drained into the right atrium instead of the left atrium.[17] One might expect that patients with the scimitar syndrome may also be susceptible to HAPE, since in this syndrome anomalous right pulmonary veins connect to the inferior vena cava with hypoplasia of the right pulmonary artery and pulmonary hypertension.[18] Patients who have had a right pneumonectomy may be susceptible to HAPE but to my knowledge no case reports have been made.

Cyanotic Congenital Heart Disease

Patients with cyanotic congenital heart disease may tolerate commercial air travel without difficulty. Harinck and associates studied twelve patients during a simulated flight of 1.5 and 7 hours in a hypobaric chamber. The maximal mean decrease in arterial oxygen saturation did not exceed 8.8 percent. The authors speculated that the lack of a greater decrease in saturation was probably due to a high concentration of 2.3 diphosphoglycerate in the red cells.[19]

References

1. DALEN J, BRUCE R, and COBB L. Interaction of chronic hypoxia of moderate altitude on pulmonary hypertension complicating defect of the atrial septum. *N. Engl. J. Med.* 1962; 266:272-77.
2. VOGEL J. Importance of mild hypoxia on abnormal pulmonary vascular beds. In *Hypoxia, high altitude*, and the heart, vol. 5 of Advances in cardiology. Basel: S. Karger, 1970:159-65.
3. VOGEL J, MCNAMARA D, and BLOUNT S, JR. The role of hypoxia in determining pulmonary vascular resistance in infants with ventricular septal defects. *Am. J. Cardiol.* 1967; 20:346-49.
4. BLOUNT S, JR. Comparison of patients with ventricular septal defect at high altitude and sea level. *Circulation* 1977; 56, Suppl. I:79-82.
5. WILLERSON J, BAGGETT A, THOMAS J, and GOLDBLATT A. Ventricular septal defect with altitude-dependent pulmonary hypertension. *N. Engl. J. Med.* 1971; 28:157-58.
6. SHETTIGAR U, HULTGREN H, SPECTER M, et al. Primary pulmonary hypertension: Favorable effect of isoproterenol. *N. Engl. J. Med.* 1976; 295:1414-15.
7. KHOURY G, and HAWES C. Primary pulmonary hypertension in children living at high altitude. *J. Pediatr.* 1963; 62:177-185.
8. VOGEL J, VOIGT G, and BLOUNT S, JR. Reversal of high altitude pulmonary hypertension. *Am. J. Cardiol.* 1966; 18:928-32.
9. CHAN K, CURRIE P, SEWARD J, et al. Comparison of three Doppler ultrasound methods in the prediction of pulmonary artery pressure. *J. Am. Coll. Cardiol.* 1987; 9:-549-54.
10. MARTICORENA E. Personal communication.
11. YU P, BEATTY D, LOVEJOY F JR, et al. Studies of pulmonary hypertension. VII: Hemodynamic effects of acute hypoxia in patients with mitral stenosis. *Am. Heart J.* 1956; 52:683-94.
12. *Rocky Mountain News*, Denver, Feb. 14, 1991.
13. HACKETT P, CREAH C, GROVER R, et al. High altitude pulmonary edema in persons without the right pulmonary artery. *N. Engl. J. Med.* 1980; 302: 1070-73.
14. FIORENZANO G, RESTELLI V, and GRECO V. Unilateral high altitude pulmonary edema in a subject with right pulmonary artery hypoplasia. *Respiration* 1994; 61:51-4.
15. LEVINE S, WHITE D, and FELS A. An abnormal chest radiograph in a patient with recurring high altitude pulmonary edema. *Chest* 1988; 94:827-28.
16. HULTGREN H, HONIGMAN B, THEIS K, and NICHOLAS D. High-altitude pulmonary edema at a ski resort. *West. J. Med.* 1996; 164:222-27.
17. BOSCH F. High altitude pulmonary edema in partial anomalous pulmonary connection of drainage with intact atrial septum. *Chest* 1993; 103:534-36.
18. GAO YANG-AN, BURROWS P, BENSON L, et al. Scimitar syndrome in infancy. *J. Am. Coll. Cardiol.* 1993; 22:873-82.
19. HARINCK E, HUTTER P, HOORNTJE T, et al: Air travel and adults with cyanotic congenital heart disease. *Circulation* 1996; 93:272-6.

CHAPTER 25

Systemic Hypertension

SUMMARY

During the first ten days at altitude, normal subjects will usually exhibit a rise in blood pressure, involving both systolic and diastolic pressures and also systemic resistance. This is largely due to increased sympathetic activity due to norepinephrine which acts on the alpha receptors. The rise in blood pressure may be greater in patients with hypertension. Since beta blockers may not prevent the rise in blood pressure, patients with hypertension who are planning to go to high altitude should see their physician to obtain appropriate medications. The dose of antihypertensive medication should probably be increased during the first ten days at high altitude. Alpha blockers, ACE inhibitors, and calcium channel blockers may be more effective than beta blockers and diuretics during this period. Prolonged residence at high altitude is not associated with an increase in blood pressure, but may on the contrary over several months or years result in a decrease in pressure or at least the absence of the usual rise in systolic pressure seen with advancing age.

• • •

Systemic hypertension is defined as a systolic blood pressure exceeding 140 mm Hg or a diastolic pressure above 90 mm Hg. Patients with pressures between 140/80 and 160/95 mm Hg are classified as borderline or mild hypertensives. In males 45 to 54 years the prevalence of hypertension is around 26 percent; in women it is slightly less, at 19 percent. The prevalence increases with advancing age.[1] Hypertension is thus one of the major cardiovascular health problems in the United States. In normal persons, ascent to high altitude is usually accompanied by a rise in blood pressure. In patients with systemic hypertension the rise in blood pressure may be substantial.

Normal Persons

Several studies have indicated an elevation of both systolic and diastolic pressures as well as an increase in heart rate during exposure to high altitude. Systemic vascular resistance is increased. Kamat and Banerji observed a rise in blood pressure in 31 of 32 subjects who ascended to an altitude between 11,500 and 13,000 feet (3,500-4,000 m). Systolic pressure rose from 115 mm Hg to 125 mm Hg and diastolic pressure rose from 78 mm Hg to 93 mm Hg (see Fig. 25.1).[2] Wolfel and his associates reported significant elevations in blood pressure and peripheral vascular resistance in seven young men exposed to 14,110 feet (4,300 m) for 21 days. Mean blood pressure rose from 124/71 mm Hg to 145/88 mm Hg, and estimated systemic vascular resistance (mean values) rose from 17 to 28 Wood units (mm Hg/L/min). Pressures during exercise were higher than at sea level. Arterial norepinephrine levels were increased.[3] Japanese studies have shown striking elevations of blood pressure in some normal subjects. On a Japanese expedition to Mount Everest,

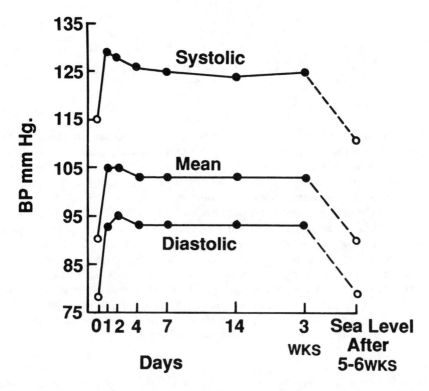

Figure 25.1. Changes in blood pressure in 32 subjects during a stay at an altitude of between 11,500 and 13,000 feet (3,500-4,000 m). From Kamat and Banerji, ref. 2.

systolic blood pressures in two subjects rose from 128 and 125 mm Hg at Katmandu 4,382 feet (1,336 m) to 178 and 163 mm Hg respectively at base camp 17,712 feet (5,400 m)[4] In a study of fourteen men, aged 22 to 55 years, during a 22-day sojourn at altitudes of 14,000-23,000 feet (4,270-7,015 m) on Mount Aconcagua diastolic blood pressures increased until the end of the second week to levels that were 10-25 mm Hg higher than at sea level. Systolic pressure was either unchanged or only slightly higher.[5] Seven normal subjects, after a three week graded ascent to 18,000 feet (5,400 m) in a hypobaric chamber, exhibited an increase in blood pressure at rest and during exercise. Systolic pressure (rest) increased from 105 mm Hg to 119 mm Hg, and during exercise from 119 mm Hg to 146 mm Hg. Diastolic pressures (rest) increased from 59 mm Hg to 66 mm Hg.[6]

A study of telescope workers who work at 13,780 feet (4,200 m) on Mauna Kea in Hawaii showed a rise in diastolic blood pressure of about 10 percent above the pre-ascent level, which was persistent during a 40-day stay on the mountain. Systolic pressure was increased on the second day. On descent, both pressures returned to pre-ascent levels.[7] Both systolic and diastolic pressures are higher during exercise at high altitude than at sea level for similar work levels.[6,8] Recent studies by Wolfel and his associates confirmed earlier observations, evaluated the time course of the

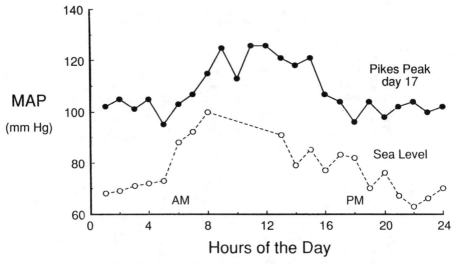

Figure 25.2. Systemic blood pressure in 11 normal subjects during a 17 day stay on Pikes Peak. Ambulatory monitoring was employed. From Wolfel, ref. 9.

changes in blood pressure and concluded that the rise in pressure was probably related to increased sympathetic activity from norepinephrine.[9] The time course of the blood pressure in 11 healthy men over 21 days on Pikes Peak is shown in Figure 25.2.

The incidence of pregnancy-associated hypertension is more common at 10,168 feet (3,100 m) 12 percent than at 7,904 feet (2,410 m) 4 percent or at 5,248 feet (1,600 m) 3 percent. The degree of hypertension is inversely related to the arterial oxygen saturation.[10]

Systemic Hypertension

Few studies have been made of patients with systemic hypertension who travel to high altitude. One study examined the effect of ascent to an intermediate altitude of 4,000 feet (1,200 m) in twelve subjects with untreated borderline hypertension (140/80-160/95 mm Hg). Using 24-hour ambulatory blood pressure monitoring, the investigators found that the maximum increase in systolic pressure was 17 mm Hg, and 16 mm Hg in diastolic pressure, both being greatest during the waking hours. Plasma levels of epinephrine and norepinephrine were also higher. The magnitude of the blood pressure elevation was, however, similar to that in twelve normal nonhypertensive control subjects.[11]

In a study of the blood pressure in 95 elderly men (mean age 69 years) who travelled from low altitude to a Colorado resort at 8,200 feet (2,500 m) the following observations were made: in 62 normotensive subjects both systolic and diastolic pressures rose at altitude with the highest reading 24 hours after arrival and a decrease thereafter but not to low altitude levels. In 33 hypertensive subjects a substantially greater rise in both systolic and diastolic pressures occurred with a similar time course. (Fig. 25.3) Very high blood pressures (183/78-218/105 mm Hg) were present on day 1 or day 2 in seven subjects who did not report the presence of

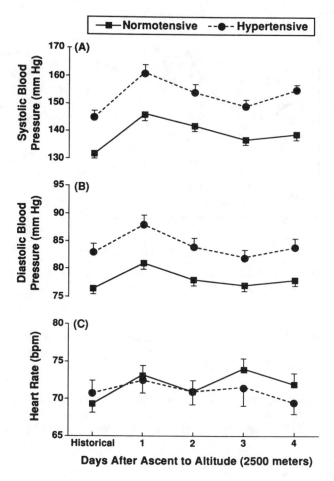

Figure 25.3. Blood pressures in 62 normotensive elderly men before and after ascent to 8,200 feet (2,500 m) compared to the response of 33 hypertensives. From Roach, ref. 12.

an elevated blood pressure at a lower altitude. None experienced symptoms or a decrease in physical activity.[12] Scholing carried out a study of the effect of ascent and a longer stay at 5,576-6,560 feet (1,700-2,000 m) in 31 hypertensives and 8 normal subjects who resided in Munich, 1,700 feet (520 m). Studies were made at rest and during exercise. The mean resting systolic blood pressure in hypertensive patients rose from 146 mm Hg to 156 mm Hg by the second day at altitude. After 13 days the blood pressure had decreased to 141 mm Hg, and it remained at that level for the 30-day duration of altitude exposure. A surprising finding was that the blood pressure decreased further upon descent and this decrease persisted for three months after descent (mean blood pressure, 136 mm Hg). Blood pressures recorded during exercise showed a similar change. These variations were not seen in normotensive subjects.[13]

Similar results were obtained by Halhuber and his colleagues, who found that in 593 patients with mild hypertension who moved to altitudes up to 9,900 feet (3,000 m), systolic and diastolic pressures decreased after acclimatization. The decrease in blood pressure persisted for four to eight months after descent. No instances of cerebrovascular accidents or cardiac problems occurred during the altitude stay.[14] These results are comparable to the effect of continued residence at high altitude on blood pressure seen in normal subjects.[15]

Case report. An example of hypertension aggravated by high altitude exposure is the case of a 77-year-old woman who had borderline hypertension for six years, with pressures varying from 135/76 mm Hg to 150/80 mm Hg. In a routine examination before a skiing trip to Colorado, she was told that her blood pressure was "slightly elevated". She was given no medication. A month later she went to Aspen, Colorado (8,000 feet/2,440 m), where she went cross-country skiing. On the third day she did not feel well and saw a doctor. Her blood pressure was 200/125 mm Hg. She was hospitalized; nifedipine and hydrochlorothiazide were started and oxygen was administered with a decrease in blood pressure. After hospital discharge, she used oxygen from a portable tank while she went down to Grand Junction, Colorado (4,600 feet/1,403 m), where she felt better. She has since maintained her pressure at 130/70 mm Hg with medication. She is asymptomatic.

A close relationship between altitude and blood pressure is illustrated by the case of a middle-aged physician who had mild, uncomplicated hypertension at sea level with pressures of 120/82-134/92 mm Hg while on propranolol 40 mg daily. He went on an auto tour of the Rocky Mountains and continued his daily medication. He recorded his own blood pressure twice daily. Figure 25.4 illustrates the changes in blood pressure during the trip. Both systolic and diastolic pressures rose and fell in relation to the altitude. The highest readings were obtained in Dillon, Colorado, at 9,300 feet (2,836 m), where his pressure was 160/105 mm Hg. Lower readings of 155/100 mm Hg occurred at Denver, at 5,400 feet (1,635 m). At Dillon, the morning blood pressures were higher than evening blood pressures. This is a reversal of the usual diurnal variation and it could be related to a greater degree of hypoxemia during sleep. The mean blood pressure at sea level was 130/83 mm Hg before the high altitude sojourn and 110/75 mm Hg after returning to sea level. The heart rate remained slow, 50/min, at all elevations probably because of the beta blockade, although the dose of propranolol was moderate.[16] The fact that the subject's blood pressure was lower at sea level after the high altitude sojourn than before is interesting, and it corresponds with similar findings reported by Scholing[13] and by Halhuber.[14]

Mechanism of Blood Pressure Rise

Increased sympathetic stimulation mediated by hypoxemia via the carotid body chemoreceptors is the most likely cause of the rise in blood pressure.

The chemoreceptor response to hypoxia by the carotid body may be enhanced in hypertensives. Somers studied eight borderline hypertensives and eight normal subjects exposed to short periods of isocapneic hypoxia—five minutes of 10 percent oxygen. There was no difference in the increase in heart rate, blood pressure, or ventilation between the two groups. During hypoxia, however, sympathetic activity in the hypertensives increased by 41 ± 5 percent compared with an increase of 21 ± 5 percent in the control subjects. Sympathetic activity was obtained from

444

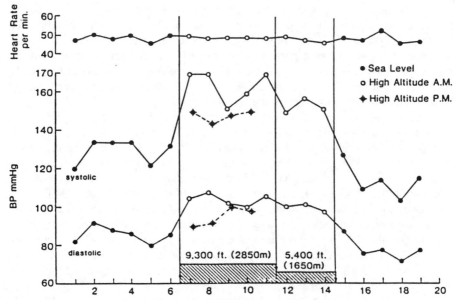

Figure 25.4. Heart rate and systolic and diastolic blood pressure in a 64-year-old physician at sea level and during an auto tour of the Rocky Mountains. Data from Penrod, ref. 16.

direct multi-unit recordings from a nerve fascicle to muscle in the peroneal nerve posterior to the fibular head. It was concluded that the chemoreceptor reflex is enhanced in borderline hypertensives and results in an increase in sympathetic nerve activity during hypoxia. The chemoreceptor stimulus is sensed by the carotid body. It is not known whether this phenomenon is present in persons with established hypertension.[17]

Several workers have demonstrated a rise in norepinephrine and epinephrine blood levels following ascent to high altitude with an associated rise in blood pressure.[3,9,18] The effect of hypoxemia upon catecholamine release and blood pressure is further illustrated by the studies of Bärtsch and associates, who showed that persons who developed acute mountain sickness or high altitude pulmonary edema had higher plasma levels of norepinephrine and epinephrine than subjects who did not develop symptoms.[19] An analysis of 136 cases of high altitude pulmonary edema at Keystone, Colorado, 9,300 feet (2,840 m), revealed that 46 (32 percent) had systolic blood pressures of 140 mm Hg or higher, with a mean arterial oxygen saturation of 76 percent.[20] Blood pressures decreased to normal with oxygen or hyperbaric bag therapy.[21]

The principal effect upon blood pressure appears to be alpha stimulation and resulting systemic vasoconstriction. The mechanism of the rise in heart rate and blood pressure at high altitude has been investigated by Reeves and his associates. They concluded that altitude activates both the beta-adrenergics and alpha sympathetics. Beta adrenergic stimulation increases the heart rate and myocardial contractility. Alpha sympathetic stimulation increases systemic arterial pressure and peripheral vascular resistance, and this effect can be blocked by phentolamine.[23] The increase in heart rate can be blocked by propranolol. The rise in blood norepinephrine concentration is accompanied by a rise in peripheral vascular resistance and blood pressure.[9,22,24] Although increased sympathetic stimulation is probably an important factor in the rise in peripheral resistance, other factors may also be involved.

Atrial natriuretic peptide (ANF) may play a role in regulating angiotensin production as well as having a direct effect on systemic vascular resistance, since it can antagonize arterial constriction due to both angiotensin and norepinephrine.[25] A diminished secretion of ANF would enhance the vasoconstrictive effect of these agents. The initial decrease in plasma volume during ascent to high altitude may be a stimulus to a decrease in ANF secretion with a resulting increase in vasoconstrictive activity of both angiotensin and norepinephrine. Plasma ANF levels have been shown to be increased during acute altitude exposure in normal subjects.[19] Plasma renin activity and plasma aldosterone are not increased by altitude exposure.[17] No studies have been done on hypertensives at high altitude.

It is clear that these questions can only be answered by studies of normal and hypertensive subjects exposed to high altitude.

Practical Clinical Considerations

Patients with hypertension may expect an increase in blood pressure to occur during the first week or two after ascent to high altitude. Since systemic hypertension is usually asymptomatic, symptoms experienced at high altitude, such as

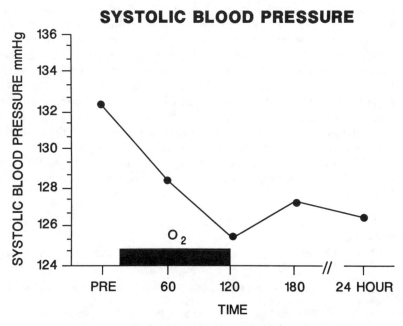

Figure 25.5. Effect of 100 percent oxygen upon systolic blood pressure in fifteen patients with acute mountain sickness at 9,300 feet (2,850 m). All were recent arrivals from sea level (<3 days at altitude). Oxygen was given via a plastic face mask at a flow rate of 4 L/min. Arterial oxygen saturation increased from 88 percent to 97 percent. Systolic blood pressure decreased during oxygen breathing. From Kasic et al., ref. 21.

headache, will probably be due to acute mountain sickness rather than to the increase in blood pressure. Patients on antihypertensive medications should be prepared to increase the dose after ascent depending upon the blood pressure measurements. Postural hypotension or weakness may be experienced during the first week of altitude exposure especially if diuretic drugs are used. Blood pressure measurements at high altitude may be made with either a mercury or an aneroid sphygmomanometer. Mercury sphygmomanometers give slightly higher readings at high altitude, but the effect is small, 5 mm Hg, and is only apparent at altitudes of 9,750-16,900 feet (3,000-5,200 m).[26]

Special attention should be paid to hypertensives who are on diuretic therapy. Potassium supplements should be continued if they are taken daily at sea level, and in some instances they should be increased, since at high altitude there is a possibility of a potassium diuresis with an accompanying decrease in total body potassium and serum potassium.[27,28] I have seen one patient on diuretic therapy who had an inadequate potassium intake on a trek between 7,000 and 9,000 feet (2,120-2,725 m) in the Sierra Nevada in California. During two walks of six to eight miles on hot days he developed severe muscular weakness and was barely able to continue. When the problem was recognized and potassium supplements were administered, he had no further difficulty.

It is possible, as one of the cases described above indicates, that beta blockers may not be effective in controlling elevations of blood pressure at high altitude, because beta blockade lowers blood pressure primarily by reductions in cardiac output and plasma renin activity. Clonidine may be a more effective means of controlling altitude hypertension in that it produces a diffuse inhibition of sympathetic neural outflow of the central nervous system.[29] Terazosin is a long-acting selective alpha[1] receptor antagonist which may be useful in controlling altitude-induced hypertension. The usual dose is 5 to 20 mg daily.[30] Doxazosin mesylate is another alpha blocking agent which has been used in the treatment of hypertension. The half life is 22 hours. An initial daily dose of 2 mg is recommended.[31] Labetalol, an alpha and beta receptor blocker has been used to treat hypertension. It may, because of its alpha-blocking properties, also be useful in the control of altitude-induced hypertension.[32] Calcium channel blockers may also be effective. Nifedipine has been shown to lower to normal levels a blood presure of 250/125 mm at high altitude.[33] Nifedipine has also been shown to be effective in the treatment and prevention of high altitude pulmonary edema presumably by lowering pulmonary artery pressure.[34]

References

1. WELTON P, and RUSSELL P. Systemic hypertension. In *The principles and practice of medicine*, ed. A Harvey, R Johns, H McKusick, A Owens, and R Ross. Norwalk, Conn.: Appleton-Century-Crofts, 1984: 278-80.
2. KAMAT S, and BANERJI B. Study of cardiopulmonary function on exposure to high altitude. *Am. Rev. Resp. Dis.* 1972; 106:404-13.
3. WOLFEL E, GROVES B, BROOKS G, et al. Oxygen transport during steady state submaximal exercise in chronic hypoxia. *J. Appl. Physiol.* 1991; 70:1129-36.
4. NAKASHIMA M. High altitude medical research in Japan. In *Hypoxia, exercise, and altitude*, ed. J Sutton, C Houston, and N Jones, New York: A.R. Liss, 1985: 175.
5. NAGASAKA T, ANDO S, and TAKAGI K. Studies on adaptation to high altitudes with special references to changes in cardiovascular functions. *Nagoya J. Med. Sci.* 1967; 29:231-37.

6. SUAREZ J, ALEXANDER J, and HOUSTON C. Enhanced left ventricular systolic performance at high altitude during Operation Everest II. *Am. J. Cardiol.* 1987; 60:137-42.

7. FORSTER P. Telescopes in high places. In D Heath, ed., *Aspects of hypoxia* Liverpool: Liverpool University Press, 1986.

8. ALEXANDER J, HARTLEY H, MODELSKI M, and GROVER R. Reduction of stroke volume during exercise in man following ascent to 3,100 m altitude. *J. Appl. Physiol.* 1967; 23:849-58.

9. WOLFEL E, SELLAND M, MAZZEO R, et al. Systemic hypertenison at 4,300 m is related to sympathoadrenal activity. *J. Appl. Physiol.* 1994; 76:1643- 50.

10. MOORE LG, HERSEY DW, JAHNIGAN D, and BOWES W. The incidence of pregnancy-induced hypertension is increased among Colorado residents at high altitude. *Am. J. Obst. and Gyn.* 1982; 144:423-29.

11. PALATINI P, BUSINARO R, BERTON G, et al. Effects of low altitude exposure on 24-hour blood pressure and adrenergic activity. *Am. J. Cardiol.* 1989; 64: 1379-82.

12. ROACH R, HOUSTON C, HONIGMAN B, et al. How well do the older persons tolerate moderate altitudes? *West. J. Med.* 1995; 162:32-36.

13. SCHOLING W. High altitude climate: Adaption processes of healthy individuals and hypertensive patients. *Medizinische Klinik* 1981; 76:519-25.

14. HALHUBER M, HUMPELER E, INAMA A, and JUNGMAN H. Does altitude cause exhaustion of the heart and circulatory system? Indications and contraindications for cardiac patients at altitudes. In *High Altitude Deterioration*, ed. R Rivoher, P Cerretelli, J Foray, and P Segatini. Basel: S. Karger, 1985: 192-202.

15. HULTGREN H. Reduction of systemic arterial blood pressure at high altitude. In J Vogel, ed., *Hypoxia, high altitude, and the heart*. New York: S. Karger, 1970; 49-55.

16. PENROD K. Personal communication.

17. SOMERS V, MARK A, and ABBOUD A. Potentiation of sympathetic nerve responses to hypoxia in borderline hypertensive subjects. *Hypertension* 1988; 11:608-12.

18. BROOKS G, BUTTERFIELD G, WOLFEL R, et al. Decreased reliance on lactate during exercise after acclimatization to 4,300 m. *J. Appl. Physiol.* 1991; 71:333- 41.

19. BÄRTSCH P, MAGGIORINI M, SCHOBERSBERGER W, et al. Enhanced exercise-induced rise of aldosterone and vasopressin preceding mountain sickness. *J. Appl. Physiol.* 1991;71:134-43.

20. HULTGREN H, HONIGMAN B, THEIS K, and NICHOLAS R. High altitude pulmonary edema in a ski resort. *West. J. Med.* (in press).

21. KASIC J, YARON M, NICHOLAS R, et al. Treatment of acute mountain sickness: Hyperbaric versus oxygen therapy. *Ann. Emerg. Med.* 1991; 20:1109-12.

22. REEVES J, MOORE L, WOLFEL E, et al. Activation of the sympatho-adrenal system at high altitude. In G. Ueda, R. Reeves and M. Sekiguchi, eds., *High altitude medicine*. Matsumoto Japan Shinshu University, 1992; 10-23.

23. MOUE Y, SMITH P, CLANCY R and GONZALEZ N. Role of vasoconstrictors in the systemic hypertension of rats acclimatized to hypoxia. *J. Appl. Physiol.* 1995; 79:1657-67.

24. REEVES J. Sympathetics and hypoxia: a brief overview. In J. Sutton, C. Houston and G. Coates, eds, *Hypoxia and Molecular Medicine*. Burlington, VT: Queen City Printers Inc. 1993; 1-6.

25. deBOLD A. Atrial naturetic factor: A hormone produced by the heart. Science, 1985; 230:767-70.

26. DASGUPTA D, DHAWAN A, SHARMA A, et al. Do mercury and aneroid sphygmomanometers give identical readings at high altitude? *J. Indian Med. Assn.* 1989; 87:20. Correspondence.

27. WATERLOW J, and BUNJE H. Observations on mountain sickness in the Colombian Andes. *Lancet* 1966; 2: 651-55.

28. MALHOTRA M, BRAHMACHARI K, SRIDHARAN T, et al. Electrolyte changes at 3,500 m in males with and without high altitude pulmonary edema. *Aviat. Space Environ. Med.* 1975; 46:409-21.

29. TUCK M. The sympathetic nervous system in essential hypertension. *Am. Heart J.* 1985; 112:877-86. Proceedings of a symposium on New Considerations in Mild Hypertension.

30. TITMARSH S, and MONK J. Terazosin: A review of its pharmacodynamic and pharmacokinetic properties and therapeutic efficacy in essential hypertension. *Drugs* 1987; 33:461-77.

31. The Treatment of Mild Hypertension Research Group. The Treatment of Mild Hypertension Study: a randomized placebo-controlled trial of a nutritional-hygienic regimen along with various drug monotherapies. *Arch. Int. Med.* 1991; 151: 1413-23.

32. NASH T. Alpha-adrenergic blockers: Mechanism of action, blood pressure control, and effects on lipoprotein metabolism. *Clin. Cardiol.* 1990; 13:764-72.

33. WINNIFORD M, FILIPCHUCK N, and HILLIS D. Alpha adrenergic blockade for variant angina: A long-term, double-blind, randomized trial. *Circulation* 1983: 67:1185-88.

34. OELZ O, MAGGIORINI M, RITTER M, et al. Nifedipine for high altitude pulmonary edema. *Lancet* 1989; 2:1241-44.

CHAPTER 26

Sickle Cell Disease

SUMMARY

Sickle cell disease is present in about 6-8 percent of blacks in the United States. The majority of those so afflicted are not anemic but only have the sickle cell trait, a condition that results in deformation or "sickling" of red cells when exposed to hypoxia or high altitude. The most common complication is acute abdominal pain caused by splenic infarction—a "splenic crisis." This occurs usually only above altitudes of 8,000-10,000 feet (2,440-3,050 m). The onset may occur within a few hours after ascent, or it may be delayed until several days after descent. Some persons with sickle cell disease have experienced crises during prolonged aircraft flights, but this seems to be a rare occurrence. Persons with the sickle cell trait should be cautious about traveling to high altitude, and once a crisis has occurred, a return to a similar altitude is inadvisable. Patients with sickle cell anemia should not travel to high altitude and caution should be observed during long aircraft flights. A physician's advice should be followed. Supplementary oxygen during the flight may be indicated.

· · ·

Sickle cell disease refers to several abnormalities of hemoglobin that cause red blood cells to become deformed and inflexible when exposed to a low oxygen tension. Normally the biconcave disc-shaped red cells are flexible and can easily squeeze through capillaries and quickly regain their original shape. "Sickle cells" are rigid, crescent-shaped structures that cannot pass through small vessels and capillaries and therefore clump into masses that obstruct the circulation, most commonly in the spleen and microcirculation. This uncommon form of anemia can be easily diagnosed by microscopic examination of red blood cells.

Hundreds of mutant types of hemoglobin occur in man, with many varieties occurring in different races and in many parts of the world; but only about 0.5 percent of human beings carry hemoglobin S, which is the type associated with sickle cell disease. The abnormality of the cells is genetically determined. The severity of the disorder is related to the concentration of S hemoglobin in the red cell.[1-4] The concentration of hemoglobin S in four common types of sickle cell disorders is shown in Table 26.1.

Hemoglobin S may occur in other types of anemia as well as in sickle cell anemia and the sickle cell trait. The most severe problem occurs in B°-thalassemia, which contains no hemoglobin A and results in a condition similar to sickle cell anemia. B+-thalassemia, less severe, contains about 50 percent hemoglobin A, which dilutes the hemoglobin S in the red cell and therefore results in less sickling. The type of thalassemia can only be determined by a careful family history and special studies of the hemoglobin.

Table 26.1
Sickle Cell Disease and Sickle Cell Disorders

Type	Genotype	%S	Severity
Sickle cell anemia	SS	96	Most
Sickle cell B⁰-thalassemia	SA	96	
Sickle cell B⁺-thalassemia	SA	70	
Sickle cell trait	AS	40	Least

SOURCE: Harvey et al., ref. 1.

NOTES: SS is the hemozygous form, in which both genes carry the disorder; SA and AS are heterozygous, with only one gene affected. The severity is correlated with the amount of hemoglobin S in the blood.

Occurrence

The common variety of sickle cell anemia and sickle cell trait occurs largely in blacks or those with a degree of black ancestry. Rare cases may occur in Caucasians. Thalassemia occurs commonly in those of Mediterranean, Asian, or Indian ancestry. About 6-8 percent of blacks and persons with a black ancestry have sickle cell disease, but the majority have only the sickle cell trait. Patients with a high concentration of hemoglobin S are anemic, and most of these patients have had some complications, including infarction of the spleen, by the end of the first decade of life.

Sickle Cell Crises

Patients with the sickle cell trait, however, are usually asymptomatic and may be unaware of their disease unless routine testing is employed. Such persons may experience symptoms resulting from increased sickling of their red cells when exposed to high altitude or when traveling in a non-pressurized aircraft. The symptoms are commonly related to splenic crises (infarction of the spleen) or vaso-occlusive nonsplenic crises. Splenic sequestration of red cells without infarction has been reported by Githens.[5] Splenic crises are manifested by abdominal pain and tenderness, usually located in the left upper quadrant. The pain may be intense and aggravated by motion, breathing, or coughing. The pain is due to infarction or swelling of the spleen by clumps of red cells with associated inflammatory changes. Fever, sweats, and malaise are common. Non-splenic crises occur commonly in persons who have sickle cell anemia or sickle cell trait and have experienced previous episodes of splenic crises with resultant splenic fibrosis or who have had splenectomy. Severe pain in the abdomen, back, or extremities may occur along with malaise and fever.

Symptoms

Symptoms usually appear within a few hours of altitude exposure and may persist for up to fourteen days after returning to a lower elevation. In some persons the onset of pain may not occur until a day or two after returning from high altitude.[6,7,8] Several conditions other than hypoxemia may lead to sickle cell crises, including dehydration, pulmonary disease, alkalosis, and exposure to cold.[9,10]

So far as high altitude exposure is concerned, the persons most at risk are those who carry the sickle cell trait but are not aware of it; the smaller number of persons who have sickle cell anemia are usually aware of their condition and for that reason avoid high altitude. Patients with sickle cell anemia usually have infarcted, fibrotic spleens and therefore rarely have a splenic syndrome. Goldberg and his colleagues, for example, found only two reported cases of altitude-related splenic infarction in patients with sickle cell anemia.[11]

The sickle cell trait affects about 2 million people in the United States. It does not shorten life, and aside from exposure to altitude, it does not result in an increased incidence of illness. Heavy exercise at lower elevations is probably not harmful.[12]

A recent report based upon a review of all deaths occurring among 2 million recruits during basic training in the U.S. Armed Forces from 1977 to 1981 indicated that in black recruits with hemoglobin AS rates for sudden unexplained deaths were 32.2 per 100,000 compared with 1.2 among black recruits who did not have hemoglobin S (p <0.001). The relative risk increased from ages 17-18 compared with 26-30 years.[12] These results should be kept in perspective, as pointed out in an accompanying editorial.[13] Although only one in 3,200 black recruits with sickle cell trait died suddenly, the deaths occurred during or after the considerable exertion associated with basic training, some of it at moderate altitudes and during extreme heat. These data are not applicable to the 8 percent of blacks in the United States who do not carry out heavy physical exertion under similar adverse circumstances, but clearly caution should be exercised.[14]

Patients with sickle cell disease range from individuals with blond hair and blue eyes to those with olive skin and straight black hair to those with dark skin and curly black hair. Nearly 10 percent of patients with various sickling disorders identify themselves as non-black.[15]

The Effect of High Altitude

Splenic crises occur usually at altitudes greater than 8,000 feet (2,440 m), either during surface travel or occasionally during long flights in a nonpressurized aircraft. Sickle cell crises occurring at moderate altitudes are rare. In the 1968 Olympic Games in Mexico City at an altitude of 7,200 feet (2,200 m), no problems were encountered by black athletes, including two long-distance runners who had the sickle cell trait.[7] Similar observations have been made in black football players.[15]

Sickle Cell Disease in Non-Blacks

Sickle cell crises may occur in persons who are not black. Lane and Githens described six phenotypically non-black men who experienced the acute onset of severe left upper quadrant abdominal pain within 48 hours of arrival in Colorado from lower altitudes. Three of these patients had symptoms at moderate altitudes of 5,280-7,000 feet (1,609-2,134 m). All recovered with medical management and none required splenectomy. Functional hyposplenia was a late sequel in one patient. The authors suggested that non-black persons with the sickle cell trait may be more susceptible to the splenic syndrome at altitude.[16] Goldberg reported two additional cases of non-blacks, a father and son who both developed splenic infarction in Santa Fe, New Mexico, at an altitude of 7,000 feet (2,134 m).[11] Both had the sickle cell trait. The son had Hgb A 51 percent, Hgb A_2 2.8 percent, and Hgb S 46 percent. The father had Hgb A 55 percent, Hgb A_2, 3.4 percent, Hgb S 41 percent, and Hgb CA

0.6 percent. A splenectomy was performed in the both patients. The spleens were grossly infarcted, with arterial occlusions.

Retrospective studies of patients with sickle cell disease who have traveled to high altitude have suggested a higher incidence of crises occurring at lower altitudes than previously reported.[9,17] One study reported symptoms suggesting crises occurring in 58 percent of patients who ascended above 10,500 feet (3,200 m).[17] Retrospective reports must be accepted with caution, however, because they are based upon a patient's recollection of symptoms that could be inaccurate, and because no controls had been employed. In all retrospective reports, the incidence of crises is far higher than that reported by other investigators.[15,18]

Exposure to very high altitudes is dangerous. Massive splenic necrosis with pseudocyst formation has been reported in a 19-year-old Peruvian who ascended to 14,990 feet (4,570 m) in the Andes.[19] A case of pulmonary infarction occurring in a patient with sickle cell disease while flying in an unpressurized aircraft at 15,830 feet (4,827 m) has been reported by Heffner and Sohn.[20]

Aircraft Flights

Modern pressurized aircraft maintain cabin pressures usually equivalent to no more than 8,000 feet (2,440 m). There are several reports of sickle cell crises occurring under these conditions. Green described seven cases occurring during aircraft flights. One patient had thalassemia and one had sickle cell C trait.[8] Diggs collected fifteen cases of sickle cell crisis occurring during coast-to-coast flights in a nonpressurized aircraft at altitudes between 10,000 feet (3,050 m) and 15,000 feet (4,575 m). Eleven patients had the sickle cell trait, three had sickle cell anemia, and one had thalassemia.[7] Smith and Conley described fifteen cases of splenic crises occurring in non-blacks in an aircraft with a cabin pressure simulating an altitude of greater than 5,000 feet (1,525 m) one patient had sickle cell C disease.[21] Short exposures of patients with the sickle cell trait to simulated altitudes of 5,000 feet (1,525 m) to 25,000 feet (7,625 m) in a hypobaric chamber have shown no deterioration in pulmonary function as measured by diffusing capacity or spirometry.[22] In other chamber studies sickling has not been observed unless the simulated altitude exceeded 15,000 feet (4,575).[2] The relation between the sickle cell trait and aviation has been reviewed by Long.[23]

On the basis of the studies reviewed, one can summarize the generally accepted guidelines regarding travel to high altitude by patients with sickle cell disease.

1. Complications occur primarily in those who have the sickle cell trait, and this may be undetected if hematologic studies have not been performed.

2. Ascent to altitudes exceeding 8,000-10,000 feet (2,440-3,050 m) is dangerous, and the occurrence of abdominal pain or other symptoms is an indication for prompt descent and oxygen therapy.

3. Patients who have had symptoms during a single ascent to any altitude should avoid return ascents.

4. Patients with sickle cell anemia (SS hemoglobin) and those who have had symptoms at elevations below 10,000 feet (3,050 m) should arrange for supplemental oxygen during aircraft flights. The presence of pulmonary disease with a decreased arterial PO_2 may result in symptoms at even modest altitudes. Dehydration should be avoided. Whether acetazolamide provides some protection against sickle cell crisis by preventing alkalosis has not been examined.

5. Sickle cell trait is not a contraindication to travel to altitudes less than 8,000 feet (2,440 m) or prolonged flights in pressurized aircraft unless clearly documented crises have occurred before at these altitudes.

Diagnosis of Acute Episodes

The diagnosis of altitude-related splenic crisis is not difficult. Acute pain and tenderness in the left upper quadrant and flank during a recent trip to high altitude in a black is the classic picture. Fever and leucocytosis may be present. Crises may occur in non-blacks and crises may occur within a few days after descent from high altitude. Atypical presentations may simulate other more common medical conditions, including: (1) bone pain simulating osteomyelitis (more common in children), (2) pulmonary infarction simulating pleurisy, (3) acute cholecystitis due to pigment stones, (4) mesenteric artery obstruction simulating an acute abdomen, (5) thrombotic stroke, and (6) secondary gout.

Common diagnostic findings are anemia, nucleated and sickled red cells in peripheral blood, a positive sickledex screening test, leucocytosis, fever, and an elevated level of S hemoglobin by electrophoresis. The sedimentation rate may be normal. Splenic infarction may result in splenic rupture or pseudocyst formation. Congestive splenomegaly may occur without rupture.[5] Abdominal films, CT scans of the abdomen, and nuclear scans of the spleen and liver are useful diagnostic methods.

Treatment of Acute Episodes

At altitude, high-flow oxygen followed by prompt pharmacological pain relief and descent are indicated if splenic rupture can be excluded. Oral hydration with carbonated beverages is preferable to IV fluids. Narcotics are usually required for pain relief. Meperidine hydrochloride 25-125 mg and hydroxyzine hydrochloride 25-75 mg may be used initially. If pleuritic chest pain is present a lung scan should be done to exclude pulmonary infarction. Pulmonary infarction will often be associated with a very low arterial oxygen saturation.[24] Splenic rupture or mesenteric infarction are indications for emergency surgery. Many antisickling agents have been used in the past, but none has proved efficacious.

References

1. HARVEY A, JOHNS R, MCKUSICK V, et al. In *The principles and practice of medicine*, ed. A Harvey, R Johns, H McKusick, A Owens, and R Ross. Norwalk, Conn.: Appleton-Century-Crofts, 1984: chap 50, pp 488-93.
2. SEARS D. The morbidity of the sickle cell trait. *Am. J. Med.* 1978; 64:1021-35.
3. FRANKLIN V. Sickle cell crises in hypoxia. In *Man at altitude*, ed. J Sutton, N Jones, and C Houston. New York: Thieme-Stratton, 1982: 177-79.
4. WINSLOW R. Notes on sickle cell disease. In *Man at altitude*, ed. J Sutton, N Jones, and C Houston. New York: Thieme-Stratton, 1982: 178-81.
5. GITHENS J, GROSS G, EIFE R, and WALLNER S. Splenic sequestration syndrome at mountain altitudes in sickle/hemoglobin C disease. *J. Pediatr.* 1977; 90:203-10.
6. DIGGS L. The sickle cell trait in relation to the training and assignment of duties in the Armed Forces: I, Policies, observations, and studies. *Aviat. Space Environ. Med.* 1984; 55:180-85.
7. DIGGS L. The sickle cell trait in relation to the training and assignment of duties in the Armed Forces: II, Aseptic splenic neurosis. *Aviat. Space Environ. Med.* 1984; 55:271-76.
8. GREEN R, HUNTSMAN R, and SERJEANT G. The sickle-cell and altitude. *Brit. Med. J.* 1971; 4:593-95.

9. CLUSTER S, GODWIN M, and EMBURY S. Risk of altitude exposure in sickle cell disease. *West. J. Med.* 1981; 135:364-67.

10. RATNER S, and ATHANASIAN E. Water sports and sickle cell anemia. *Ann. Int. Med.* 1986; 105:971. Letter to the Editor.

11. GOLDBERG N, DORMAN J, RILEY C, and ARMBRUSTER E. Altitude-related splenic infarction in sickle cell trait: Case reports of a father and son. *West. J. Med.* 1985; 143:670-72.

12. KARK J, POSEY D, SCHUMACKER H, and RUEHLE C. Sickle cell trait as a risk factor for sudden death in physical training. *N. Engl. J. Med.* 1987; 317:781- 86.

13. SULLIVAN L. The risks of sickle-cell trait. *N. Engl. J. Med.* 1987; 317:831-32.

14. POWARS D. Sickle cell disease in non-black persons. *JAMA* 1994; 271:1885. Questions and Answers.

15. MURPHY J. Sickle cell hemoglobin (H6AS) in black football players. *JAMA* 1973; 225:981-82.

16. LANE P, and GITHENS J. Splenic syndrome at mountain altitudes in sickle cell trait: Its occurrence in non-black persons. *JAMA* 1985; 253:2251-54.

17. MAHONY B, and GITHENS J. Sickling crises and altitude: Occurrence in the Colorado patient population. *Clin. Pediatr.* 1979; 18:431-38.

18. KONDLAPOODI P. Sickling crises at high altitude. *West. J. Med.* 1982; 137:139. Letter to the Editor.

19. RYWLIN A, and BENSON J. Massive neurosis of the spleen with formation of a pseudocyst: Report of a case in a white man with the sickle cell trait. *Am. J. Clin. Path.* 1961; 36:142-44.

20. HEFFNER J, and SOHN S. High altitude pulmonary infarction. *Arch. Int. Med.* 1981; 141:1721-28.

21. SMITH E, and CONLEY L. Sicklemia and infarction of the spleen during aerial flight - electrophoresis of the hemoglobin in 15 cases. *Bull. Johns Hopkins Hosp.* 1955; 96:35-41.

22. DILLARD T, KARK J, RAJAGOPAL K, et al. Pulmonary function in sickle cell trait. *Ann. Int. Med.* 1987; 106:191-96.

23. LONG I. Sickle cell trait and aviation. *Aviat. Space Environ. Med.* 1982; 53:1021-29.

24. HAMILTON G. Anemia. In *Emergency medicine*, vol. 2, ed. P Rosen et al. St. Louis: C. V. Mosby Co, 1988: 1240-58.

CHAPTER 27

Pulmonary Disease

SUMMARY

Patients with chronic obstructive pulmonary disease whose primary problem is airway obstruction without significant blood gas abnormalities will tolerate moderate high altitude exposure and aircraft travel without an increase in symptoms. Patients with pulmonary disease associated with a decreased arterial PO_2 or an elevated PCO_2 may become more symptomatic even at moderate altitudes. Simple clinical evaluation of the degree of physical disability combined with blood gas studies can usually identify these patients. In general, a resting arterial PO_2 of less than 50 mm is a sign of poor altitude tolerance. In such patients even aircraft flights may be uncomfortable and supplementary oxygen should be arranged in advance with the airline. A prolonged stay or continued residence at high altitude in such patients not only may increase the severity of symptoms due to increased hypoxemia but also may enhance right ventricular failure by a rise in pulmonary artery pressure. A move to a lower altitude may result in improvement and is advisable, especially if the patient is clearly improved after a trial period of living at a lower altitude.

During expeditionary climbs to very high and extreme altitudes, drying of the throat and upper airways often results in irritation, with an associated painful throat and a persistent cough, usually noninfectious. Symptomatic treatment measures without antibiotics are indicated.

• • •

Chronic Obstructive Disease

Chronic obstructive pulmonary disease (COPD) may be adversely affected by exposure to even modest elevations. It is important to recognize two types of chronic pulmonary disease. A substantial percentage of patients can be roughly characterized as "pink puffers." These patients have airway obstruction and are markedly dyspneic on exertion but exhibit only a modest decrease in arterial saturation. They have relatively normal arterial PCO_2 levels. Severe pulmonary hypertension, polycythemia, and right ventricular failure are rare. Such patients are not usually benefited by oxygen therapy but rely on bronchodilators, diuretics, and occasionally steroids to minimize symptoms. A smaller percentage of patients can be designated as "blue bloaters," a condition characterized by arterial unsaturation and carbon dioxide retention, and also frequently by polycythemia, clubbing of the digits, pulmonary hypertension, and right ventricular failure. These patients are usually benefited by oxygen therapy, which must be adjusted to avoid undue CO_2 retention and acidosis. They may experience varying degrees of sleep hypoxemia. Diuretics and digitalis are needed to treat right ventricular failure and edema.[1,2] Many patients will, however, fall somewhere in between the typical pink puffer and blue bloater.

Patients in the pink puffer category may tolerate exposure to high altitude with only a slight increase in symptoms. Graham and Houston exposed eight patients with COPD for three days a 6,400 feet (1,950 m). No significant increase in symptoms was noted despite a slight fall in arterial PO_2 from 66 mm to 52 mm. The arterial PCO_2 fell from 38 mm to 34 mm. Subjective discomfort during exercise was experienced on the second day, but was improved on the third day.[3] Matthys and his co-workers used a hypobaric chamber at a simulated altitude of 6,300 feet (1,922 m) to study ten patients with COPD. Arterial blood gases after 90 minutes of exposure revealed a fall in the mean arterial PO_2 and PCO_2 of approximately 15 and 6 mm Hg, respectively.[4]

The patients in both these studies were probably in the pink puffer group and arterial PCO_2 values were normal. In such patients the reduced density of inspired air at high altitude may relieve some symptoms of airway obstruction and reduce the work of breathing. In normal subjects maximum flow velocities are increased in proportion to the altitude.[5] Since high altitude air may contain fewer pollens, patients who have allergic asthma may not have episodes of acute obstruction. Earlier studies have suggested that the following factors are important predictors of physiological changes at high altitude in patients with COPD: (1) exertional dyspnea, (2) cor pulmonale and cyanosis, (3) vital capacity of less than 50 percent of predicted, (4) maximum voluntary ventilation of less than 40 L/min, (5) respiratory acidosis, and (6) arterial PO_2 of less than 50 mm Hg. Exertional dyspnea should be defined and preferably evaluated by a treadmill test in order to arrive at an accurate evaluation of the degree of physical limitation that is due to dyspnea. Spirometric variables may not predict symptoms at altitude.

Aircraft Travel

Physicians are frequently asked by patients with pulmonary disease whether or not they can tolerate long aircraft flights. It should be noted that because present-day aircraft fly at higher elevations than ever before, cabin altitudes may also be higher, especially when climbing to avoid turbulence. In sixteen different aircraft flown by twenty-eight airlines, the median cabin altitude was 6,214 feet (1,894 m), and some cabin altitudes were as high as 8,915 feet (2,717 m).[6] To evaluate predictors for the need of supplemental oxygen in flight, Dillard and his associates exposed eighteen patients with severe chronic obstructive pulmonary disease to a simulated altitude of 8,000 feet (2,438 m) in a hypobaric chamber.[7] Similar studies were performed in nine healthy normal subjects. The mean arterial PO_2 of the patients at sea level was 72 ± 9 mm, and during hypobaria, 47 ± 6 mm. Four patients had arterial PO_2 values as low as ≤ 40 mm. Arterial PCO_2 fell from 38 ± 5 mm to 35 ± 4 mm. No patient developed severe symptoms. The authors concluded that the arterial PO_2 at sea level and the FEV_1 were useful predictors of the degree of fall in PO_2 during hypobaria. All patients had a low FEV_1 (mean 0.97 ± 0.32 liters or 31 ± 10 percent of predicted). Dillard and his associates performed a meta-analysis of five studies totaling 71 patients with chronic obstructive pulmonary disease. The data supported previous conclusions that the FEV_1 and the arterial PO_2 at sea level are useful predictors of the PO_2 during altitude exposure.[8]

Schwartz studied thirteen patients during a flight in an unpressurized aircraft at an altitude of 5,300 feet (1,616 m). Mean arterial PO_2 decreased from 68 mm ± 9 (SD) to 61 mm ± 9 and mean arterial PCO_2 decreased from 41 ± 1 mm to 37 mm $\pm$

6. At 7,300 feet (2,227 m), mean arterial PO_2 was 45 mm ± 9 and PCO_2 was 37 mm ± 6. No symptoms were experienced. It was also found that the arterial PO_2 measured in patients breathing room air several weeks before the flight did not correlate with values measured at 5,300 feet (1,616 m), but arterial PO_2 measured within two hours of the flight or while breathing a 17.2 percent oxygen measure did predict the decrease during the flight.[6] Schwartz later recommended that the arterial PO_2 obtained while breathing a 15 percent oxygen mixture in nitrogen can predict who may become significantly hypoxemic during a flight with a cabin altitude of 8,000 feet (2,440 m).[9]

Gong has recently discussed advice given to patients with pulmonary disease during air travel.[10] He points out that both a hypoxia test (15 percent oxygen) and an FEV_1 measured within two weeks before a flight are useful predictors of significant in-flight hypoxemia. Apte and Karnad, however, believe that a preflight arterial blood gas estimation will suffice to predict arterial PO_2 at 8,000 feet (2,438 m) and that no additional benefit is obtained by pulmonary function testing, which is expensive and inconvenient.[11]

Patients with severe pulmonary disease who must travel by air may require oxygen during the flight. Airlines do not permit a passenger to carry on board a personal oxygen supply,[9,10] but supplemental oxygen during aircraft travel can be ordered by a physician and arrangements can be made with the airline several days before traveling. I once asked a stewardess whether low-flow oxygen could be made available during a flight if a passenger required it in an emergency. I was shown a face mask connected to a chemical oxygen candle in which flow rate could not be determined. The only alternative would have been to activate the emergency oxygen equipment, and oxygen masks would have fallen into the laps of all the passengers. The stewardess correctly estimated that this might have caused some anxiety throughout the aircraft.

Clinical Considerations

Patients with pulmonary hypertension, cyanosis, right heart failure, polycythemia, carbon dioxide retention, and an arterial PO_2 of less than 50 mm Hg with significant limitation of physical activity (Canadian Heart Association Class III or IV) should probably not go to high altitude. If a trip to even a modest altitude is necessary or if travel by aircraft is absolutely necessary, supplemental low-flow oxygen should be provided during the trip. Such patients may exhibit several responses to even modest decreases in inspired PO_2 that can result in more severe symptoms and may be dangerous.

1. If sea-level arterial PO_2 values are less than 50 mm at even modest altitudes of 5,000-7,200 feet (1,525-2,200 m), arterial PO_2 would fall below 40 mm and cause impairment of physical and mental function.

2. The fall in arterial PO_2 may be even greater than the 10-15 mm decreases observed in the two studies by Schwartz cited above, since blue bloaters may have a decreased respiratory response to hypoxia.

3. If arterial PO_2 is less than 50 mm, one is on the steep part of the oxygen hemoglobin dissociation curve where even small changes in altitude will result in significant changes in arterial oxygen saturation, upon which oxygen delivery depends.

4. Hypoxia will result in an increased pulmonary artery pressure due to pulmonary arteriolar constriction, and this in turn will increase right ventricular work and accentuate or precipitate right ventricular failure. Oxygen delivery to the exercising muscles and other tissues will be impaired because of the lessening of the ability of the right ventricle to increase cardiac output.

5. Oxygen administration to compensate for the lowered inspired PO_2 may result in a further increase in arterial PCO_2 by damping the carotid body response. This increases respiratory acidosis.

Appropriate oxygen equipment during auto travel and during a sojourn at higher altitude can be recommended and provided by a patient's physician.

Primary Pulmonary Hypertension

Patients with symptomatic primary pulmonary hypertension should be cautious about trips to high altitude or prolonged aircraft travel. Many patients with primary pulmonary hypertension show an increase in pulmonary artery pressure at high altitude resulting from hypoxic pulmonary arteriolar constriction.[12] This may result in an increase in symptoms of dyspnea, fatigue, and exertional light-headedness or syncope. Symptoms may be exacerbated even at very modest altitudes of 4,000-5,000 feet (1,220-1,525 m). Since primary pulmonary hypertension is a serious, usually fatal disease with a high prevalence of sudden death, anyone who has such a condition should consult an experienced physician before traveling to high altitude or before taking any trip by air. Recommendations may include an increased use of pulmonary vasodilators, limitation of activity, and the use of low-flow oxygen.

Residence at Sea Level or High Altitude

Patients with COPD and arterial unsaturation as well as patients with primary pulmonary hypertension who reside at high altitude should be encouraged to move to sea level, and sea-level patients with these problems should not move to altitude.[12,13] There is evidence that COPD patients who live at high altitude have increased mortality compared with similar patients who live at sea level.[13,14] The cause of death in such patients is most commonly cor pulmonale at high altitude and pneumonia at sea level.[14] Elderly patients who leave high altitude areas in Colorado do so primarily because of pulmonary and cardiac disease; patients who moved away from lower altitude areas usually did so for nonmedical reasons such as wanting to be closer to family members, preferring a better climate, and the like.[15]

The physician is often consulted by patients with pulmonary disease or heart disease regarding possible permanent moves to a low or high elevation, not necessarily for reasons of health and long-term prognosis. It is wise to suggest that the patient live in the new area for several weeks or months on a trial basis and carefully observe symptoms, physical working capacity, and medication requirements. This may be more effective in helping the patient make a decision than advice by the doctor. A move to a lower altitude may involve a serious disruption of life style. Most COPD patients are disabled, unemployed, elderly, and dependent for their medical care on the community. A move to a different area may not only involve leaving relatives and friends but may also create problems regarding continued medical care.

High Altitude Throat

A common problem at very high altitudes is irritation of the throat and upper airways as a result of dehydration of the tissues by hyperventilation of the cold, dry air. During ordinary breathing, which uses the nasal pathways, air is sufficiently moistened and warmed to prevent dehydration and injury of the throat and upper airways. During exertion at high altitude mouth breathing is employed as well, with resulting damage to mucous membranes. Many remedies have been employed, including various troches, mouthwashes, gargles, and steam inhalations. It has even been suggested that covering one's nose and mouth with a cotton surgical mask would be useful in preventing dehydration and cold injury, but because a mask substantially decreases maximum airflow velocity, it is impractical for use during heavy effort.

High Altitude Cough and Bronchitis

Bronchitis with persistent coughing is a common problem at very high and extreme altitudes. Coughing may be severe enough to fracture ribs,[16] and it may also cause retinal hemorrhages. There are only a few references to this problem.[16,17,18] One observational study has been published by a physician-climber who reported on 19 climbers during a climb on Aconcagua (22,834 feet/6,964 m).[19] Thirteen of the climbers (68 percent) complained of a bothersome, persistent cough beginning above 14,000 feet (4,270 m). All subjects reached at least 21,500 feet (6,560 m). All 13 noted that the cough was preceded by a period of hyperventilation during strenuous activity; 8 of the 13 noted cough at rest, and 5 noted a modest amount (six teaspoons per day) of yellow-green, occasionally blood-tinged sputum. Symptoms improved with descent. None had rales or evidence of infection.

The probable mechanism is similar to that of high altitude throat, that is, a sterile, inflammatory process resulting from high levels of ventilation of cold, dry air. The high ventilation may be more important than the humidity and temperature of the inspired air. Subjects in Operation Everest II also experienced sore throats and cough despite the maintenance of warm, humidified air in the chamber.[19] Prevention and treatment consist of the same measures used for high altitude throat. High altitude cough and bronchitis must be differentiated from high altitude pulmonary edema.

Patients who have a chronic cough at sea level should be aware of the probability that the cough will be worse at high altitude, especially during heavy physical exertion. They should consult their physician before such a trip for medications that will diminish their discomfort.

References

1. DEMARCO F, JR., WYNNE J, BLOCK J, BOYSEN P, and TAASAN V. Oxygen desaturation during sleep as a determinant of the "Blue and Bloated" syndrome. *Chest* 1981; 79:621-25.
2. WYNNE J, BLOCK A, and BOYSEN P. Oxygen desaturation in sleep: Sleep apnea and COPD. *Practitioner* 1980; 15:77-85.
3. GRAHAM W, and HOUSTON C. Short-term adaptation to moderate altitude by patients with chronic obstructive pulmonary disease. *JAMA* 1978; 240:1491-94.
4. MATTHYS H, VOLZ H, KONIETZKO H, and KLEEBERG H. Kardiopulmonale Belastung von Flugpassagieren mit Obstructive Ventilationsstörungen. *Schweiz Med. Wochenschn.* 1974; 104:1786-89.

5. KRYGER M, ALDRICH F, REEVES J, and GROVER R. Diagnosis of airflow obstruction at altitude. *Am. Rev. Resp. Dis.* 1978; 117:1055-58.

6. SCHWARTZ J, BENCOWITZ H, and MOSER K. Air travel hypoxemia with chronic obstructive pulmonary disease. *Ann. Int. Med.* 1984; 100:473-77.

7. DILLARD T, BERG B, et al. Hypoxemia during air travel in patients with chronic obstructive pulmonary disease. *Ann. Int. Med.* 1989; 111: 362-67.

8. DILLARD T, ROSENBERG A, BERG B, et al. Hypoxemia during altitude exposure. A meta-analysis of chronic obstructive pulmonary disease. *Chest* 1993; 103:422-25.

9. SCHWARTZ J. Hypoxemia during air travel. *Ann. Int. Med.* 1990; 112:147-48. Letters and Corrections.

10. GONG H. Advising patients with pulmonary disease on air travel. *Ann. Int. Med.* 1989; 111: 349-51. Editorial.

11. APTE N, and KARNAD D. *Ann. Int. Med.* 1990; 112:547. Letters and Corrections.

12. SHETTIGAR U, HULTGREN H, SPECTER M, MARTIN R, and DAVIES H. Primary pulmonary hypertension: Favorable effect of isoproterenol. *N. Engl. J. Med.* 1976; 295:1414-15.

13. RENZETTI A, MCCLEMENT J, and LITT B. Veterans Administration Cooperative Study of Pulmonary Function: III. Mortality in relation to respiratory function in chronic obstructive pulmonary disease. *Am. J. Med.* 1966; 41:115-29.

14. MOORE L, ROHR A, MAISENBACH J, and REEVES J. Emphysema mortality is increased in Colorado residents at high altitude. *Am. Rev. Resp. Dis.* 1982; 126:225-28.

15. MOORE L, and REGENSTEINER J. Migration of the elderly from high altitudes in Colorado. *JAMA* 1985; 253:3124-28.

16. STEELE P. *Doctor on Everest*. Newton Abbot, Devon, Engl.: Readers Union, 1973: 82, 186, 199.

17. CLARK C. The care of the mountaineer. *Practitioner* 1986; 217:235-39.

CHAPTER 28

Migraine

SUMMARY

Migraine attacks may be precipitated by exposure to high altitude, but the actual incidence in patients with a history of migraine is unknown. Cerebral events very similar to migraine equivalents have been reported at high altitude, including transient visual loss, scintillating scotomata, and visual hallucinations. Transient ischemic attacks and cerebrovascular accidents at high altitude have also been reported in patients with a history of migraine. Patients with migraine should carry appropriate medications, as recommended by their physician, when going to high altitude. Patients with a history of migraine attacks on previous visits to high altitude should use prophylactic medications. The headache of acute mountain sickness appears to be different from the common migraine headache, although both may have a vascular origin.

• • •

Clinical Features

Migraine attacks occur in a significant proportion of our population. One author estimates that the incidence may be as high as 23-29 percent largely occurring under the age of 40.[1] Migraine is more common in women than in men. There is little objective evidence that the frequency and severity of migraine attacks are increased by acute exposure to altitude, but this may be due to a lack of appropriate studies.

Mountaineering literature contains many accounts of episodes that are compatible with migraine attacks. Houston has described several examples of episodes compatible with migraine associated with blackouts and scotomata occurring at high altitude.[2,3] A 29-year-old man during a descent from Mount Rainier experienced a total loss of vision that lasted about 30 seconds and occurred every 10 minutes. The same man had similar episodes during a climb on Mount McKinley at an altitude of 14,500 feet (4,423 m). A 40-year-old man experienced repeated attacks of scintillating scotomota accompanied by dysarthria and episodes of complete blindness. The attacks occurred several times a month, usually on a mountain. A neurologist made a diagnosis of migraine equivalents.

Walter Alvarez, who suffered from frequent episodes of migraine and scintillating scotomata, in a scholarly review of the literature, described 618 patients with migrainous scotomata.[4] Carroll described fifteen patients with what he termed "retinal migraine" occurring in migraine patients who experienced recurrent episodes of complete loss or dimness of vision in one or both eyes. The duration of the visual disturbance was usually fleeting and rarely lasted more than ten minutes. In rare cases an episode may last up to one hour. A noteworthy feature was the lack of a headache during the attack.[5] Whitty described sixteen patients with migraine and visual disturbances. Nine had headache but seven had only visual or other neurological abnormalities.[6]

Transient ischemic attacks may also represent migraine equivalents. Three episodes described in Chapter 18 consisted of: (1) recurrent left and right hemiparesis of two days' duration, (2) hemiplegia and dysphasia of three days' duration, and (3) dysphasia and headache in a patient with a history of migraine. One woman in her 60's who died of a cerebrovascular accident at 17,500 feet (5,340 m) had a history of migraine. Whether these episodes were related to vascular spasm or migraine equivalents is speculative, but physicians should be aware of the possibility of such attacks in patients with a history of migraine.[7,8,9,10]

Diagnosis

Diagnostic features of migraine consist of a history of recurrent headaches beginning in childhood and a positive family history of similar attacks (this is true in about 75 percent of cases). Psychological stress often precipitates attacks. Neurological examination between attacks is normal. Attacks tend to diminish or disappear after the age of 40. Three general types of migraine are recognized:

1. *Common migraine.* Vascular headache unaccompanied by visual or neurological symptoms. Occurs in about 12 percent of patients.

2. *Classic migraine.* Vascular headache preceded by painless sensory experience most often consisting of scotomata, field defects, or scintillating flashes of light. About two-thirds of patients will experience this type of migraine.

3. *Complicated migraine or migraine equivalents.* The remainder of patients may experience transient sensory or neurological impairment without headache.

Mechanisms

The cause of migraine is probably a result of the movement of wavelike areas of vasoconstriction and cortical excitation across the outer cortex followed by subsequent vasodilation in the same areas. The vasoconstriction or spasm does not cause headache, but it is presumably responsible for the focal neurological symptoms.[11]

The process begins gradually, in a slow progression that may increase over 5 to 30 minutes and last from 15 to 60 minutes. Isotope studies have shown a wavelike area of reduced superficial blood flow extending over the cortex during the initial phase. This is followed by vasodilation, which is accompanied by headache. The duration may be hours or a day or even two days. A sterile inflammation of the vascular walls may occur. When vasodilation subsides, either spontaneously or by the use of vasoconstrictors such as ergotamine tartrate, the headache disappears. Although transient neurological deficits in the vasoconstrictive phase of migraine may simulate transient ischemic attacks, the latter are usually due to vascular occlusions deep within the brain, whereas migraine affects primarily the outer cortex.[1,11] Common symptoms of migraine are summarized in Tables 28.1 and 28.2.

Platelet embolism may play a role in some of the visual symptoms of migraine. O'Connor reported that in 61 patients with migraine without headache, 34 had homonymous hemianopsia and 8 had classic amaurosis fugax suggesting platelet embolism.[12] Whity described sixteen patients without headache.[6] Houston reported two cases of recurrent transient blindness at high altitude that did not recur after the prophylactic use of aspirin.[3] D'Andrea reported that platelet activation in migraine was decreased by aspirin.[13] Aspirin prophylaxis for migraine has been reviewed by Dalessio, who concluded that low-dose aspirin prophylaxis might be beneficial for men with migrainous attacks occurring at least weekly.[14] Altitude probably precipitates episodes of migraine by the resulting cerebral hypoxia.[15]

Table 28.1
Characteristics of Migraine Headache

Often unilateral
May involve eye, ear, neck, or face
Pounding; throbbing may be dull, boring, or expanding
Sudden movement of the head, coughing, sneezing, straining, or
      bright lights and loud noises may increase the intensity
Nausea and vomiting common, especially in children
Onset in childhood; diminishes after 40
Positive family history
More common in women
Psychological stress may precipitate attacks
Relief by ergotamine tartrate

Table 28.2
Symptoms of Migraine

Symptom	Incidence
Headache	100%
Nausea	87
Photophobia	82
Vomiting	56
Visual disturbances	36
Vertigo	33
Syncope	10
Seizures	4
Confused state	4

Classic migraine consists of:
1. Headache
2. Vomiting
3. Focal neurological symptoms

There is some evidence that migraine may be more common in high altitude residents. An epidemiological survey of 1,226 persons living at 14,200 feet (4,331 m) in Peru and 1,031 persons at sea level revealed a prevalence of migraine of 22.3 percent at altitude and 14.5 percent at sea level. Women were more commonly affected than men. There was no difference in the prevalence of tension headaches between altitude and sea-level residents.[16]

Treatment and Prevention

For many years the standard treatment of a migraine attack has been the use of ergotamine tartrate, which acts by causing cerebral vasoconstriction. Immediate relief in most cases occurs within a few minutes of giving 0.25 to 0.50 mg intravenously. Ergotamine can also be given by means of a medihaler and sublingually for rapid action. Suppositories for rectal administration in patients with nausea and vomiting are also available. Ergotamine tartrate (Cafergot) can also be given orally.

The usual dose is two 1 mg tablets at the onset of the headache repeated each half-hour to a maximum dose of six in 24 hours.

The prevention of migraine attacks includes the elimination of factors that may precipitate or increase the frequency of episodes as well as the use of pharmacological agents. Factors that may adversely affect migraine include oral contraceptives, psychological stress, and the ingestion of foods that are high in tyramine, such as pods of broad beans, aged cheese, beer, wines, pickled herring, yogurt, liver, and yeast extracts. Migraine headaches may be intensified by certain drugs, including nitrates, histamine, reserpine, hydralazine, and estrogens, and by the withdrawal of steroids.

Calcium channel-blocking drugs and beta blockers have been shown to reduce the frequency of migraine attacks.[17-20] These include nifedipine, verapamil, diltiazem, propranolol, and timolol. Most of these preparations have been reported to reduce the frequency of migraine attacks by 50 percent or more and also to reduce the duration of episodes to a similar degree. Sublingual nifedipine (10 mg) has been reported to be effective in terminating a migraine attack, and daily administration of 10 mg every six hours may prevent attacks.[17] However, a recent, carefully controlled study of nifedipine (3 capsules, 3 times daily) showed no advantage over a placebo in the monthly frequency of migraine headaches. The incidence of side effects was 54 percent in the nifidipine-treated patients.[21] Timolol, a beta-blocking drug, has been reported to reduce the frequency of attacks of migraine.[22] I have seen one patient who had severe migraine attacks during visits to high altitude areas. The use of propranolol, 20 mg three times daily, completely prevented subsequent attacks. A meta analysis of data from 53 studies of 2,403 patients with migraine treated with propranolol (80 to 300 mg; mean daily dose 146 mg) yielded a reduction of 44 percent in migraine activity. Subjects were improved but not headache-free. About one in 18 patients stopped the drug because of side effects.[23] Cady and his associates reported that sumatriptan (6 mg subcutaneously) provided rapid relief of symptoms of migraine including headache, nausea, and photophobia. Side effects were minor.[24] Chest pain may occur in 3-5 percent of patients but the pain is probably not cardiac in origin but due to increased esophageal contractions.[25] Recently intranasal lidocaine has been shown to provide rapid relief of headache in about 55 percent of patients with migraine.[26]

It is important for patients who have a history of migraine to bring appropriate medication for the treatment of an attack when going to high altitude; and patients who have had previous attacks of migraine precipitated by high altitude exposures should certainly consult their physician regarding appropriate medications that may prevent attacks. Patients who experience recurrent scotomatas or transient visual impairment at high altitude should consider using low-dose aspirin as a preventive measure if their physician agrees.

References

1. SACKS O. *Migraine: Understanding a common disorder*, 2d ed. Berkeley: University of California Press, 1985.
2. HOUSTON C. *Going higher*. Boston: Little, Brown, 1987: 192-93.
3. HOUSTON C. Transient visual disturbance at high altitude. In *Hypoxia and Cold*, ed. J Sutton, C Houston and G Coates. New York: Praeger, 1987: 536. Abstract.

4. ALVAREZ W. The migrainous scotoma as studied in 618 persons. *Am. J. Ophthalmal.* 1960; 49: 489-504.
5. CARROLL D. Retinal migraine. *Headache* 1970; April.
6. WHITTY C. Migraine without headache. *Lancet* 1967; 2: 283-85.
7. BARTLESON J. Transient and persistent neurological manifestations of migraine. *Current Concepts Cerebrovasc. Dis.* 1983; 18:21-25.
8. JENZER G, BÄRTSCH P. Migraine with aura at high altitude. *J. Wild. Med.* 1993; 4:412-5.
9. MURDOCH D. Focal neurological deficits and migraine at high altitude. *J. Neurol. Neurosurg. Psychiat.* 1995; 58:637-43.
10. WOHNS R. Transient ischemic attacks at high altitude. *Crit. Care Med.* 1986; 14:517-18.
11. OLESEN J, LARSON B, and LAURITZEN M. Focal hyperemia followed by spreading oligemia and impaired activation of RCBF in classic migraine. *Ann. Neurol.* 1981; 9:344-52.
12. O'CONNOR P. Acephalic migraine. *Opthalmology* 1981; 88:999-1002.
13. D'ANDREA G, TOLDO M, CANANZI A, and FERRO-MILONE F. Study of platelet activation in migraine: Control by low doses of aspirin. *Stroke* 1984; 15:271-75.
14. DALESSIO D. Aspirin prophylaxis for migraine. *JAMA* 1990; 264:1721. Editorial.
15. AMERY W. The oxygen theory of migraine. In Blau J, ed. *Migraine: Clinical and research aspects.* Baltimore: The Johns Hopkins University Press. 1987; 403-31.
16. ARREGOI A, CABRERA F, LEONVELARDE S, et al. High prevalence of migraine in a high altitude population. *Neurology* 1991; 41:1668-70.
17. KAHAN A, WEBER S, AMOR B, et al: Nifedipine in the treatment of migraine in patients with Raynauld's phenomenon. *N. Engl. J. Med.* 1983; 308:1102-3.
18. GELMERS H. Calcium channel blockers in the treatment of migraine. *Am. J. Cardiol.* 1985; 55:139B- 143B.
19. SOLOMON G, STEELE J, and SPACCAVENTO L. Verapamil prophylaxis of migraine: A double-blind placebo-controlled study. *JAMA* 1983; 250:2500-2502.
20. MARKLEY H. Verapamil and migraine prophylaxis: Mechanisms and efficacy. *Am. J. Med.* 1991; 90, Suppl. 5A:485-535.
21. MCARTHUR J, MAREK K, PESTRONK A, et al. Nifedipine in the prophylaxis of classic migraine: A crossover double-masked, placebo-controlled study of headache frequency and side effects. *Neurology* 1989; 39: 284-86.
22. STELLAR S, AHRENS S, MEIBOHM M, and REMES S. Migraine prevention with timolol: A double-blind crossover study. *JAMA* 1984; 252:2574-80.
23. HOLROYD K, PENZIEN D, and CORDINGLEY G. Propranolol in the management of recurrent migraine: A metaanalytic review. *Headache* 1991; 265:2831-35.
24. CADY R, WEND T, KIRCHNER J, et al. Treatment of acute migraine with subcutaneous sumatriptan. *JAMA* 1991; 265:2831-35.
25. HOUGHTON L, FOSTER J, WHORWELL P, et al. Is chest pain after sumatriptan oesophageal in origin? *Lancet* 1994; 344:985-6.
26. MAIZELS M, SCOTT B, COHEN W and CHEN W. Intranasal lidocaine for treatment of migraine. A randomized double-blind, controlled trial. *JAMA* 1996; 276:319-21.

CHAPTER 29

Miscellaneous Sea Level Conditions

SUMMARY

Today many persons can enjoy trekking and climbing at high altitude who previously would have been advised to stay at home. Despite the inevitable physiological changes that occur with advancing years, many physically fit individuals in their 70's and even 80's may go to high altitude without adverse effects. Diabetics may participate in treks and climbs if careful attention is paid to diet and insulin requirements. High altitude does not have any adverse effect upon epilepsy provided appropriate medication is continued. Pregnancy at high altitude should not entail any additional risks, provided the mother is acclimatized; however, delivery at a lower elevation is usually desirable. Pregnant women should not go to high altitude during the first trimester. Asthmatics may tolerate altitude without problems if attention is paid to appropriate medications and avoidance of exposure to allergens. Persons who are obese may experience discomfort at high altitude owing to a greater degree of hypoxemia especially during sleep. Oxygen, acetazolamide, or progesterone may provide relief from sleeplessness and dyspnea. Smokers and persons who continue to smoke at high altitude will have more symptoms than nonsmokers and in some instances may need to descend. Persons who plan to participate in a trek or a visit to a high altitude area should consult their physician regarding potential risks and appropriate preventive measures.

• • •

Age and Altitude

There is no chronological age limit to enjoying high altitude. Many 70-year-olds have walked or climbed safely to altitudes higher than 18,000 feet (5,490 m). Recently, a 91-year-old woman climbed Mount Fuji in Japan (12,395 feet/3,780 m); a few days later, a 100-year-old man reached the summit! Ed Stuhl of Mount Shasta, California, climbed Popocatepetl (17,900 feet/5,460 m) at the age of 76. Julius Boehm, an 80-year-old member of the American Alpine Club, climbed Mount Rainier, 14,500 feet (4,422 m), and Hulda Crooks made the summit of Mount Whitney, 14,495 feet (4,421 m), at 93. Orvis Agee of Woodland, California, was leading climbs of Mount Shasta, 14,162 feet (4,320 m), at the age of 81.[1] There are some risks to the elderly because diminished coordination, impaired eyesight, and lapses of memory may cause falls or other mishaps, and elderly climbers on treks walk and climb more slowly and have difficulty carrying heavy packs. Trip leaders should be careful not to force older climbers to go faster than they can, or make them feel that they are a burden to the group.

Most of the few studies of the elderly at high altitude have had to do with physiological responses. Dill and his associates studied six subjects, aged 58 to 71 years, at an altitude of 14,235 feet (4,340 m).[2,3] In four of the subjects, vital capacity decreased by more than 10 percent compared with sea-level values. One subject showed a decrease of 32 percent after a strenuous climb, and a decrease in vital capacity of 30 percent was seen in another subject after an exercise test. These decreases are larger than the normal (the usual decrease in vital capacity with ascent is about 4 to 8 percent)[4] and suggest the presence of subclinical pulmonary edema. The two subjects were asymptomatic. Aerobic capacity decreased with ascent to about 75-85 percent of sea-level values, but a similar decrease was observed in young subjects. In one subject the arterial oxygen saturation was 79 percent and decreased to 74 percent during exercise. The alveolar-arterial oxygen gradient was 12.4 mm Hg. The two subjects who had the greatest decrease in vital capacity had higher gradients than the other subjects (14 mm Hg and 18 mm Hg), suggesting the possibility of mild pulmonary edema. These studies indicate no adverse effects of altitude upon healthy elderly subjects except the possibility of asymptomatic pulmonary edema following heavy exercise.

Elderly subjects who are free of symptoms at sea level can tolerate a stay at moderate altitude with minimal symptoms and no adverse effects upon the pulmonary or cardiovascular systems. A study was made of 77 men and 20 women aged 59 to 83 years (mean 69 years) who spent five days at Vail, Colorado (8,200 feet - 2,500 m). Sixteen percent had mild symptoms of AMS. A higher incidence has been found in younger subjects.[5] Twenty percent had a history of coronary artery disease and 34 percent had a history of hypertension. Neither symptoms or ECGs changed during the five days at altitude. All subjects had an increase in systemic blood pressure on the first day at altitude which then decreased to normal. No untoward clinical events occurred despite vigorous physical activity (tennis, mountain climbing) by many subjects. No electrocardiographic evidence of ischemia was seen. The authors suggested that persons with preexisting, generally asymptomatic cardiovascular disease can safely visit moderate altitudes.[6,7] While ventricular and supraventricular ectopy are common in the elderly, there is little information regarding the effect of altitude upon these arrhythmias. Alexander published a report of ambulatory monitoring of his cardiac arrhythmias during a climb of Kilimanjaro 19,335 feet (5,895 m) at 65 years of age. Above 15,000 feet marked ventricular ectopy, runs of ventricular bigeminy and a short run of supraventricular tachycardiac occurred. The arrhythmias ceased upon descent. At sea level a treadmill test, thallium scan, and a coronary arteriogram were normal. No ventricular ectopy occurred during treadmill exercise.[8] Further studies of cardiac arrhythmias and altitude are clearly indicated.

Little information is available regarding the response of the pulmonary circulation to high altitude in the elderly. In normal subjects at sea level, pulmonary vascular resistance probably increases with advancing age. Davidson and Fee studied 14 clinically normal subjects aged 60 to 69 years (mean 64 ± 3) and 33 subjects aged 24 to 55 years (mean 42 ± 8) to determine systemic and pulmonary hemodynamics and blood gases. Pulmonary artery pressures were higher in the elderly subjects (16 ± 3 mm Hg versus 12 ± 2 mm Hg in the younger group), and pulmonary vascular resistance was also increased in the elderly subjects (124 ± 32 dynes cm^{-5}m^2 compared with 70 ± 25 dynes cm^{-5}m^2 in younger subjects).[9] Similar studies at altitude would be of interest.

The hypoxic ventilatory response (HVR) decreases with age,[10] but this may be of little clinical significance. Honigman and his associates reported that subjects over 60 years actually had a lower incidence of acute mountain sickness than persons under 40 years.[5] Infants and small children do not tolerate altitude well and may become somnolent and cyanotic upon ascending to altitudes greater than 8,000 feet (2,440 m). Upper respiratory infections or a pneumonitis may increase hypoxemia. Children and teenagers have higher susceptibility to high altitude pulmonary edema than do adults, and physical activity should be limited for a day or two after arrival at high altitude.

Some trekkers and trek leaders bring infants and small children into remote high altitude areas. In my opinion, this is unwise, and certainly dangerous unless a physician and an adequate medical kit are available. Infants and small children are susceptible to many infectious diseases, and in remote areas like Nepal, where infectious diseases are common in children, the danger is particularly great.[11] Illnesses such as meningitis may strike suddenly and progress rapidly, and unless the trek physician is an experienced pediatrician, diagnosis of childhood diseases with an atypical presentation may be difficult.

Obesity

Moderately overweight persons should not be discouraged from going to high altitude—indeed, a prolonged trek may be an excellent way to reduce weight—but physicians should be aware that obese persons seem to have a greater susceptibility than persons of normal weight to acute mountain sickness and probably also to high altitude cerebral edema.[5,12-14] Obese persons who contemplate high altitude travel should have a careful study of their history and a physical examination to detect sleep disturbances, for if sleep abnormalities are present at sea level, they will probably be worse at high altitude. Obese persons appear to have higher pulmonary artery pressures than normal subjects at 7,392 feet (2,240 m). A study by Lupi-Herrera and his colleagues of 20 obese persons who resided at that altitude showed a mean pulmonary artery pressure of 30 mm Hg + 13. This is a higher pressure than the 15 mm Hg pressure reported in normal subjects at the same altitude, and even higher than pressures of 22 mm Hg in Peruvians living at the higher altitude of 12,300 feet (3,750 m).[15] Also, among persons without pulmonary disease at sea level, the incidence of sleep hypoxemia is more common in obese subjects.[16] Sleep hypoxemia may increase the susceptibility to acute mountain sickness, high altitude pulmonary edema, and high altitude cerebral edema. Acetazolamide should be recommended if sleep is significantly disturbed at high altitude.

Diabetes

Diabetes is not a contraindication to high altitude travel, although diabetics who require insulin should be aware that great variations in energy expenditure, in which strenuous all-day climbs are interrupted by days of inactivity, may significantly change insulin needs. During heavy activity, insulin requirements may decrease by up to 30 percent because exercising muscles increase the utilization of glucose. To compensate for these variations, a diabetic climber should probably use only quick-acting (regular) insulin, taking 3-4 injections daily as blood or urine sugar tests determine. The control of blood sugar can be evaluated by the use of Tes-Tape, which requires only a few drops of urine and is a good system for a cold climate.

The finger-prick glucometer test that many diabetics commonly use is less convenient in the field because it requires a clean finger, a stop watch, a wash bottle, and reagent strips.

The trip doctor should carry an extra supply of insulin in his first aid kit. It should be noted that insulin loses very little of its potency even when it has been frozen and thawed several times. Frozen insulin may precipitate into small visible particles, but it is still acceptable to use, although it may require a larger bore needle.[17] Two diabetics on Mount McKinley developed ketoacidosis because of loss of an insulin supply or freezing of the insulin.[18]

Serious insulin reactions may require placing glucose paste (glutose) in the buccal pouch, introducing sugar solutions via a nasogastric tube, or giving an intramuscular injection of an insulin antagonist (glucagon). The diabetic should also carry sugar in the form of candy bars or glucose tablets in the event of an insulin reaction. The trip leader or physician should carry glucose and glucagon available for intravenous use in the event of a serious insulin reaction. Patients on oral medications are not subject to these difficulties.

Patients on Steroids

It has been suggested that patients on steroids should double the daily dose at altitudes above 10,000 feet (3,050 m) since hypoxia causes release of corticotrophin.[19]

Epilepsy

In view of the effect of hypoxemia and respiratory alkalosis upon the central nervous system, one might expect exposure to high altitude to provoke seizures in epileptics, but this is apparently not the case. There is no evidence that epileptic seizures are more frequent at high altitude than at sea level. Indeed, Clarke has stated that in 25 years of experience in mountain medicine, he has found epilepsy to be distinctly uncommon at high altitude, and furthermore, patients with established epilepsy whose attacks are well controlled at sea level are not at particular risk of seizures at altitude.[20] For the same reasons that some epileptics are not allowed to drive and are discouraged to swim, one should not recommend that an epileptic undertake a technical climb, but if an epileptic is on adequate medication and has not had a seizure for the previous six months, a nonhazardous trek does not pose any extraordinary risk.

Pregnancy

Complications of pregnancy, such as toxemia, uterine hemorrhage, and miscarriages, are more common in women living above 9,000 feet (2,745 m), as noted in Chapter 12. However, most of the data on pregnancy at high altitude have come from a Peruvian native population, where social and economic factors may have been important in addition to altitude. Where excellent medical facilities are available and prenatal care is good, the risk of pregnancy at high altitude is probably no greater than at sea level. This conclusion is supported by the experience at Chulec General Hospital in La Oroya, Peru, at 12,230 feet (3,730 m). Newborn birth weight is lower at high altitude, however, and perinatal morbidity and mortality are slightly greater.[21] For unacclimatized women particularly, if pregnancy occurs at high altitude, it is advisable to return to sea level, especially during the last trimester when the fetus is vulnerable to hypoxemia. For the same reason, it is probably not advisable for a woman pregnant at sea level to go to an altitude of over 8,000 feet (2,440 m), especially during the third trimester.[22,23]

Aircraft flights with cabin pressures equivalent to 5,000-7,000 feet (1,525 m-2,135 m) are apparently safe.[22] Cautious obstetricians advise pregnant lowlanders to avoid visits to high altitudes and even to avoid crossing high mountain passes.[21] Exercise at high altitude may have particularly bad consequences because ischemic uterine contractions may temporarily decrease the blood supply to the fetus. This has been shown by experiences of U.S. State Department employees in La Paz, Bolivia, at 11,880 feet (3,623 m). Six women who traveled to La Paz during the first and second trimesters underwent numerous complications, including eclampsia, threatened abortion, and premature delivery. Not only were birth weights of the infants on the average one pound less than those of infants delivered to six women who arrived at La Paz before conception, but also none of those six women had any complications of pregnancy.[24]

Pregnant women should be careful about traveling to remote areas where there may not be skilled and prompt medical care facilities and where an accident during pregnancy could prove fatal. The use of oral contraceptives is usually discouraged during high altitude treks or climbs because of the increased risk of venous thrombosis, pulmonary embolism, migraine, and hypertension; oral contraceptives may also aggravate systemic edema and pulmonary hypertension, because they decrease the synthesis of prostaglandin E, which is a potent dilator of pulmonary arterioles.[20,25] Clearly, the use of oral contraceptives at altitude is a matter of personal choice, but the physician should point out the possible hazards.

Asthma

Extrinsic or allergic asthma is in no way a contraindication to visiting high altitude, where, in fact, breathing is usually easier because of fewer pollens and allergenic substances and a reduced air density. Many asthmatics find that they need less medication and fewer steroids at high altitude than they do at sea level.[26] The difference is due in part to the fact that exposure to high altitude increases serum cortisol and norepinephrine levels, and both these substances decrease bronchoconstriction. Some persons may suffer from exercise-induced asthma brought on by bronchospasm.[27] In such cases, it may be necessary to limit exercise and employ bronchodilators.

Hemorrhoids

Persons who have problems with hemorrhoids may find that the condition is aggravated during a trek or climb when squatting during bowel movements. The explanation is that the intra-ampullar pressure is higher when squatting and straining than when seated on a toilet.[28] The best advice, obviously, is to use a seated position whenever possible.

Smoking

Smoking at high altitude reduces the already diminished oxygen-carrying capacity of the blood because of the formation of carbon monoxide hemoglobin. Brewer and his associates studied smokers and nonsmokers in Leadville, Colorado, at 10,168 feet (3,100 m). Smokers had a carbon monoxide hemoglobin level of 6.6

± 2.7 percent. Sea-level smokers had a significantly lower level, 4.7 ± 2.2 percent. The arterial PO_2 in the Leadville smokers was 53.4 ± 5.8 mm compared with 58.6 ± 4.2 mm in nonsmokers.[29] In another study, smokers also had a higher red cell mass, indicating the presence of a greater degree of tissue hypoxia.[30] At 9,840 feet (3,000 m), smokers have a higher mean corpuscular volume and mean corpuscular hemoglobin concentration than nonsmokers. Smoking is associated with a reduction in the predicted forced expiratory flow at sea level but not at high altitude.[30] Smokers are less tolerant than nonsmokers to a prolonged stay at high altitude, and persons who continue smoking after arrival at high altitude tolerate the altitude poorly, compared with nonsmokers. A study was made of workers recruited to work on an irrigation program at 10,500 feet (3,200 m) in southern Peru. Of 51 Swedish employees, 25 smokers and 26 nonsmokers, 14 had to terminate their contract. All 10 who had to return to a lower altitude for nonmedical reasons were smokers. Smokers had a higher hematocrit and hemoglobin level than nonsmokers.[31] Honigman and his associates, however, found no difference in the incidence of acute mountain sickness between smokers and nonsmokers in visitors to a Colorado ski resort at 9,300 feet (2,840 m).[5]

References

1. HULTGREN H. Personal observations.
2. DILL D, HILLYARD S, and MILLER J. Vital capacity, exercise performance, and blood gases at altitude as related to age. *J. Appl. Physiol.* 1980; 48:6-9.
3. TERMAN J, and NEWTON J. Changes in alveolar and arterial gas tensions as related to altitude and age. *J. Appl. Physiol.* 1964; 19:21-24.
4. TENNEY S, RAHN H, STROUD R, and MITHOEFER J. Adaptation to high altitude: Changes in lung volumes during the first seven days at Mount Evans, Colorado. *J. Appl. Physiol.* 1953; 5: 607-13.
5. HONIGMAN B, THEIS M, KOZIOL-MCLAIN J, et al. Acute mountain sickness in a general tourist population at moderate altitudes. *Annals Int. Med.* 1993; 118:587-92.
6. ROACH R, HOUSTON C, HONIGMAN B, et al. How well do older persons tolerate moderate altitude? *West. J. Med.* 1995; 162:32-6.
7. YARON M, HULTGREN H, and ALEXANDER J. Low risk of myocardial ischemia in the elderly visiting moderate altitude. *J. Wild. Environ. Med.* 1995; 6:20-8.
8. ALEXANDER J. Age, altitude and arrhythmia. *Texas Heart Inst. J.* 1995; 22:3098-16.
9. DAVIDSON W, JR., and FEE E. Influence of aging on pulmonary hemodynamics in a population free of coronary artery disease. *Am. J. Cardiol.* 1990; 65: 1454-58.
10. WEIL J, BYRNE-QUINN E, SODAL I, et al. Hypoxic ventilatory drive in normal man. *J. Clin. Invest.* 1970; 49:1061-72.
11. SHLIM D. Personal communication.
12. HIRATA K, MASUYAMA S, and SAITO A. Obesity as a risk factor for acute mountain sickness. *Lancet* 1989; 2:1040-41.
13. KAYSER B. Acute mountain sickness in western tourists around the Thorong pass (5,400 m) in Nepal. *J. Wilderness Med.* 1991; 2: 110-17.
14. DICKINSON J. High altitude cerebral edema: Cerebral acute mountain sickness. *Sem. Resp. Med.* 1983; 5:151-58.
15. LUPI-HERRERA E, SEOANE M, SANDOVAL J, et al. Behavior of the pulmonary circulation in the grossly obese patient: Pathogenesis of pulmonary arterial hypertension at an altitude of 2,240 meters. *Chest* 1980; 78:553-58.
16. ZWILLICH C, SUTTON F, PIERSON D, et al. Decreased hypoxic ventilatory drive in the obesity-hypoventilation syndrome. *Am. J. Med.* 1975; 59:343-48.
17. RENNIE D, and WILSON R. Who should not go high. In *Hypoxia: Man at altitude*, ed, J Sutton, N Jones, and C Houston. New York: Thieme-Stratton, 1982; 186-90.
18. WILSON R, MILLS W, ROGERS D, and PROPST M. Death on Denali. *West. J. Med.* 1978l 128:471-6.

19. WESTENDORP, RGJ, FROLICH M, and MEINDERS AE. What to tell steroid-substituted patients about the effects of high altitude? *Lancet* 1993; 342:310-11.
20. CLARKE C. The incidence of epilepsy at high altitude. *Proceedings*, Internal Congress of Mountain Medicine, 1991: 63. Abstract.
21. YIP R. Altitude and birth weight. *J. Pediatr.* 1987; 111:869-76.
22. CAMERON R. Should air hostesses continue flight duty during the first trimester of pregnancy? *Aerospace Med.* 1973; 44:552-56.
23. TAYLOR E. Management of normal pregnancy, labor and puerperium. In *Obstet. Gynecol. Survey* 1973; 28:802.
24. MOORE L. Altitude-aggravated illness: Examples from pregnancy and prenatal life. *Ann. Emerg. Med.* 1987; 16:965-73.
25. DAS U. Possible role of prostaglandins in the pathogenesis of pulmonary hypertension. *Prostaglandins Med.* 1980; 4:163-70.
26. WILTNER W, and SZABOLSCI L. Letter to editor. *JAMA* 1979; 241.
27. MCFADDEN E, and INGRAM R. Exercise-induced asthma: Observations on the initiating stimulus. *N. Engl. J. Med.* 1979; 301:763-69.
28. SKRICKA T. Cited in *Newsletter, Internat. Soc. Mountain Med.* 1991; 1:6.
29. BREWER G, EATON J, GROVER R, and WEIL J. Cigarette smoking as a cause of hypoxemia in man at altitude. *Chest* 1971; 59:305-18.
30. RAMIREZ G, BITTLE P, COLICE G, et al. The effect of cigarette smoking upon hematological adaptations to moderately high altitude. *J. Wilderness Med.* 1991; 2:274-86.
31. LINDGARDE F, and LILJEKVIST R. Failure of long-term acclimatization in smokers moving to high altitude. *Acta Med. Scand.* 1984; 216:317-22.

CHAPTER 30

Women and Altitude

SUMMARY

Few studies have been made of the physiological responses of women to high altitude compared with those of men. Hannon's classic studies of men and women on Pikes Peak, 14,104 feet (4,300 m), showed that women had a higher food intake and lost less weight than men during the first two weeks on the mountain. Arterial PCO_2 was lower and PO_2 was higher in women. Presumably this was related to an increase in ventilation due to the effect of female hormones, especially progesterone and estrogen. Hannon also reported that women had a lower hematocrit than men throughout the altitude stay. This was corrected by daily oral iron supplements given for six weeks before the ascent. These results suggest that if iron stores are low, as evidenced by a low ferritin level, there may be a diminished response to erythropoietin at high altitude.

Women have a significantly lower incidence of high altitude pulmonary edema, chronic mountain sickness and high altitude polycythemia than men. Acute mountain sickness and retinal hemorrhages appear to be equally distributed between men and women. Systemic edema of high altitude appears to be more common in women, but more studies are needed. Although high altitude cerebral edema and thromboembolism seem mostly to affect males, this may simply be the consequence of the greater number of men exposed to the conditions that lead to these problems. The decreased susceptibility of women to high altitude pulmonary edema is probably due to their higher ventilatory response to hypoxia. This factor, as well as a greater blood loss and iron deficiency, may in part explain the low incidence of chronic mountain sickness and high altitude polycythemia in women.

• • •

Too little attention has been given to the subject of women and altitude, especially the difference between men and women in their responses to altitude. Most altitude studies have been confined to men, usually young and physically fit; for various reasons, women, who constitute 51 percent of the population, have historically been omitted from altitude studies. It is therefore appropriate to review briefly the physiological effects of acute altitude exposure in women and to examine the differences between women and men in susceptibility to short-term altitude illnesses. The effects of long-term altitude exposure will not be examined.

Food Intake and Weight Loss.

Hannon compared the response of young men and young women who were transported to the summit of Pikes Peak, Colorado, 14,110 feet (4,300 m), under controlled conditions for a stay of three to eleven weeks.[1,2] During the first few days after arrival, both men and women experienced a loss of appetite, with consequent decreased food intake. However, the women increased their food intake more

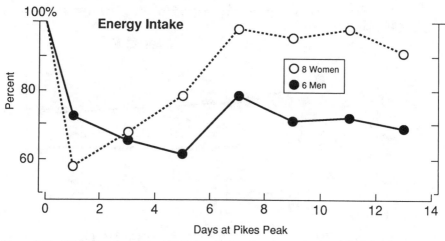

Figure 30.1. Effect of high altitude, 14,110 feet (4,300 m) on energy intake of food. Levels are percent of low altitude values of 2,980 K cal/24 hr. for men and 1,980 for women. From Hannon, ref. 1.

rapidly than the men, and therefore over a two-week sojourn lost only 1.49 percent of their body weight compared to a loss of 4.86 percent in the men (Fig. 30.1). The decreased food intake resulted in an increase in plasma-free fatty acids that was greater in the men than in the women. It is possible that part of this difference could have been due to a lower incidence of acute mountain sickness in women.

Arterial PO$_2$ and PCO$_2$

Arterial PCO$_2$ and arterial HCO$_3^-$ were lower in women than in men and arterial PO$_2$ was higher in women. The difference in PO$_2$ ranged from 2 to 6 mm Hg with the greatest difference beginning about seven days after arrival (Figs. 30.2, 30.3). The increase in ventilation and resulting higher PO$_2$ could have resulted in a theoretical altitude reduction of about 540-1,640 feet (165-500 m) at the summit. This may be the reason food intake increased more rapidly in women and weight loss was less. The effect of female hormones, especially progesterone and estrogen, which are ventilatory stimulants, probably is the basis for the higher ventilation in women. Progesterone and estrogen have a combination of peripheral (carotid body) and central sites of action. The two hormones together have a more consistent stimulatory effect upon the ventilatory response to hypoxia than does either hormone alone.[3]

Blood Volume

Women experience a greater degree of hemoconcentration upon ascent, as evidenced by a greater rise in hemoglobin, hematocrit, and arterial oxygen content (Fig. 30.4). This is accompanied by a greater decrease in extracellular fluid volume and plasma volume. Red cell mass is not increased.[1,2] The effect is primarily due to a decrease in plasma volume that results not from dehydration but from loss of plasma from the vascular bed. This more prolonged decrease in plasma volume probably explains why women probably achieve hemoconcentration over a longer period of time than men, who have a fairly rapid initial decrease in plasma volume

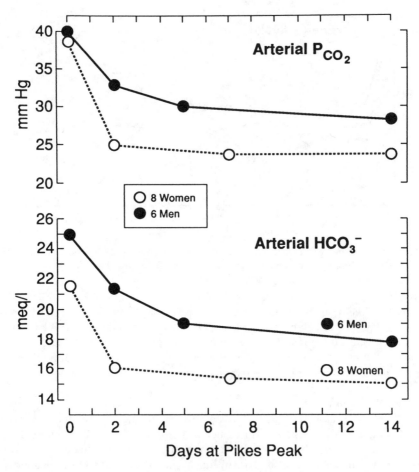

Figure 30.2. Effect of high altitude, 14,110 feet (4,300 m) on arterial PCO_2 and HCO_3- concentration. From Hannon, ref. 1.

accompanied by a more rapid increase in red cell mass. Zamudio and her associates reported that women living at 10,168 feet (3,100 m) had a normal red cell mass but a lower plasma volume and a lower total blood volume than women living at 5,248 feet (1,600 m).[4] It is well known that men living permanently at higher altitudes have about a 15 percent increase in total blood volume owing to an almost doubling of red cell mass with a normal or slightly reduced plasma volume.[5,6]

Heart Rate

Increases in resting heart rate are higher in women than in men upon ascent to high altitude (Fig. 30.5). A possible explanation is that women have a greater activation of the sympathetic nervous system with hypoxia.[7] Zamudio has shown that long-term female residents of high altitudes have higher heart rates than their low-altitude counterparts.[4] Palmer has suggested that enhanced sympathetic respon-

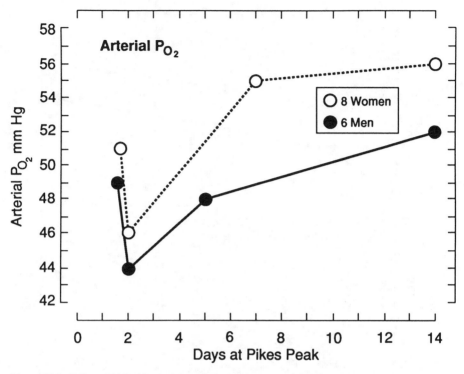

Figure 30.3. Effect of high altitude, 14,110 feet (4,300 m) on arterial PO$_2$. From Hannon, ref. 1.

siveness may be present in some women at high altitude.[8] A lower hemoglobin concentration may also be a factor, since cardiac output and heart rate must be higher to maintain tissue oxygen delivery.[9]

Pulmonary Function

The effect of altitude acclimatization upon pulmonary function was studied in eight women after ascent to the summit of Pikes Peak, 14,104 feet (4,300 m), and after a 65-day stay at the summit.[10] The following changes were similar to those obtained from eight men studied under similar conditions: an initial decrease in vital capacity, an initial increase in one second vital capacity, an increase in maximum breathing capacity and maximum midexpiratory flow and a decrease in breath-holding time. Women increased their maximum breathing capacity by only 10 to 13.4 percent, compared with an increase in men of 42 to 50 percent (Fig. 30. 6). The explanation for this difference is not clear.

Maximum Exercise Capacity

Drinkwater evaluates the response of eight experienced women mountaineers to maximum exercise during hypoxia.[11] Normoxic values for VO$_{2max}$ were above average for all subjects and did not decline with age (range, 20-49 years). The mean decrease in VO$_{2max}$ of 26.7 percent during breathing 12.58 percent oxygen

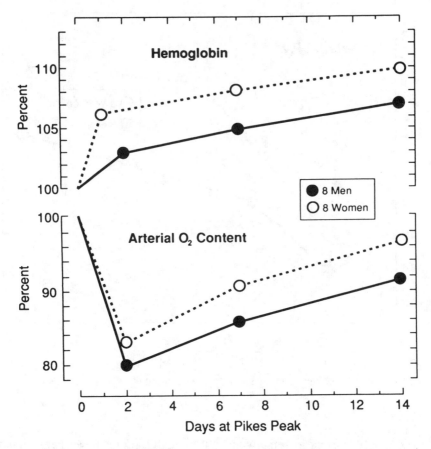

Figure 30.4. Effect of high altitude exposure, 14,110 feet (4,300 m), on hemoglobin and arterial oxygen content. Levels are expressed as percent of low altitude control value: hemoglobin 14.9 g/100 ml for men, 13.7 for women, and oxygen content 19.4 ml O_2/100 ml blood for men and 17.3 for women. From Hannon, ref. 1.

was equivalent to that reported for younger males. Four of these women successfully climbed Annapurna, 26,500 feet (8,080 m). Elliott and Atterbom compared the effect of cycle ergometer exercise at 5,169 feet (1,576 m), 8,111 feet (2,473 m), and 13,000 feet (3,962 m) in 17 men and 20 women in a hypobaric chamber. For submaximal and maximal exercise women had a smaller increase in ventilation, but no other significant differences were observed.[12] Similar studies of women without male controls in a hypobaric chamber have shown that women can perform quite as well as men at simulated altitudes of 6,986 feet (2,130 m) and 10,000 feet (3,050 m).[13] Women have been successful in climbing the highest summits in the world, including Mount Everest. In 1975 the first woman climbed Mount Everest and in 1988 Stacy Allison was the first American woman to reach the summit. Women from Tibet, Germany, Poland, India, China, Japan, and Canada have also reached the summit.

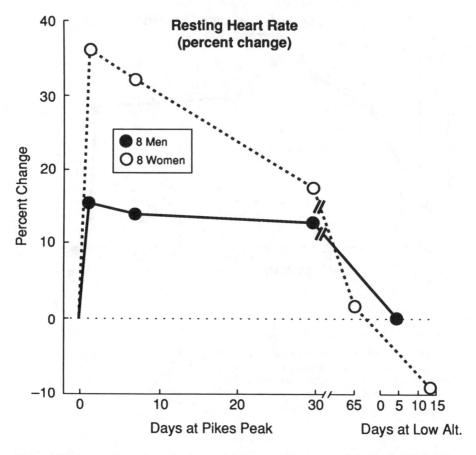

Figure 30.5. Percent change in resting heart rate in 8 men and 8 women at low altitude (700 ft, 214 m) and during sojourn on Pikes Peak (14,110 ft, 4,300 m). From Hannon, Shields, and Harris, ref. 20.

Extreme Altitudes

Few systematic studies have been made of women on expeditionary climbs to extreme altitudes. Drinkwater and associates studied six women before and during an expedition to a 22,300 foot (6,798 m) Himalayan peak. The responses of the women to spending one month above 13,940 feet (4,250 m) were similar to those of men. Results of exercise studies before the climb were also similar to those in men.[14,15,16]

Red Cell Mass

It has long been recognized that women have a lower hemoglobin and hematocrit than men. Premenopausal women frequently have low iron stores. Some women do not respond to high altitude with an appropriate increase in hemoglobin. Richalet and his associates studied four women and six men during an altitude expo-

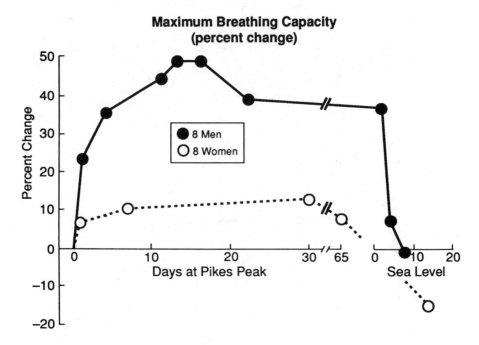

Figure 30.6. Relative changes in maximum breathing capacity of men and women during exposure to 14,110 feet (4,300 m). Maximum breathing capacity expressed as liters/Kg body weight were, in men, 3.33 at sea level and 5.04 at altitude. In women the sea level value was 4.33 and at altitude the value was 4.89. From Shields et al., ref. 10.

sure to 21,458 feet (6,542 m). Two women had a decrease in hemoglobin during the altitude stay despite an increase in erythropoietin.[17] Ferritin levels were decreased and dietary iron was low. All women had amenorrhea during the altitude stay. It is quite likely that the women had low iron stores; this would explain the lack of response to erythropoietin, which is known to be ineffective in the presence of low iron stores.[18,19] Iron supplements before and during an altitude stay would seem indicated by this experience.

These findings are supported by Hannon's observations in eight women brought to Pikes Peak.[2,20] Starting three months before the ascent, each subject took iron supplements in the form of one 5-grain tablet of $FeSO_4$ daily. The average hematocrit increased from 40.3 percent to 43.0 percent, indicating a relative iron deficiency state. Upon exposure to Pikes Peak, these women exhibited a rapid increase in hematocrit and hemoglobin that was qualitatively similar to the increases observed in male subjects. Eight women who did not take iron supplements before ascent, however, had lower hematocrits prior to ascent and a lesser increase in hematocrit during the altitude stay (Fig. 30.7). Evaluation of iron stores before ascent would seem appropriate. Iron deficiency is characterized by a reduced serum iron and ferritin and an increased iron binding capacity. Free erythrocyte protoporphyrin is decreased.[21]

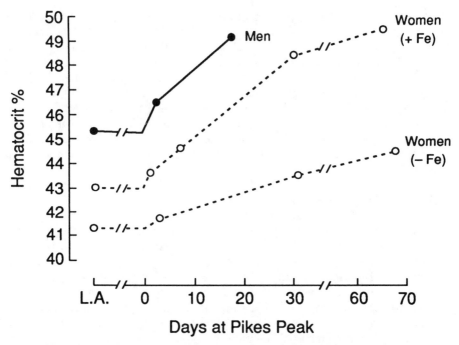

Figure 30.7. Effect of high altitude exposure to 14,110 feet (4,300 m) on hematocrit levels of men and women. Women (±Fe) were on iron supplementation for three months prior to ascent and received 5 grains of FE SO₄ daily. LA = low altitude. From Hannon et al., ref. 20.

Menstrual Abnormalities

Menstrual abnormalities at high altitude are not uncommon, but scant attention has been directed to systematic studies of this phenomenon.[16,17,20] Since many factors are probably involved in addition to altitude, studies would be difficult.

Susceptibility to Altitude Illness

Little information is available regarding the male-female ratio in various forms of altitude illness, mainly because only small numbers have been evaluated and most expeditionary climbing groups consist primarily of males. Opinions differ regarding the susceptibility of women to acute mountain sickness (AMS) and high altitude pulmonary edema (HAPE). For example, it was at first thought that HAPE was rare in women. An editorial in the *British Medical Journal* in 1972 stated, "Women have not so far been recorded as victims of this disease."[22] In a reply to the editorial, Steele pointed out that he had seen three cases of HAPE in women in the Himalayas.[23] A difference in incidence of certain altitude illnesses between the sexes may provide information regarding etiologic mechanisms.

Acute Mountain Sickness

A recent questionnaire survey of 3,158 adult visitors to mountain resorts in Colorado at levels between 6,300 and 9,700 feet (1,922 and 2,959 m) revealed that 25 percent developed three or more symptoms of AMS, including loss of appetite, vomiting, dyspnea, dizziness or light-headedness, unusual fatigue, sleep disturbance, and headache. Fifty-one percent of the patients with AMS had a moderate reduction of activity and 5 percent stayed in bed. Of 2,159 males, 23.6 percent had AMS, compared with 27.9 of 981 females (p = <0.01).[24] These results agree with those of Hackett's studies of 278 trekkers in Nepal. AMS occurred in both sexes in approximately equal numbers: 53 percent in males and 51 percent in females.[25] An additional study of 200 trekkers revealed AMS to occur in 70 percent of males and 71 percent in females.[26] Hannon suggested that women brought to the summit of Pikes Peak, 14,104 feet (4,300 m), had less severe symptoms of AMS than men, but only eight men and eight women were studied.[12] In a recent study by Honigman and his colleagues, the severity and number of symptoms were the same in men and women.[24]

High Altitude Pulmonary Edema

Unlike AMS, there appears to be a clear predilection in males for HAPE. In a study of 150 patients with HAPE seen at Keystone, Colorado, over a 39-month period 84 percent were males.[27] Sophocles described 46 patients with HAPE in Summit County, Colorado, 9,000-11,000 feet (2,743-3,354 m). Ninety-three percent were males.[28] Hochstrasser and his colleagues described 50 patients with HAPE who were evacuated to a lower altitude in the Swiss Alps. All but one were males.[29]

It is of interest that there is a lesser predilection for HAPE in male children in Peru. Sixty percent of 200 patients under sixteen years of age were male.[30] Similar observations have been made in Colorado.[31]

The lower incidence of HAPE in females may be due to a hormonal increase in ventilation and thus a higher arterial PO_2. It is of interest that in the study of HAPE at Keystone, Colorado, 21 percent of women with HAPE were 50 years old or older, compared with only 13 percent of men. Decreased hormonal activity may have increased the susceptibility to HAPE in older women.

Chronic Mountain Sickness

Chronic mountain sickness occurs largely in older males. Thirty-nine cases reported from the Western Himalaya were all males.[32,33] In Lhasa, high altitude polycythemia, and presumably chronic mountain sickness, was reported to occur only in males.[34] Wu reported 26 cases from China of whom 22 were males.[35] Fifty-one cases reported from the Quinhai region of China were all males.[36] Thirty cases reported from Peru were all males.[37]

High Altitude Polycythemia

High altitude polycythemia, a condition also known as excessive polycythemia of high altitude, is largely confined to older males, especially to miners and men who are obese.[38] This is the same group that is usually afflicted with chronic mountain sickness.

High Altitude Cerebral Edema

High altitude cerebral edema is not rare in women and occurred in 6 of 19 cases (32 percent) not accompanied by HAPE, pneumonia, or pulmonary embolism.[39] The higher percentage in males is probably linked to the fact that most of these cases occurred at altitudes exceeding 16,000 feet (4,880 m), where far more men than women were exposed. Dickinson has observed that most episodes of HACE occur in obese males.[40]

Systemic Edema

Systemic edema occurring at high altitude appears to be more common in women. Hackett and Rennie reported that systemic edema occurred in 36 of 200 trekkers in Nepal. Edema was about twice as frequent in women (28 percent) as in men (14 percent). Of 12 trekkers with multiple areas of edema, 9 were women. Systemic edema was more common in trekkers with AMS (27 percent) than in those without symptoms (11 percent).[26] Most episodes of altitude related systemic edema that I have observed have been in women.

Thromboembolism

Thromboembolism appears to be rare in women. Of 31 cases of pulmonary embolism, completed strokes, and transient ischemic attacks collected by the author, all were men.[39] Here again, however, these statistics may have been skewed by the fact that all cases occurred during expeditionary climbs where most of the members were men.

Retinal Hemorrhages

There does not seem to be a gender predisposition of retinal hemorrhages. Of 13 cases of retinal hemorrhages observed in 340 trekkers, 8 were women (62 percent).[26] McFadden and his colleagues reported a 56 percent incidence of retinal hemorrhages in 39 healthy subjects on Mount Logan. The hemorrhages were present equally in men and women.[41] Gender differences in the incidence of four altitude illnesses are shown in Figure 30.8.

Conclusions

The results here reported are largely preliminary and incomplete, but certain general assumptions may be made regarding mechanisms that may be the basis for sex differences in altitude illnesses. The lower prevalence of adult females with HAPE and the possibility that postmenopausal women do not have a similar low prevalence suggests that premenopausal women have a physiologic mechanism that lowers their susceptibility. The most likely mechanism is a higher ventilation and arterial PO_2 mediated by hormonal mechanisms, probably largely by progesterone. It appears that unlike AMS, the occurrence of HAPE is more closely related to the degree of hyperventilation following ascent to high altitude. Matsuzawa and Hackett have shown that a blunted hypoxic ventilatory drive is present in subjects susceptible to HAPE.[42,43]

Chronic mountain sickness and high altitude polycythemia has a large male predominance, and older men are most susceptible. This appears to be related to the decline in ventilation, vital capacity, and other aspects of respiratory function with advancing age that is more prevalent in men.[44] Postmenopausal women resemble men in response to disordered breathing during sleep and nocturnal oxygen desaturation. Protection from these disorders in premenopausal women might be afforded by the respiratory stimulating effects of circulating progesterone.[3] It is well known that men are more susceptible than women to sleep apnea and desaturation.[45] Another possibility is that most men at high altitude do manual labor, such as working in mines and may work at higher altitudes than women.

High altitude systemic edema appears to be more common in women, but further studies of the mechanism are clearly indicated. It is likely that hormonal factors that

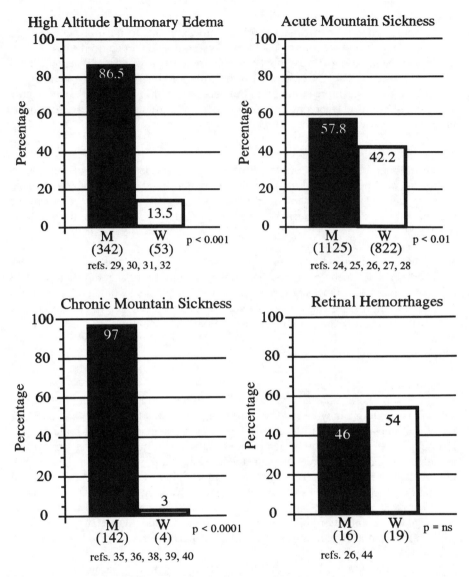

Figure 30.8. Gender differences in four common high altitude medical conditions as reported in the literature. The proportion of men and women at risk is not reported.

facilitate sodium and water retention are involved. Some studies have indicated that systemic edema does not appear to be related to the use of birth control pills or to the phase of the menstrual cycle.[25,26]

High altitude cerebral edema not associated with edema occurs less frequently in women than in men. Their higher ventilatory response to altitude may be involved, but more data are needed to examine this possibility.

The rarity of thromboembolism in women remains to be explained by further studies. It is likely that men are more frequently exposed to extreme altitudes and poor weather conditions than women.

Retinal hemorrhages show little gender difference, but more data are needed. Additional studies of male-female susceptibility to all types of altitude illnesses are clearly indicated, as well as studies of the mechanisms involved where clear gender differences are present.

[Note: The author is indebted to John Hannon for permission to reproduce illustrations from his publications.]

References

1. HANNON J. Comparative adaptability of young men and women. In L Folinsbee, J Wagner, J Borgia, B Drinkwater, J Gliner, and J Bedi, eds., *Environmental stress: Individual human adaptations*. New York: Academic Press, 1978; 335-50.
2. HANNON J. High altitude acclimatization in women. In R. Goddard, ed., *The effects of altitude on physical performance*. Chicago: Athletic Institute, 1966; 37-44.
3. REGENSTEINER J, WOODARD W, HAGERMAN D, et al. Combined effects of female hormones and metabolic rate on ventilatory drives in women. *J. Appl. Physiol.* 1989; 66:808-13.
4. ZAMUDIO S, MONGE C, SUN S, and MOORE L. Ventilatory characteristics of Peruvian and Tibetan women and men native to high altitude. To be published.
5. HURTADO A. Studies at high altitude Blood observations on the Indian natives of the Peruvian Andes. *Am. J. Physiol.* 1932; 100:487-505.
6. SANCHEZ C, MERINO C, FIGALLO M. Simultaneous measurement of plasma volume and cell mass in polycythemia of altitude. *J. Appl. Physiol.* 1970; 28: 775-78.
7. REEVES J, MOORE L, WOLFEL E, et al. Activation of the sympathoadrenal system at high altitude. In G Ueda, J Reeves, and M. Segiguchi, eds., *High altitude medicine*. Matsumoto Japan Shinshu University Press. 1992, pp. 10-23.
8. PALMER S, BERMAN J, ZAMUDIO S, et al. Altered heart rate response to hypoxia in women who develop preeclampsia. *Anesthesiology* 1992; 77:A1000. Abstract.
9. BANCHERO H, SIME F, PEÑALOZA D, et al. Pulmonary pressure, cardiac output, and arterial oxygen saturation during exercise at high altitude and at sea level. *Circulation* 1966; 33:249-62.
10. SHIELDS JL, HANNON JP, HARRIS CW, PLATNER WS. Effects of altitude acclimatization on pulmonary function in women. *J. Appl. Physiol.* 1968; 25:606-09.
11. DRINKWATER B. Responses of women mountaineers to maximal exercise during hypoxia. *Aviat. Space Environ. Med.* 1979; 50:657-62.
12. ELLIOTT PR, and ATTERBOM HA. Comparison of exercise responses of males and females during acute exposure to hypobaria. *Aviat. Space Environ. Med.* 1978; 49:415-18.
13. WAGNER JA, MILES DS, HORVATH SM, and REYBURN JA. Maximal work capacity of women during acute hypoxia. *J. Appl. Physiol.* 1979; 47:1223-27.
14. DRINKWATER BL, KRAMAR PO, BEDI JF, and FOLINSBEE LJ. Women at altitude: cardiovascular response to hypoxia. *Aviat. Space Environ. Med.* 1982; 53:472- 77.
15. MILES DS, WAGNER JA, HORVATH SM, and REYBURN JA. Absolute and relative work capacity in women at 758, 586, and 523 Torr barometric pressure. *Aviat. Space Environ. Med.* 1980; 51:439-44.
16. KRAMAR PO, DRINKWATER BL, FOLINSBEE LJ, and BEDI JF. Ocular functions and incidence of acute mountain sickness in women at altitude. *Aviat. Space Environ. Med.* 1983; 54:116-20.
17. RICHALET J, SOUBERBIEL J, BIENVENU A, et al. Variability of altitude-induced erythropoises. *Proceedings Eighth International Hypoxia Symposium*, 1983: 23. Abstract.
18. FINCH C. Erythropoiesis, erythropoietin and iron. *Blood* 1982; 60:1241-46.
19. ESCHBACH J, EGRIE J, DOWNING R, et al. Correction of the anemia of end-stage renal disease with recombinant human erythroietin. Results of a combined phase I and II clinical trial. *N. Engl. J. Med.* 1987; 316:73-8.
20. HANNON J, SHIELDS J, and HARRIS C. A comparative review of certain responses of men and women to high altitude. In *Proceedings of the Symposia on Arctic Biology and Medicine, VI: The physiology of work in cold and altitude*, ed. C Helffereich. Fort Wainwright, Alaska: Arctic Aeromedical Laboratory, 1966.

484

21. OSKI F. Iron deficiency in infancy and childhood. *N. Engl. J. Med.* 1993; 329:190-93.
22. Pulmonary oedema of mountains. *Br. Med. J.* July 8, 1972: 65-66. (Editorial)
23. STEELE P. Pulmonary oedema of mountains. *Br. Med. J.*, July 22, 1972: 231-32. (Correspondence)
24. HONIGMAN B, THEIS M, KOZIAL-MCLAIN J, et al. Acute mountain sickness in a general tourist population at moderate altitudes. *Ann. Int. Med.* 1993; 118: 587-92.
25. HACKETT P and RENNIE D. The incidence, importance, and prophylaxis of acute mountain sickness. *Lancet* 1976; 2:1149-55.
26. HACKETT P and RENNIE D. Rales, peripheral edema, retinal hemorrhage, and acute mountain sickness. *Am. J. Med.* 1979; 67:214-18.
27. HULTGREN H, HONIGMAN B, THEIS K, et al. High altitude pulmonary edema in a ski resort. *West. J. Medicine* 1996; 164:222-27.
28. SOPHOCLES A. High-altitude pulmonary edema in Vail, Colorado, 1975-1982. *West. J. Med* 1986; 144:569-73.
29. HOCHSTRASSER J, NANZER A, and OELZ O. Altitude edema in the Swiss Alps. Observations on the incidence and clinical course in 50 patients 1980-1984. *Schweiz Med. Wochenscr.* 1986; 116:866-73.
30. LOPEZ DIAZ C. Edema agudo pulmonar de altura en ninos. Doctoral thesis, Lima, Peru, 1972.
31. SCOGGIN C, HYERS T, REEVES J, and GROVER R. High altitude pulmonary edema in the children and young adults of Leadville, Colorado. *N. Engl. J. Med.* 1977; 297:1269-72.
32. NATH C, KASHYAP S and SUBRAMANIAN A. Chronic mountain sickness. Probang type. *Armed Forces Med. J.* India 1983; 39:131-40.
33. NATH C, KASHYAP S and SUBRAMANIAN. Chronic mountain sickness. Probang type. *Defense Sci J.* 1984; 34:443-50.
34. WU S. Hypoxia in China. An overview. In *Hypoxia, exercise and altitude*, ed. J Sutton, C Houston, and N Jones. New York, A. R. Liss, 1983: 157-82.
35. WU T, ZHANG Q, JIN B, et al. Chronic mountain sickness (Monge's disease). An observation in Quinghai, Tibet plateau. In *High altitude medicine*, ed. G Ueda, J Reeves, and M Segiguchi. Matsumoto, Japan: Shinshu University Press, 1992: 314-24.
36. MIAO C, ZHANG Y, BAY Z, et al. Studies on chronic mountain sickness in recent years in Qinghai, China. In *High altitude medicine*, ed. G Ueda, J Reeves, and M Segiguchi. Matsumoto, Japan: Shinshu University Press, 1992: 265-74.
37. REATEGUI-LOPEZ. Soroche cronico: observaciones realizada en la Cuzco en 30 casos. *Rev. Peruana Cardiol.* 1969; 15:45-59.
38. TUFTS D, HAAS J, BEARD J, and SPIELVOGEL H. Distribution of hemoglobin and functional consequences of anemia in adult males at high altitude. *Am. J. Clin. Nut.* 1985; 42:1-10.
39. HULTGREN H. Personal observations.
40. DICKINSON J. High altitude cerebral edema: Cerebral acute mountain sickness. *Seminars in Resp. Med.* 1983; 5:151-58.
41. MCFADDEN D, HOUSTON C, SUTTON J, et al. High-altitude retinopathy. *JAMA* 1981; 245: 581-86.
42. MATSUZAWA Y, FUJIMOTO K, KOBAYASHI T, et al. Blunted hypoxic ventilatory drive in subjects susceptible to high altitude pulmonary edema. *J. App. Physiol* 1989; 66:1152-55.
43. HACKETT P, ROACH R. The Denali medical research project; 1982-1985. *Am. Alpine J.* 1986; 28:129-137.
44. MONGE C, LEON-VELARDE F, and ARREGUI A. Increasing prevalence of excessive erythrocytosis with age among healthy high altitude miners. *N. Engl. J. Med.* 1989; 321:1271. (Correspondence)
45. BLOCK A, BOYSEN P, WYNNE J, and HUNT L. Sleep apnea, hypopnea, and oxygen desaturation in normal subjects. A strong male predominance. *N. Engl. J. Med.* 1979; 300:513-17.

APPENDIX 1

Medicolegal Aspects of Wilderness Travel

SUMMARY

Physicians who participate in a trek or an expedition should realize that they may be exposed to a risk of liability in the event of an accident or an illness in any member of the party. Although the probability of a claim is small, since group members are usually in good health and have accepted the risks inherent in the trip, in the event of a lawsuit the cost and time involved in one's defense could be dev-astating, especially if malpractice insurance does not include actions by the physician on the trip. For these reasons it is useful to review the various medicolegal problems that may arise on a trek or expedition.

Medicolegal problems may be involved in several possible situations:

1. Life-threatening high altitude illness, including pulmonary edema, cerebral edema, and the thromboembolism
2. Aggravation of sea-level medical conditions, including coronary artery disease, systemic hypertension, pulmonary hypertension, congenital, valvular heart disease, and sickle cell disease
3. Accidental injuries such as falls, blows from falling rocks, frostbite, insect stings
4. Death of a member of the group for any cause.
   Legal action may be brought by clients against any of the following:
   a. The corporation or trekking company that organizes and carries out the activity
   b. Trek leaders
   c. Designated trip physicians
   d. Physicians participating in the trek as clients but not as trip physicians
   e. Physicians who give instructions to trek leaders and trip personnel before the trek
   f. The personal physician of the trekkers, who gives advice on the possible risks of a trek.

• • •

The Organization

The organization that sponsors or conducts the trip is responsible for the health and safety of the participants and will usually be liable for damages in lawsuits resulting from inappropriate decisions or actions by any of its employees, including the trip leaders. Potential participants should be informed in advance of the nature and physical requirements of the trek, the terrain and obstacles to be encountered, proper clothing, foot-gear, equipment, and possible health hazards, including altitude illness. Extensive treks far from adequate medical care usually require participants to have their own personal physician fill out a form that attests to the health of the participant and indicates any special precautions that the participant should observe. If an applicant has a dangerous medical condition, he may be required to sign a waiver absolving the organization from liability in the event of illness or accident. Participants should be advised to supply whatever medications they are accustomed to use or are recommended by their personal physician. Most trekking organizations ask potential clients to sign a waiver attesting to the client's understanding and acceptance of the potential risks involved in the expedition.

For its part, the organization is supposed to state whether or not a trip physician will accompany the group, and what sort of methods of evacuation and definite medical care via hospitals or first aid facilities are provided. Any trekking or expedition organization should be equipped with an appropriate first aid kit. Statements by the organization regarding the first aid equipment and medical care are not legally binding, however, and may have little value in court if the expedition fails to meet the conditions that are described by the organization whose headquarters are in the United States. Such action is not possible against a foreign-based company unless it is working under contract to a U.S. company or is conducting business on its own in the United States.

The Trip Leader

The trip leader is the person delegated by the organization to be responsible for the health and safety of the clients. He is responsible also for any action by other trip employees that may cause injury or illness to any member of the group. If there is no trip physician, the leader may delegate a member of the trip to act as a "first-aider" or he may assume this duty alone. In either case, the person so delegated must possess appropriate training, skill, and experience to handle common medical and accidental emergencies. He need not have the knowledge of a physician, but he ought to have completed a standard first aid course.

Trip Physician

A designated trip physician is considered an employee of the organization. He will not, in most cases, be a salaried employee, but he will probably receive reimbursement in the form of reduced trip expenses or transportation costs. In any event, if a medical problem occurs, the trip physician is held to a standard of competence far above that of the good samaritan standard. Before the trip, the physician should check the contents of the medical kit and make sure that adequate supplies are available for usual medical problems. He should also be informed of the health status of the participants. He should know the exact route of the projected trip and be aware of the location of hospitals, medical facilities, and methods of evacuation that are available along the route. He should fulfill the standard of competence that is accepted by his profession as being appropriate for his specialty status. A dermatologist, for example, should not be expected to manage complicated fractures or extensive lacerations that require suturing. If the physician is involved in the planning of the expedition, he bears responsibility for the selection of the trip participants.

The question of malpractice insurance is particularly important. Usually the physician should carry personal malpractice insurance, since in most cases the organization does not provide it, and the physician should ascertain in advance whether the coverage includes travel situations when the physician is acting as a trip physician. Many insurance policies cover only physicians' duties when they are confined to a clinic, HMO, or hospital. If coverage is extended to the duties of trek physician, one should be sure to get a letter from the insurance company certifying that such coverage is provided, and if there is any question, one should review the policy, not with the company but with an experienced attorney who has a broad background in interpreting liability insurance policies.

Physicians should be familiar with the elements that can arise in a malpractice suit:

1. Presence of knowledge, skill, and experience appropriate to the situation. A psychiatrist, for example, would not be expected to reduce correctly a dislocated shoulder nor should he attempt to do so.

2. Informed consent. This applies to treatment by the physician as well as by nonmedical personnel. A patient may refuse medical treatment. If this should happen, the physician must explain to the patient, in the presence of witnesses, the consequences of the refusal. Bear in mind that lawsuits have been successfully prosecuted where the physician has not explained the consequences of a patient's refusal to accept medical treatment or a recommended referral to a specialist and the patient's refusal has resulted in adverse consequences.

3. The treatment applied should be whatever meets reasonable and prudent standards for the physician's type of practice or speciality.

4. Abandonment of the patient. After the physician has provided appropriate treatment, it is a legal duty to see that continued care is provided. This usually means staying with the patient until more definitive care is provided, but may mean turning the patient over to emergency medical personnel for transport to a hospital. Even in this circumstance, the physician must take all reasonable precautions to ensure that the patient is properly cared for during transport. In critical cases the physician may need to accompany the patient — for example, to be sure an airway remains patent.

It is extremely important, whenever a physician renders medical care, to keep accurate notes of the circumstances of the disability, the condition of the patient, the care rendered, and the referral to continuing medical care. Such notes are essential in the event of a lawsuit.

Physician-clients

A physician who has paid the full cost of the trip and is not designated as the trip physician has no more duty to his fellow passengers than any other member of the group. However, before the trip begins, the physician should always ask the leaders, "Am I the trip physician?" He should discuss with the trip leader or the designated trip physician whether or not he would be willing to assist in medical emergencies, and he should define his expertise, in the event that his knowledge and experience are needed. It is wise to have a written contract prepared in advance, clearly stating that the physician is not the trip physician and that he waives all liability for any actions in a good samaritan emergency. It is to be expected that in an emergency, when there is no designated trip physician, a physician client may decide to render aid as necessary; in such cases he will usually be protected by the good samaritan rule. But the fact that the physician possesses special skills and training does not convey automatic responsibility to provide medical care in an emergency.

When they apply, good samaritan statutes usually offer total immunity from liability, even if the physician fails the community standard. The theory of the good samaritan immunity has been accepted in all fifty states of the United States, but because every state's statute is different, the physician should review the statute in his own state so that he is aware of the limitations and exceptions in the law. In the event of any emergency, the physician must perform the service gratuitously, with no preexisting patient-doctor relationship or subsequent fee.

Few would refuse to provide first aid or assistance to anyone who is injured or in distress, but there is no law that *requires* one to do so. If assistance is given, the victim must consent to the assistance, whether it is only simple first aid, administration of medication, the performance of minor surgery or transport to a medical facility. In most situations, the fact that the victim consciously allows assistance to be undertaken implies consent. In special situations, such as a helicopter evacuation, the victim's verbal consent should be documented by witnesses to prevent any subsequent legal action. Treatment of a minor requires consent from a parent or guardian; if the parent or guardian is not going on the trip, the permission should be stated in writing before the trip begins. In some situations the injured or ill person may be so incapacitated that informed consent cannot be obtained. Under these conditions a universally recognized "emergency doctrine" comes into effect. This means that any reasonable person would want assistance to be provided if a delay in such assistance would result in serious harm, injury, or death. The assistance provided must be performed in a reasonable and careful manner, and must be that which an ordinarily prudent person under such circumstances would provide. Anyone who provides medical assistance is legally liable for harm caused to the patient, if the harm could have been avoided by reasonable precautions. Therefore the care that is provided must be whatever is reasonable *under the circumstances*. Such care rarely results in legal action. The usual legal action for mismanagement of an accident or medical problem is a lawsuit against the trip leader and organization for negligence or failure to warn.

It is wise for any physician on a trip to keep a diary, especially if any medical care is given or if an accident or a fatality occurs. One should remember that in case of a legal action the diary may be used as evidence, and therefore one must be careful to state the simple facts and not enter any biased statements or accusations.

The Personal Physician of the Trip Client

Most trekking or climbing organizations require the prospective client to provide some evidence of good health and suitable physical conditioning, usually by filling out a simple medical questionnaire. For older clients, a statement by the client's personal physician may be required, and in some cases the company may ask for an electrocardiogram, a treadmill exercise test, or a chest x-ray.

A special problem exists when the prospective client has a known medical condition that may be adversely affected by trekking or high altitude — coronary artery disease, for example, or systemic hypertension, pulmonary hypertension, congenital or valvular heart disease, or sickle cell anemia. The personal physician should perform any tests that are indicated and inform the patient of the potential risks of the proposed trip. In general, this means three categories of medical conditions: (a) conditions that make a trip dangerous because of an unacceptable risk; (b) a moderate but acceptable risk but not dangerous, provided that acclimatization, appropriate medications, and adequate rest are observed; (c) medical conditions that are stable and are unlikely to be affected by the proposed activity. Consultation with a specialist may be necessary in the case of medical conditions that are not frequently encountered by the general practitioner or internist.

Organizations and physicians should be aware that a prospective client may conceal symptoms or evidence of significant medical problems in order to join a trip. A physician who signs a medical certificate without taking a history, examining the patient, or performing indicated tests may be liable in a lawsuit if a medical condition that was not detected, or not reported, becomes a hazard on a trip.

Fatalities

In rare instances, a trek leader or the trip physician will be faced with the death of a trekking client. Such an event is usually the result of an accident such as a fall, being struck by falling rock, hypothermia or avalanches. Less common are deaths due to medical conditions, including myocardial infarction, dissecting aneurysm, or a cerebral hemorrhage. Fatal episodes of high altitude pulmonary edema or cerebral edema may occur. In the event of a fatality, the leader and/or the trip physician must assume several responsibilities. The determination of death is primarily the responsibility of a physician. If a physician is not available, the evidence of death — absent pulses, absent heart beat, and cessation of breathing — should be noted and several witnesses should attest to the findings. Written notes, including the names of witnesses, the existence and extent of trauma, and the circumstances of the death are important for future evidence. In accidental deaths photographs of the location of the accident, as well as photographs of the deceased, provide important documentation in the event of possible future legal action. If death is due to a medical condition, written notes regarding any symptoms preceding the event may be important in determining the cause of death. Occasionally suicide may simulate accidental death. Witnesses should be interviewed by the trip leader and the trip physician to obtain as much information as possible. Since a fatality that occurs on a trip may result in a legal action, any physician on the trip should be very careful about pub-lic statements that may be seized upon by the media and adversely affect the litigation. In one instance a trip physician made so many allegations regarding a fatality that it probably influenced the outcome of the trial and resulted in a slander suit against the physician.

Disappearance does not constitute evidence of death unless the circumstances have made it impossible for the person to survive, such as someone who is lost in a storm at extreme altitude, where survival for more than a few hours is impossible. In other situations a reasonable time must elapse before a legal "presumption" of death can be established. In many jurisdictions, this is seven years.

Estates and Life Insurance

For the administration of an estate and to carry out provision of a will the fact of death must be established, but not necessarily the cause or mode of death. For ordinary life insurance, the fact of death as attested by witnesses is sufficient evidence for the payment of insurance. However, exclusions or special provisions in the insurance policy may require the cause or mode of death to be documented accurately. For example, suicide or hazardous activities such as mountaineering or hang gliding may be exclusions. Double-indemnity life insurance policies pay double the value of the policy for accidental death. A person who has a heart attack may fall as the result of a medical condition and death may be due to the medical condition and not the fall; in such a case the double-indemnity provision would not apply. But if a person had a nonfatal heart attack and fell, and as result suffered fatal injuries, the death would be accidental, because if the fall had not occurred the person would have survived. In some circumstances a court may need to decide whether or not death was due to an accident: for example, are deaths due to high altitude pulmonary or cerebral edema accidents?

Disposal of the Body

The next of kin must be informed of the death as soon as possible, because only the next of kin has the legal right to determine what should be done with the body. Should burial or cremation be performed? Should the body be returned to the place of residence of the deceased for burial? What ceremonies should be observed? Many difficult legal problems have resulted from a hasty burial or cremation of a body before the next of kin was notified.

Law enforcement agencies also have a legal interest in the cause of death in order to ascertain whether a crime has been committed or whether death was due to a contagious disease that might pose a health hazard. In extremely remote areas, the members of the group are not legally responsible for recovery of the body. This decision rests with the local officials and the next of kin.

Medicolegal Cases

The following are summaries of medicolegal cases with which the author is familiar that illustrate some of the problems discussed in this chapter. The descriptions have been changed slightly to preserve anonymity.

Case 1. A 46-year-old woman went on a safari in an African country. The safari was organized by a U. S. company but actually conducted by an African company. The trip company in printed brochures that were sent out before the trip warned clients about leaving the safari camp alone, because of the danger of wild animals. The warning was repeated at the briefing before the trip, and during the trip the warning was again emphasized. Nonetheless, the woman ventured near a river and was mauled by a hippopotamus. She sued the African safari company in an African court. The judge threw the case out of court, saying that the woman had been adequately warned, had not heeded the warning, and the mauling was therefore her own fault. The woman then sued the U.S. company that had organized the trip. A financial settlement was made before the trial.

Comment. Written and verbal warnings or signed waivers regarding possible dangers on a trek or safari may not always be sufficient to prevent legal action. The sponsor of a trip or the trekking company may be sued for negligence, and also the trip leader or trip doctor. Financial settlements before a trial are common in the U.S., since the accused avoids the expense of a jury trial and attorney's fees, but settlements do not imply liability.

Case 2. J.B., a 50-year-old active man in good physical condition, joined a trek sponsored by a college to visit ruins in the South American Andes. He was accompanied by his wife. Before leaving the United States they attended a briefing for the tour group that described the country and the route of trek. There was no discussion of altitude illness. The group traveled by air to 11,500 feet (3,500 m) and visited several ruins for six days and then returned to sea level for several days. The group then went to 11,650 feet (3,551 m) and began a four day walking tour that involved climbing a 15,300 foot (4,663 m) pass and descending to a camp at 13,450 feet (4,100 m). On arrival at the camp J.B. was tired, felt weak, had chest tightness, and complained of a pain in his legs. The following day J.B. was still weak and spent most of the day in his tent. He required assistance to walk. He had a continuous cough and produced a clear sputum. He appeared lethargic and he was incoordinate. He was examined by a physician member of the group who noted no dyspnea. In the evening J.B. died. During resuscitation of a bloody, frothy fluid was expressed from the airways. An autopsy two days later at a village mortuary revealed extensive pulmonary and cerebral edema. The heart was normal. A lawsuit charging negligence was brought by J.B.'s widow against the sponsor of the trip, the physician, and the trek leader. The suit alleged that the group received no information regarding altitude illness before or during the trek, that the trek leader did not examine J.B., and that neither he nor the physician arranged for J.B.'s descent to a lower altitude. Shortly before the trial a financial settlement was made.

Comment. There was some uncertainty about the diagnosis in this case. High altitude pulmonary edema was most likely, but an acute coronary thrombosis with myocardial infarction or pulmonary embolism could not be excluded, since apparently the coronary arteries and the branches of the pulmonary artery were not opened to look for a thrombus or an embolus. An autopsy performed by an experienced forensic pathologist would probably have clarified the diagnosis.

Case 3. R.B., a 29-year-old man, joined an expedition to visit the headwaters of a river in China. Before the trip, the expedition members were assured in writing that a trip physician would accompany the group and that in the event of an emergency helicopters would be available and radio contact would be possible. The expedition traveled by vehicle to 10,000 feet (3,048 m) where they spent several days acclimatizing. They then traveled on foot to a base camp at 14,000 feet (4,268 m) to prepare for the climb to 18,000 feet (5,490 m). At that camp R.B. developed a "patch of pneumonia," according to the trip doctor, and descended to a lower altitude where he recovered after two or three weeks of rest. He then rejoined the expedition. The trip doctor, an emergency room physician with little experience in high altitude illness, advised him to rest for a few days after arrival at the higher altitude of 14,500 feet (4,420 m). All members of the group were performing heavy work including pulling rafts and carrying heavy loads. Despite the doctor's advice, R.B. was encouraged by the trip leader to work with the other members. R.B. developed pulmonary edema and probably cerebral edema. Attempts by radio to obtain help failed. R.B.'s condition deteriorated rapidly, and he died in a coma three days after the onset of his illness.

A lawsuit charging negligence was brought by the parents of the deceased against the U.S. company that organized the expedition. A jury trial was held and the company was absolved. The jury consisted of local ranchers and hunters, and their opinion was that the defendant was innocent, because the victim assumed the risk by going on the trip.

Comment. It is of interest that such a heavily financed expedition to an area far from medical facilities would hire a physician who had little experience in the diagnosis and management of altitude illness. The trip physician did not recognize the serious nature of high altitude pulmonary edema. High altitude pulmonary edema may recur after recovery at a lower altitude. An important precipitating factor is heavy physical activity. Failure to recognize the symptoms of recurrent pulmonary edema and failure to descend contributed to death. Descent by litter as soon as the diagnosis is made is preferable to wasting time seeking a helicopter rescue. An inexperienced attorney may have lost a jury trial decision.

Case 4. R.S was a 46-year-old man who had experienced an uncomplicated myocardial infarct five years earlier. He had resumed full activity and had no symptoms with even strenuous activity and was on no medication. He saw his personal physician regarding a hiking trip to the mountains with a youth group. R.S had been a very active hiker for the past two years and had led youth groups to altitudes as high as 11,000 feet (3,353 m) four or five times each year Previous electrocardiograms and treadmill tests had been normal. Three days before his last hike his physician performed another treadmill test; that was also normal. His heart rate increased to 161 beats/min and there was no chest pain or EKG changes. His physician cleared him for the trip, but said he should acclimatize at an intermediate altitude. R.S. drove to 7,600 feet (2,316 m) where the group camped for the night. The next day they hiked to 10,400 feet (3,170 m) for a second camp. R.S. had no symptoms. The following morning after about one hour of level walking R.S. collapsed and died. At autopsy a healed infarct was present, but there was no evidence of recent infarction. The cause of death was a probable cardiac arrest.

A suit for malpractice was brought against the cardiologist by the widow. The charge was that the cardiologist failed to tell the patient that he should not go to 10,400 feet (3,170 m), because of the possibility that such an altitude could result in a heart attack. The defense claimed that R.S. had previously gone to 10,400 feet (3,170 m) without difficulty and that there was no evidence in the medical literature that moderate altitude posed a threat to a patient with a healed myocardial infarct and an excellent exercise tolerance. The advice that was given was appropriate, namely, to avoid overexertion and to spend at least one night at an intermediate altitude.

The case went to trial and the jury voted unanimously in favor of the defense.

Comment. The cardiologist was familiar with the patient's activity, his absence of symptoms, and previously normal treadmill tests. The performance of an additional treadmill test and the advice given was probably correct. Sudden death without warning is a recognized occurrence in patients with coronary disease, and a normal treadmill test cannot exclude the possibility of sudden death.[1] There is no evidence that ascent to 10,400 feet (3,170 m) would have been any more dangerous for R.S. than performing the same level of exercise at sea level.

Case 5. A 38-year-old lawyer had a quarrel with his girlfriend. She left him and went to a Colorado ski resort. He drove to the resort in two days from Southern California and attempted a reconciliation. This was unsuccessful and another quarrel resulted. The rejected lawyer drove his camper to a remote campground at an altitude of 8,750 feet (2,650 m). He did not return and two days later he was found dead in his sleeping bag. An autopsy revealed severe bilateral pulmonary edema. There was no evidence of cardiovascular disease or trauma. There was no carbon monoxide in the blood or tissues, but alcohol and cold may have been contributing factors. There was gasoline in the fuel tank and the engine had been switched off. An autopsy revealed extensive bilateral pulmonary edema. There was no evidence of cardiac disease. A physician who was an expert in high altitude medicine and physiology testified that in his opinion death was due to high altitude pulmonary edema. The insurance company listed the cause of death as an accident and the beneficiaries were reimbursed.

Comment. The most logical cause of death in this case was high altitude pulmonary edema. It is not uncommon for death due to this illness to occur during the night especially when a companion is not present to seek medical aid. It is interesting that in this instance high altitude pulmonary edema was considered an accident and not an ordinary illness like pneumonia. Did the deceased have an insurance policy that paid a double indemnity for accidental death?

Case 6. J.M. was a 42-year-old real estate developer whose hobby was trophy game hunting in various parts of the world. He went on a Marco Polo sheep hunt in Afghanistan, organized and arranged by a U.S. organization. He had always been in excellent health. He traveled by air to Kabul, 6,400 feet (1,951 m), where he met his guides and trip assistants, and stayed for three days. They then traveled by air to Fazibad, 6,000 feet (1,829 m), and by car to a roadhead at 9,000 feet (2,743 m). By horseback he and the guides crossed a pass at 17,000 feet (5,182 m). They camped for the night at 16,000 feet (4,877 m) and then descended to a base camp at 13,500 feet (4,115 m). J.M. did not feel well on arrival at the camp, but on the following two days he hunted by yak and on foot up to 17,000 feet (5,182 m). On the afternoon of the second day, he felt very weak, tired, and groggy. There were several oxygen tanks at the base camp and oxygen was administered, but the tanks became empty in a few minutes. Other tanks were either empty or had inappropriate fittings. The following day J.M. was still groggy and breathing heavily. He became comatose in the afternoon and died during the night. An autopsy 68 hours later revealed bilateral pulmonary edema and no evidence of cardiac disease. The deceased had a large insurance policy with a double indemnity clause of accidental death. The insurance company refused to pay the double indemnity amount, claiming that death was due to natural causes and not to an accident. The widow's attorney claimed that high altitude pulmonary edema is an accident, and furthermore it was accidental that the oxygen bottles were not usable. The trial date was set, but an out-of-court settlement was made.

Comment. This is another example of a fatality from high altitude pulmonary edema resulting from failure to descend promptly upon the onset of symptoms. No physician was on the trip and it is possible that neither the trip leader nor the victim recognized the possibility of pulmonary edema and the need for descent. Descent would have been difficult, since it involved climbing over a 17,000 foot (5,182 m) pass, but if the oxygen had been usable, the patient might have improved enough so that descent could have been carried out. A court decision on whether or not high altitude pulmonary edema is an accident would have set a useful precedent. To my knowledge this question has not yet been decided. The decision may be dependent upon the circumstances. Death due to HAPE in a patient who cannot descend because of a storm or a broken leg may be considered an accidental death. Death from HAPE in someone who has been warned of the possibility of HAPE and disregards advice about acclimatization and prompt descent and then dies may not be considered an accidental death.

The proposed instruction of the widow's attorneys to the trial judge stated that a jury must decide whether or not death due to HAPE is an accident and whether or not a predisposition to HAPE can be held by law to be an illness or disease or physical defect or physical infirmity. Double indemnity for accidental death does not exist in the case of deaths resulting directly or indirectly from illness or disease or any kind of physical or mental defect or infirmity.

Lawsuits unfortunately are a way of life in the United States. Trekking companies, trek leaders, and physicians may be sued for almost any mishap, injury, or death that occurs on a trip. Although the chances of a physician's being sued are relatively small, any lawsuit may have a devastating effect upon the physician's time and resources. Pertinent references should be reviewed by any physician who joins a trekking or climbing group.

Herr has recently reviewed this problem and presents some interesting observations. He points out that most illnesses or injuries that occur on a trek or a climb do not require the services of a physician but can be handled by any capable trip leader or staff member who has had basic first aid training.[2,3] The availability of rapid rescue by helicopters has delegated the role of the physician in the event of a serious accident principally to applying clinical judgment. Helicopter rescue crews trained as nurses, paramedics, or emergency medical technicians are likely to have more experience in handling serious injuries than the average physician. Thus a physician's most important contribution to a trek or climb may be in advance of the trip, in the organization of appropriate immunizations, health precautions, and individual methods of preventing and treating simple medical problems. A trip leader and a staff trained in first aid may then make a trip physician unnecessary.

General references regarding physicians and emergency medical technicians are available.[4-8]

References

1. HULTGREN H. Coronary heart disease and trekking. *J. Wilderness Med.* 1990; 1:154-61.
2. HERR R. The climb physician: An endangered species. *J. Wilderness Med.* 1990; 1:144-46. Editorial.
3. HENRY G, and STEIN E. Medical liability in wilderness emergencies. In P Auerbach and E Geehr, eds, *Management of wilderness and environmental emergencies.* St. Louis: C.V. Mosby, 1989: 1041-47.
4. ALTON W. *Malpractice: A trial lawyer's advice of physicians. (How to avoid, how to win).* Boston: Little, Brown, 1977.
5. BELLI M, and CARLEVA J. *Belli for your malpractice defense.* Oradell, N.J.: Medical Economics Books, 1986.
6. FREUR W. *Medical malpractice law.* Irvine, Calif. Lawprep Pres, 1990.
7. BERNSTEIN A. *Avoiding medical malpractice.* Chicago: Pluribus Press, 1987.
8. FREW S. *Street Law: Rights and responsibilities of the EMT.* Reston, VA: Prentice-Hall, 1983.

APPENDIX 2

Selected Monographs and Reviews on High Altitude Physiology and Medicine

1. *Life of Man on the High Alps*. A. Mosso; English trans., T. Fisher. London: Unwin, 1898. 342 pages. Describes Mosso's researches and concepts of the effect of high altitude on man.
2. *Barometric Pressure*. P. Bert; English trans., F. Hitchock and M. Hitchock. Columbus, Ohio: College Book, 1943; reprinted 1978, Undersea Medical Soc., Bethesda, Md. 1,053 pages. The classic book on early observations on hypoxia and altitude. Contains description of many experiments conducted by Paul Bert.
3. *Respiration*. J. Haldane. New Haven, Conn.: Yale University Press, 1922. 427 pages. Reviews physiology pertinent to high altitude including regulation of respiration, blood as a carrier of O_2 and CO_2, effects of hypoxemia, causes of hypoxemia, gas secretion in the lungs, and effects of low atmospheric pressure.
4. *The Respiratory Function of the Blood. Part 1: Lessons from High Altitudes*. J. Barcroft. Cambridge: Cambridge University Press, 1925. 207 pages. An excellent summary of altitude research to that date as well as a description of Barcroft's visit to Cerro de Pasco, Peru, and the studies performed during his stay there.
5. *Adventures in Respiration*. Y. Henderson. Baltimore: Williams & Wilkins, 1938. 316 pages. A series of essays on early researches by Haldane and Barcroft.
6. *Life, Heat, and Altitude: Physiologic Effects of Hot Climates and Great Heights*. D. B. Dill. Cambridge, Mass: Harvard University Press, 1938. 211 pages. This contains chapters on high altitude, including animal life, man, and high altitude flights. An excellent historical account of altitude research in the 1930's.
7. *A Bibliography of Aviation Medicine*. C. Hoff and C. Fulton. Springfield, Ill.: Charles C. Thomas, 1942. 237 pages. A valuable source of references on various aspects of aviation medicine and altitude hypoxia.
8. *Acclimatization in the Andes: Historical Confirmations of Climatic Aggression in the Development of Andean Man*. C. Monge. Baltimore: Johns Hopkins University Press, 1948. 130 pages. A historical account of the effects of high altitude on the Indians and Spanish in the days of the Spanish conquest of Peru as well as an account of military operations during Peru's war of independence.

9. *Anoxia: Its Effect on the Body*. E. Van Liere and J. Stickney. Chicago: University of Chicago Press, 1963. 269 pages. A reprint of the 1942 edition. Reviews the effect of anoxia on many organ systems.

10. *Americans on Everest*. J. Ullman. Philadelphia: Lippincott, 1964. 429 pages. A well-written account of the 1963 American Everest Expedition with chapters on health and medicine, oxygen, and physiology.

11. *Mountain Sickness*. B. Bhattacharjyta. Bristol: John Wright and Sons, 1964. 58 pages. A brief summary of high altitude physiology, acute mountain sickness, pulmonary edema, and pulmonary hypertension.

12. *The Physiologic Effects of High Altitude*. Ed. W. Weihe. New York: Macmillan, 1964. 351 pages. Proceedings of a symposium held at Interlaken, Switzerland, September 1962. Thirty-two presentations on the physiological effects of high altitude.

13. *The Physiology of Human Survival*. Ed. O. Edholm and A. Bacharach. New York: Academic Press, 1965. 581 pages. Seventeen chapters including "High Altitude" by L. G. Pugh.

14. *The Effects of Altitude on Physical Performance*. Albuquerque, N. Mex.: Athletic Institute, 1966. 208 pages. A collection of 26 papers presented at an international symposium. Topics primarily related to exercise and competitive sports at high altitude.

15. *International Symposium on the Cardiovascular and Respiratory Effects of Hypoxia*. J. Hatcher and D. Jennings. New York: Hafner, 1966. 407 pages. Fifty sections of papers including discussions of physiological aspects of hypoxia and high altitude.

16. *Proceedings of a Symposia on Arctic Biology and Medicine*. Ed. C. Helfferich. Fort Wainwright, Alaska: Arctic Aeromedical Laboratory, 1966. 529 pages. Ten sections on physiological responses to cold and altitude.

17. *Exercise at Altitude*. R. Margaria. Amsterdam, NY: Exerpta Medica Foundation, 1967. 215 pages. Twenty-one papers presented at an international symposium in Milan, September 1966. Topics included related to energetics and oxygen uptake, respiration, cardiovascular system, blood, and adaptation.

18. *Exercise and Altitude*. Ed. E. Jokl and P. Jokl. S. New York: S. Karger, 1968. 195 pages. Thirteen chapters primarily related to exercise at high altitude, including competitive running.

19. *Physiological Factors Relating to Terrestrial Altitudes*. L. Wulff, I. Braden, F. Shillito, and J. Tomashefski. Columbus: Ohio State University Press, 1968. 738 pages. A collection of 4,000 references related to high altitude.

20. *Biomedical Problems of High Terrestrial Elevations*. Ed. A. Hegnauer. Natick, Mass: U.S. Army Research Institute of Environmental Medicine, 1969. 323 pages. Twenty-four chapters of presentations on high altitude medical problems, pulmonary and systemic circulations, respiratory control, and behavior and performance.

21. *Effects of High Altitude on Human Birth: Observations on Mothers, Placentas, and the Newborn in Two Peruvian Populations*. J. McClung. Cambridge, Mass.: Harvard University Press, 1969. 150 pages. A review of previous studies in this field and a report of original studies carried out by the author in Cuzco and Lima.

22. *Proceedings of the International Symposium on Altitude and Cold.* Federation Proceedings, and Federation of American Societies of Experimental Biology, 1969. 402 pages. This contains 127 sections including discussions of various aspects of acute and chronic altitude exposure as well as physiological effects of cold.

23. *Hypoxia, High Altitude, and the Heart.* Ed. J. Vogel. New York: S. Karger, 1970. 195 pages. Twenty-six papers presented at the first conference on Cardiovascular Disease in Snowmass-at-Aspen, Colorado. Sections include physiological changes at altitude, coronary circulation, respiratory control, and the pulmonary circulation.

24. *High Altitude Physiology.* R. Porter and J. Knight. Edinburgh: Churchill, Livingston, 1971. 196 pages. Twelve chapters of presentations at a Ciba Foundation symposium in honor of Professor Alberto Hurtado. Respiratory control, pulmonary and systemic circulation, and altitude illness are reviewed.

25. *Physiological Adaptations: Desert and Mountains.* Ed. M. Yousef, S. Horvath, and R. Bullard. New York: Academic Press, 1972. 258 pages. Excellent sections on altitude exposure.

26. *Doctor on Everest.* P. Steele. Newton Abbot, Devon, Engl: Readers Union, 1973. 222 pages. A personal account of experiences as a physician to the International Himalayan Expedition of 1971 and a description of miscellaneous medical problems and hardships of an Everest expedition.

27. *Mountain Medicine.* M. Ward. London: Crosby, Lockwood, Staples, 1975. 376 pages. Twenty-nine chapters on the effect of high altitude upon physiological functions in man. Also has discussions of high altitude medical problems, including cold injury, hypothermia, frostbite, and accidents.

28. *Mountain Medicine and Physiology.* C. Clarke, M. Ward, and E. Williams. London: Alpine Club, 1975. 142 pages. Eighteen chapters of presentations at a symposium for mountaineers, expedition doctors, and physiologists sponsored by the Alpine Club. Reviews practical problems of mountaineering including cold injury, effects of high altitude, fitness, and fatigue.

29. *Proceedings, Mountain Medicine Symposium.* Ed. C. Houston and S. Cummings. Yosemite, Calif.: Yosemite Institute, 1975. 104 pages. Presentations and discussions during a three-and-a-half-day symposium on various topics of mountain medicine, including cold, nutrition, injuries, altitude illness, and environmental health.

30. *Man in the Andes.* Ed. P. Baker and M. Little. Stroudsberg, Pa.,: Dowden, Hutchinson, and Ross, 1976. 482 pages. Results of many studies of the Peruvian highlanders.

31. *Man at High Altitude.* D. Heath and D. Williams. Edinburgh: Churchill, Livingston, 1977. 292 pages. Twenty-seven chapters review the effects of acute and chronic high altitude exposure upon physiological functions in man. Discusses acute mountain sickness, pulmonary edema, Monge's disease, and pulmonary hypertension.

32. *The Biology of High-Altitude Peoples.* Ed. P. Baker. Cambridge: Cambridge University Press, 1978. 357 pages. Reviews a varied number of aspects of high altitude residents in the altiplano of Peru.

33. *Environmental Stress: Individual Human Adaptations.* L. Folinsbee, J. Wagner, J. Borgia, B. Drinkwater, J. Gliner, and J. Bedi. New York: Academic Press, 1978. 393 pages. A multiauthored review of the effects of heat, air pollution, work physiology, cold stress, and altitude on man. Five sections on altitude relate to historical aspects of altitude physiology by Kellogg, adaptation by Grover, adaptation of men and women by Hannon, exercise by Blatteis, and sleep hypoxemia by Powles and others.

34. *High Altitude Physiology Study.* C. Houston. Burlington, Vt.: Queen City Printers, 1980. 72 pages. A collection of papers published between 1968 and 1980 concerning research done on Mount Logan, Canada.

35. *Mountain Sickness: Prevention, Recognition, and Treatment.* P. Hackett. New York: American Alpine Club, 1980. 77 pages. A handy booklet on major mountain medical problems with practical suggestions for recognition, management, and prevention by an experienced mountaineer.

36. *Environmental Physiology: Aging, Heat, and Altitude.* Ed. S. Horvath and M. Yousef. Haarlem: Elsevier, 1981. 468 pages. A multiauthored volume with sections on adaptations to heat and altitude and advances in the biology of aging. The section on altitude contains historical perspectives and chapters on acid base balance, nutrition, biochemical adaptations, respiration, neuroendocrine changes, and extreme altitudes.

37. *High Altitude Physiology.* Ed. J. West. Stroudsburg, Pa.: Hutchinson, Ross, 1981. 461 pages. A collection of important papers on altitude physiology going back to Acosta.

38. *Man at High Altitude.* D. Heath and D. Williams. London: Churchill, Livingston, 1981. 347 pages. A second edition, with additional new material, of the volume first published in 1977.

39. *High Altitude Physiology and Medicine.* Ed. W. Brendel and R. Zink. New York: Springer-Verlag, 1982. 310 pages. Forty-nine chapters on physiological aspects of hypoxia and altitude and sections on high altitude medical problems.

40. *Hypoxia: Man at Altitude.* Ed. J. Sutton, N. Jones, and C. Houston. New York: Thieme-Stratton, 1982. 213 pages. Proceedings of the 1981 Hypoxia symposium at Banff. Thirty-six chapters cover physiological aspects of hypoxia and medical and mountaineering problems.

41. *Oxygen Transport to Human Tissues.* J. Loeppky and M. Riedesel. New York: Elsevier Biomedical, 1982. 377 pages. Proceedings of a symposium honoring Dr. U. Luft, Albuquerque, N. Mex., June 1981. Thirty-one papers and 11 abstracts, with sections on alveolar capillary gas equilibration, cardiovascular adjustments, altitude and oxygen transport, and clinical problems.

42. *Hypoxia, Exercise, and Altitude. Proceedings of the Third Banff International Hypoxia Symposium.* Ed. J. Sutton, C. Houston, and N. Jones. New York: A. R. Liss, 1983. 495 pages. Thirty-nine papers and 51 abstracts covering a wide variety of topics relating to hypoxia and altitude including discussions.

43. "Man at Altitude." Ed. J. Sutton. *Seminars in Respiratory Medicine*, 1983. 5:103-201. Reviews articles on various aspects of altitude exposure and acclimatization.

44. *High Altitude and Man*. Ed. J. West and S. Lahiri. Bethesda, Md.: American Physiological Society, 1984. 199 pages. A summary of 16 presentations at a symposium on man at high altitude sponsored by the American Physiological Society. Topics covered are man at extreme altitude, sleep, respiration, and the physiology of Sherpas.

45. *High Altitude Deterioration*. Ed. J. Rivolier, P. Cerretelli, J. Foray, and P. Segantini. Basel: S. Karger, 1984. 228 pages. Proceedings of the International Congress on Mountain Medicine, Chamonix, Switzerland, 1984. Twenty-one chapters on various medical and physiological problems of high altitude including exercise.

46. *Surviving Denali*. J. Waterman. New York: American Alpine Club, 1984. 192 pages. This book, by a Denali guide, describes all types of accidents that occurred between 1910 and 1982 on this dangerous mountain.

47. *Adaptation to Altitude Hypoxia in Vertebrates*. P. Bouverot. Berlin: Springer-Verlag, 1985. 176 pages. Written by a respiratory physiologist, this book reviews available data on adaptations to high altitude in man and numerous animal species. Especially useful for comparative physiologists, since no previous publication has summarized animal studies.

48. *Everest: The Testing Place*. J. West. New York: McGraw-Hill, 1985. 187 pages. A personal account, written in nontechnical language, of the American Research Expedition to Mount Everest in 1981. Includes an appendix on medical problems by F. Sarnquist, M.D.

49. *Aspects of Hypoxia*. Ed. D. Heath. Liverpool: Liverpool University Press, 1986. 264 pages. Contributions of 16 speakers at a symposium on hypoxia in April 1986. Topics covered were pulmonary endocrine cells, effects of hypoxia on the endocrine system, structure of the carotid bodies, long-term oxygen therapy, pulmonary hypertension, and effects of hypoxia upon telescope workers in Hawaii.

50. "Cardiovascular Adaptation to Exercise at High Altitude." J. Weil and J. Reeves. In K. Pandolf, ed., *Exercise and Sports Sciences Reviews*, vol. 14. New York: Macmillan, 1986. A 33-page review of the major factors that effect exercise performance at high altitude. Contains many observations made by the authors.

51. *Human Performance Physiology and Environmental Medicine at Terrestrial Extremes*. K. Pandolph, M. Sawka, R. Gonzalez. Dubuque, Ia., Brown & Benchmark, 1988. 637 pages.

52. *Going Higher: The Story of Man and Altitude*. C. Houston. Rev. ed. Boston: Little, Brown, 1987. 324 pages. Historical summary of early researches on oxygen, the atmosphere, and high elevations; contains sections on respiration, the cell, hemoglobin, and altitude illness.

53. *Hypoxia, Polycythemia, and Chronic Mountain Sickness*. R. Winslow and C. Monge, Jr. Baltimore: Johns Hopkins University Press, 1987. 251 pages. A comprehensive review of chronic mountain sickness with an excellent historical introduction, description of physiological abnormalities, and the effect of venesection.

54. *Aviation Medicine*. Ed. J. Ernsting and P. King. 2d ed. London: Butterworth's, 1988. 738 pages. A review of the physiological aspects of aircraft flight, including sections on health problems, sleep, and wakefulness, and on gas laws and blood gas effects.

55. *High Altitude Medical Science*. Ed. G. Ueda, S. Kusama, and N. Voelkel. Matsumoto, Japan: Shinshu University, 1988. 466 pages. A collection of 77 abstracts of papers presented at the Matsumoto International Symposium on High Altitude Medical Science, November 1987.

56. *High Altitude Medicine and Pathology*. D. Heath and D. Williams. London: Butterworth's, 1989. 352 pages. A revised and updated third edition with additional new information.

57. *High Altitude Medicine*. M. Ward, J. Milledge, and J. West. Philadelphia: University of Pennsylvania Press, 1990. 352 pages. An excellent comprehensive monograph on physiological effects of high altitude with a review of high altitude medical problems. Physiological aspects of respiration and blood gas exchange are particularly well covered.

58. *Hypoxia: The Adaptations*. Ed. J. Sutton, G. Coates, and J. Remmers. Toronto: B. C. Decker, 1990. 344 pages. A collection of 42 papers and 92 abstracts presented at the Sixth international Hypoxia Symposium held at Lake Louise, Canada, in 1989. Topics include avian physiology, high altitude populations, metabolic rate, chemoreceptors, gas exchange, brain, muscle, heart, and lung.

59. *Adaptación humana a la extrema altura*. J. Ferrer. Vitoria-Gasteiz, Alava, Spain: Pradells, 1991. 155 pages. A detailed, illustrated report of the 1985 expedition to Cho-Oyu. Topics covered are respiratory function, electrocardiography, functional aerobic capacity, and hematology.

60. *Color Atlas of Mountain Medicine*. Ed. F. Dubas and J. Vallotton. St. Louis: Mosby Yearbook, 1991. 223 pages. Forty-six chapters by various authors on mountain rescue, effects of altitude, solar radiation, cold, ice and snow, lightning, and injuries associated with hiking, skiing, and mountaineering. Abundantly illustrated.

61. *Response and Adaptation to Hypoxia: Organ to Organelle*. S. Lahiri, N. Cherniack, and R. Fitzgerald. New York: Oxford University Press, 1991. 232 pages. A multiauthored review of physiological responses and adaptations to hypoxia; sponsored by the American Physiological Society. Responses from mitochondria to organ systems and to the entire man or animal are discussed with emphasis on molecular and cellular mechanisms.

62. *Bibliography of High Altitude Medicine*. Ed. R. Roach, P. Hackett, and C. Houston. Keystone, Colo.: Colorado Altitude Research Institute, 1992. 179 pages. An alphabetical listing by first authors of 3,024 references to high altitude topics published largely during the past 30 years. This publication will be updated annually.

63. *High Altitude Medicine*. Ed. G. Ueda, J. Reeves, and M. Sekiguchi. Matsumoto, Japan: Shinshu University, 1992. 540 pages. Proceedings of the 4th Matsumoto International Symposium on High Altitude Medical Science, Matsumoto, Japan, August 30-September 1, 1991. Contains 87 presentations on physiological and clinical aspects of high altitude.

64. *Hypoxia and Mountain Medicine.* Ed. J. Sutton, G. Coates, and C. Houston. Burlington, Vt.: Queen City Printers, 1992. 330 pages. Proceedings of the Seventh International Hypoxia Symposium held at Lake Louise, Canada, February 1991. Twenty-five chapters on psychomotor effects of hypoxia, hormonal changes, clinical aspects, muscle metabolism, and high altitude illness. Contains 117 abstracts and a consensus report on the definition and quantification of altitude illness.

65. *Pathologie et Altitude.* J-P. Richalet and C. Rathat. Paris: Masson, 1991. 211 pages. Eleven chapters on general problems of high altitude medicine, practical advice for doctors on trekking groups or high altitude expeditions and a bibliography of nearly 700 references dating up to 1990.

66. *Hypoxia, Metabolic Acidosis, and the Circulation.* Ed. A. Arieff. New York: Oxford University Press, 1992. 215 pages. Ten chapters discuss physiological and clinical manifestations of hypoxia.

67. *Hypoxia and Molecular Medicine.* Ed. J. Sutton, G. Coates, and C. Houston. Burlington, Vt.: Queen City Printers, 1993. Proceedings of the Eighth International Hypoxia Symposium, February 1993. Twenty-seven chapters on the autonomic nervous system, hypoxic regulation and gene expression, science and Mount Everest and mountain medicine. Contains 106 abstracts.

68. *High Altitude Medicine and Physiology,* Second Edition. M. Ward, J. Milledge, and J. West. N.Y.: Chapman and Hall, 1994. 640 pages. An updated edition with a separate chapter on high altitude populations and management of emergencies at altitude.

69. *High Altitude. Illness and Wellness.* C. Houston. Merrillvile, In.: ICS Books, 1993. 72 pages. A brief review of the physiology of hypoxia followed by a description of a few of the more common medical problems of high altitude.

70. *Altitude Illness. Prevention and Treatment.* S. Besruchka, Seattle, Wa.: The Mountaineers, 1994. 93 pages. A brief review of common medical problems of high altitude including prevention, diagnosis and treatment.

71. *Hypoxia: Investifaciones basica y clinica.* A. Arregui and F. Leon-Velarde. Lima: IFEA-UPCH, 1993. 374 pages. Written in honor of Carlos Monge. Contains five chapters and 28 contributors. Biomedical problems of acute and chronic high altitude exposure as well as experimental work.

72. *Acclimatization to Altitude.* Ulrich Luft 1941. Translated by Friedrich Luft 1993. Lovelace Medical Foundation. 95 pages. A review of acclimatization containing many results of studies performed by Ulrich Luft.

73. *Desadaptation a la Vida en las Grandes Alturas.* F. Leon-Velarde and A. Arregui. Lima: IFEA-UPCH, 1994. 145 pages. Epidemiologic studies done at Cerro de Pasco on clinical and experimental aspects of chronic mountain sickness and adaptation to high altitude.

74. *Biomedicina Andina: Compendio Bibliogràfico.* D. Lerner de Bigio and L. Huicho. Lima: IFEA-IBBA- UPCH, 1994. 430 pages. A compendium of 1,350 summaries of papers on chronic hypoxia representing work done primarily in Peru and Bolivia.

Index

Italic type is used to denote an illustration; the letter "t" following a page reference denotes a table.

A

B

C

D

F

G

hemodynamics, 473-474, *476*
high altitude cerebral edema, 332, 480
high altitude polycythemia, 472, 480, 481
high altitude pulmonary edema, 285, 472, 479, 480, 481
high altitude studies, 472, 477
high altitude systemic edema, 472, 480-481
pulmonary function, 475, *478*
systemic edema, 472, 480-481
thromboembolism, 472, 481, 482
Genton, E., 99
Gill, M., 151
Gillette, Ned, 177
Glaisher, J., 119
Glucose tolerance curve, at high altitude, 145
Goiter, in high altitude locations, 125, 135
Gong, H., 456
Good samaritan rule, 487
Graded ascent, 174, 283, 315
Graham, W., 454-455
Grawitz, E., 101
Gray, G., 237, 242
Graybiel, A., 47
Great Headache Mountain, 213, 398
Greene, C., 235
Grover, R., 20, 47, 59, 151, 185, 361, 425
Grunt breathing, 312

H

HACE. *See* High altitude cerebral edema
Hackett, P., 200, 215, 220, 228, 229, 231, 245, 247, 283, 305, 307, 308, 310, 311, 331, 342, 344, 368, 393, 398, 402, 480-481
Haldane, F., 5, 28, 167
Haldane, J., 215
Halhuber, M., 443
Hallucinations, 118, 323
Han Chinese
    heart rate, 128
    pulmonary hypertension, 410, 412
Hannon, J., 472
Hansen, J., 322
HAPE. *See* High altitude pulmonary edema
HARH. *See* Retinal hemorrhage
Harper, A., 322
Hartig, G., 402
Harvey, T., 235, 401
HASE. *See* High altitude systemic edema
Hawaii
    high altitude research stations, 13t
    Mauna Kea

L

M

O

P

S

T

W

X

Y

Z